T0309204

New Insights into Pulmonary Medicine

New Insights into Pulmonary Medicine

Editor: Lily Hartman

AMERICAN
MEDICAL PUBLISHERS
www.americanmedicalpublishers.com

AMERICAN
MEDICAL PUBLISHERS
www.americanmedicalpublishers.com

Cataloging-in-Publication Data

New insights into pulmonary medicine / edited by Lily Hartman.
p. cm.
Includes bibliographical references and index.
ISBN 979-8-88740-586-5
1. Lungs--Diseases--Case studies. 2. Lungs—Diseases--Treatment--Case studies.
3. Respiratory organs—Diseases--Treatment--Case studies. I. Hartman, Lily.
RC756.P85 2023
616.24--dc23

American Medical Publishers,
41 Flatbush Avenue,
1st Floor, New York,
NY 11217, USA

ISBN 979-8-88740-586-5 (Hardback)

Contents

Preface

Pulmonary medicine is the subspecialty of internal medicine that is involved with management and treatment of diseases affecting the respiratory system, which includes the thoracic cavity, lungs, chest wall and upper airways. It is aimed at treating a wide range of conditions and diseases, including asthma, severe acute respiratory syndrome (SARS), interstitial lung disease, lung cancer, acute respiratory distress syndrome (ARDS), chronic obstructive pulmonary disease (COPD), pulmonary hypertension, cystic fibrosis, lung transplant and pulmonary tuberculosis. Medicines taken orally or by inhalation is the most efficient and practical method of treating respiratory conditions. This book aims to shed light on some of the unexplored aspects of pulmonary medicine and the recent researches in this field. It covers in detail some existent theories and innovative concepts revolving around this domain. This book will prove to be immensely beneficial to students and researchers in this field.

The information contained in this book is the result of intensive hard work done by researchers in this field. All due efforts have been made to make this book serve as a complete guiding source for students and researchers. The topics in this book have been comprehensively explained to help readers understand the growing trends in the field.

I would like to thank the entire group of writers who made sincere efforts in this book and my family who supported me in my efforts of working on this book. I take this opportunity to thank all those who have been a guiding force throughout my life.

Editor

1

ALDH Expression in Angiosarcoma of the Lung: A Potential Marker of Aggressiveness?

Beatrice Aramini[1], Valentina Masciale[1], Daniel Bianchi[1], Beatrice Manfredini[1], Federico Banchelli[2], Roberto D'Amico[2], Federica Bertolini[3], Massimo Dominici[3], Uliano Morandi[1] and Antonino Maiorana[4]*

[1] Division of Thoracic Surgery, Department of Medical and Surgical Sciences, University of Modena and Reggio Emilia, Modena, Italy, [2] Department of Medical and Surgical Sciences, Center of Statistic, University of Modena and Reggio Emilia, Modena, Italy, [3] Division of Oncology, Department of Medical and Surgical Sciences, University of Modena and Reggio Emilia, Modena, Italy, [4] Department of Medical and Surgical Sciences, Institute of Pathology, University of Modena and Reggio Emilia, Modena, Italy

***Correspondence:**
Beatrice Aramini
beatrice.aramini@unimore.it

Background: Primary angiosarcoma of the lung is a very aggressive rare malignant disease resulting in a severe prognosis (1). This type of cancer represents about 2% of all soft tissue sarcomas and has a high rate of metastasis through the hematogenous route. For the rarity of this malignant vascular tumor it is still challenging to set a diagnosis (1). The diagnostic features that have thus far been considered include primarily clinical and radiological findings. In some cases, immunohistochemical characteristics based on the most common markers used in pathology have been described. The aim of this report is to present two cases of angiosarcoma of the lung in which the aldehyde dehydrogenase (ALDH) marker was analyzed by immunohistochemistry.

Methods: We report two cases of angiosarcoma of the lung in patients underwent lung surgery at our Unit. In addition to the standard histopathological analysis for this disease, immunohistochemistry using an ALDH1A1 antibody was performed in both of the cases. For ALDH quantification, a semi-quantitative method based on the positivity of the tumor cells was used: 0 (<5%), 1 (5–25%), 2 (>25–50%), 3 (>50–75%), 4 (>75%).

Results: One patient with recurrent lung disease survived, achieving complete remission after chemo- and radiotherapy. The second patient died of recurrent disease within 5 years of diagnosis. ALDH1A1 was evaluated in both of these cases using an immunohistochemistry scoring system based on the positivity for this marker. The scores were consistent with the patients' clinical outcomes, as the lower (score 1) was observed in the patient with the better clinical outcome, while the higher (score 3) was seen in the patient with the worse outcome.

Conclusion: Our data suggest that ALDH may be an important clinical marker in angiosarcoma of the lung. Although further studies need to be performed in a larger cohort of patients, we believe that, if the results will be confirmed, ALDH1A1 may be used to stratify patients in terms of prognosis and for targeted therapy.

Keywords: target therapy, aldehyde dehydrogenase (ALDH), malignant rare lung tumor, rare tumor, angiosarcoma, marker, angiogenetic process, malignant vascular tumors

BACKGROUND

Angiosarcoma is a rare form of malignant vascular tumor occurring for the 2% of soft tissue sarcoma (1–3). Clinical symptoms are similar to those observed in other pulmonary tumors (2). The radiological presentation is highly variable, ranging from a solitary nodule to multiple bilateral lesions. In addition, due to its clinicopathological similarity to metastatic angiosarcoma of the lung, a diagnosis of primary disease requires a complete clinical and radiological examination of the body in order to ensure that there are no primary lesions outside of the chest. Therefore, immunohistochemistry is the gold standard technique to make a diagnosis of angiosarcoma of the lung; in particular, the most used markers are Factor VIII, CD31, CD34, and Fli-1 (4). There is not yet a standardized therapy for this disease; however, therapy usually consists of surgical treatment, chemotherapy, and radiotherapy, depending on the clinical presentation and the number of lesions.

However, aldehyde dehydrogenase (ALDH) which is an enzyme able to detect normal and malignant stem/progenitor cells (5) is now used as marker in tumor initiating cells (TICs) especially for the two ALDH isoforms, ALDH1A1 and ALDH1A3 (6–8). In particular, ALDH1A1 has been considered the most effective markers in consideration of poor prognosis for lung cancer and it is considered a marker of stemness, promoting angiogenesis, which is one of the main characteristics in high vascularised tumor as the angiosarcoma (9–11). Moreover, ALDH1A3, which is another ALDH isoform, is mainly enrolled in the regulation of matricellular proteins promoting the vascular smooth muscle cell proliferation (12).

ALDH has also the capacity to regulate the most important cells functions as self-renewal, expansion, differentiation and drug resistance (13). A deeper knowledge of the ALDH molecular pathways will be useful in many specialties, as regenerative medicine and oncology. In particular, a current clinical trial demonstrates the importance of comparing the effects of the ALDH inhibitor dimethyl ampal thiolester (DIMATE) on normal and malignant hematopoietic cells and stem cells (9, 13). In particular, it has been shown that DIMATE could potentially be used to selectively eliminate cancer cells (9). Although these results were obtained in hematological disease, they demonstrated the importance of ALDH in oncology and suggested that ALDH may be considered not only a marker, but also a target.

In this report, we present our experience with two cases of primary angiosarcoma of the lung that had completely different clinical presentations and, therefore, completely different treatments. In particular, we found that, while both of the angiosarcomas showed ALDH expression, high and low ALDH scores were associated with worse and better prognosis, respectively. Further studies on the presence of this marker in angiosarcomas of the lung may highlight the importance of ALDH as a prognostic factor and as a potential biomarker for targeted therapies.

METHODS

Case 1

A 27-year-old man arrived at our Department in June 2016 after multiple episodes of hemoptysis followed by intense chest pain. He referred only previous episodes of inflammatory bowel disease (IBD). Chest X-rays showed multiple bilateral lesions in the lungs that were confirmed by the computed tomography (CT) scan in which multiple pseudonodular features surrounded by a ground glass halo were identified in both lungs (**Figure 1A**). The abdomen and brain CT scan were negative for atypical lesions. A PET scan was performed, revealing evidence of multiple active sites in the lungs (**Figure 1B**). In June 2016, transbronchial biopsies were non-diagnostic and the patient underwent surgical left lung biopsies performed using a video-assisted thoracic surgery (VATS) approach. The pathological exam revealed spindle cells of endothelial origin that stained positive for CD31 and partially positive for cytokeratin AE3/AE4. Staining for CD34, TTF1, and CD30 were found to be negative. An angiosarcoma of the lung was diagnosed.

The patient was sent to the oncologist. A new chest CT performed in July 2016 showed a recurrence at the level of the thoraco-abdominal passage at the cardiophrenic angle and caudally to the right lower lobar pulmonary vein; after positioning of a port-a-cath (PORT device), patient started first-line chemotherapy with epirubicin and ifosfamide. The revaluation after three cycles revealed an excellent response in the parenchymal lung lesions, a net reduction of bilateral pleural effusion, and a reduction in the lesion at the level of the D5 soma in net volumetric evolution. On October 2016, radiosurgery (18 Gy in single dose) on the D5 lesion was performed. Another three cycles with the same scheme followed. In January 2017, due to lung progression, the patient was started on second-line chemotherapy with docetaxel plus gemcitabine associated with radiotherapy until April 2017 (four total cycles given); starting in April, the therapy continued with only gemcitabine. After these treatments, in May 2017, the patient showed additional hemoptysis episodes, which drew attention to a recurrence at the level of the left lower lobe. In August 2017, he started weekly paclitaxel and achieved a complete remission of the disease, which has been confirmed in the subsequent follow-up examinations. The most recent chest CT (performed in January 2020) showed a complete remission of angiosarcoma (**Figure 2**).

Case 2

A 61-year-old woman came to our hospital for persistent cough in the last 2 years, initially treated as an allergic bronchiolitis without any improvement. Her medical history was notable only for a prior isterectomy due to fibromatosis. She denied smoking habit.

In August 2005, a chest X-ray showed a small single lesion in the left lung. At the same time, a CT scan of the chest

---

Abbreviations: ALDH, aldehyde dehydrogenase; CT, computed tomography; DAB, 3,3-diaminobenzidine; DIMATE, dimethyl ampal thiolester; PBS, phosphate buffered saline; VATS, video-assisted thoracic surgery; ^{18}F-FDG PET/CT, 18-fluorodeoxyglucose integrated with computed tomography.

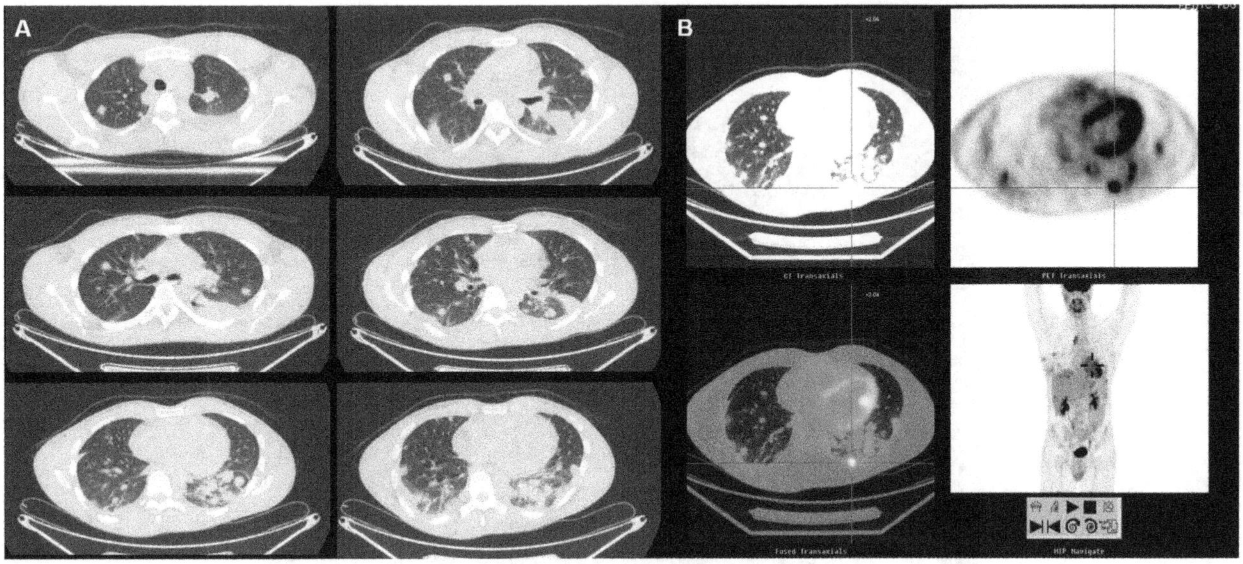

FIGURE 1 | (A) Chest CT in case 1 before treatment. The lungs showed bilateral nodules. **(B)** Total body ^{18}F-FDG PET. No hypermetabolic lesions other than the lesions in the lungs.

showed evidence of hyper-dense tissue of ~2 cm around the lower left bronchus.

In September 2005, we performed a bronchoscopy with transbronchial biopsy, leading to the diagnosis of angiosarcoma. To ensure that it was not a metastatic lesion, we performed a magnetic resonance imaging (MRI) of the abdomen followed by an 18-fluorodeoxyglucose integrated with computed tomography (^{18}F-FDG PET/CT). Neither showed evidence of any other atypical lesion. Primary angiosarcoma of the lung was diagnosed.

In October 2005, a left lower lobectomy was performed by thoracotomy, without any major complications after the surgical procedure.

The histological examination confirmed the initial diagnosis of angiosarcoma, with immunohistochemistry positive for myocyte nuclear factor (MNF116) and CD34 and partially positive for Factor VIII and CD31. A hilar lymph node was found positive for local invasion.

After 1 month from surgery, she was undergone chemotherapy with docetaxel plus gemcitabine (four total cycles given), associated with radiotherapy on the mediastinum (~50 Gy in 25 fractions). Patient performed 3 years follow up by chest and abdomen CT with contrast enhancement until 2008, which showed normal radiological findings, free from the tumor lung disease.

In 2009, the patient was admitted to our Unit for left thoracic pain and suspicious for rib fractures. She underwent to a chest CT with contrast enhancement showing a neoformation of 3.5 × 2 × 1.5 cm at the level of the left intercostal space, between the tenth and the eleventh rib. Due to the previous history of angiosarcoma of the lung, patient underwent surgery in general anesthesia to remove the mass and make a diagnosis. An excision was performed at the level of the chest neoformation with partial removal of the ninth and tenth left rib and a plastic reconstruction of the left thoracic wall. Patient stayed clinically stable and she was discharged from hospital after 6 days without complications. The oncologic team evaluated the patient after few weeks from surgery and a chemotherapy plan was set with only gemcitabine for other 4 months, with no complete remission. The patient died in early 2010 due to insufficient respiratory function caused by lung recurrence.

Immunohistochemistry

Paraffin was firstly removed from tissue section with the use of xylene, and subsequently a descending scale of ethyl alcohol (100, 90, 80, and 70°) was used to rehydrate the slices before the washing procedure with phosphate-buffered saline (PBS). The antigen retrieval was performed with a 10 mM sodium citrate buffer ad a high temperature water bath (95°C). After 15 min the slices were washed with PBS for 30 min. To suppress the interference of endogenous peroxidase a solution of 3% H_2O_2 was used to dip samples. Therefore, serum was necessary for blocking non-specific signal. At the end of this procedure primary antibodies were added for hours to tissue slices (ab-134188, Abcam, Cambridge, MA, USA), anti-CD34 (Ventana Medical Systems, Arizona, USA), and anti-CD31 (Cell Marque, California, USA). Furthermore, sections were incubated for 30 min with a secondary antibody (PK-4001; Vector Labs, USA) before three times washing with PBS. Samples were subsequently incubated with ABC-HRP (PK-4001; Vector Labs, USA), washed in PBS in order to remove the excess antibody, and stained with 3,3-diaminobenzidine (DAB). Finally, a secondary stain with Mayer's hematoxylin was applied to provide contrast in the section. At the end slices were dehydrated with an ascendant alcohol grade scale (70, 80, 90, and 100°), and then subsequently mounting media was added. Tissue sections were analyzed using a Zeiss Axioskop microscope, with a Zeiss AxioCam

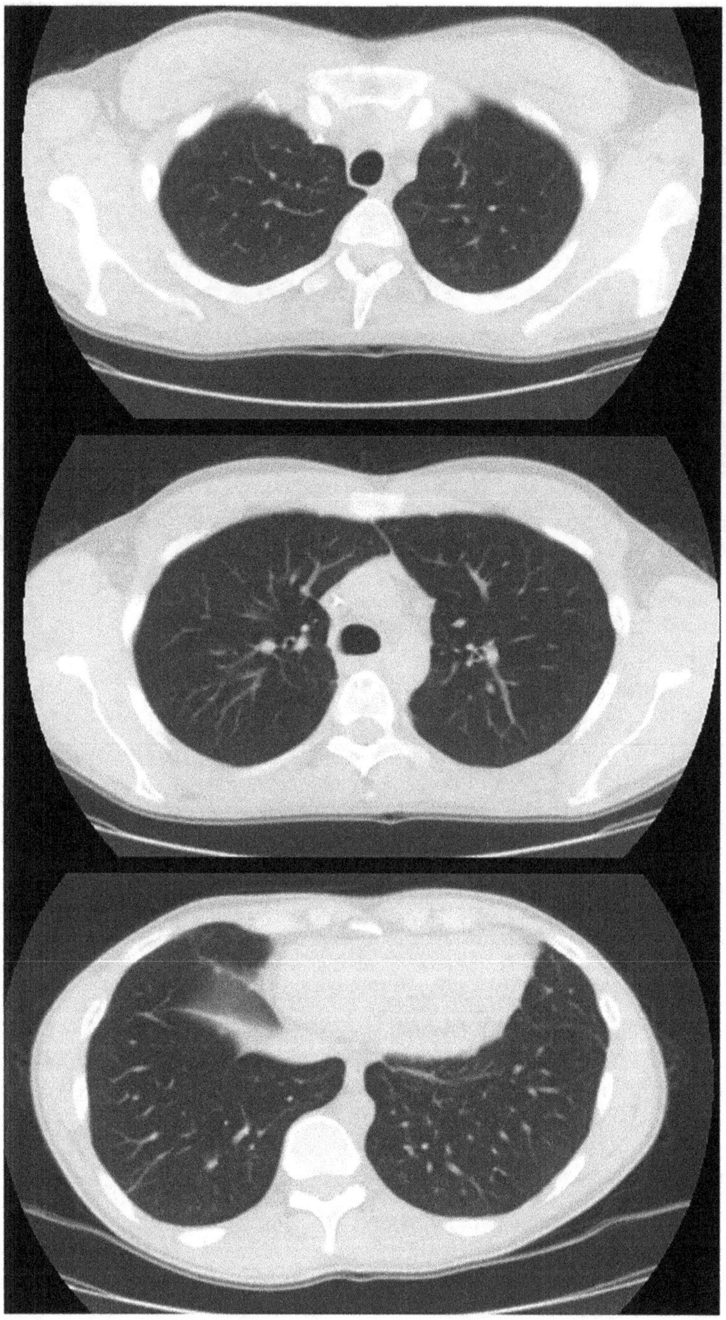

FIGURE 2 | Chest CT in case 1 after chemo- and radiotherapy treatment. After 1 year of treatment, the patient showed a complete remission of the disease.

ICc 3 High-Resolution Microscope Camera, at 10× and at 20× magnification. Blinded a and independent evaluation of the sample were performed to assign the right score for the evaluation of positive cells, in accordance to a previous score (6–8). Immunoreactivity for ALDH marker was assess by a semi-quantitative method based on this range of positivity for the tumor cells: 0 (<5% positive), 1 (5–25%), 2 (>25–50%), 3 (>50–75%), and 4 (>75%) (7).

RESULTS

Clinical Results

Case 1

After 1 year of chemotherapy and radiotherapy cycles, the patient showed a complete remission of the disease. The last chest CT performed in January 2020 showed complete remission.

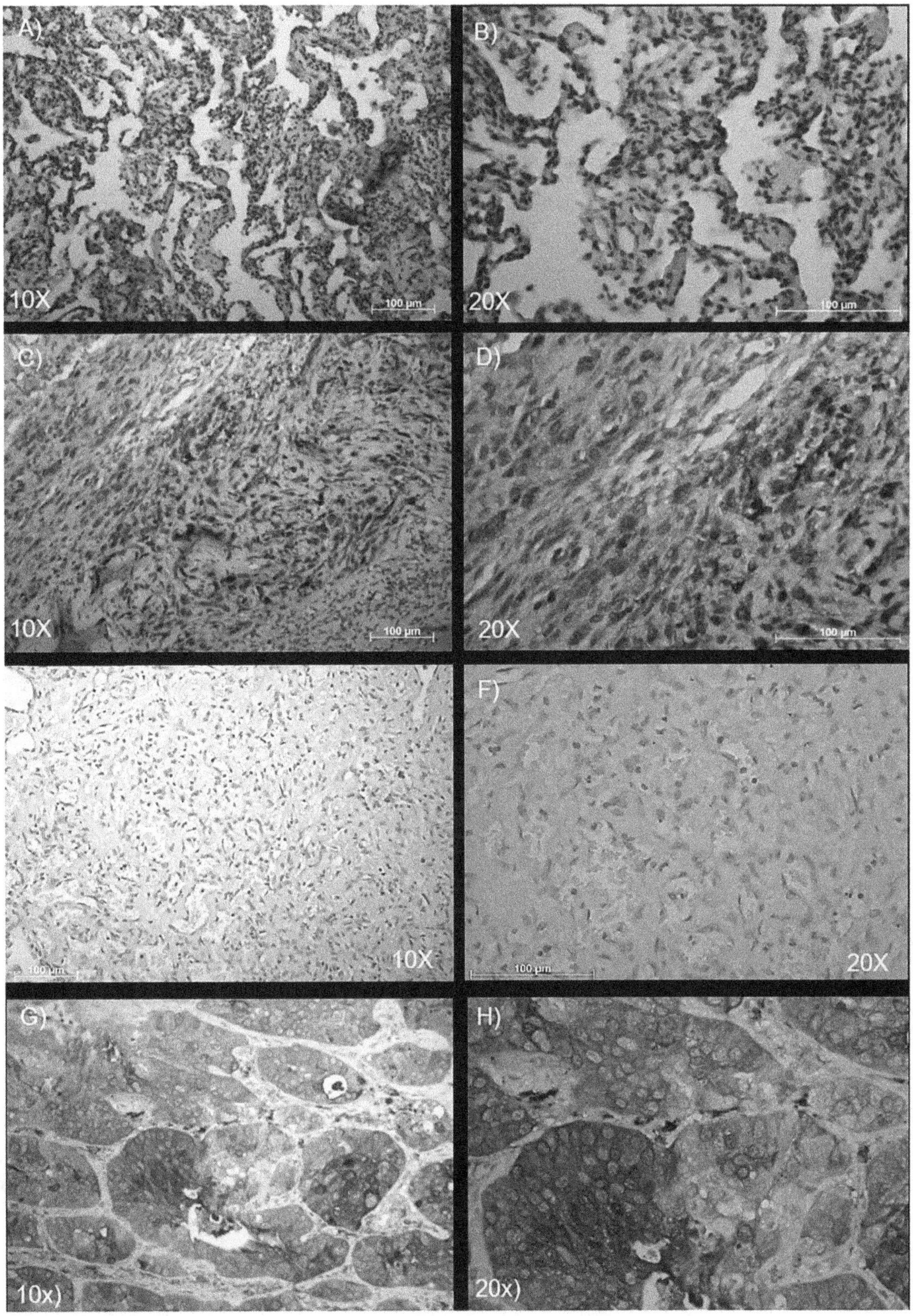

FIGURE 3 | Immunohistochemical analysis and quantification of ALDH-positive cells in two cases of angiosarcoma of the lung. Paraffin-embedded tissues were stained with an ALDH antibody to detect positive cells in these two different cases of angiosarcoma of the lung. **(A,B)** Case 1 and **(C,D)** Case 2. **(E,F)** Isotype control of anti-ALDH antibody. **(G,H)** Adenocarcinoma of the lung used as positive control of anti-ALDH antibody. Semi-quantitative method to measure ALDH based on the positivity of the tumor cells: 0 (<5% positive), 1 (5–25% positive), 2 (>25–50% positive), 3 (>50–75% positive), and 4 (>75% positive). Representative images are shown, with 10× and 20× magnification. Scale bar = 100 µm.

TABLE 1 | Angiosarcoma of the lung.

References	Patients enrolled (n)	Gender (M/F)	Age	Type of treatment (surgery and/or medical treatment)	Type of resection	Type of treatment	Immunohistochemistry (IHC) markers
Aramini et al. (19)	2	1 M 1 F	27 61	Diagnostic surgery + chemotherapy and radiotherapy 2. Surgery + chemotherapy	Surgical left lung biopsies 2. Left lower lobectomy	First line (epirubicin and ifosfamide + radiotherapy); second line (docetaxel plus gemcitabine) and then only gemcitabine 2. Four cycles gemcitabine	CD31 + CD 34 +
Carillo et al. (20)	1	M	56	Chemotherapy	Not resectable for advanced disease.	Adriamicin, II line ifosfamide	AE1/AE3 + CD31 + EMA + Vimentin + + + CD34 + + + (CEA, TTF-1, calretinin, trombomodulin, S100, HMB45, melan-A, Bcl-2, actin, desmin, CD117-)
Chen et al. (21)	2	1 F 1 M	41 50	Surgery + chemotherapy 2. Surgery + chemotherapy	Wedge resection middle lobe 2. Left lower lobectomy and lingula segmentectomy	Sorafenib 2. Four cycles Docetaxel + cisplatin	CD31 + CD 34 + Factor VIII + (CK, EMA, SMA, HMB-45, desmin, S100, ALK-)
Maglaras et al. (22)	1	M	46	Diagnostic surgery + chemotherapy	Right surgical biospy	Adriamicin + ifosfamide	Vimentin + CD31 + (EMA, CEA, S-100, pancytocheratin, cheratin, Leu-M, CD34, Factor VIII, desmin, NSE-)
Modrzewska et al. (23)	1	F	65	Diagnostic surgery	Lung surgical biopsy	/	CD31 + CD34 + (AE1/AE3, calretinin-)
Ozcelik et al. (24)	1	M	62	Surgery	Right upper lobectomy	/	CD31 + CD34 + Factor VIII + CAM 5.2 +
Palvio et al. (25)	1	M	59	Surgery	Right pneumonectomy	/	Factor VIII + Vimentin + (chetarin, desmin, EMA-)
Pandit et al. (26)	1	F	79	Surgery + chemotherapy	Wedge resection Left lower lobe	/	Factor VIII + Vimentin + CD34 +
Ng et al. (14)	1	M	60	Surgery	Left upper lobectomy	/	ERG + CD31 + (CD34, TTF-1-)
Yang et al. (27)	1	M	41	Surgery	Wedge resection left upper lobe	/	Vimentin + CD34 + CD31 + (CK7, CK5, CK20, CK8, S-100, AE1/AE3, TTF-1, Napsin-A, HMB-45, sinaptofisin, CD68, EMA, LCA, actin, desmin-)
Tanaka et al. (28)	1	M	48	Surgery + chemotherapy	Left pneumonectomy	/	ERG + CD31 + Factor VIII + FLI-1 + P53 + (CD34, C2-40, CK7, CK20, EMA, TTF-1, HMB-45, CD10)

(Continued)

TABLE 1 | Continued

References	Patients enrolled (n)	Gender (M/F)	Age	Type of treatment (surgery and/or medical treatment)	Type of resection	Type of treatment	Immunohistochemistry (IHC) markers
Shirey et al. (29)	1	M	65	Surgery + chemotherapy	Wedge resection Right upper lobe	Gemcitabin and Docetaxel	CD31 + + + Vimentin + + + AE1/AE3 + Pancytocheratin + CK7 + EMA + (CAM5.2, CK5/6, p63, S-100, desmin, SMA, Factor VIII, TTF-1, napsin-A, CD34, D2-40, CD21-)
Sheppard et al. (30)	1	M	65	Diagnostic surgery	Lung biopsy	/	CD31 + Factor VIII + CD34 + CAM 5.2 +
Zhang et al. (31)	1	M	72	Surgery for age	Left lower lobectomy	/	CD34 + CD31 + FLI-1 + Vimentin +

Review of the literature on the surgical and medical approaches in the past and at the present time. The table shows also the markers used in each study to highlight the diagnosis.

Case 2

After 5 years of treatments, the patient died in 2010 due to respiratory insufficiency caused by this malignant lung disease.

Immunohistochemical Evaluation of the ALDH Stem Cell Marker in Two Cases of Angiosarcoma of the Lung

The positivity to the ALDH marker was assessed for these pulmonary angiosarcoma cases, using a previous score system (10–12, 14). Samples were examined at 10× and at 20× magnification to assign the appropriate score value. In accordance with the literature, in the normal bronchial epithelium ALDH1A1 expression was assed (8). These two patient samples had a different expression of ALDH1A1 staining in the tumor fraction: for case 1, the score was 1 (<5–25% positive tumor cells), while in case 2 the score was 3 (>50–75% positive tumor cells) (**Figure 3**). The scores seem to be consistent with the clinical outcome of these two patients, as the lower score was observed in the patient with the better clinical outcome, while the higher score was measured in the patient with the worse clinical outcome.

DISCUSSION

Angiosarcoma of the lung is an extremely rare tumor described in only a few case reports because of its low prevalence in the population. However, it is very interesting to study because of the aggressiveness of this disease which tends to be spread in different part of the body. The rate of recurrence is very high for the intrinsic properties of this tumor with a 5-year survival rate around 20–35% (15–17), which is in contrast to the 5-year survival for all types of soft tissue sarcomas, around 65% (18).

The approaches to treat this malignancy are primarily surgery (in operable patients) and chemoradiotherapy for advanced disease. **Table 1** shows an updated information from the recent literature (10–12, 14–18, 20–29), highlighting the clinical and surgical approaches, as well as also the most frequently used markers for this disease.

It has been recently showed that ALDH identifies tumor cells with increased affinity for primary tumors, as well as a high capacity to disseminate in many organs (30–32). The scientists have recently found a correlation between ALDH and the capacity to calibrate the tumor cells dissemination into the body (30–33). In particular, different ALDH isoforms seem to be able to regulate the cells diffusion into several solid tumors (30–33). In an interesting study published in 2014 by Nicholas Greco et al. it has been demonstrated a significant correlation of aldehyde dehydrogenase (ALDH) activity and the presence/absence of distant metastases in ten consecutive cases of human bone sarcomas (34). Although angiosarcoma is more difficult to investigate for the rarity of this tumor into the population, it is important to understand the possible role that ALDH may have in this tumor for the possibility to set new target treatment against this aggressive malignant disease. Another interesting aspect recently described which needs to be considered regards the central role of ALDH into the angiogenetic process, detected into the endothelial stem-like cells in vascularized tumors (35, 36). This aspect may strongly confirm the possible presence of ALDH even in a vascularized tumor as the angiosarcoma of the lung.

In our report, we showed two cases of angiosarcoma of the lung with different scores of ALDH protein expression. In particular, in case 1, we noted a low ALDH expression (score 1). This patient had a very good outcome: he had recurrence, but achieved remission of the disease after chemo- and radiotherapeutic treatments. In case 2, the patient showed a higher ALDH expression (score 3), and the patient died due to disease recurrence. This may indicate that the severity of the ALDH score could link with the worst prognosis and viceversa. This is the first report showing the presence of the ALDH marker in angiosarcoma of the lung. Notably, this is a report of only two cases; however, although the publications in this field are limited, we believe that the current data on this marker in this disease support future studies in a larger cohort of patients to test the presence of this marker and, possibly, determine whether prognosis is correlated with the expression of this protein. If the results from this report will be confirmed in a larger population, it will be interesting to consider new targeted treatment based on ALDH, which is currently being tested in a clinical trial for hematological malignancies (9).

Limitations

Our study is the first report showing the presence of ALDH1A1 in lung angiosarcoma. We are conscious that this is a brief report of only two clinical cases, probably due to the rarity of this disease. Further multicentric studies will need to be set to confirm our data. However, we believe that our report is important to amplify the knowledge regarding possible markers which have been already studied in non-small cell lung cancer showing a high impact of this marker on the prognosis, as well as also in responses to cancer treatments (9, 10, 13, 33, 34).

In conclusion, although not confirmed in a larger cohort of patients for lung angiosarcoma, ALDH targeted therapy may be an effective treatment perspective for this malignancy, which usually appears at a high grade with an aggressive prognosis.

AUTHOR CONTRIBUTIONS

The idea for the manuscript was conceived in February 2019 by BA and was further developed by VM, DB, BM, FB, RD'A, FB, MD, UM, and AM was involved in histopathological diagnosis. BA and VM wrote the first draft of the manuscript. BA and UM had been involved in surgery and tissue collection. VM performed laboratory experiments. BA, VM, FB, MD, RD'A, AM, and UM all reviewed the manuscript and were involved in its critical revision before submission. All authors read and approved the final manuscript.

REFERENCES

1. Ren Y, Zhu M, Liu Y, Diao X, Zhang Y. Primary pulmonary angiosarcoma: three case reports and literature review: primary pulmonary angiosarcoma. *Thorac Cancer.* (2016) 7:607–13. doi: 10.1111/1759-7714.12376
2. Cao J, Wang J, He C, Fang M. Angiosarcoma: a review of diagnosis and current treatment. *Am J Cancer Res.* (2019) 9:2303–13.
3. Grafino M, Alves P, Mendes de Almeida M, Garrido P, Hasmucrai D, Teixeira E, et al. Angiosarcoma of the lung. *J Bras Pneumol.* (2016) 42:68–70. doi: 10.1590/S1806-37562016000000193
4. Hart J, Mandavilli S. Epithelioid angiosarcoma: a brief diagnostic review and differential diagnosis. *Arch Pathol Lab Med.* (2011) 135:268–72. doi: 10.1043/1543-2165-135.2.268
5. Vassalli G. Aldehyde dehydrogenases: not just markers, but functional regulators of stem cells. *Stem Cells Int.* (2019) 2019:3904645. doi: 10.1155/2019/3904645
6. Masciale V, Grisendi G, Banchelli F, D'Amico R, Maiorana A, Sighinolfi P, et al. Isolation and identification of cancer stem-like cells in adenocarcinoma and squamous cell carcinoma of the lung: a pilot study. *Front Oncol.* (2019) 9:1394. doi: 10.3389/fonc.2019.01394
7. Masciale V, Grisendi G, Banchelli F, D'Amico R, Maiorana A, Sighinolfi P, et al. Correlating tumor-infiltrating lymphocytes and lung cancer stem cells: a cross-sectional study. *Ann Transl Med.* (2019) 7:619. doi: 10.21037/atm.2019.11.27
8. Masciale V, Grisendi G, Banchelli F, D'Amico R, Maiorana A, Morandi U, et al. Cancer stem-neuroendocrine cells in an atypical carcinoid case report. *Transl Lung Cancer Res.* (2019) 8:1157–62. doi: 10.21037/tlcr.2019.12.07
9. Liu WT, Liu WB, Gao M, Zhang YY, Gu KS. Expression of ALDH1A1 and CD133 is associated with the prognosis and effect of different chemotherapeutic regimens in gastric cancer. *Oncol Lett.* (2019) 18:4573–82. doi: 10.3892/ol.2019.10798
10. Kahlert C, Bergmann F, Beck J, Welsch T, Mogler C, Herpel E, et al. Low expression of aldehyde dehydrogenase 1A1 (ALDH1A1) is a prognostic marker for poor survival in pancreatic cancer. *BMC Cancer.* (2011) 11:275. doi: 10.1186/1471-2407-11-275
11. Jiang F, Qiu Q, Khanna A, Todd NW, Deepak J, Xing L, et al. Aldehyde dehydrogenase 1 is a tumor stem cell-associated marker in lung cancer. *Mol Cancer Res.* (2009) 7:330–8. doi: 10.1158/1541-7786.MCR-08-0393
12. Xie X, Urabe G, Marcho L, Stratton M, Guo L-W, Kent CK. ALDH1A3 regulations of matricellular proteinspromote vascular smooth muscle cell proliferation. *iScience.* (2019) 19:872–82. doi: 10.1016/j.isci.2019.08.044
13. Rossi A, Voigtlaender M, Klose H, Schlüter H, Schön G, Logesl S, et al. High aldehyde dehydrogenase levels are detectable in the serum of patients with lung cancer and may be exploited as screening biomarkers. *J Oncol.* (2019) 2019:8970645. doi: 10.1155/2019/8970645
14. Ng FH, Yu SM, Wai OKH, Chan JCS. Primary epithelioid angiosarcoma of lung: radiologic and clinicopathologic correlation. *J. Clin Imaging Sci.* (2017) 7:33. doi: 10.4103/jcis.JCIS_71_16
15. Buehler D, Rice SR, Moody JS, Rush P, Hafez GR, Attia S, et al. Angiosarcoma outcomes and prognostic factors: a 25-year single institution experience. *Am J Clin Oncol.* (2014) 37:473–9. doi: 10.1097/COC.0b013e31827e4e7b
16. Singla S, Papavasiliou P, Powers B, Gaughan J, von Mehren M, Watson JC, et al. Challenges in the treatment of angiosarcoma: a single institution experience. *Am J Surg.* (2014) 208:254–9. doi: 10.1016/j.amjsurg.2014.01.007
17. Mark RJ, Poen JC, Tran LM, Fu YS, Juillard GF. Angiosarcoma. A report of 67 patients and a review of the literature. *Cancer.* (1996) 77:2400–6. doi: 10.1002/(SICI)1097-0142(19960601)77:11<2400::AID-CNCR32>3.0.CO;2-Z
18. Schottenfeld D, Fraumeni J, editors. *Cancer. Epidemiology and Prevention.* 3rd ed. New York, NY: Oxford University Press (2006).
19. Aramini B, Masciale V, Manfredini B, Bianchi D, Banchelli F, D'Amico R, et al. Expression of ALDH and SOX-2 in pulmonary sclerosing pneumocytoma (PSP) of the lung: is there a meaning behind? *Front Med.* (2020) 7:497. doi: 10.3389/fmed.2020.00497
20. Carillo GA, Carretero MA, Vazquez JE, Fontan EG, Ramos MB, Ventura JA, et al. Epithelioid angiosarcoma of the lung with pleural metastases: a rare cause of haemoptysis clinicopathological conference. *Heart Lung Circ.* (2010) 19:624–8. doi: 10.1016/j.hlc.2010.05.007
21. Chen Y-B, Guo L-C, Yang L, Feng W, Zhang X-Q, Ling C-H, et al. Angiosarcoma of the lung: 2 cases report and literature reviewed. *Lung Cancer.* (2010) 70:352–6. doi: 10.1016/j.lungcan.2010.09.002
22. Maglaras GC, Katsenos S, Kakadelis J, Katsanos C, Metafratzi Z, Stefanou DG, et al. Primary angiosarcoma of the lung and pleura. *Monaldi Arch Chest Dis.* (2004) 61:234–6. doi: 10.4081/monaldi.2004.687
23. Modrzewska K, Radzikowska E, Szołkowska M, Oniszh K, Szczesna M, Roszkowski-Sliz K. Diffuse pulmonary haemorrhage accompanied by haemothorax as a rare presentation of primary lung angiosarcoma. *Kardiochir Torakochirurgia Pol.* (2015) 12:367–71. doi: 10.5114/kitp.2015.56792

24. Ozcelik C, Onat S, Yaldiz M, Ozcelik Z. Primary epithelioid angiosarcoma of the lung presenting as pulmonary hemorrhage. *Asian Cardiovasc Thorac Ann.* (2006) 14:69–71. doi: 10.1177/021849230601400118
25. Palvio DHB, Paulsen SM, Henneberg EW. Primary angiosarcoma of the lung presenting as intractable hemoptysis. *Thorac Cardiovasc Surg.* (1987) 35:105–7. doi: 10.1055/s-2007-1020207
26. Pandit SA, Fiedler PN, Westcott JL. Primary angiosarcoma of the lung. *Ann Diagn Pathol.* (2005) 9:302–4. doi: 10.1016/j.anndiagpath.2005.04.001
27. Yang CF, Chen TW, Tseng GC, Chiang I-P. Primary pulmonary epithelioid angiosarcoma presenting as a solitary pulmonary nodule on image. *Pathol Int.* (2012) 62:424–8. doi: 10.1111/j.1440-1827.2012.02809.x
28. Tanaka H, Yorita K, Takahashi N, Usuma Y, Nakamura K, Kataoka H. Primary pulmonary angiosarcoma: a case report. *Pathol Int.* (2015) 65:554–7. doi: 10.1111/pin.12341
29. Shirey L, Coombs D, Talwar A, Mickus T. Pulmonary epithelioid angiosarcoma responsive to chemotherapy: a case report. *Radiol Case Rep.* (2018) 13:479–84. doi: 10.1016/j.radcr.2018.02.002
30. Sheppard MN, Hansell DM, Du Bois RM, Nicholson AG. Primary epithelioid angiosarcoma of the lung presenting as pulmonary haemorrhage. *Hum Pathol.* (1997) 28:383–5. doi: 10.1016/S0046-8177(97)90140-4
31. Zhang Y, Huang X, Peng C, Wang Y, Wu Q, Wu Z, et al. Primary pulmonary epithelioid angiosarcoma: a case report and literature review. *J Cancer Res Ther.* (2018) 14:533–5. doi: 10.4103/0973-1482.176419
32. Sullivan JP, Spinola M, Dodge M, Raso MG, Behrens C, Gao B, et al. Aldehyde dehydrogenase activity selects for lung adenocarcinoma stem cells dependent on Notch signaling. *Cancer Res.* (2010) 70:9937–48. doi: 10.1158/0008-5472.CAN-10-0881
33. Lohberger B, Rinner B, Stuendl N, Absenger M, Liegl-Atzwanger B, Walzer SM, et al. Aldehyde dehydrogenase 1, a potential marker for cancer stem cells in human sarcoma. *PLoS ONE.* (2012) 7:e43664. doi: 10.1371/journal.pone.0043664
34. Lei HM, Zhang KR, Wang CH, Wang Y, Zhuang GL, Lu LM, et al. Aldehyde dehydrogenase 1A1 confers erlotinib resistance via facilitating the reactive oxygen species-reactive carbonyl species metabolic pathway in lung adenocarcinomas. *Theranostics.* (2019) 9:7122–39. doi: 10.7150/thno.35729
35. Greco N, Schott T, Mu X, Rothenberg A, Voigt C, McGough RL, III, et al. ALDH activity correlates with metastatic potential in primary sarcomas of bone. *J Cancer Ther.* (2014) 5:331–8. doi: 10.4236/jct.2014.54040
36. Ohmura-Kakutani H, Akiyama K, Maishi N, Ohga N, Hida Y, Kawamoto T, et al. Identification of tumor endothelial cells with high aldehyde dehydrogenase activity and a highly angiogenic phenotype. *PLoS ONE.* (2014) 9:e113910. doi: 10.1371/journal.pone.0113910

2

Risk of Pleural Empyema in Adult Patients with Asthma

Wei-Chih Liao [1,2], Cheng-Li Lin [3], Te-Chun Shen [1,2,4], Chih-Yen Tu [1,2], Te-Chun Hsia [1] and Wu-Huei Hsu [1,2]*

[1] Division of Pulmonary and Critical Care Medicine, Department of Internal Medicine, China Medical University Hospital, Taichung, Taiwan, [2] School of Medicine, China Medical University, Taichung, Taiwan, [3] Management Office for Health Data, China Medical University Hospital, Taichung, Taiwan, [4] Intensive Care Unit, Chu Shang Show Chwan Hospital, Nantou, Taiwan

***Correspondence:**
Te-Chun Shen
chestshen@gmail.com

Background: Respiratory system infections commonly occur among individuals with asthma. However, whether asthma patients have a higher risk of pleural empyema development remains unclear.

Methods: This is a retrospective cohort study based on data from the National Health Insurance Research Database of Taiwan. The asthma cohort consisted of 48,360 newly diagnosed adult individuals from 2000 to 2012. The comparison cohort consisted of the same number of adults who did not have asthma and was matched for age, gender, comorbidity, and the year of diagnosis. The development of pleural empyema was followed up to 2013.

Results: Pleural empyema incidence was 2.03-fold higher in the asthma cohort compared to the comparison cohort (8.65 vs. 4.25 per 10,000 person-years), with an adjusted hazard ratio (HR) of 2.12 [95% confidence interval (CI) = 1.76–2.56]. Stratified analyses by age, gender, comorbidity, and corticosteroid use revealed that the crude and adjusted HRs of pleural empyema associated with asthma were all significant. Among patients with asthma, the risk of pleural empyema elevated with increased frequency of annual asthma-related emergency room visits and hospital admissions (≥1 vs. <1, aHR = 8.07, 95% CI = 4.31–15.1 and aHR = 9.31, 95% CI = 5.56–15.6).

Conclusion: An increased risk of pleural empyema occurrence was observed in adult patients with asthma than those without asthma. Furthermore, the risk of pleural empyema may increase with poor control of asthma.

Keywords: empyema, asthma, pneumonia, cohort study, retrospective study

INTRODUCTION

Asthma is a heterogeneous disease manifesting with airway inflammation (1). This disease is defined by the presence of respiratory symptoms that vary over time and in intensity, together with variable expiratory airflow limitation (2). Inadequate control of asthma may lead to frequent exacerbations, worse health status, and poor quality of life (3). Asthma is also found to be associated with respiratory system infections, but information on the underlying mechanism of this predisposition is limited (4). Altered epithelial microenvironment and impaired immune function may contribute to the susceptibility of respiratory system infections (5, 6).

Pleural empyema indicates the occurrence of frank pus within the pleural space (7). It is most commonly caused by respiratory system infections, such as pneumonia (8). Mortality rate among individuals having pneumonia with pleural empyema is far higher than in patients who do not have pleural empyema (9, 10). The crucial nature of pleural empyema and the need for removal have been identified for several centuries (11). Delayed diagnosis and poor drainage have been found to be linked with high mortality (12). Alcohol consumption, substance use, diabetes mellitus, immunosuppression, malignancy, pulmonary disease, and prior occurrence of pleural effusion are predictors of the development of pleural empyema (13, 14).

Several studies have investigated the association between asthma and respiratory system infections (15–18). However, the studies did not examine the incidence of pleural empyema in asthma patients. Pleural empyema is a noticeable infection of the respiratory system and requires timely treatments, such as antibiotic therapy, pleural drainage, intrapleural fibrinolysis, and surgery. Thus, investigating the risk of pleural empyema in patients with asthma is necessary. This study aimed to examine whether patients with asthma have a higher risk of pleural empyema development. In addition, we attempted to assess the effect of asthma control on the occurrence of pleural empyema.

MATERIALS AND METHODS

Data Source

The Taiwan National Health Insurance (NHI) program was established in 1995. The National Health Insurance Research Database (NHIRD) is a nationwide database housing medical claims data of over 99.5% of people living in Taiwan (https://nhird.nhri.org.tw/en/). The database is updated and maintained by the National Health Research Institutes. The Longitudinal Health Insurance Database 2000 (LHID2000, a subset data of NHIRD) was used for this study. The database contains medical claims data of one million persons randomly selected from users registered in 2000. Data on their demographic characteristics, diagnostic codes, procedure claims, and medication claims were available from 1995 to 2013. All data were deidentified to protect their privacy; therefore, written informed consent from the participants involved was unnecessary. This study was approved by the Research Ethics Committee of the China Medical University and Hospital (CMUH-104-REC2-115).

Study Cohorts

Patients with newly diagnosed asthma [International Classification of Disease, 9th Revision, Clinical Modification (ICD-9-CM) code 493 and asthma medication (bronchodilator or corticosteroid)] from January 1, 2000, to December 31, 2012, were selected in the asthma cohort. The date of the diagnosis was defined as the index date. Individuals with a diagnosis of pleural empyema before the index date and those with incomplete data were excluded from the analysis. The individuals in the comparison cohort included people free from asthma. The exclusion criteria for the comparison cohort were the same as for the asthma cohort. The comparison cohort was 1:1 frequency-matched with the asthma cohort by age, gender, comorbidity, and index year. All subjects were monitored until any of the following occurred: (1) development of pleural empyema, (2) withdrawal from NHI system, (3) death, and (4) the date of 31st of December 2013.

Outcome and Variables

All diseases were recorded in accordance with the ICD-9-CM in the NHIRD. The primary outcome was pleural empyema (based on ICD-9-CM code 510 and related antibiotic treatment). We also determined the related baseline comorbidities between 1995 and index date, including chronic obstructive pulmonary disease (COPD, ICD-9-CM code 496), diabetes mellitus (ICD-9-CM code 250), chronic kidney disease (CKD, ICD-9-CM code 585), chronic liver disease and cirrhosis (CLD, ICD-9-CM code 571), rheumatic disease (ICD-9-CM codes 446.5, 710.0–710.4, 714.0–714.2, 714.8, and 725), stroke (ICD-9-CM codes 433–438), cancer (ICD-9-CM codes 140–209), and malnutrition (ICD-9-CM codes 260–269). We selected only diagnoses from the outpatient department that appeared at least twice within 1 year or had a diagnosis of hospitalization to increase the accuracy for asthma, pleural empyema, and all comorbidities. In addition, we evaluated the related medication, corticosteroid use.

Statistical Analysis

We used the Chi-squared test to examine the proportion distribution of age group, gender, comorbidity, and medication between asthma and comparison cohorts. The means of age in the two cohorts were compared using a student's *t*-test. The estimation of cumulative incidence of pleural empyema in asthma and comparison cohorts was performed by the Kaplan–Meier method. A log-rank test was utilized to determine the significance. The incidence rates of pleural empyema were calculated by asthma, age group, gender, comorbidities, and medication. Univariable and multivariable Cox proportional hazard regression models were used to estimate hazard ratios (HRs) and 95% confidence intervals (CIs). Moreover, we calculated the incidence rates and relative risk of pleural empyema by stratification with age, gender, comorbidities, and medication between asthma and comparison cohorts. Among patients with asthma, we further evaluated the impact of the annual number of asthma-related emergency room visits and hospital admissions and cumulative corticosteroid doses on pleural empyema development. Data analysis was performed with the SAS statistical software (Version 9.4 for Windows; SAS Institute, Inc., Cary, NC, USA). Statistical significance was considered at a p-value < 0.05.

RESULTS

We recruited an asthma group comprising 48,360 patients and a comparator group of 48,360 individuals (**Table 1**). Age and gender did not significantly differ between asthma and comparator group. The mean age $\pm$ standard division of asthma and comparator group was 54.9 $\pm$ 18.7 and 54.1 $\pm$ 18.5 years, respectively. Approximately 52% of the individuals were women in both groups. The major comorbidities of the asthma group were COPD (24.8%), CLD (21.7%), followed by diabetes mellitus

TABLE 1 | Baseline characteristics between asthma and non-asthma cohorts.

	Asthma				*p*-value
	No		Yes		
	N = 48,360		*N* = 48,360		
	n	%	*n*	%	
Age					0.63
20–49	19,720	40.8	19,680	40.7	
50–64	11,918	24.6	11,826	24.5	
≥65	16,722	34.6	16,854	34.9	
Mean ± SD	54.1	±18.5	54.9	±18.7	0.001
Gender					0.46
Women	24,873	51.4	24,988	51.7	
Men	23,487	48.6	23,372	48.3	
Comorbidity					
Diabetes mellitus	5,254	10.9	5,269	10.9	0.88
CKD	1,195	2.47	1,066	2.20	0.01
CLD	10,337	21.4	10,513	21.7	0.17
COPD	11,880	24.6	11,988	24.8	0.42
Rheumatic disease	1,360	2.81	1,346	2.78	0.78
Stroke	3,549	7.34	3,350	6.93	0.01
Cancer	1,598	3.30	1,527	3.16	0.20
Malnutrition	401	0.83	339	0.70	0.02
Medication					
Corticosteroid	7,355	15.2	11,392	23.6	<0.001

CKD, chronic kidney disease; CLD, chronic liver disease and cirrhosis; COPD, chronic obstructive pulmonary disease; SD, standard deviation.

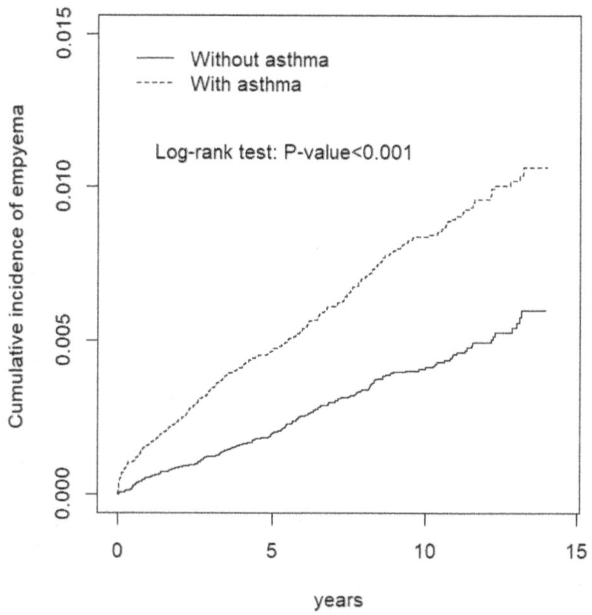

FIGURE 1 | Cumulative incidence of pleural empyema in the asthma group (dashed line) and in the comparison group (solid line).

(10.9%), stroke (6.93%), and cancer (3.16%). The mean follow-up periods were 7.72 ± 4.15 years in the asthma group and 8.03 ± 4.02 years in the comparator group. The proportion of corticosteroid use were 23.6% in the asthma group and 15.2% in the comparator group. **Figure 1** showed that patients with asthma had a higher cumulative incidence of pleural empyema than individuals without asthma throughout the 14-year study period.

The overall incidence density rates of pleural empyema were 8.65 and 4.25 per 10,000 person-years in asthma and comparator groups, respectively (**Table 2**). Compared with the comparator group, the corresponding adjusted HR (aHR) of pleural empyema was 2.12 (95% CI = 1.76–2.56) in the asthma group after adjusting for age, gender, COPD, diabetes mellitus, CKD, CLD, stroke, cancer, and corticosteroid use. Compared with persons aged 20–49, the aHRs of pleural empyema were 2.43-fold higher in those aged 50–64 (95% CI = 1.80–3.29) and 4.10-fold higher in those aged ≥65 (95% CI = 3.09–5.44). The aHR of pleural empyema was 2.55-fold higher for men relative to women (95% CI = 2.09–3.12). Moreover, the risk of pleural empyema was higher in persons with stroke (aHR = 2.68, 95% CI = 2.12–3.38), diabetes mellitus (aHR = 1.86, 95% CI = 1.50–2.31), and COPD (aHR = 1.48, 95% CI = 1.22–1.79) compared with subjects without these comorbidities.

Further analyses revealed that the incidences and aHRs of pleural empyema for the asthma group were all significantly higher compared with the comparator group after stratification for age, gender, presence of comorbidities, and corticosteroid use (**Table 3**). In addition, we assessed the impact of the frequency of asthma-related emergency room visits and hospital admissions on the development of pleural empyema among the asthma group (**Table 4**). A higher frequency of annual asthma-related emergency room visits and hospital admissions raised the risk of pleural empyema development (both p for trend <0.001). Moreover, we analyzed cumulative corticosteroid doses on pleural empyema development among the asthma group (**Table 4**). The incidence of pleural empyema was higher in those with corticosteroid use; however, the p value for trend was not significant ($p = 0.25$).

DISCUSSION

We believed that this investigation is the first population-based retrospective cohort study to evaluate the incidence of pleural empyema in patients with asthma. Our findings revealed that patients with asthma have a significantly higher risk of developing pleural empyema than those without asthma. The risk of pleural empyema was also larger in older people, in males, those with comorbidities. Furthermore, the hazards of pleural empyema were significantly larger in the asthma cohort compared with the comparison cohort under stratification by age, gender, comorbidity, and corticosteroid use. Moreover, we found that the risk of pleural empyema was higher in asthma patients with an increased number of asthma-related emergency medical demands and hospital admissions, indicating that the level of asthma control may influence the occurrence of pleural empyema.

TABLE 2 | Incidences and hazard ratios of pleural empyema by asthma, age, gender, comorbidity, and corticosteroid use among all participants.

	Event	PY	Rate[#]	Crude HR (95% CI)	Adjusted HR[†] (95% CI)
Asthma					
No	165	388,334	4.25	1.00	1.00
Yes	323	373,337	8.65	2.03 (1.68–2.45)***	2.12 (1.76–2.56)***
Age					
20–49	69	347,688	1.98	1.00	1.00
50–64	121	196,168	6.17	3.10 (2.31–4.16)***	2.43 (1.80–3.29)***
≥65	298	217,815	13.7	6.76 (5.20–8.79)***	4.10 (3.09–5.44)***
Gender					
Women	135	404,727	3.34	1.00	1.00
Men	353	356,945	9.89	2.95 (2.42–3.60)***	2.55 (2.09–3.12)***
Comorbidity					
COPD					
No	278	569,143	4.66	1.00	1.00
Yes	210	165,529	12.7	2.68 (2.24–3.21)***	1.48 (1.22–1.79)***
Diabetes mellitus					
No	372	694,873	5.35	1.00	1.00
Yes	116	66,799	17.4	3.17 (2.57–3.91)***	1.86 (1.50–2.31)***
CKD					
No	470	749,761	6.27	1.00	1.00
Yes	18	11,911	15.1	2.30 (1.43–3.68)***	1.22 (0.75–1.96)
CLD					
No	350	599,220	5.84	1.00	1.00
Yes	138	162,451	8.49	1.45 (1.19–1.77)***	1.16 (0.95–1.41)
Rheumatic disease					
No	471	743,383	6.34	1.00	
Yes	17	18,288	9.30	1.44 (0.89–2.33)	
Stroke					
No	390	727,905	5.36	1.00	1.00
Yes	98	33,766	29.0	5.19 (4.15–6.49)***	2.68 (2.12–3.38)***
Cancer					
No	466	746,246	6.24	1.00	1.00
Yes	22	15,425	14.3	2.17 (1.41–3.33)***	1.39 (0.91–2.14)
Malnutrition					
No	484	756,482	6.40	1.00	
Yes	4	5,189	7.71	1.19 (0.45–3.18)	
Medication					
Corticosteroid					
No	370	634,551	5.83	1.00	1.00
Yes	118	127,120	9.28	1.56 (1.27–1.92)***	1.02 (0.82–1.26)

CI, confidence interval; CKD, chronic kidney disease; CLD, chronic liver disease and cirrhosis; COPD, chronic obstructive pulmonary disease; HR, hazard ratio; PY, person-years.
[#]Incidence rate per 10,000 person-years.
*[†]Multivariable analysis including age, gender, COPD, diabetes mellitus, CKD, CLD, stroke, cancer, and corticosteroid use. ***$p < 0.001$.*

The mechanism between asthma and pleural empyema remains largely unknown. Patients with asthma who are susceptible to pneumonia may still play a major role. This condition may be driven by the following: (1) a large prevalence of carriage of the bacteria, (2) a disordered immune response from exposure to the bacteria, (3) impaired bacterial clearance, and (4) a suboptimal response to vaccination (5). Parapneumonic pleural effusions are known to represent a common complication of pneumonia and can be found in approximately 40% of bacterial pneumonia cases (11). In addition, inhaled or systemic corticosteroid use, shared comorbidities, cigarette smoking, alcohol consumption, unhealthy lifestyle, poor self-care, and poor physical health are commonly noted among asthma patients. These factors are also related to the development of pneumonia and pleural empyema (9).

Inconsistent evidence was found between chronic inflammatory airway disease and the development of pleural empyema. Lu et al. (19) conducted a case-control study to

TABLE 3 | Incidences and hazard ratios of pleural empyema by age, gender, comorbidity, and corticosteroid use between asthma and non-asthma cohorts.

	Asthma						Crude HR (95% CI)	Adjusted HR† (95% CI)
	No			Yes				
	Event	PY	Rate#	Event	PY	Rate#		
Age								
20–49	23	174,025	1.32	46	173,662	2.65	2.01 (1.22–3.31)**	1.98 (1.20–3.27)**
50–64	31	99,658	3.11	90	96,510	9.33	3.00 (1.99–4.51)***	3.06 (2.03–4.62)***
≥65	111	114,651	9.68	187	103,164	18.1	1.86 (1.47–2.36)***	1.91 (1.51–2.43)***
Gender								
Women	36	205,289	1.75	99	199,437	4.96	2.83 (1.93–4.14)***	2.78 (1.89–4.08)***
Men	129	183,045	7.05	224	173,900	12.9	1.82 (1.47–2.26)***	1.94 (1.56–2.42)***
Comorbidity§								
No	34	212,837	1.60	98	210,361	4.66	2.92 (1.98–4.31)***	2.95 (1.99–4.36)***
Yes	131	175,497	7.46	225	162,975	13.8	1.84 (1.48–2.28)***	1.91 (1.54–2.37)***
Corticosteroid								
No	139	338,472	4.11	231	296,079	7.80	1.90 (1.54–2.34)***	2.05 (1.66–2.53)***
Yes	26	49,862	5.21	92	77,258	11.9	2.28 (1.48–3.53)***	2.43 (1.61–3.86)***

CI, confidence interval; HR, hazard ratio; PY, person-years.
#Incidence rate per 10,000 person-years.
†Multivariable analysis including age, gender, COPD, diabetes mellitus, CKD, CLD, stroke, cancer, and corticosteroid use.
§Individuals with any comorbidity of COPD, diabetes mellitus, CKD, CLD, rheumatic disease, stroke, cancer, and malnutrition were classified into the comorbidity group.
$^{**}p < 0.01$, $^{***}p < 0.001$.

TABLE 4 | Incidences and hazard ratios of pleural empyema by emergency room visits, hospital admissions, and cumulative corticosteroid doses among asthma cohort.

	Event	Incidence#	Crude HR (95% CI)	Adjusted HR† (95% CI)
Annual emergency room visits				
<1	311	8.34	1.00	1.00
≥1	12	334.9	19.7 (10.6–36.4)***	8.07 (4.31–15.1)***
p for trend				<0.001
Annual hospital admissions				
<1	302	8.10	1.00	1.00
≥1	21	362.7	24.6 (15.0–40.5)***	9.31 (5.56–15.6)***
p for trend				<0.001
Cumulative corticosteroid doses (mg)				
None	231	7.80	1.00	1.00
<115	9	10.3	1.31 (0.67–2.55)	0.98 (0.50–1.91)
115–335	35	15.4	1.93 (1.35–2.75)***	1.53 (1.07–2.19)*
≥335	48	10.6	1.30 (0.95–1.78)	0.93 (0.68–1.28)
p for trend				0.25

CI, confidence interval; HR, hazard ratio.
#Incidence rate per 10,000 person-years.
†Multivariable analysis including age, gender, COPD, diabetes mellitus, CKD, CLD, stroke, cancer, and corticosteroid use.
$^{*}p < 0.05$, $^{***}p < 0.001$.

evaluate the potential risk factors of pleural empyema. They enrolled 1,851 pleural empyema cases and 7,404 non-empyema controls and found significant factors that lead to pleural empyema include the following: aspiration history [odds ratio (OR) = 7.28, 95% CI = 5.00–10.6)], human immunodeficiency virus infection (OR = 5.66, 95% CI = 1.38–23.2), malnutrition (OR = 2.86, 95% CI = 2.07–3.95), cancer (OR = 2.74, 95% CI = 2.28–3.30), diabetes mellitus (OR = 2.25, 95% CI = 1.96–2.59), stroke (OR = 1.99, 95% CI = 1.70–2.34), CKD (OR = 1.78, 95% CI = 1.42–2.25), chronic obstructive pulmonary disease (COPD, OR = 1.72, 95% CI = 1.47–2.01), asthma (OR

= 1.34, 95% CI = 1.15–1.57), and CLD (OR = 1.20, 95% CI = 1.06–1.35). In another study, Lu et al. evaluated COPD and the subsequent development of pleural empyema (20). They enrolled 55,136 COPD cases and 98,769 non-COPD controls and found that the incidence of pleural empyema was 3.64-fold higher in the COPD cohort than in the comparison cohort (15.8 vs. 4.34 per 10,000 person-years), with a corresponding aHR of 3.25 (95% CI = 2.73–3.87). These findings may suggest that chronic inflammatory airway disease may contribute to the development of pleural empyema. By contrast, Dusemund et al. (21) performed a case-control study in Switzerland to investigate outcomes of community-acquired pneumonia in patients with chronic lung disease. They found that the incidence of pleural empyema was insignificant in asthma [0.5% (asthma) vs. 0.9% (controls), $p = 0.141$] and COPD [0.5% (COPD) vs. 0.5% (controls), $p = 0.817$]. In addition, Elemraid et al. (22) assessed predictors of pleural empyema development in children. They found that age, sex, mother's age, smoking among the child's parents, poverty, nursery attendance, asthma, and household characteristics (bedrooms and number of occupants) were not significantly related. Therefore, we may need additional investigations to clarify this issue.

Strength

The strength of this study lies in the establishment of a population-based asthma cohort to assess the risk of developing pleural empyema. Conducting a prospective cohort study is expensive. Therefore, a retrospective cohort study based on insurance claims data may be a suitable and economical alternative. Regardless of socioeconomic background and/or residential location, the universal coverage by the NHI program lowers access barriers to health care all citizens (23). This study was able to reflect a "real world" scenario in which asthma, pleural empyema, and comorbidities were assessed during medical evaluation.

Limitation

Several limitations exist and need to be considered in interpreting the study findings. First, the ICD-9-CM algorithm was used to define asthma, pleural empyema, and comorbidities. All diagnoses were dependent on the competence of clinical physicians in diagnosing; however, asthma has been carefully validated in the NHIRD (24). In addition, an *ad hoc* committee established by the insurance authority monitored the evaluation of claims data to prevent errors and violations. We selected only diagnoses from the outpatient department that appeared at least twice within 1 year or had a diagnosis of hospitalization to increase the accuracy. In addition, we applied the medication used to improve the diagnosis of asthma and empyema. Second, the NHIRD does not provide detailed information regarding smoking habits, drinking habits, and other environmental factors, which are potentially confounding factors in the current study. In addition, relevant clinical variables, such as serum laboratory data, image reports, and culture results, were unavailable in the database.

CONCLUSION

An increased risk of pleural empyema occurrence was observed in adult patients with asthma compared to those without asthma. Furthermore, the risk of pleural empyema may increase with the degree of asthma control.

AUTHOR CONTRIBUTIONS

W-CL, T-CS, C-YT, T-CH, and W-HH: conception and design. C-YT, T-CH, and W-HH: administrative support. W-CL, C-LL, and T-CS: collection and assembly of data and data analysis and interpretation. All authors: manuscript writing and final approval of manuscript.

REFERENCES

1. Borish L, Culp JA. Asthma: a syndrome composed of heterogeneous diseases. *Ann Allergy Asthma Immunol.* (2008) 101:1–8. doi: 10.1016/S1081-1206(10)60826-5
2. Menzies-Gow A, McBrien CN, Baker JR, Donnelly LE, Cohen RT. Update in asthma and airway inflammation 2018. *Am J Respir Crit Care Med.* (2019) 200:14–9. doi: 10.1164/rccm.201902-0321UP
3. Stanescu S, Kirby SE, Thomas M, Yardley L, Ainsworth B. A systematic review of psychological, physical health factors, and quality of life in adult asthma. *NPJ Prim Care Respir Med.* (2019) 29:37. doi: 10.1038/s41533-019-0149-3
4. Tracy MC, Mathew R. Complicated pneumonia: current concepts and state of the art. *Curr Opin Pediatr.* (2018) 30:384–92. doi: 10.1097/MOP.0000000000000619
5. Zaidi SR, Blakey JD. Why are people with asthma susceptible to pneumonia? a review of factors related to upper airway bacteria. *Respirology.* (2019) 24:423–30. doi: 10.1111/resp.13528
6. Christou EAA, Giardino G, Stefanaki E, Ladomenou F. Asthma: an undermined state of immunodeficiency. *Int Rev Immunol.* (2019) 38:70–8. doi: 10.1080/08830185.2019.1588267
7. Redden MD, Chin TY, van Driel ML. Surgical versus non-surgical management for pleural empyema. *Cochrane Database Syst Rev.* (2017) 3:CD010651. doi: 10.1002/14651858.CD010651.pub2
8. Bedawi EO, Hassan M, Rahman NM. Recent developments in the management of pleural infection: a comprehensive review. *Clin Respir J.* (2018) 12:2309–20. doi: 10.1111/crj.12941
9. Hasley PB, Albaum MN, Li YH, Fuhrman CR, Britton CA, Marrie TJ, et al. Do pulmonary radiographic findings at presentation predict mortality in patients with community-acquired pneumonia? *Arch Intern Med.* (1996) 156:2206–12. doi: 10.1001/archinte.156.19.2206
10. Menéndez R, Torres A, Zalacaín R, Aspa J, Martín Villasclaras JJ, Borderías L, et al. Risk factors of treatment failure in community acquired pneumonia: implications for disease outcome. *Thorax.* (2004) 59:960–5. doi: 10.1136/thx.2003.017756
11. Feller-Kopman D, Light R. Pleural disease. *N Engl J Med.* (2018) 378:740–51. doi: 10.1056/NEJMra1403503
12. Ashbaugh DG. Empyema thoracis. factors influencing morbidity and mortality. *Chest.* (1991) 99:1162–5. doi: 10.1378/chest.99.5.1162
13. Strange C, Sahn SA. The definitions and epidemiology of pleural space infection. *Semin Respir Infect.* (1999) 14:3–8.
14. Sahn SA. Diagnosis and management of parapneumonic effusions and empyema. *Clin Infect Dis.* (2007) 45:1480–6. doi: 10.1086/522996
15. Talbot TR, Hartert TV, Mitchel E, Halasa NB, Arbogast PG, Poehling KA, et al. Asthma as a risk factor for invasive pneumococcal disease. *N Engl J Med.* (2005) 352:2082–90. doi: 10.1056/NEJMoa044113
16. Juhn YJ, Kita H, Yawn BP, Boyce TG, Yoo KH, McGree ME, et al. Increased

risk of serious pneumococcal disease in patients with asthma. *J Allergy Clin Immunol.* (2008) 122:719–23. doi: 10.1016/j.jaci.2008.07.029
17. Klemets P, Lyytikainen O, Ruutu P, Ollgren J, Kaijalainen T, Leinonen M, et al. Risk of invasive pneumococcal infections among working age adults with asthma. *Thorax.* (2010) 65:698–702. doi: 10.1136/thx.2009.132670
18. Almirall J, Serra-Prat M, Bolíbar I, Balasso V. Risk factors for community-acquired pneumonia in adults: a systematic review of observational studies. *Respiration.* (2017) 94:299–311. doi: 10.1159/000479089
19. Lu TC, Shen TC, Lin CL, Yen CC, Wu HS. Risk factors of empyema and their impacts on the prognosis in Taiwan. *J Intern Med Taiwan.* (2020) 31:276–83. doi: 10.6314/JIMT.202008_31(4).08
20. Lu HY, Liao KM. Risk of empyema in patients with COPD. *Int J Chron Obstruct Pulmon Dis.* (2018) 13:317–24. doi: 10.2147/COPD.S149835
21. Dusemund F, Chronis J, Baty F, Albrich WC, Brutsche MH. The outcome of community-acquired pneumonia in patients with chronic lung disease: a case-control study. *Swiss Med Wkly.* (2014) 144:w14013. doi: 10.4414/smw.2014.14013
22. Elemraid MA, Thomas MF, Blain AP, Rushton SP, Spencer DA, Gennery AR, et al. Risk factors for the development of pleural empyema in children. *Pediatr Pulmonol.* (2015) 50:721–6. doi: 10.1002/ppul.23041
23. Hsing AW, Ioannidis JP. Nationwide population science: lessons from the Taiwan national health insurance research database. *JAMA Intern Med.* (2015) 175:1527–9. doi: 10.1001/jamainternmed.2015.3540
24. Su VY, Yang KY, Yang YH, Tsai YH, Perng DW, Su WJ, et al. Use of ICS/LABA combinations or LAMA is associated with a lower risk of acute exacerbation in patients with coexistent COPD and asthma. *J Allergy Clin Immunol Pract.* (2018) 6:1927–35. doi: 10.1016/j.jaip.2018.01.035

3

Radio-Histological Correlation of Lung Features in Severe COVID-19 Through CT-Scan and Lung Ultrasound Evaluation

*Pere Trias-Sabrià [1,2], Eduard Dorca Duch [3], Maria Molina-Molina [1,2], Samantha Aso [1], Marta Díez-Ferrer [1], Alfredo Marín Muñiz [1], Jaume Bordas-Martínez [1], Joan Sabater [2,4], Patricio Luburich [5], Belén del Rio [5], Xavier Solanich [5], Jordi Dorca [1,2], Salud Santos [1,2] and Guillermo Suárez-Cuartin [1,2]**

[1] Respiratory Department, Hospital Universitari de Bellvitge, Institut d'Investigació Biomèdica de Bellvitge (IDIBELL), L'Hospitalet de Llobregat, Spain, [2] Universitat de Barcelona-Campus Bellvitge, L'Hospitalet de Llobregat, Spain, [3] Pathology Department, Hospital Universitari de Bellvitge, Institut d'Investigació Biomèdica de Bellvitge (IDIBELL), L'Hospitalet de Llobregat, Spain, [4] Critical Care Department, Hospital Universitari de Bellvitge, Institut d'Investigació Biomèdica de Bellvitge (IDIBELL), L'Hospitalet de Llobregat, Spain, [5] Radiology Department, Hospital Universitari de Bellvitge, Institut d'Investigació Biomèdica de Bellvitge (IDIBELL), L'Hospitalet de Llobregat, Spain

***Correspondence:**
Guillermo Suárez-Cuartin
gsuarezc@bellvitgehospital.cat

Background: Patients with coronavirus disease 2019 (COVID-19) can develop severe bilateral pneumonia leading to respiratory failure. Lung histological samples were scarce due to the high risk of contamination during autopsies. We aimed to correlate histological COVID-19 features with radiological findings through lung ultrasound (LU)-guided postmortem core needle biopsies (CNBs) and computerized tomography (CT) scans.

Methodology: We performed an observational prospective study, including 30 consecutive patients with severe COVID-19. The thorax was divided into 12 explorations regions to correlate LU and CT-scan features. Histological findings were also related to radiological features through CNBs.

Results: Mean age was 62.56 ± 13.27 years old, with 96.7% male patients. Postmortem LU-guided CNBs were performed in 13 patients. Thirty patients were evaluated with both thoracic LU and chest CT scan, representing a total of 279 thoracic regions explored. The most frequent LU finding was B2-lines (49.1%). The most CT-scan finding was ground-glass opacity (GGO, 29%). Pathological CT-scan findings were commonly observed when B2-lines or C-lines were identified through LU (positive predictive value, PPV, 87.1%). Twenty-five postmortem echo-guided histological samples were obtained from 12 patients. Histological samples showed diffuse alveolar damage (DAD) (75%) and chronic interstitial inflammation (25%). The observed DAD was heterogeneous, showing multiple evolving patterns of damage, including exudative (33.3%), fibrotic (33.3%), and organizing (8.3%) phases. In those patients with acute or exudative pattern, two lesions were distinguished: classic hyaline membrane; fibrin "plug" in alveolar space (acute fibrinous organizing pneumonia, AFOP). C-profile was described in 33.3% and presented histological signs of DAD and lung fibrosis. The predominant findings were collagen deposition (50%) and AFOP (50%). B2-lines were identified in 66.7%; the presence of hyaline membrane was the predominant finding (37.5%), then organizing pneumonia (12.5%) and fibrosis (37.5%). No A-lines or B1-lines were observed in these patients.

Conclusion: LU B2-lines and C-profile are predominantly identified in patients with severe COVID-19 with respiratory worsening, which correspond to different CT patterns and histological findings of DAD and lung fibrosis.

Keywords: COVID-19, lung ultrasonography (LU), biopsy, pathology, radiology

INTRODUCTION

Coronavirus disease 2019 (COVID-19) is a viral infection by novel severe acute respiratory syndrome coronavirus 2 (SARS-CoV-2). Patients with COVID-19 develop interstitial pneumonia, which can lead to respiratory failure (54%) and acute respiratory distress syndrome (ARDS) (31%) (1). The COVID-19 has a global spread all around the globe (2). Monitoring and therapeutic protocols are being modified regarding growing research evidence.

Chest imaging is a valuable tool for diagnosis, clinical management, and guiding therapy. Chest radiography is initially performed for identifying pneumonia and computerized tomography (CT) is recommended for better evaluating ARDS and other potential complications (3). The main radiological findings are multi-lobar asymmetric ground-glass opacity (GGO) and bilateral peripheral consolidations (4–6). When ARDS develops, other findings might be present, such as organizing pneumonia and traction bronchiectasis (7–9). Although chest CT gives relevant information for therapeutic approach, some challenges have been found during the COVID-19 pandemic, including the risk of infection for healthcare workers, the need of space and surface cleaning and disinfection, the life-threatening for critical patients of their transfer, and the inconvenience for monitoring disease progression or worsening in respiratory critical conditions that make difficult the mobilization of patient (3). Lung ultrasound (LU) has been developed as an important tool in monitoring patients with COVID-19, both in intermediate respiratory care units (IMCUs) and in intensive care units (ICUs) (10, 11). LU is easy to use, repeatable, and reproducible, and allows an immediate bedside application which drives to rapid decision-making (12). LU has the ability to identify and monitor an alveolar–interstitial pattern, defined by the presence of convalescents B-lines, white lung, or subpleural consolidations (13–15). Some initial correlations between LU and CT patterns have been described (3). However, the pathological findings behind this radiological imaging of COVID-19-induced lung damage remain elusive.

Histopathological understanding of the disease would be relevant for better targeting therapeutic options. However, performing lung biopsy in severe COVID-19 infection may associate clinical deterioration and potential life-threatening complications. Most pathological findings from autopsies or postmortem biopsies describe diffuse alveolar damage (DAD) with cellular interstitial pattern and fibromyxoid interstitial deposition as well as microthrombi in small vessels (16–19). The different histomorphological patterns of damage could correspond to specific ultrasound and/or tomographic patterns. Characterizing the lung images that correspond to the different histological findings could help in prognostication and optimizing treatments. We aimed to correlate histological COVID-19 features with LU findings and CT-scan features by performing LU-guided transthoracic immediately postmortem core needle biopsy (CNB). Furthermore, we looked for the CT radiological features that were present in the different LU patterns using both as complementary radiological tools.

MATERIALS AND METHODS

Data Collection and Design

This observational prospective study included 30 consecutive patients with severe COVID-19 with progressive worsening despite supportive care who were evaluated through CT scan and LU. All of them were hospitalized in the IMCU or ICU of the University Hospital of Bellvitge, Barcelona, Spain, in April 2020. LU-guided CNB immediately postmortem was performed in 13 patients.

The study protocol was approved by the local ethics committee (N° PR122/20). All procedures performed in this study involving human participants were in accordance with the ethical standards of the institution, and with the 1964 Helsinki Declaration. The inclusion criteria were confirmed COVID-19 diagnosis with a positive polymerase chain reaction (PCR) for SARS-CoV-2, having informed consent by the family for transthoracic biopsy in case of death. The exclusion criteria included a clinical worsening due to other reasons different than COVID-19 lung injury and/or extrapulmonary complications. Demographic, clinical, radiological, and laboratory data were collected, including previous medical conditions, time from the onset of symptoms, blood test analysis, and treatment received. LU findings were described following the international evidence-based recommendations (13).

LU Exploration

A targeted LU examination was performed by a trained pulmonologist. A Philips Lumify C5-2 transducer was used, equipped with a portable Samsung tablet and the Lumify APP. LU examination was performed with the convex transducer set into lung configuration. During the examination, the portable tablet device and the transducer were wrapped in single-use plastic protection to reduce contamination and improve sterilization.

Wireless transducers may be indicated for assessing LU in highly infectious diseases as COVID-19 (3, 13). At the end of the exploration, the tablet and the transducer were sterilized following recent recommendations (20). Ultrasound findings were assessed using the LU score (LUS) as described in the previous studies (11, 13). Briefly, LUS evaluates lung parenchyma following a twelve-zone examination of the thorax (11, 14, 21). Anterior (midclavicular line), lateral (midaxillary line), and posterior (paravertebral line) chest wall regions were divided in two (superior and inferior). Posterior exploration was performed when subjects were able to sit or tilt sideways. When posterior access was not possible, it was substituted with posterior axillary line exploration. The transducer was placed longitudinally to the ribs to enhance pleural and lung exploration. Each region was then scored following recommendations for point-of-care LU (14, 22–24): lung sliding with A-lines or fewer than three isolated B-lines scored 0; multiple well-defined B-lines (B1) scored 1; multiple coalescent B-lines (B2) or white lung scored 2; and subpleural consolidation scored 3. The sum of the scores defined the LUS, ranging from 0 to 36 points (14, 24). Data were directly recorded and saved in video format.

Computerized Tomography of the Chest

In 30 patients, both LU and CT scan (Aquilion ONE / GENESIS, Toshiba, Barcelona, Spain) were done at the moment of patient worsening. From them, two trained thoracic radiologists described lung parenchyma in all the 12 regions used in LUS. Both radiologists were blinded to LUS and to histological information. CT scans were individually analyzed and then agreed. Endovenous contrast was used in 37%. A total of 279 exploration regions were assessed. GGO, consolidation, organizing pneumonia, septal thickening, and fibrosis were identified. Radiological findings were matched with the LU findings.

Postmortem CNB of Lung

In those cases that finally died (13 patients), after exploring both hemithoraxes through ultrasound, immediately postmortem CNB guided by LU was performed. All of them were taken from third anterior intercostal space at midclavicular line. A 16G semiautomatic biopsy needle for soft tissue biopsy was used. Between 4 and 6 biopsies were collected in the same intercostal space from each lung.

Histological Processing of CNB

Biopsies were fixed with formaldehyde 4% during 24 h, and then paraffin-embedded. From each block, 7 cuts of 2.5 μm thick were performed. Histological preparations were stained using Hematoxylin and Eosine, Masson's trichrome (for assessing fibrosis and collagen deposition), and Weigert-Van-Giesson (for the architectural evaluation of elastic fibers). The slides were scanned using a 3D Histech P-1000 scanner, at 40x resolution, obtaining whole slide images. Histological diagnosis was performed by two experienced pulmonary pathologists (blinded to clinical and radiological findings).

Statistical Analysis

Categorical data were described as frequency and percentages. Continuous variables were expressed as mean and standard deviation for normally distributed variables or median and interquartile range otherwise. Positive and negative predictive values (PPV and NPV) were calculated. Data were analyzed by using SPSS 24 (SPSS, IBM Corp) and R (Software Version 3.6.2).

RESULTS

Thirty consecutive patients admitted into the IMCU that presented disease worsening were included in the study. The median time between CT scan and LU was 5 days (IQR, 12.5 days) and between CT scan and histology was 8.4 days (IQR, 9 days). Histological samples were taken LU-guided. The mean age was 62.56 ± 13.27 years old, with 29 (96.7%) male patients. Patients received complete COVID-19 treatment, following the approved protocol. Thirteen patients died after 30 ± 16.8 days of inclusion. Those who died were older than those who recovered and presented a higher prevalence of smoking history and comorbidity.

TABLE 1 | Demographic and clinical characteristics of patients at the time of evaluation according to lung ultrasound score.

	Total of patients (*n* = 30)	Progressive worsening and death (*n* = 13)
Patient background		
Age, mean (SD)	62.56 (13.27)	67.92 (12.96)
Male, *n* (%)	29 (96.7%)	9 (69.23%)
Smoking history, *n* (%)	9 (30%)	5 (38.48%)
Hypertension, *n* (%)	21 (70%)	9 (69.23%)
Dyslipidemia, *n* (%)	16 (53.3%)	5 (38.48%)
Diabetes, *n* (%)	9 (22.50%)	4 (30.77%)
Obesity, *n* (%)	15 (30%)	4 (30.77%)
COPD, *n* (%)	3 (10%)	1 (7.69%)
Asthma, *n* (%)	2 (6.7%)	1 (7.69%)
Cardiopathy, *n* (%)	2 (6.7%)	1 (7.69%)
Hepatopathy, *n* (%)	2 (6.7%)	0
History of malignancies, *n* (%)	8 (40%)	5 (38.48%)
Chronic kidney disease, *n* (%)	3 (10%)	1 (7.69%)
Laboratory blood test on LU initial assessment		
Lactate dehydrogenase (U/L), median (IQR)	409 (205.50)	426 (136)
C-Reactive protein (mg/L), median (IQR)	66.90 (146.60)	159.5 (219.50)
Ferritin (μg/L), median (IQR)	985.90 (932.10)	1,237 (2,198.50)
Leukocyte count (x10^9/L), median (IQR)	12.25 (10.75)	15.4 (15.60)
Lymphocyte count (x10^9/L), median (IQR)	0.93 (0.89)	0.73 (0.68)
D-dimer (μg/L), median (IQR)	707 (641.50)	735 (1,480)

LUS, lung ultrasound score; COPD, chronic obstructive pulmonary disease; SD, standard deviation; IQR, interquartile range.

The most frequent comorbidities were hypertension (70%), dyslipidemia (53.3%), and history of malignancies (40%). The mean time from hospitalization to death was 30 ± 16.89 days. The main cause of death was respiratory failure (n = 11; 84.61%), multiple organ dysfunction (n = 1; 7.69%), and refractory septic shock (n = 1; 7.69%). The demographic and clinical characteristics of included patients are described in **Table 1**.

LU and CT Scan Comparative

Lung ultrasound and CT scan were both performed in 30 patients, with a total of 279 thoracic regions explored. In 4 (13.33%) patients, the complete twelve-zone ultrasonographic exploration was not possible. The most frequent LU finding was B2-lines (137/279 thoracic regions; 49.1%), followed by C-profile (76/279; 27.2%), B1-lines (42/279; 15.1%), and A-lines (24/279; 8.6%). Average LUS was 23.5 ± 6.2 points, which reveals a moderate–severe alveolar–interstitial pattern. The most frequent CT-scan finding was GGO (81/279 thoracic regions; 29%), followed by consolidation (79/279; 28.3%), and crazy paving (66/279; 23.7%). Interestingly, the type of LU finding in the different regions may predict CT-scan abnormalities; while A-lines were associated with areas of normal lung aeration in 10/24 of observation regions (41.7%), pathological CT-scan findings were commonly observed when B2-lines or C-lines were identified through LU (189/213; 88.7%). The type of radiological CT pattern was variable in those cases that presented C-profile: consolidation (35/76; 46.1%), GGO (20/76; 26.3%), and crazy paving (11/76; 14.5%); instead, some area of the normal lung was only observed in 6/76 (7%). LU and CT-scan findings are shown in **Table 2** and **Figure 1**.

TABLE 2 | Description of all thoracic regions explored by LU and CT scan.

		CT-SCAN						
		Normal	GGO	C	CP	PT	PE	Total explored regions (%)
LU	A-Lines *N* (%)	10 (41.7%)	10 (41.7%)	1 (4.2%)	3 (12.5%)	0	0	24 (8.6%)
	B1-Lines *N* (%)	9 (21.4%)	12 (28.6%)	9 (21.4%)	9 (21.4%)	1 (2.4%)	2 (4.8%)	42 (15.1%)
	B2-Lines *N* (%)	18 (13.1%)	39 (28.5%)	34 (24.8%)	43 (31.4%)	0	3 (2.2%)	137 (49.1%)
	C-Profile *N* (%)	6 (7.9%)	20 (26.3%)	35 (46.1%)	11 (14.5%)	0	4 (5.3%)	76 (27.2%)
	Total explored regions (%)	43 (15.4%)	81 (29.0%)	79 (28.3%)	66 (23.7%)	1 (0.4%)	9 (3.2%)	279 (100%)

The proportion of CT-scan findings in relation to LU findings in the same explored regions. CT scan, computerized tomography scan; GGO, ground-glass opacity; C, consolidation; CP, crazy paving; PT, pneumothorax; PE, pleural effusion; LU, lung ultrasound.

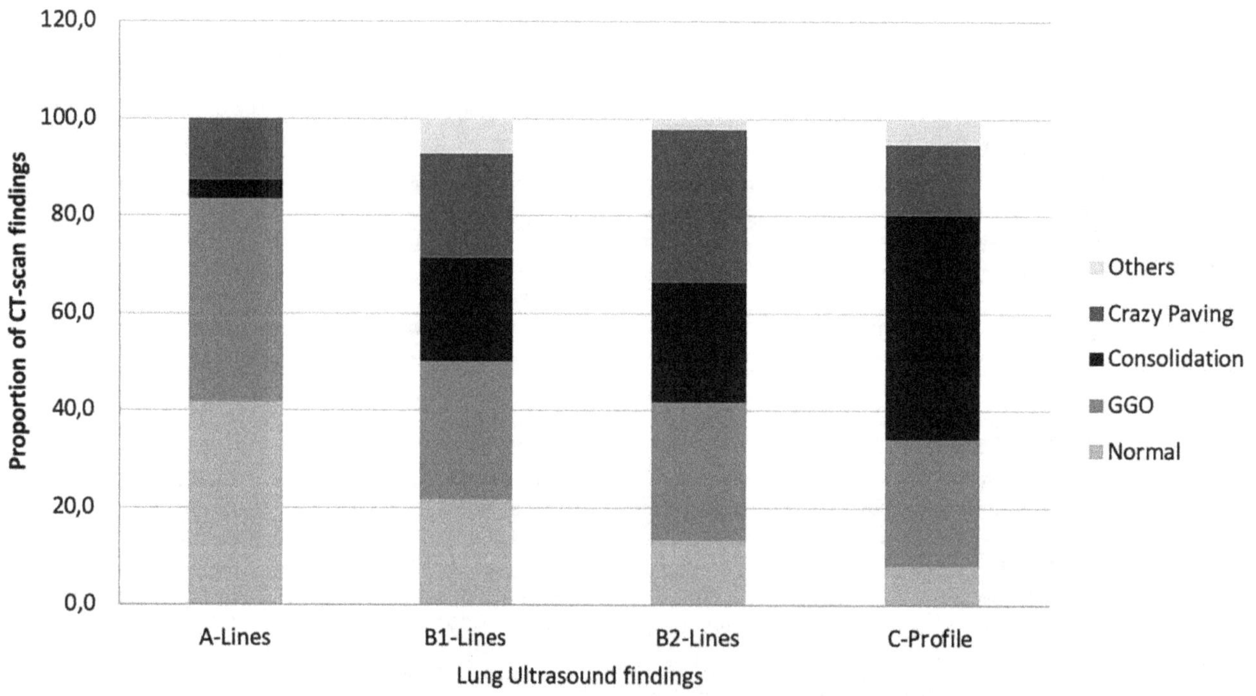

FIGURE 1 | Proportion of CT-scan findings in the function of LU images. CT scan, computerized tomography scan; LU, lung ultrasound; GGO, ground-glass opacity.

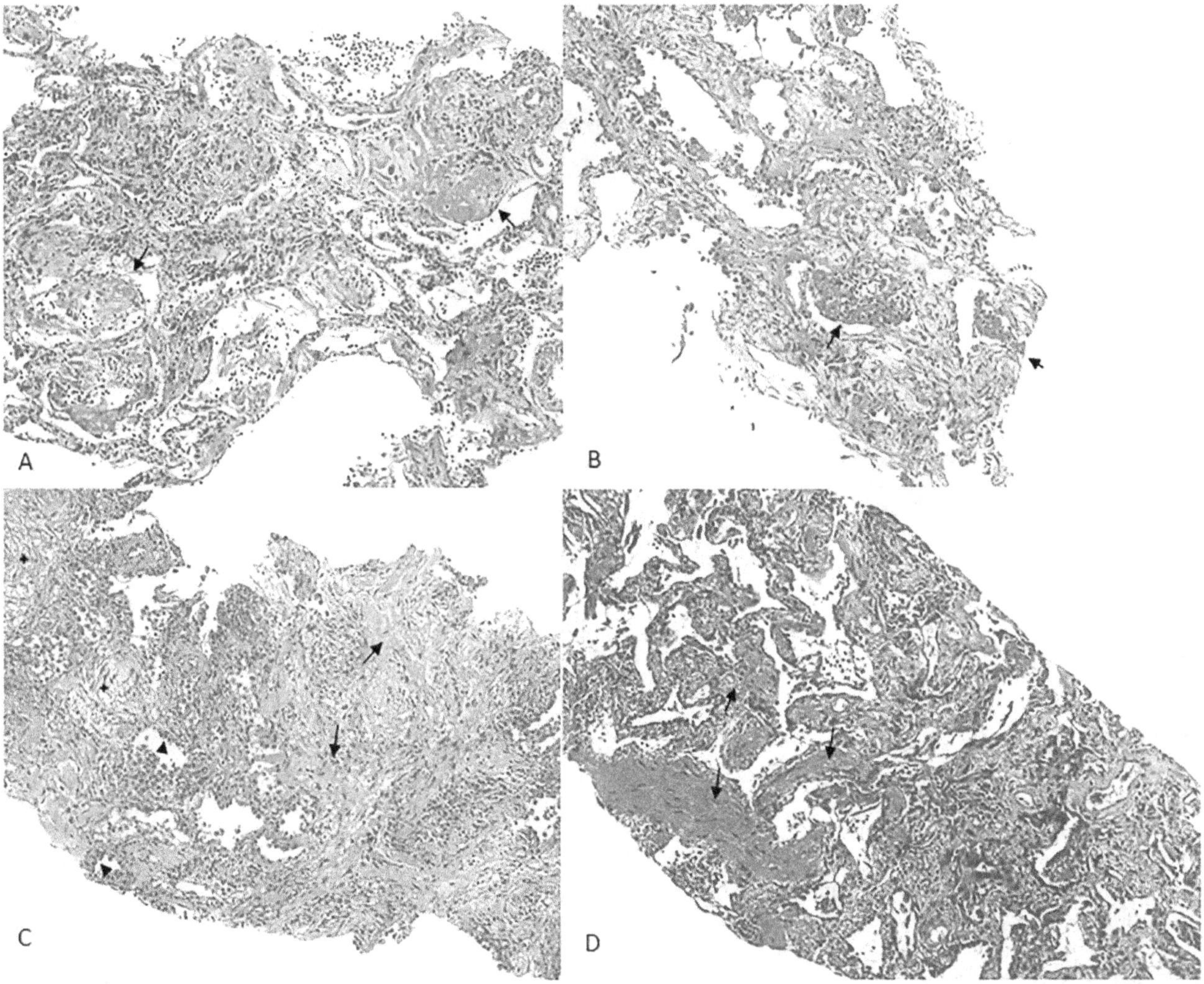

FIGURE 2 | Examples of CNB. **(A)**: AFOP-like DAD: (arrows: deposition of fibrin plugs filling the alveolar space); **(B)**: AFOP-like organizing DAD (arrows: fibrin plugs deposited in the alveoli and focal organization changes in the interstitium); **(C)**: AFOP-like fibrotic DAD [focal organizational changes (star), interstitial deposition of collagen (arrow) accompanied by pneumocyte type II hyperplasia (arrowhead)]. **(D)**: Fibrotic DAD (arrows: thickening of the alveolar septa with mature collagen deposition in the interstitium). CNB, core needle biopsy; DAD, diffuse alveolar damage; AFOP, acute fibrinous organizing pneumonia.

Histological Findings

Twenty-five echo-guided histological samples were obtained from 13 patients. All patients presented the same LU findings in both hemithoraxes. Samples obtained from one patient were not representative of lung parenchyma. From the remaining 24 samples, 18 (75%) showed DAD, whereas 6 (25%) showed chronic interstitial inflammation. The observed DAD was heterogeneous, showing multiple evolving patterns of damage, including exudative (8/24, 33.3%), fibrotic (8/24, 33.3%), and organizing (2/24, 8.3%) phases. In those patients with acute or exudative pattern, two lesions were distinguished: classic hyaline membrane and fibrin "plug" in alveolar space (acute fibrinous organizing pneumonia, AFOP). Regarding fibrotic findings, collagen fibrosis was predominant, frequently associated to pneumocyte hyperplasia. Consistent fibrosis with architectural remodeling was seen in only two samples (8.3%). Neither microangiopathy nor microthrombi was found. Examples of CNB are shown in **Figure 2.**

Lung Ultrasound and Histological Findings

Lung ultrasound and histological findings were matched in the 12 patients with representative lung biopsy samples. In these cases, only C-profile and B2-lines were identified. C-profile was described in 4 patients (33.3%). These cases presented histological signs of DAD and lung fibrosis. The predominant finding in 2 (50%) of them was collagen deposition and AFOP in the other two cases. B2-lines were identified in 16 regions (66.7%); the presence of hyaline membrane was the predominant finding in 6 of them (37.5%), organizing pneumonia in 2 samples (12.5%), and fibrosis in 6 samples (37.5%). No A-lines or B1-lines were observed in these patients (see **Figure 3**).

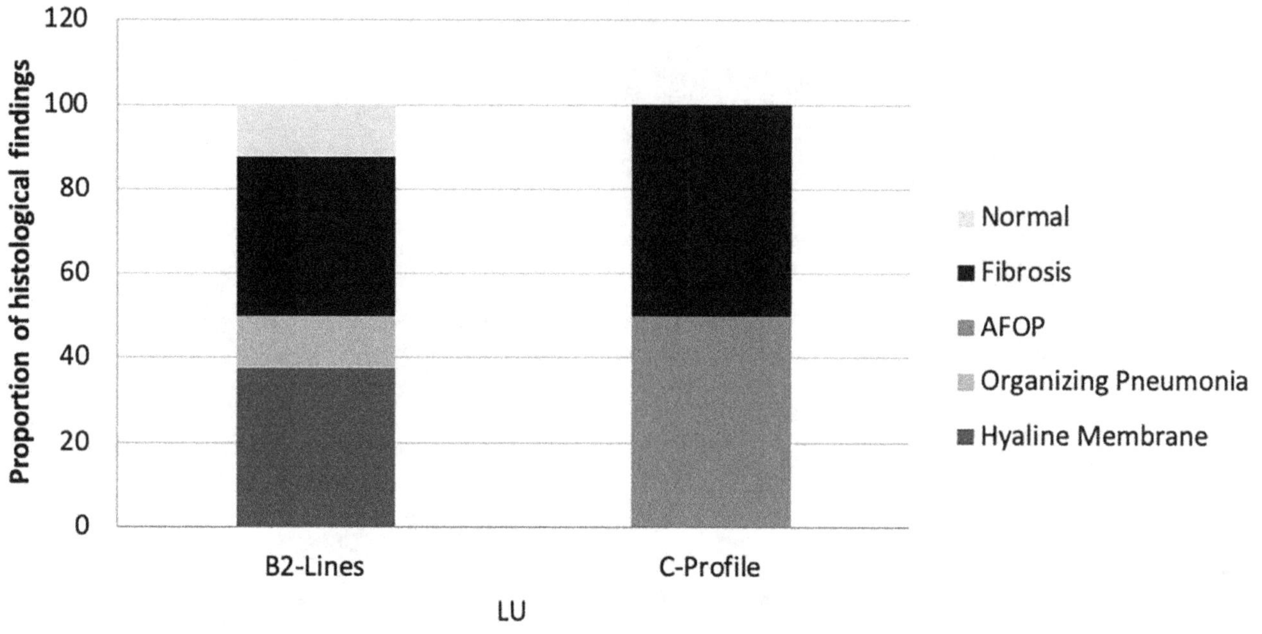

FIGURE 3 | Proportion of histological findings in function of LU images. AFOP, Acute Fibrinous Organizing Pneumonia; LU, Lung ultrasound.

DISCUSSION

The present results show that a majority of patients with severe COVID-19 with worsening of respiratory failure present B2-lines and C-lines in LU, which histologically correspond to different signs of DAD, including hyaline membranes and AFOP areas, and lung fibrosis. GGOs and crazy-paving areas in the CT had no specific LU imaging correlation since both were found in all LU patterns. However, CT areas of consolidation were more predominant in LU B2-lines and C-lines. Those patients who died because of respiratory failure only presented LU B2-lines and C-lines at the time of death.

In 2008, an LU protocol was introduced in the examination of acute respiratory failure: the BLUE (Bedside Lung Ultrasound in Emergency) protocol (25, 26). The accuracy of this protocol in diagnosing the cause of acute respiratory failure in critical care patients was 90.5%, with higher sensitivity, specificity, and diagnostic accuracy for pleural effusions, alveolar consolidation, and interstitial syndromes (12). Using the BLUE protocol features, COVID-19 causes clear and typical ultrasonographic patterns. B-lines in COVID-19 are predominant; both in separate (B1) and coalescent (B2) forms, and can give the appearance of a shining white lung. Irregularity of the pleural line and subpleural consolidations (C-profile) also occur in bilateral patchy clusters, and are mainly visible in the posterior and inferior areas (24, 26–28). According to published data, our results show that B2-lines were predominant in patients with severe COVID-19 followed by C-profile. These findings were able to predict the clinical outcome in patients admitted into the IMCU (28): Furthermore, the present data agree with previous findings which indicated that the higher the LUS, the worse clinical outcome is expected, but it also correlates with more pathological CT findings. Therefore, LUS could help in monitoring the patient clinical evolution in a bedside setting and help in the CT-scan indication.

Yang et al. (29) performed a two-centered retrospective comparison between LU and CT-scan imaging in hospitalized patients with COVID-19. In total, 63% of positive regions were detected by LU. In contrast, CT scan showed 38.7% of regions with abnormalities. Both LU and CT-scan findings showed the lesions of COVID-19 were more likely to occur in the posterior regions of the lung with bilateral distribution. In our study, LU detected alveolar–interstitial disorders in 91% (255/279), whereas CT scan detected in 84% (236/279). Our study shows higher radiological abnormalities because only patients with severe COVID-19 were included. When A-lines were described in LU, pathological CT-scan findings were observed in 58.3% of regions. Therefore, the finding of A-lines in patients with COVID-19 should not be interpreted as normal aeration of the lung but the probability of pathological CT-scan findings is lower than that for B-lines or C-profile. A-lines had an NPV of 87.1%. However, it has a PPV of 41.7% for normal lung aeration. Though, when C-profile is seen in LU, it is mainly associated with consolidation in CT-scan, but also with GGO and crazy paving. However, it is almost never associated with normal healthy lung (PPV 76% and NPV 18.3% for abnormal CT scan).

The initial recommendations for biosafety control required during specimen collection and handling have strongly limited the practice of autopsies of the COVID-19 at the beginning of this pandemic. The first autopsy study published by a Chinese group in February 2020 reported a case of postmortem CNB (18). Since then, the number of autopsies has increased. The main reported pathological findings were exudative DAD, as well

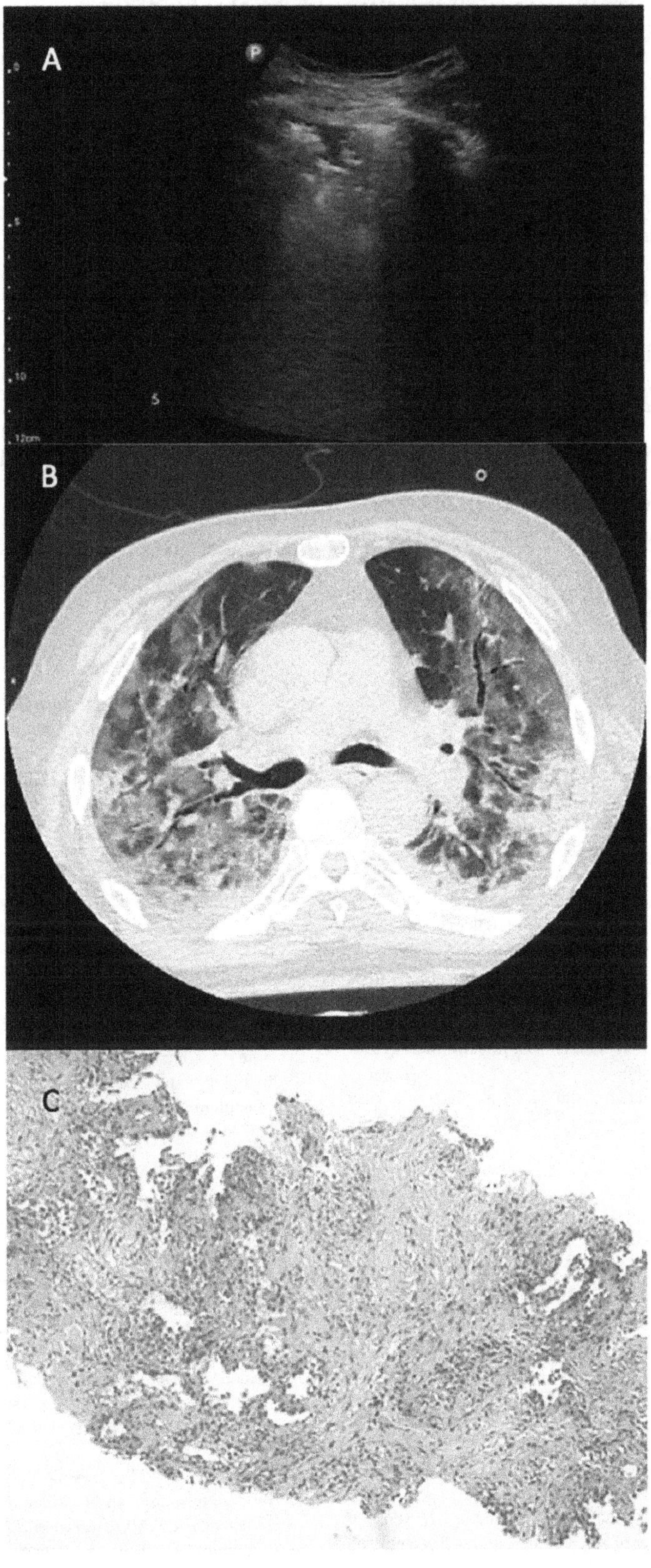

FIGURE 4 | LU–CT–histology from the same region. LU **(A)**, CT-scan **(B)**, and histological **(C)** images of the same patient. The LU exploration **(A)** shows a C-profile pattern, seen in the anterior left region of the thorax; CT scan **(B)** shows areas of ground-glass opacity in the same region. In the histological sample **(C)**, we observe an AFOP-like fibrotic DAD (focal organizational changes, interstitial deposition of collagen accompanied by pneumocyte type II hyperplasia).

as organizing pneumonia (OP), reactive type II pneumocytes, and chronic interstitial pneumonia (30, 31). The results of our CNB specimens are consistent with published data: the main histological finding was DAD (75%), including different pathological findings, such as AFOP areas together with collagen fibrotic areas and chronic interstitial inflammation (25%) (see **Figure 4**).

To date, there are no published data concerning the association between LU and histological findings in COVID-19. In our study, the LU exploration of only progressive severe COVID-19 cases showed B2-lines and C-profile. Recently, a high LUS (predominant B2-lines and C-profile) has been related to poor clinical outcomes (28). The present data show that the histological findings associated with C-profile are predominantly AFOP and collagen fibrosis, both findings associated with a poor prognosis and lack of response to glucocorticoid or immunomodulators (32).

The main limitation of our study is the reduced number of patients due to the difficulties in achieving both LU and CT images at the proper timeline of respiratory worsening in patients with COVID-19 and the challenges of the immediately postmortem LU-guided CNBs.

CONCLUSION

LU B2-lines and C-profile are predominantly identified in patients with severe COVID-19 with respiratory worsening, which correspond to different CT patterns and histological findings of DAD and lung fibrosis. LU could help in optimizing CT requirements and anticipating prognosis or treatment response.

AUTHOR CONTRIBUTIONS

PT-S, ED, MM-M, and GS-C conceptualized the study and investigated the study. PT-S, ED, and GS-C contributed to data curation. GS-C contributed to formal analysis. PT-S, ED, MM-M, JD, SS, and GS-C contributed to methodology. PT-S, MM-M, and GS-C contributed to project administration. ED, SA, MD-F, JB-M, AM, JS, BR, XS, and PL contributed to resources. PT-S wrote the original draft. ED, MM-M, and GS-C contributed to writing, reviewing, and editing the manuscript. All authors contributed to the article and approved the submitted version.

REFERENCES

1. Huang C, Wang Y, Li X, Ren L, Zhao J, Hu Y, et al. Clinical features of patients infected with 2019 novel coronavirus in Wuhan, China. *Lancet.* (2020) 395:497–506. doi: 10.1016/S0140-6736(20)30183-5
2. *WHO Coronavirus Disease (COVID-19) Dashboard.* Available online at: https://covid19.who.int/ (accessed May 11, 2020).
3. Rubin GD, Ryerson CJ, Haramati LB, Sverzellati N, Kanne JP, Raoof S, et al. The role of chest imaging in patient management during the covid-19 pandemic: a multinational consensus statement from the fleischner society. *Radiology.* (2020) 296:172–80. doi: 10.1148/radiol.2020201365
4. Blaivas M. Lung ultrasound in evaluation of pneumonia. *J Ultrasound Med.* (2012) 31:823–6. doi: 10.7863/jum.2012.31.6.823
5. Soldati G, Demi M, Inchingolo R, Smargiassi A, Demi L. On the physical basis of pulmonary sonographic interstitial syndrome. *J Ultrasound Med.* (2016) 35:2075–86. doi: 10.7863/ultra.15.08023
6. Song F, Shi N, Shan F, Zhang Z, Shen J, Lu H, et al. Emerging 2019 novel Coronavirus (2019-nCoV) pneumonia. *Radiology.* (2020) 295:210–7. doi: 10.1148/radiol.2020200274
7. Pan F, Ye T, Sun P, Gui S, Liang B, Li L, et al. Time course of lung changes on chest CT during recovery from 2019 novel Coronavirus (COVID-19) pneumonia. *Radiology.* (2020) 13:200370. doi: 10.1148/radiol.2020200370
8. Bernheim A, Mei X, Huang M, Yang Y, Fayad ZA, Zhang N, et al. Chest CT Findings in Coronavirus disease-19 (COVID-19): relationship to duration of infection. *Radiology.* (2020) 20:200463. doi: 10.1148/radiol.2020200463
9. Kong W, Agarwal PP. Chest imaging appearance of COVID-19 infection. *Radiol Cardiothorac Imaging.* (2020) 2:e200028. doi: 10.1148/ryct.2020200028
10. Lichtenstein DA. BLUE-protocol and FALLS-protocol: two applications of lung ultrasound in the critically ill. *Chest.* (2015) 147:1659–70. doi: 10.1378/chest.14-1313
11. Bouhemad B, Mongodi S, Via G, Rouquette I. Ultrasound for "lung monitoring" of ventilated patients. *Anesthesiology.* (2015) 122:437–47. doi: 10.1097/ALN.0000000000000558
12. Lichtenstein D, Goldstein I, Mourgeon E, Cluzel P, Grenier P, Rouby JJ. Comparative diagnostic performances of auscultation, chest radiography, and lung ultrasonography in acute respiratory distress syndrome. *Anesthesiology.* (2004) 100:9–15. doi: 10.1097/00000542-200401000-00006
13. Moore S, Gardiner E. Point of care and intensive care lung ultrasound: a reference guide for practitioners during COVID-19. *Radiography.* (2020) 26:e297–302. doi: 10.1016/j.radi.2020.04.005
14. Soldati G, Smargiassi A, Inchingolo R, Buonsenso D, Perrone T, Briganti DF, et al. Proposal for international standardization of the use of lung ultrasound for COVID-19 patients; a simple, quantitative, reproducible method. *J Ultrasound Med.* (2020) 39:1413–9. doi: 10.1002/jum.15285
15. Copetti R, Soldati G, Copetti P. Chest sonography: a useful tool to differentiate acute cardiogenic pulmonary edema from acute respiratory distress syndrome. *Cardiovasc Ultrasound.* (2008) 29:16. doi: 10.1186/1476-7120-6-16
16. Sapino A, Facchetti F, Bonoldi E, Gianatti A, Barbareschi M. Società Italiana di Anatomia Patologica e Citologia - SIAPEC. The autopsy debate during the COVID-19 emergency: the Italian experience. *Virchows Arch.* (2020) 29:1–3. doi: 10.1007/s00428-020-02828-2
17. Xu Z, Shi L, Wang Y, Zhang J, Huang L, Zhang C, et al. Pathological findings of COVID-19 associated with acute respiratory distress syndrome. *Lancet Respir Med.* (2020) 8:420–2. doi: 10.1016/S2213-2600(20)30076-X
18. Tian S, Hu W, Niu L, Liu H, Xu H, Xiao SY. Pulmonary pathology of early-phase 2019 novel Coronavirus (COVID-19) pneumonia in two patients with lung cancer. *J Thorac Oncol.* (2020) 15:700–4. doi: 10.20944/preprints202002.0220.v2
19. Hanley B, Lucas SB, Youd E, Swift B, Osborn M. Autopsy in suspected COVID-19 cases. *J Clin Pathol.* (2020) 73:239–42. doi: 10.1136/jclinpath-2020-206522
20. Kampf G, Todt D, Pfaender S, Steinmann E. Persistence of coronaviruses on inanimate surfaces and their inactivation with biocidal agents. *J Hosp Infect.* (2020) 104:246–51. doi: 10.1016/j.jhin.2020.01.022
21. Yin W, Zou T, Qin Y, Yang J, Li Y, Zeng X, et al. Poor lung ultrasound score in shock patients admitted to the ICU is associated with worse outcome. *BMC Pulm Med.* (2019) 19:1. doi: 10.1186/s12890-018-0755-9
22. Soldati G, Demi M, Smargiassi A, Inchingolo R, Demi L. The role of ultrasound lung artifacts in the diagnosis of respiratory diseases. *Expert Rev Respir Med.* (2019) 13:163–72. doi: 10.1080/17476348.2019.1565997
23. Singh AK, Mayo PH, Koenig S, Talwar A, Narasimhan M. The use of M-mode ultrasonography to differentiate the causes of b lines. *Chest.* (2018) 153:689–96. doi: 10.1016/j.chest.2017.10.019
24. Buonsenso D, Piano A, Raffaelli F, Bonadia N, de Gaetano Donati K, Franceschi F. Point-of-care lung ultrasound findings in novel coronavirus disease-19 pnemoniae: a case report and potential applications during COVID-19 outbreak. *Eur Rev Med Pharmacol Sci.* (2020) 24:2776–80. doi: 10.26355/eurrev_202003_20549

25. Lichtenstein DA, Mezière GA. Relevance of lung ultrasound in the diagnosis of acute respiratory failure the BLUE protocol. *Chest.* (2008) 134:117–25. doi: 10.1378/chest.07-2800
26. Jackson K, Butler R, Aujayeb A. Lung ultrasound in the COVID-19 pandemic. *Postgrad Med J.* (2021) 97:34–9. doi: 10.1136/postgradmedj-2020-138137
27. Huang Y, Wang S, Liu Y, Zhang Y, Zheng C, Zheng Y, et al. A preliminary study on the ultrasonic manifestations of peripulmonary lesions of non-critical novel Coronavirus pneumonia (COVID-19). *SSRN Electron J.* (2020). doi: 10.2139/ssrn.3544750
28. Trias-Sabrià P, Molina-Molina M, Aso S, Argudo MH, Diez-Ferrer M, Sabater J, et al. Lung ultrasound score to predict outcomes in COVID-19. *Respir Care.* (2021) 66:1263–70. doi: 10.4187/respcare.08648
29. Yang Y, Huang Y, Gao F, Yuan L, Wang Z. Lung ultrasonography versus chest CT in COVID-19 pneumonia: a two-centered retrospective comparison study from China. *Intensive Care Med.* (2020) 46:1761–3. doi: 10.1007/s00134-020-06096-1
30. Sellarés J, Guerrero C, Martínez D, Benegas M, Cuerpo S, Hernández-González F, et al. Estudio histológico mediante biopsia pulmonar post mortem en pacientes con neumonía por COVID-19. *Arch Bronconeumol.* (2021). doi: 10.1016/j.arbres.2021.09.009. [Epub ahead of print].
31. Calabrese F, Pezzuto F, Fortarezza F, Hofman P, Kern I, Panizo A, et al. Pulmonary pathology and COVID-19: lessons from autopsy. The experience of European pulmonary pathologists. *Virchows Arch.* (2020) 477:359–72. doi: 10.1007/s00428-020-02886-6
32. Collard HR, Ryerson CJ, Corte TJ, Jenkins G, Kondoh Y, Lederer DJ, et al. Acute exacerbation of idiopathic pulmonary fibrosis an international working group report. *Am J Respir Crit Care Med.* (2016) 194:265–75. doi: 10.1164/rccm.201604-0801CI

4

A Simple-to-Use Web-Based Calculator for Survival Prediction in Acute Respiratory Distress Syndrome

Yong Liu[†], *Jian Liu*[†] *and Liang Huang*[*]

Department of Emergency, The First Affiliated Hospital of Nanchang University, Nanchang, China

***Correspondence:**
Liang Huang
huangliang6312@sina.com

[†]*These authors have contributed equally to this work*

Background: The aim of this study was to construct and validate a simple-to-use model to predict the survival of patients with acute respiratory distress syndrome.

Methods: A total of 197 patients with acute respiratory distress syndrome were selected from the Dryad Digital Repository. All eligible individuals were randomly stratified into the training set (n=133) and the validation set (n=64) as 2: 1 ratio. LASSO regression analysis was used to select the optimal predictors, and receiver operating characteristic and calibration curves were used to evaluate accuracy and discrimination of the model. Clinical usefulness of the model was also assessed using decision curve analysis and Kaplan-Meier analysis.

Results: Age, albumin, platelet count, PaO_2/FiO_2, lactate dehydrogenase, high-resolution computed tomography score, and etiology were identified as independent prognostic factors based on LASSO regression analysis; these factors were integrated for the construction of the nomogram. Results of calibration plots, decision curve analysis, and receiver operating characteristic analysis showed that this model has good predictive ability of patient survival in acute respiratory distress syndrome. Moreover, a significant difference in the 28-day survival was shown between the patients stratified into different risk groups ($P < 0.001$). For convenient application, we also established a web-based calculator (https://huangl.shinyapps.io/ARDSprognosis/).

Conclusions: We satisfactorily constructed a simple-to-use model based on seven relevant factors to predict survival and prognosis of patients with acute respiratory distress syndrome. This model can aid personalized treatment and clinical decision-making.

Keywords: acute respiratory distress syndrome, LASSO regression, nomogram, model, survival

INTRODUCTION

Acute respiratory distress syndrome (ARDS) is a clinically and pathophysiologically complex syndrome characterized by rapid progression and devastating hypoxemic respiratory failure (1). Many risk factors, such as sepsis, pneumonia, pancreatitis, and major trauma, are associated with the development of ARDS (2). Although there has been some progress in ARDS treatment in the last several decades, the prognosis of patients with ARDS are still not satisfactory. The in-hospital mortality rate of ARDS patients remains between 34 and 60% (3). At present, the treatment of ARDS predominantly includes mechanical ventilation therapy (4). Therefore, identification of

TABLE 1 | Baseline characteristics of included patients in training and validation sets.

Characteristic	Entire cohort (n = 197)	Training set (n = 133)	Validation set (n = 64)	P-value
Age, years	73.94 ± 11.92	74.41 ± 11.95	72.97 ± 11.90	0.427
Sex				0.647
Female	74(37.6%)	48(36.1%)	26(40.6%)	
Male	123(62.4%)	85(63.9%)	38(59.4%)	
Alb, g/Dl	2.84 ± 0.58	2.81 ± 0.58	2.90 ± 0.59	0.317
PLT, per mm^3	19.23 ± 10.56	19.18 ± 10.50	19.32 ± 10.75	0.927
WBC, per mm^3	11010.66 ± 7255.91	10600.75 ± 7076.02	11862.50 ± 7602.22	0.254
CRP, mg/dl	17.42 ± 10.66	16.77 ± 10.83	18.77 ± 10.26	0.219
SOFA score	7.71 ± 3.47	8.09 ± 3.63	6.91 ± 2.98	0.024
McCabe score				0.474
1	174 (88.3%)	115 (86.5%)	59 (92.2%)	
2	11 (5.6%)	9 (6.8%)	2 (3.1%)	
3	12 (6.1%)	9 (6.8%)	3 (4.7%)	
PaO2/FiO2	116.11 ± 50.96	117.66 ± 50.57	112.89 ± 52.01	0.540
LDH, IU/L	390.57 ± 231.73	386.68 ± 199.63	398.64 ± 288.90	0.735
HRCT score	236.69 ± 66.70	233.46 ± 64.94	243.41 ± 70.27	0.328
PEEP, cmH$_2$O	10.40 ± 5.23	10.14 ± 5.22	10.92 ± 5.25	0.329
ARDS etiology				0.036
DARDS	170(86.3%)	120(90.2%)	50(78.1%)	
Non-DARDS	27(13.7%)	13(9.8%)	14(21.9%)	
Vital status				0.212
Living	128(65.0%)	82(61.7%)	46(71.9%)	
Deceased	69(35.0%)	51(38.3%)	18(28.1%)	

Alb, albumin; PLT, platelet count; WBC, white cell count; CRP, C reactive protein; SOFA, sequential organ failure assessment; LDH, lactate dehydrogenase; HRCT, high-resolution computed tomography; DARDS, drug-associated ARDS.

novel and effective treatment strategies is crucial for patients with ARDS. Moreover, a simple-to-use clinical prediction model is also required to provide adequate care to patients with ARDS.

The severity of ARDS is often assessed using the PaO_2/FiO_2 ratio, although this variable has a low-to-moderate prognostic value (5). Recently, several biomarkers including inflammation cytokines, epithelial or endothelial damage, and coagulation have been established to evaluated prognosis and therapeutic response of patients with ARDS. For example, a meta-analysis reported that elevated plasma levels of angiopoietin-2 strongly correlate with diagnosis and mortality in populations at high risk of ARDS (6). Moreover, various clinical biomarkers including lung inflammatory mediators (soluble suppression of tumorigenicity-2 and interleukin-6) (7) and products of epithelial and endothelial injury (the soluble form of the receptor for advanced glycation end products) (8, 9) were developed to monitor pathophysiologic changes and outcomes of ARDS. Unfortunately, although several lung-specific biomarkers have been validated to assess ARDS; however, none of them have been applied into clinical practice. Currently, there is no favorable prognosis prediction model for ARDS.

Nomograms (visualized graphs of a predictive model) are widely applied for prognosis and prediction of various diseases (10, 11). To date, no nomogram and corresponding web-based calculator has been developed to predict the prognosis of ARDS patients. Therefore, a refined model is needed to predict the prognosis of ARDS and guide clinical treatment. In this study, we aimed to construct a web-based calculator to predict the 28-day survival of patients with ARDS using several clinical parameters that are routinely used and readily available. This simple-to-use calculator might serve as an early warning and prediction system for patients with ARDS.

Abbreviations: Alb, albumin; PLT, platelet count; WBC, white cell count; CRP, C reactive protein; SOFA, sequential organ failure assessment; APACHE, acute physiology and chronic health evaluation; LDH, lactate dehydrogenase; HRCT, high-resolution computed tomography; DARDS, drug-associated ARDS.

METHODS

Patients

A total of 197 patients with ARDS were extracted from the Dryad Digital Repository (http://www.datadryad.org/), which was shared by Anan et al. (12). All ARDS patients were diagnosed according to the Berlin definition (5). Patients with chronic interstitial lung disease (idiopathic pulmonary fibrosis), vasculitis or alveolar hemorrhage, hypersensitivity pneumonitis were excluded. All eligible patients were randomly stratified into two groups in a 2:1 ratio (training set and validation set, respectively). The extracted clinical data included age, gender, white cell count (WBC), C-reactive protein (CRP), lactate dehydrogenase (LDH), albumin (Alb), platelet count (PLT), PEEP, SOFA score, high-resolution computed tomography (HRCT) score, McCabe score, PaO2/FiO2, ARDS etiology, survival time, and survival status. Institutional ethical approval was not necessary because all the data were obtained from an online database.

Development of the Nomogram

To obtain the subset of predictors, the LASSO regression analysis was used to select the optimal predictors from the risk factors in the training cohort. The "glmnet" package was used to perform the LASSO regression analysis (13, 14). Finally, using the selected predictors from the LASSO regression, a nomogram was developed using the "rms," "survival," "foreign," and "openxlsx" R packages (15–18). A dynamic web-based calculator was constructed using "DynNom" package (19).

Validation of the Nomogram

To validate the constructed nomogram, the corresponding calibration map and receiver operating characteristic (ROC) analysis were performed in the training and validation sets to assess the prognostic accuracy of the nomogram by using the "rms," "survival," "foreign," and "timeROC" R packages (20).

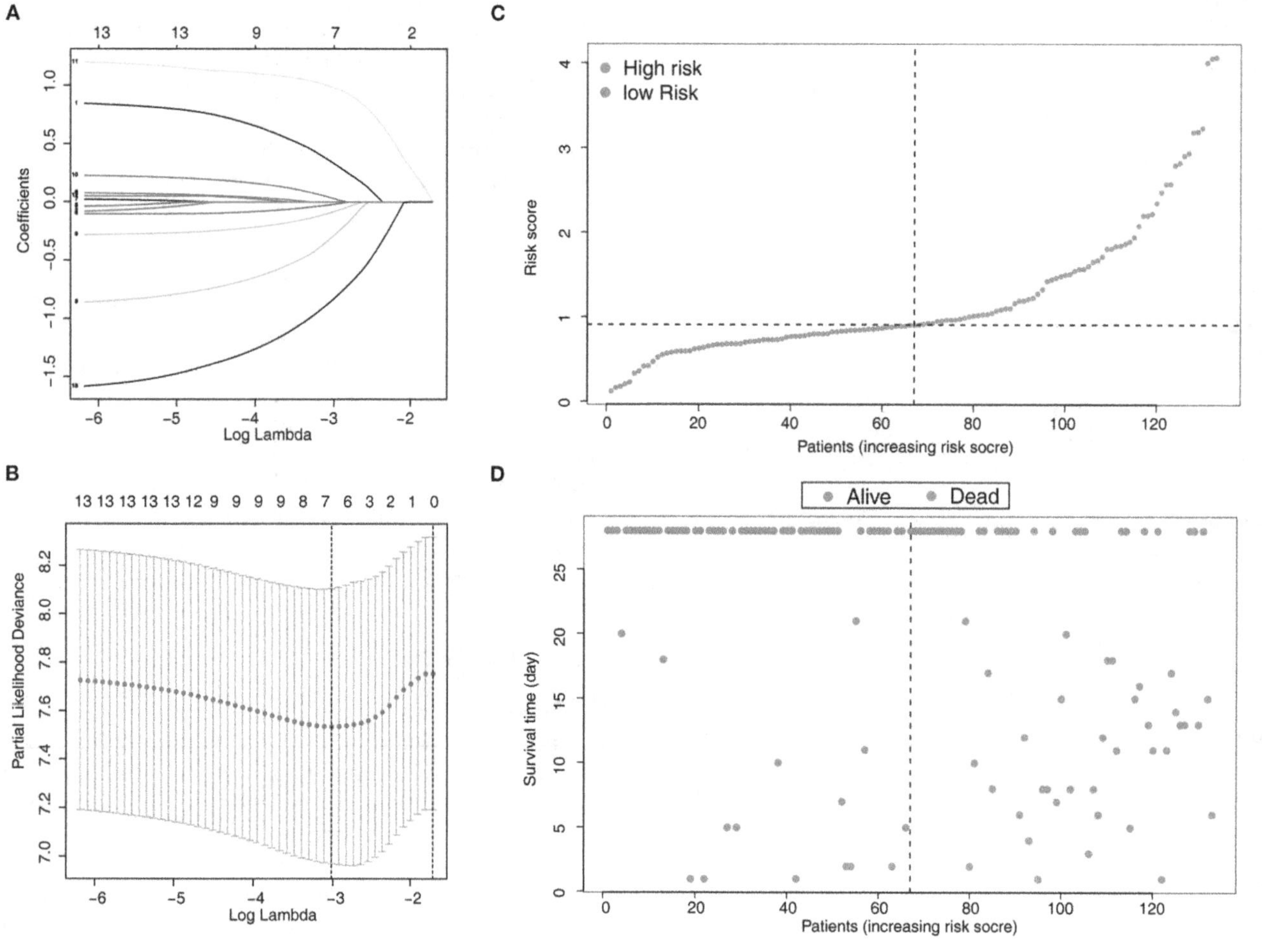

FIGURE 1 | Parameter selection using LASSO regression. **(A)** LASSO coefficient profiles of the 13 features. A coefficient profile plot is produced against the log(λ) sequence. **(B)** Variables selected through LASSO with 10-fold cross-validation. **(C)** Distribution of the risk score. **(D)** Relationships between survival status and survival times of ARDS patients ranked by risk score. The black dotted line represents the optimum cut-off point dividing patients into low- and high-risk groups. LASSO, least absolute shrinkage and selection operator.

In addition, decision curve analysis (DCA) was performed to quantify the clinical applicability of the nomogram.

Statistical Analysis

The raw data were expressed as mean ± standard deviation when normally distributed, while expressed as median (interquartile range) when non-normally distributed. Differences between two groups were analyzed using chi-square tests for categorical variables and t-tests for continuous variables. The Kaplan–Meier method and the log-rank test were used to estimate survival. All statistical analyses were performed using R software (Version 3.6.2; http://www.Rproject.org). A two-sided P-value < 0.05 was considered to indicate statistical significance.

RESULTS

Baseline Characteristics

In total, 197 eligible ARDS patients with integrated information were randomly stratified into two independent cohorts (training set, $n = 133$; validation set, $n = 64$). Patients' baseline clinical characteristics are shown in **Table 1**. A total of 123 male patients and 74 female patients were enrolled in this study. The average age of the patients was 73.94 ± 11.92 years. After 28 days of follow-up, 69 (35.0%) patients died during the entire study population.

Construction of the Model

A total of 13 parameters were used for LASSO regression, and seven parameters were selected as the optimal predictors by LASSO (**Figures 1A,B**). The seven retained variables were then used to construct the predictive model. The risk-score for each individual was calculated based on the model coefficients combined with the corresponding value of the identified seven clinical parameters. Thereafter, the patients were classified into low- and high-risk groups in both cohorts according to the median risk-score. **Figures 1C,D** show the risk-score distribution and the survival status of individual in the high- and low-risk cluster. The variables including Age, Alb, PLT, PaO_2/FiO_2,

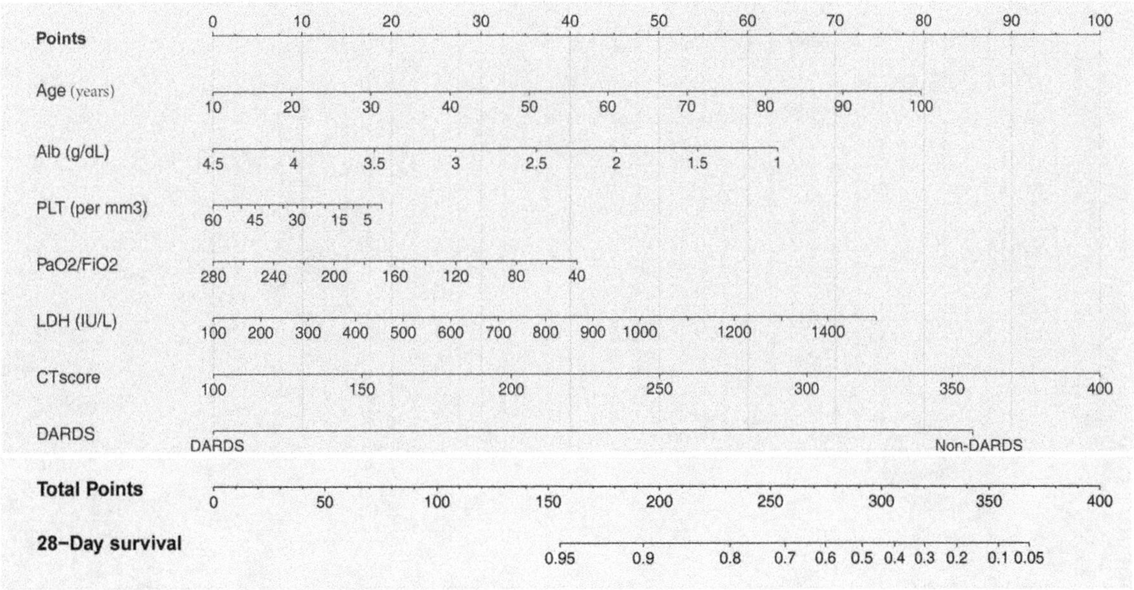

FIGURE 2 | Construction of a nomogram with clinical indices to predict ARDS-related survival (based on the training set). The score for each value is assigned by drawing a line upward to the points line, and the sum of the seven scores is plotted on the Total points line. ARDS, acute respiratory distress syndrome.

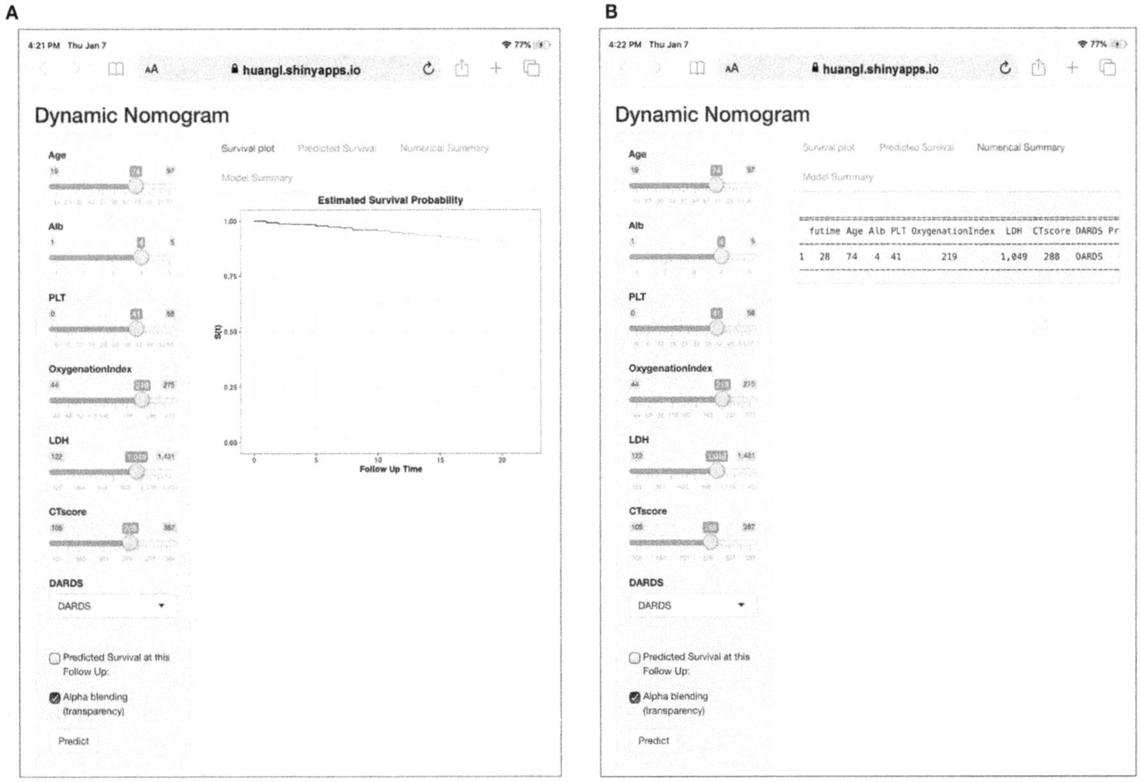

FIGURE 3 | A dynamic web-based calculator to predict ARDS-related survival (https://huangl.shinyapps.io/ARDSprognosis/). **(A)** Web survival rate calculator. **(B)** 95% confidence interval of the web survival rate calculator.

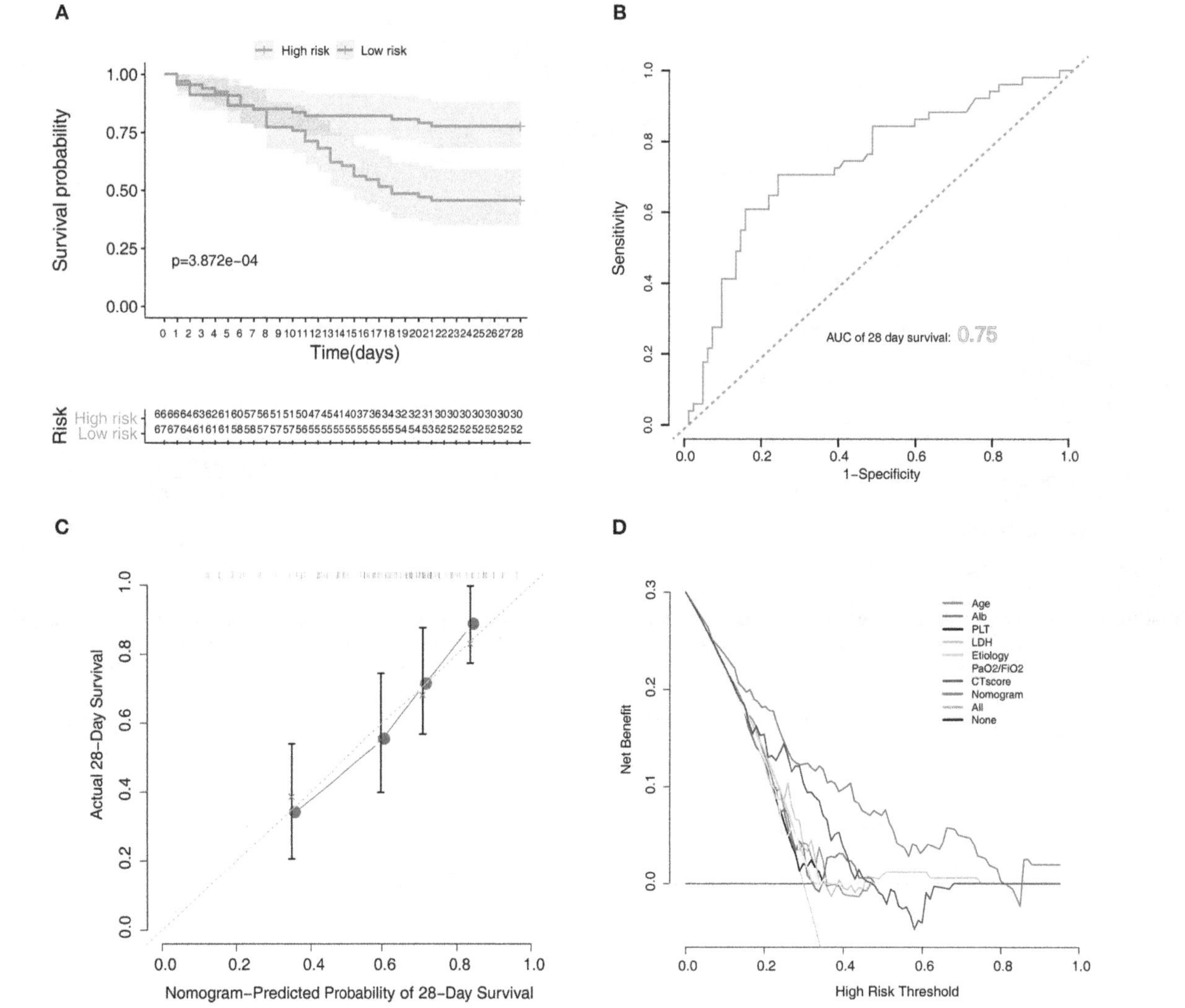

FIGURE 4 | Assessment of the model in the training set. **(A)** Kaplan–Meier survival analysis between the high- and low-risk groups. **(B)** ROC curves of predictive models at 28 days. **(C)** Calibration plot for the training set that show the predicted and observed (with 95% confidence intervals) overall survival rates at 28 days. Model performance is shown by the plot, relative to the 45-degree line, which represents perfect prediction. **(D)** Decision curve of the model. The gray line represents the treat-all-patients scheme. The dotted line represents the treat-none scheme. The red line represents prediction nomogram scheme in training dataset. The X axis represents threshold probability. The Y axis represents net benefit. ROC, receiver operator characteristic.

LDH, HRCT, and etiology were incorporated into the nomogram (**Figure 2**). To facilitate the clinical application of our findings, we developed a web-based calculator (https://huangl.shinyapps.io/ARDSprognosis/) to predict prognosis of ARDS patients according to the nomogram (**Figures 3A,B**). The estimated 28-day survival probabilities could be obtained by drawing a perpendicular line from the total point axis to the outcome axis.

Performance of the Model

The Kaplan–Meier survival curves revealed significantly poor overall survival in the high-risk group (p = 3.872e-04; **Figure 4A**). Thereafter, we performed ROC analysis to assess the discriminability of the model. The area under the ROC curve (AUC) indicative of the 28-day survival prediction was 0.75 (**Figure 4B**), which implied an efficacious performance of the model to predict prognosis. The calibration plots based on the training set showed that the model could accurately predict the 28-day survival (**Figure 4C**). The results of DCA also exhibited that the model could help clinicians to obtain maximum benefit when making clinical decisions (**Figure 4D**).

To further study the predictive value of each parameter included in the model, we performed ROC analysis for each of them (**Figures 5A–G**). The AUC values of all parameters were lower than that of the complete nomogram model. These results demonstrated that the model had superior predictive performance and clinical value than any single factor.

Performance Validation of the Model

To verify the reliability of the constructed novel model, risk-scores were calculated in the validation set with the same formula

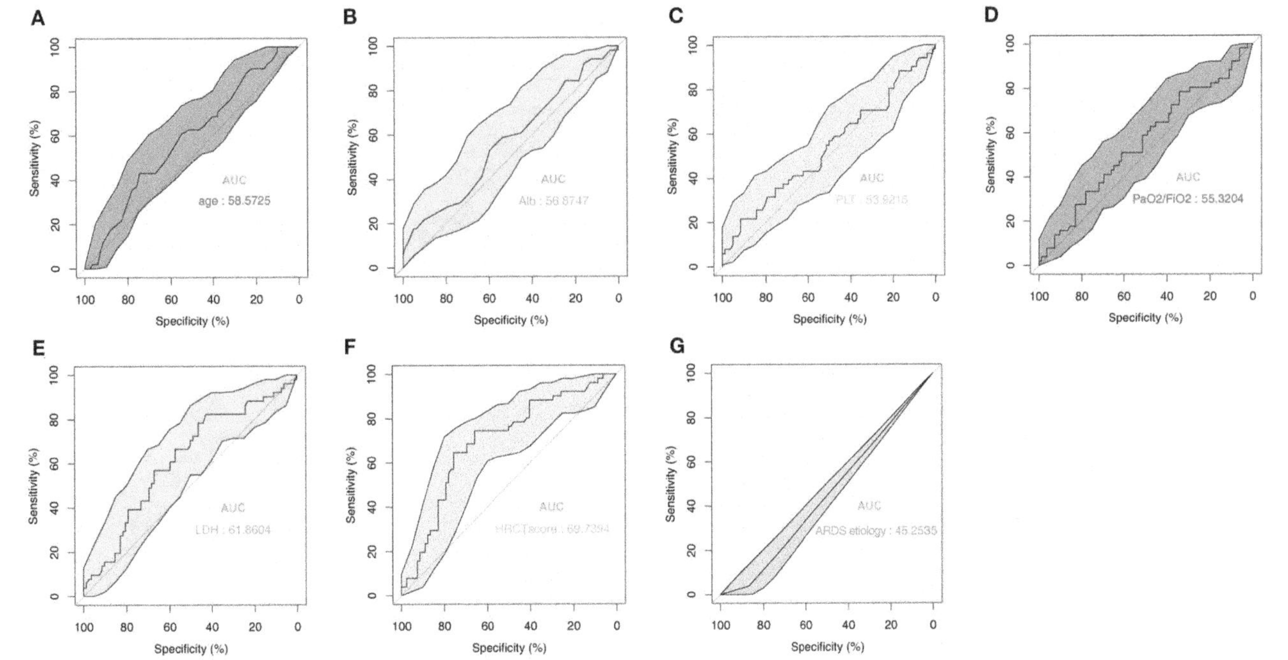

FIGURE 5 | Predictive value of the seven parameters included in the model from the training set. ROC analysis of **(A)** Age, **(B)** Alb, **(C)** PLT, **(D)** PaO_2/FiO_2, **(E)** LDH, **(F)** HRCT score, and **(G)** ARDS etiology. ROC, receiver operator characteristic; Alb, albumin; PLT, platelet; LDH, lactate dehydrogenase; HRCT, high-resolution computed tomography; ARDS, acute respiratory distress syndrome.

that was used for calculating the risk-scores of patients in the training set. In the validation set, the distribution of risk-scores and the survival status (**Figures 6A,B**) had a trend similar to that in the training set between high- and low-risk groups. Also, survival analysis indicated that low-risk patients had significantly favor prognosis than high-risk patients (**Figure 6C**). ROC curves were used to assess the prognostic value of the risk-scores; the analysis results suggested that risk-scores could accurately predict the survival rate in patients (AUC = 0.776, **Figure 6D**). The calibration plot in the validation set also showed that the model could accurately predict the 28-day survival (**Figure 6E**).

DISCUSSION

ARDS, one of the main critical diseases encountered in intensive care units, is a clinically and pathophysiologically complex syndrome of acute lung inflammation. Despite substantial progress in respiratory support strategies for critically ill patients, including the incorporation of a small tidal volume (21), high positive end-expiratory pressure (22), prone position ventilation (23), lung recruitment (24), use of neuromuscular blockers (25), high-frequency oscillatory ventilation (26, 27), and extracorporeal membrane oxygenation (28, 29), the mortality rate among patients with ARDS remains unacceptably high (30). However, to our knowledge, no study has previously developed a nomogram to predict the prognosis of patients with ARDS.

Herein, we first developed a nomogram using simple and easily available variables to evaluate the 28-day survival probabilities of ARDS patients whose information were extracted from an online database. Thereafter, we tested the performance of the nomogram in training and validation cohorts. Seven risk factors were identified in this model: age, Alb, PLT, PaO_2/FiO_2, LDH, CT score, and ARDS etiologies. Additionally, our results showed that PaO_2/FiO_2, and CT score could, albeit less accurately, predict the survival probability of ARDS patients compared to our novel model. These results suggest that the nomogram could be used as a cost-effective tool to predict the prognosis of ARDS and assist with clinical decision-making.

In 2012, the Berlin ARDS Society defined the severity of ARDS according to the oxygenation index (5). The oxygenation index (PaO_2/FiO_2) was helpful to categorize ARDS patients with different severity, and the mortality was reported to be higher in more severe stages of ARDS (mild, moderate, or severe) (5, 31). However, these severity categories have a low-to-moderate prognostic value to predict respiratory failure (32). Kamo and colleagues (33) reported that the severity stratification of the Berlin ARDS criteria may have a low capacity to differentiate between mild and moderate ARDS. In this study, the results of ROC curve analysis also indicated that the oxygenation index had low prognostic power (AUC, 55.3204%), which was consistent with previous studies.

CT or other lung imaging techniques have been used as diagnostic tools to optimize lung assessment and ventilator management in patients with ARDS; however, it is still controversial whether CT findings can predict ARDS outcomes (34–36). HRCT scores have been reported to correlate with the pathological stage of diffuse alveolar damage (37). Ichikado

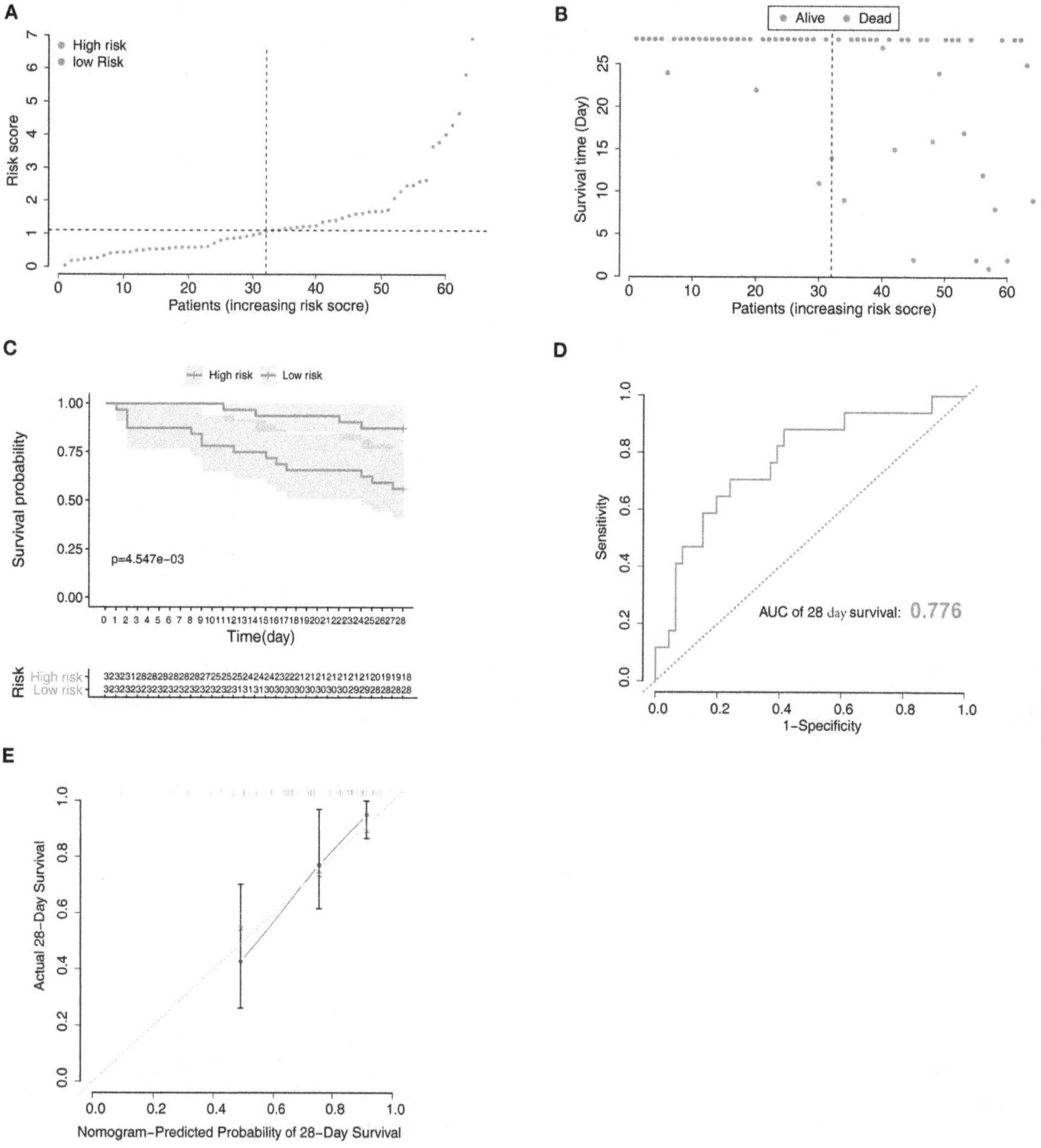

FIGURE 6 | Verification of the model in the validation set. **(A)** Distribution of the risk score. **(B)** Relationships between survival status and survival times of ARDS patients ranked by risk score. The black dotted line represents the optimum cut-off point dividing patients into low- and high-risk groups. **(C)** Kaplan–Meier survival analysis between high- and low-risk groups. **(D)** ROC curves of predictive models at 28 days. **(E)** Calibration plot for the training set that show the predicted and observed (with 95% confidence intervals) overall survival rates at 28 days. Model performance is shown by the plot, relative to the 45-degree line, which represents perfect prediction. ROC, receiver operator characteristic.

and colleagues (38) noted that HRCT score was one of the independent predictors of death and ventilator dependency in ARDS patients. Simultaneously, HRCT score was also found to be associated with multiorgan failure and ventilator-associated complications (38). In the present study, to increase model accuracy, HRCT score was incorporated into the nomogram. To evaluate the performance of HRCT score as a prognostic biomarker for the survival of ARDS patients, we performed ROC analysis. Our results showed that the model fit was significantly better than that of the one-factor HRCT model.

APACHE II score can be used as indicators to evaluate the prognosis among critically ill patients; it has been used worldwide to measure ICU performance (39). As APACHE II score included age and other factors in the calculation process, and repeated operations would be generated if the model was built again, APACHE II was not included in the LASSO regression analysis. The APACHE II score is calculated based on acute physiological parameters and chronic health conditions, all of which have significant effects on the predictive prognosis of ICU patients (40). Hwang and colleagues (41) revealed that APACHE II score was a mortality predictor for ARDS patients, but that the accuracy was not high. Lesur and colleagues (42) reported that APACHE II score may be less predictive value when applied for ARDS patients, and that in those patients, it might be less accurate than other indicators, such as age. In the present study, it was also found that the prediction accuracy of this model was better than APACHE II score when compared to the results of precious study (AUC = 0.623) (41).

Certain drugs have also been reported to have the potential to cause ARDS. It has been proved that molecular targeted therapy, such as methotrexate and certain herbal medicines, can cause severe respiratory failure or ARDS (43–45). However, only few studies have focused on the prognostic role of different etiologies of ARDS. In the present study, our results indicated that there is a lower risk of death if ARDS is caused by drugs. However, these discrepancies may be partly related to differences in the dose and duration of drug treatments.

Our study has some limitations. Firstly, the model was developed mainly based on the seven variables. As these factors were unstable throughout the whole follow-up period, which may partly influence the precision of the model. Secondly, only 197 patients were included in this study; further studies with bigger sample sizes are needed. Thirdly, the lack of external validation may limit the extrapolation of the nomogram.

To summarize, we identified eight variables and developed a novel model to predict prognosis in patients with ARDS. These results may help to further improve clinical decision-making and individualized treatment of ARDS patients. Also, this model could distinguish patients with high-risk of ARDS, and further help to perform a careful follow-up among those patients.

AUTHOR CONTRIBUTIONS

YL and LH designed the study. YL and JL performed the data analysis statistical analysis. YL prepared the manuscript. LH contributed funding for the project. All authors read and approved the final manuscript.

ACKNOWLEDGMENTS

We thank the Anan et al. for-data collection and sharing.

REFERENCES

1. Urner M, Jüni P, Hansen B, Wettstein MS, Ferguson ND, Fan E. Time-varying intensity of mechanical ventilation and mortality in patients with acute respiratory failure: a registry-based, prospective cohort study. *Lancet Respir Med.* (2020) 8:905–13. doi: 10.1016/S2213-2600(20)30325-8
2. Suresh R, Kupfer Y, Tessler S. Acute respiratory distress syndrome. *N Engl J Med.* (2000) 343:660–1. doi: 10.1056/NEJM200008313430914
3. Ware LB, Matthay MA. The acute respiratory distress syndrome. *N Engl J Med.* (2000) 342:1334–49. doi: 10.1056/NEJM200005043421806
4. Kim JS, Kim YJ, Kim M, Ryoo SM, Sohn CH, Ahn S, et al. Impact of lung compliance on neurological outcome in patients with acute respiratory distress syndrome following out-of-hospital cardiac arrest. *J Clin Med.* (2020) 9:527. doi: 10.3390/jcm9020527
5. Ranieri VM, Rubenfeld GD, Thompson BT, Ferguson ND, Caldwell E, Fan E, et al. Acute respiratory distress syndrome: the Berlin Definition. *JAMA.* (2012) 307:2526–33. doi: 10.1001/jama.2012.5669
6. Terpstra ML, Aman J, van Nieuw Amerongen GP, Groeneveld AB. Plasma biomarkers for acute respiratory distress syndrome: a systematic review and meta-analysis*. *Crit Care Med.* (2014) 42:691–700. doi: 10.1097/01.ccm.0000435669.60811.24
7. Yehya N, Thomas NJ, Meyer NJ, Christie JD, Berg RA, Margulies SS. Circulating markers of endothelial and alveolar epithelial dysfunction are associated with mortality in pediatric acute respiratory distress syndrome. *Intensive Care Med.* (2016) 42:1137–45. doi: 10.1007/s00134-016-4352-1
8. Levitt JE, Gould MK, Ware LB, Matthay MA. The pathogenetic and prognostic value of biologic markers in acute lung injury. *J Intensive Care Med.* (2009) 24:151–67. doi: 10.1177/0885066609332603
9. Jones TK, Feng R, Kerchberger VE, Reilly JP, Anderson BJ, Shashaty MGS, et al. Plasma sRAGE acts as a genetically regulated causal intermediate in sepsis-associated acute respiratory distress syndrome. *Am J Respir Crit Care Med.* (2020) 201:47–56. doi: 10.1164/rccm.201810-2033OC
10. Graesslin O, Abdulkarim BS, Coutant C, Huguet F, Gabos Z, Hsu L, et al. Nomogram to predict subsequent brain metastasis in patients with metastatic breast cancer. *J Clin Oncol.* (2010) 28:2032–7. doi: 10.1200/JCO.2009.24.6314
11. Wang J, He L, Tang Y, Li D, Yang Y, Zeng Z. Development and validation of a nomogram with an epigenetic signature for predicting survival in patients with lung adenocarcinoma. *Aging.* (2020) 12:23200–16. doi: 10.18632/aging.104090
12. Anan K, Ichikado K, Kawamura K, Johkoh T, Fujimoto K, Suga M. Clinical characteristics and prognosis of drug-associated acute respiratory distress syndrome compared with non-drug-associated acute respiratory distress syndrome: a single-centre retrospective study in Japan. *BMJ Open.* (2017) 7:e015330. doi: 10.1136/bmjopen-2016-015330
13. Friedman J, Hastie T, Tibshirani R. Regularization paths for generalized linear models via coordinate descent. *J Stat Softw.* (2010) 33:1–22. doi: 10.18637/jss.v033.i01
14. Simon N, Friedman J, Hastie T, Tibshirani R. Regularization paths for cox's proportional hazards model via coordinate descent. *J Stat Softw.* (2011) 39:1–13. doi: 10.18637/jss.v039.i05
15. Frank E Harrell Jr. *RMS: Regression Modeling Strategies. R Package Version 6.0-1.* (2020).
16. Therneau T. *A Package for Survival Analysis in R. R Package Version 3.1-12.* (2020).
17. R Core Team. *Foreign: Read Data Stored by 'Minitab', 'S','SAS', 'SPSS', 'Stata', 'Systat', 'Weka', 'dBase', R Package Version 0.8-76.* R Core Team (2020).
18. Schauberger P, Walker A. *Openxlsx: Read, Write and Edit xlsx Files. R Package Version 4.1.5.* (2020).
19. Jalali A, Roshan D, Alvarez-Iglesias A, Newell J. *DynNom: Visualising Statistical Models Using Dynamic Nomograms. R Package Version 5.0.1.* (2019). doi: 10.1371/journal.pone.0225253
20. Kamarudin AN, Cox T, Kolamunnage-Dona R. Time-dependent ROC curve analysis inmedical research: current methods and applications. *BMC Med Res Methodol.* (2017) 17:53. doi: 10.1186/s12874-017-0332-6
21. Brower RG, Matthay MA, Morris A, Schoenfeld D, Thompson BT, Wheeler A. Ventilation with lower tidal volumes as compared with traditional tidal volumes for acute lung injury and the acute respiratory distress syndrome. *N Engl J Med.* (2000) 342:1301–8. doi: 10.1056/NEJM200005043421801
22. Brower RG, Lanken PN, MacIntyre N, Matthay MA, Morris A, Ancukiewicz M, et al. Higher versus lower positive end-expiratory pressures in patients with the acute respiratory distress syndrome. *N Engl J Med.* (2004) 351:327–36. doi: 10.1056/NEJMoa032193
23. Guérin C, Reignier J, Richard JC, Beuret P, Gacouin A, Boulain T, et al. Prone positioning in severe acute respiratory distress syndrome. *N Engl J Med.* (2013) 368:2159–68. doi: 10.1056/NEJMoa1214103

24. Meade MO, Cook DJ, Guyatt GH, Slutsky AS, Arabi YM, Cooper DJ, et al. Ventilation strategy using low tidal volumes, recruitment maneuvers, and high positive end-expiratory pressure for acute lung injury and acute respiratory distress syndrome: a randomized controlled trial. *JAMA.* (2008) 299:637–45. doi: 10.1001/jama.299.6.637
25. Papazian L, Forel JM, Gacouin A, Penot-Ragon C, Perrin G, Loundou A, et al. Neuromuscular blockers in early acute respiratory distress syndrome. *N Engl J Med.* (2010) 363:1107–16. doi: 10.1056/NEJMoa1005372
26. Young NH, Andrews PJ. High-frequency oscillation as a rescue strategy for brain-injured adult patients with acute lung injury and acute respiratory distress syndrome. *Neurocrit Care.* (2011) 15:623–33. doi: 10.1007/s12028-011-9550-7
27. Ferguson ND, Cook DJ, Guyatt GH, Mehta S, Hand L, Austin P, et al. High-frequency oscillation in early acute respiratory distress syndrome. *N Engl J Med.* (2013) 368:795–805. doi: 10.1056/NEJMoa1215554
28. Zampieri FG, Mendes PV, Ranzani OT, Taniguchi LU, Pontes Azevedo LC, Vieira Costa EL, et al. Extracorporeal membrane oxygenation for severe respiratory failure in adult patients: a systematic review and meta-analysis of current evidence. *J Crit Care.* (2013) 28:998–1005. doi: 10.1016/j.jcrc.2013.07.047
29. Peek GJ, Clemens F, Elbourne D, Firmin R, Hardy P, Hibbert C, et al. CESAR: conventional ventilatory support vs extracorporeal membrane oxygenation for severe adult respiratory failure. *BMC Health Serv Res.* (2006) 6:163. doi: 10.1186/1472-6963-6-163
30. Chen X, Wu S, Tang L, Ma L, Wang F, Feng H, et al. Mesenchymal stem cells overexpressing heme oxygenase-1 ameliorate lipopolysaccharide-induced acute lung injury in rats. *J Cell Physiol.* (2019) 234:7301–19. doi: 10.1002/jcp.27488
31. Ferguson ND, Fan E, Camporota L, Antonelli M, Anzueto A, Beale R, et al. The Berlin definition of ARDS: an expanded rationale, justification, and supplementary material. *Intensive Care Med.* (2012) 38:1573–82. doi: 10.1007/s00134-012-2682-1
32. Hernu R, Wallet F, Thiollière F, Martin O, Richard JC, Schmitt Z, et al. An attempt to validate the modification of the American-European consensus definition of acute lung injury/acute respiratory distress syndrome by the Berlin definition in a University hospital. *Intensive Care Med.* (2013) 39:2161–70. doi: 10.1007/s00134-013-3122-6
33. Kamo T, Tasaka S, Suzuki T, Asakura T, Suzuki S, Yagi K, et al. Prognostic values of the Berlin definition criteria, blood lactate level, and fibroproliferative changes on high-resolution computed tomography in ARDS patients. *BMC Pulm Med.* (2019) 19:37. doi: 10.1186/s12890-019-0803-0
34. Chiumello D, Taccone P, Berto V, Marino A, Migliara G, Lazzerini M, et al. Long-term outcomes in survivors of acute respiratory distress syndrome ventilated in supine or prone position. *Intensive Care Med.* (2012) 38:221–9. doi: 10.1007/s00134-011-2445-4
35. Chung JH, Kradin RL, Greene RE, Shepard JA, Digumarthy SR. CT predictors of mortality in pathology confirmed ARDS. *Eur Radiol.* (2011) 21:730–7. doi: 10.1007/s00330-010-1979-0
36. Chiumello D, Froio S, Bouhemad B, Camporota L, Coppola S. Clinical review: lung imaging in acute respiratory distress syndrome patients—an update. *Crit Care.* (2013) 17:243. doi: 10.1186/cc13114
37. Anan K, Kawamura K, Suga M, Ichikado K. Clinical differences between pulmonary and extrapulmonary acute respiratory distress syndrome: a retrospective cohort study of prospectively collected data in Japan. *J Thorac Dis.* (2018) 10:5796–803. doi: 10.21037/jtd.2018.09.73
38. Ichikado K, Muranaka H, Gushima Y, Kotani T, Nader HM, Fujimoto K, et al. Fibroproliferative changes on high-resolution CT in the acute respiratory distress syndrome predict mortality and ventilator dependency: a prospective observational cohort study. *BMJ Open.* (2012) 2:e000545. doi: 10.1136/bmjopen-2011-000545
39. Giamarellos-Bourboulis EJ, Norrby-Teglund A, Mylona V, Savva A, Tsangaris I, Dimopoulou I, et al. Risk assessment in sepsis: a new prognostication rule by APACHE II score and serum soluble urokinase plasminogen activator receptor. *Crit Care.* (2012) 16:R149. doi: 10.1186/cc11463
40. Hsu YT, He YT, Ting CK, Tsou MY, Tang GJ, Pu C. Administrative and claims data help predict patient mortality in intensive care units by logistic regression: a nationwide database study. *Biomed Res Int.* (2020) 2020:9076739. doi: 10.1155/2020/9076739
41. Hwang H, Choi SM, Lee J, Park YS, Lee CH, Yoo CG, et al. Validation of age, PaO(2)/FIO(2) and plateau pressure score in Korean patients with acute respiratory distress syndrome: a retrospective cohort study. *Respir Res.* (2020) 21:94. doi: 10.1186/s12931-020-01357-5
42. Lesur O, Langevin S, Berthiaume Y, Légaré M, Skrobik Y, Bellemare JF, et al. Outcome value of Clara cell protein in serum of patients with acute respiratory distress syndrome. *Intensive Care Med.* (2006) 32:1167–74. doi: 10.1007/s00134-006-0235-1
43. Wolkove N, Baltzan M. Amiodarone pulmonary toxicity. *Can Respir J.* (2009) 16:43–8. doi: 10.1155/2009/282540
44. Imokawa S, Colby TV, Leslie KO, Helmers RA. Methotrexate pneumonitis: review of the literature and histopathological findings in nine patients. *Eur Respir J.* (2000) 15:373–81. doi: 10.1034/j.1399-3003.2000.15b25.x
45. Enomoto YM, Nakamura YMP, Enomoto NMP, Fujisawa TMP, Inui NMP and Suda T. Japanese herbal medicine-induced pneumonitis: a review of 73 patients. *Respir Investig.* (2017) 55:138–44. doi: 10.1016/j.resinv.2016.11.007

5

Diagnostic Significance of Metagenomic Next-Generation Sequencing for Community-Acquired Pneumonia in Southern China

Hanying Liu[1†], Ying Zhang[2†], Guiyang Chen[3], Shenghua Sun[1], Jiangang Wang[4], Fengyi Chen[5], Chun Liu[1] and Quan Zhuang[2,6*]*

[1] Department of Respiratory Diseases, The 3rd Xiangya Hospital, Central South University, Changsha, China, [2] Transplantation Center, The 3rd Xiangya Hospital, Central South University, Changsha, China, [3] Department of Cardiology, Hunan Aerospace Hospital, Changsha, China, [4] Department of Health Management, The 3rd Xiangya Hospital, Central South University, Changsha, China, [5] Vision Medicals Co. Ltd, Guangzhou, China, [6] Research Center of National Health Ministry on Transplantation Medicine, Changsha, China

***Correspondence:**
Chun Liu
liuchun7322@163.com
Quan Zhuang
zhuangquansteven@163.com

† These authors have contributed equally to this work

Background: The morbidity and mortality of community-acquired pneumonia are relatively high, but many pneumonia pathogens cannot be identified accurately. As a new pathogen detection technology, metagenomic next-generation sequencing (mNGS) has been applied more and more clinically. We aimed to evaluate the diagnostic significance of mNGS for community-acquired pneumonia (CAP) in the south of China.

Methods: Our study selected CAP patients who visited the 3rd Xiangya Hospital from May 2019 to April 2021. Pathogens in bronchoalveolar lavage fluid (BALF) specimens were detected using mNGS and traditional microbiological culture. mNGS group: detected by both mNGS and BALF culture; control group: detected only by BALF or sputum culture. The diagnostic performance of pathogens and the antibiotic adjustments were compared within mNGS group.

Results: The incidence of acute respiratory distress syndrome (ARDS) was 28.3% in the mNGS group and 17.3% in the control group. Within the mNGS group, the positive rate of pathogens detected by mNGS was 64%, thus by BALF culture was only 28%. Pathogens detected by mNGS were consisted of bacteria (55%), fungi (18%), special pathogens (18%), and viruses (9%). The most detected pathogen by mNGS was *Chlamydia psittaci*. Among the pathogen-positive cases, 26% was not pathogen-covered by empirical antibiotics, so most of which were made an antibiotic adjustment.

Conclusions: mNGS can detect pathogens in a more timely and accurate manner and assist clinicians to adjust antibiotics in time. Therefore, we recommend mNGS as the complementary diagnosis of severe pneumonia or complicated infections.

Keywords: mNGS, pneumonia, diagnostic significance, pathogen, BALF

INTRODUCTION

Community-acquired pneumonia (CAP) is a common disease with high mortality (1). According to the clinical phenotype, the pathogens for up to 60% of infectious diseases were still unknown (2, 3), and the mortality of CAP in need of emergency treatment exceeds 40% (4). Pathogens that cause pneumonia include common bacteria (such as *Streptococcus pneumoniae*), fungi, viruses, and some atypical pathogens such as *Mycoplasma pneumoniae*, *Chlamydia*, and *Legionella* (1). In a study of 329 clinical samples, it was found that the main pathogens of patients with different immune status were diverse. Among patients with normal immunity, the pathogens are mainly *S. pneumoniae*, *rhinovirus*, and *influenza*. The main pathogens in immunocompromised patients are *Pneumocystis*, *Klebsiella pneumonia*, *S. pneumoniae*, *Haemophilus influenza*, and *Pseudomonas aeruginosa* (5). In recent years, rare and atypical pathogens have been continuously detected, such as *Mycobacterium abscessus*, *Mycobacterium kansas*, etc. These pathogens may cause pneumonia, multiple-organ disorders and even acute respiratory distress syndrome (ARDS). Due to the limitations of current traditional pathogen detection methods in terms of sensitivity, detection speed and detection spectrum, rapid and accurate diagnosis of pneumonia pathogens are a big challenge (6, 7). Therefore, early and effective identification of the pathogens are essential for the precise treatment of pneumonia patients.

mNGS is the second-generation sequencing technology of metagenomics, which can identify bacteria, fungi, parasites, and viruses without much guidance from clinical experience. mNGS can identify the pathogens deeply and rapidly without culturing, and even have higher sensitivity than traditional cultivation methods (8). Another advantage of mNGS is the diversity of samples which could detect almost all pathogens in clinical samples (9) such as bronchoalveolar lavage fluid (BALF), tissue, sputum, pleural effusion, cerebrospinal fluid, pus, bone marrow, and nasal swabs (10–12), etc. Since the sensitivity and specificity of mNGS are less perturbative by the antibiotic treatment presently (13). mNGS may become a routine diagnostic test, partially replacing the traditional sputum culture method (14). However, the interpretation of the mNGS reports, especially the identification of pathogenic bacteria, colonizing bacteria, and the mixture of normal oral microbiota in respiratory tract samples in pneumonia patients need further study (15). The pathogenicity of microorganisms in different regions is generally different. There are few large-scale analysis research with respiratory samples studying the correlation between the detection efficiency of mNGS and the antibiotic therapy. Thus, our study aimed to explore the advantages of mNGS in the detection of pneumonia pathogens and its guiding significance for diagnosis and antibiotic treatment of CAP.

PATIENTS AND METHODS

Patient Selection and Study Design

We retrospectively reviewed 346 cases diagnosed as CAP at the 3rd Xiangya Hospital of Central South University from May 2019 to April 2021. With our inclusion/exclusion criteria (**Figure 1**), 346 samples were included for analysis and categorized into two groups defined as mNGS group and control group. mNGS group was subjected to regular BALF culture as well as mNGS testing (ID: PRJNA756706, https://www.ncbi.nlm.nih.gov/sra/PRJNA756706) in a pairwise manner, and control group only did the BALF or sputum culture. This study was approved by Institutional Review Board of the 3rd Xiangya Hospital of Central South University (No. 21030).

Sample Processing and Nucleic Acid Extraction

BALF were collected from patients according to standard procedures. DNA was extracted using a QIAamp® UCP Pathogen DNA Kit (Qiagen) following the manufacturer's instructions and 600 μL of the processed specimens was mixed with glass beads of 0.1–0.2 mm diameter. A vortex mixer (Crystal, TX, United States) was used to disrupt the bacterial cell wall at 1,600 g for 10 min. The tubes were then heated at 99°C for 10 min before DNA extraction. Human DNA was removed using Benzonase (Qiagen) and Tween20 (Sigma) (16). The differential lysis method was used to remove host DNA. we first use physical hypotonic lysis and chemical lysis to break human cells, and then obtain microbial cells by enzymatic hydrolysis, followed by wall breaking and nucleic acid extraction. Total RNA was extracted with a QIAamp® Viral RNA Kit (Qiagen) and ribosomal RNA was removed by a Ribo-Zero rRNA Removal Kit (Illumina). The concentration of extracted DNA/RNA was measured using a Qubit Fluorometer before library preparation. cDNA was generated using reverse transcriptase and dNTPs (Thermo Fisher).

Library Preparation and Sequencing

Libraries were constructed for the DNA and cDNA samples using a Nextera XT DNA Library Prep Kit (Illumina, San Diego, CA) (17). The initial input of DNA is 5–100 ng. Firstly, DNA needs to be fragmented to obtain 150–250 bp inserts, followed by terminal repair and adapter connection, and finally, library amplification to construct a library that meets the requirements of sequencing. Library was quality assessed by Qubit dsDNA HS Assay kit followed by High Sensitivity DNA kit (Agilent) on an Agilent 2100 Bioanalyzer. Library pools were then loaded onto an Illumina Nextseq 550Dx sequencer for 75 cycles of single-end sequencing to generate ~20 million reads for each library. For negative controls, we also prepared PBMC samples with 10^5 cells/mL from healthy donors in parallel with each batch, using the same protocol, and sterile deionized water was extracted alongside the specimens to serve as non-template controls (NTC).

Bioinformatics Analyses

Trimmomatic was used to remove low quality reads, adapter contamination, and duplicate reads, as well as those shorter than 50 bp (18). Low complexity reads were removed by Kcomplexity with default parameters (19). Human sequence data were identified and excluded by mapping to a human reference genome (hg38) using Burrows-Wheeler Aligner software.

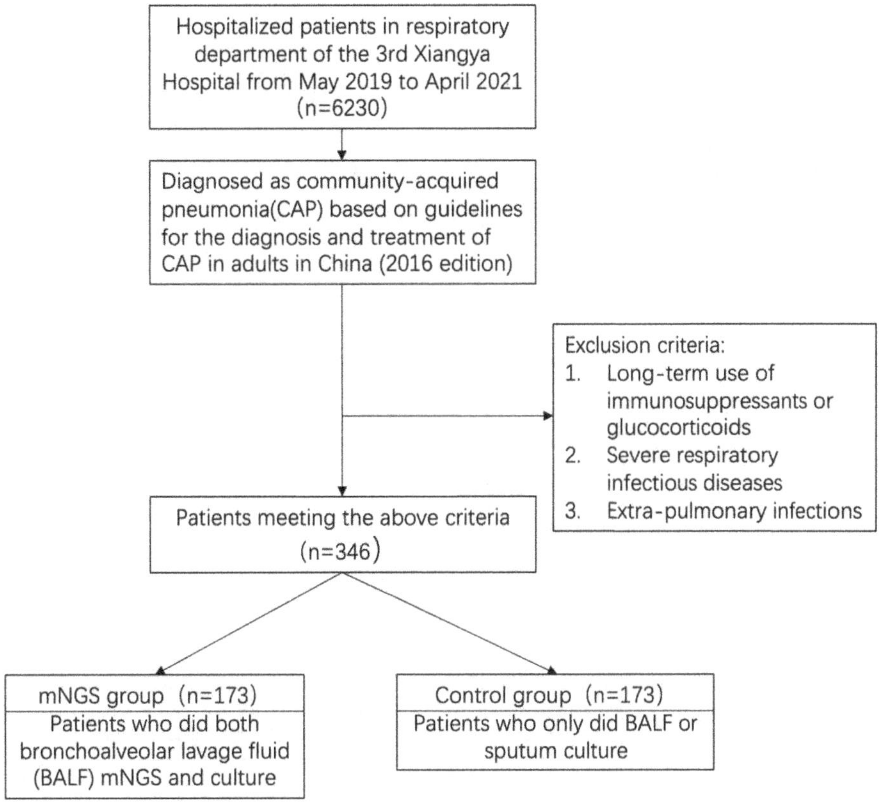

FIGURE 1 | Flowchart of case selection. From 6230 cases, a total of 370 community-acquired pneumonia cases were selected for further analysis. Patients in mNGS group did the mNGS and BALF culture at the same time. Patients in control group only did the BALF or sputum culture. mNGS, metagenomic next-generation sequencing.

We designed a set of criteria similar to the National Center for Biotechnology Information (NCBI) criteria for selecting representative assembly for microorganisms (bacteria, viruses, fungi, protozoa, and other multicellular eukaryotic pathogens) from the NCBI Nucleotide and Genome databases. Pathogen lists was selected according to three references: (1) Johns Hopkins ABX Guide (https://www.hopkinsguides.com/hopkins/index/Johns_Hopkins_ABX_Guide/Pathogens), (2) Manual of Clinical Microbiology (https://www.clinmicronow.org/doi/book/10.1128/9781683670438.MCM), and (3) clinical case reports or research articles published in current peer-reviewed journals. The final database consisted of about 18,562 genomes. Microbial reads were aligned to database with SNAP v1.0beta.18. Virus-positive detection results (DNA or RNA viruses) were defined as the coverage of three or more non-overlapping regions on the genome. A positive detection was reported for a given species or genus if the reads per million (RPM) ratio, or RPM-r was ≥ 5, where the RPM-r was defined as the RPM_{sample} / RPM_{NC} (i.e., the RPM corresponding to a given species or genus in the clinical sample divided by the RPM in the NC/negative control). In addition, to minimize cross-species misalignments among closely related microorganisms, we penalized (reduced) the RPM of microorganisms sharing a genus or family designation, if the species or genus appeared in non-template controls. A penalty of 5% was used for species (12) (**Figure 2**).

Statistical Analysis

Continuous variables were compared using the Mann–Whitney *U*-test; categorical variables were compared using the chi-square test. $P < 0.05$ was considered significant. Statistical analyses were performed using SPSS version 23.0 (SPSS, Inc., Chicago, IL, USA).

RESULTS

Clinical Characteristics of Patients With CAP

Finally, a total of 346 patients with CAP was enrolled. One hundred and seventy-three patients were in the mNGS group, and the rest 173 patients were in the control group. The clinical characteristics of patients between these two groups were different as follows (**Tables 1, 2**). The rates of patients with comorbidities including hypertension, neoplastic, diabetic, renal, and cerebrovascular diseases were relatively lower in the mNGS group, but they did not reach statistical significance. However, the incidence of ARDS was significantly higher in the mNGS group ($P = 0.021$). Not unexpectedly, the average hospital stay

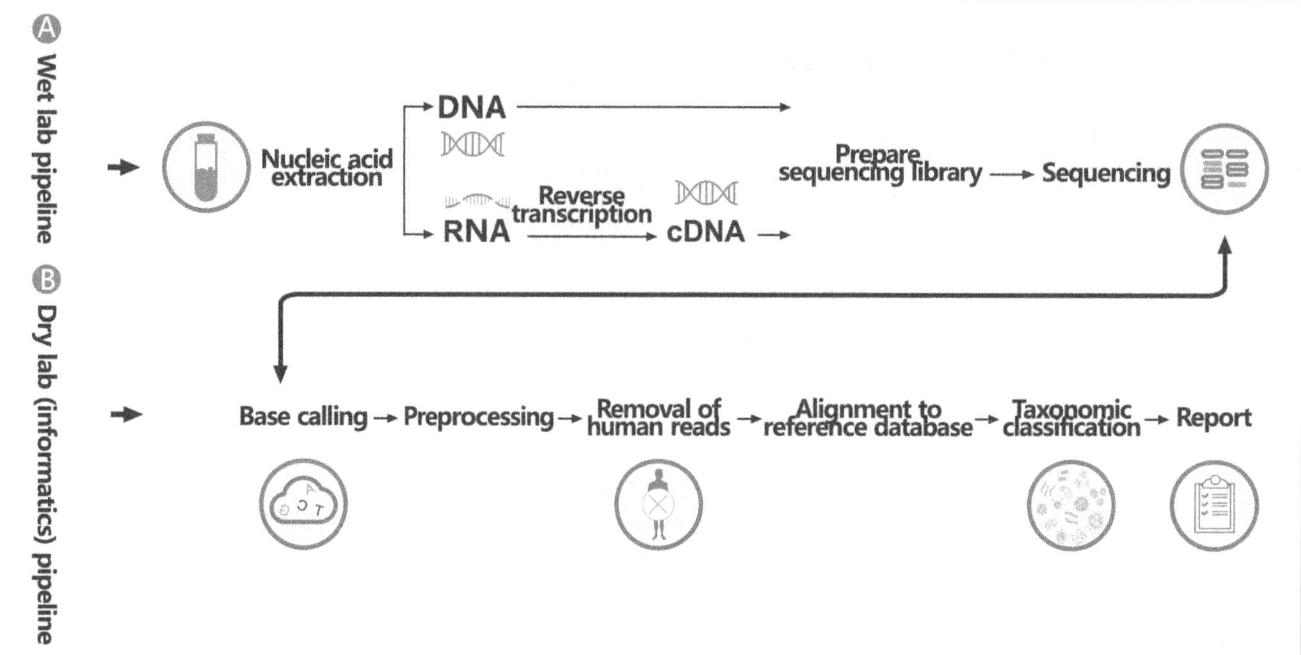

FIGURE 2 | The generalized workflow of mNGS for clinical pathogen diagnosis. The workflow has two components: **(A)** a wet lab protocol in which samples are collected, processed, extracted for nucleic acids, prepared into a sequencing library, and sequenced, and **(B)** a dry lab computational pipeline that includes microbial identification, statistical analysis, and interpretation. The sequencing library may be targeted, undergo DNA amplification, or both.

was longer in the mNGS group ($P = 0.001$). But the empirical use of antibiotics in two groups were roughly the same. The acute physiology and chronic health evaluation (Apache) II score in two groups were not very different, either. The laboratory test results were 5–7 days after the mNGS and BALF or sputum culture did. Except for the platelet-to-lymphocyte (PTL) ratio and erythrocyte sedimentation rate (ESR), there were several significant differences between the two groups, indicating that the patients in mNGS group were relatively severer. Defined daily dose (DDD) represented the strength of antibiotic application and the antibiotics use density, which was higher in the mNGS group ($P = 0.013$) indicating the use of advanced antibiotics was more frequent.

Comparison of Diagnostic Performance Between BALF mNGS and Culture

Within the mNGS group (both tested by mNGS and BALF culture), through BALF mNGS, 110 (64%) were detected positively with pathogens, and 20 (11%) were completely negative; 43 (25%) were detected with colonizing pathogens or contaminating pathogens, which we also considered as negative detection according to our experience. Furthermore, 92 (55%) were detected with bacteria, 30 (18%) with fungi, 15 (9%) with viruses, and 31 (18%) were detected with other special pathogens (**Figure 3A**). Conversely, BALF culture done at the same time with mNGS only showed 28% positive rate. Within this positive detection by BALF culture, only bacteria (91%) and fungi (9%) could be cultured, so the virus and other special pathogens could not be recognized by traditional cultures (**Figure 3B**). Thus, the sensitivity of mNGS was much higher than traditional microbiological culture. Within the mNGS group, we detected 24 cases of *Chlamydia psittaci* by mNGS, including eight female patients and 16 male patients, with the average age of 65 years old. In addition to *C. psittaci*, some of these patients were also infected with other pathogens, among which *Candida albicans* was the most (10/24). The reads of *C. psittaci* matched in these patients ranged from 16 to 270670. The relative abundance refers to the proportion of pathogen in the same type of microorganism, and the relative abundance of *Chlamydia* was: 0.1–97.9%. A higher relative abundance indicated a higher proportion of the species in the sample. Relative abundance was only a parameter that indicates the amount of pathogens, and it could not be directly judged whether it was pathogenic or not based on the value of relative abundance. Therefore, we did not compare the relative abundance of detected pathogens. In the process of clinical diagnosis, the value of relative abundance was only for reference. Sixteen out of 24 patients adjusted the use of antibiotics based on the reports of mNGS. The white blood cells and neutrophils of most patients did not increase significantly, but the increase of PCT and D-dimer and the decrease of blood calcium were related to the severity of the condition (**Supplementary Table 1**).

Comparison of Pathogens Detected by BALF mNGS and Culture

Among the 168 kinds of morbigenous microorganism, *C. psittaci* (24/168) was the most detected pathogen by mNGS, followed by *Hemophilus parainfluenzae* (19/168). We also detected virus (15/168), and other special pathogens (31/168).

TABLE 1 | Demographic and baseline characteristics of patients.

Characteristics	mNGS group (n = 173)	Control group (n = 173)	P
Age, mean (range), years	60 (15–87)	64 (18–90)	0.045
Sex, female, n (%)	47 (27.2)	67 (38.7)	0.030
Hospital, mean (range), days	16 (1–66)	11 (0–70)	0.001
Comorbidity, n (%)			
Cardiovascular disease	34 (20.0)	35 (20.2)	1.000
Hypertension	43 (24.9)	51 (29.5)	0.398
Chronic obstructive pulmonary disease	19 (11.0)	17 (9.8)	0.860
Neoplastic disease	17 (9.8)	25 (14.5)	0.249
Diabetes	27 (15.6)	30 (17.3)	0.772
Kidney disease	8 (4.6)	12 (6.9)	0.490
Bronchiectasis	16 (9.2)	16 (9.2)	1.000
Cerebrovascular disease	22 (12.7)	26 (15.0)	0.641
ARDS, n (%)	49 (28.3)	30 (17.3)	0.021
On empiric antibiotics at time of sample collection, n (%)	173 (100)	171 (98.8)	0.499
Apache II score, mean ± standard deviation	14.0 ± 5.4	12.2 ± 6.4	0.051
30-day mortality, n (%)	14 (8.1)	12 (6.9)	0.839

mNGS, metagenomic next generation sequencing; ARDS, acute respiratory distress syndrome.

TABLE 2 | Laboratory findings of patients.

	mNGS group (n = 173)	Control group (n = 185)	P
White blood cell count, x 10^9/L	9.41 (0.56–57.27)	8.44 (1.68-29.47)	0.035
Percentage of neutrophils, %	77.9 (9.8–97)	72.5 (38.5–98.4)	0.001
Lymphocyte count, x 10^9/L	1.07 (0.11–4.14)	1.28 (0.12–9.51)	0.005
NLR	11.18 (0.21–86.47)	9.05 (0.82–121.20)	0.001
PLR	282.82 (9.42–1925.00)	270.68 (6.00–1103.80)	0.803
Cre, umol/L	89 (30–855)	79 (26–527)	0.027
PCT, ng/mL	2.40 (0.01–75.57)	1.51 (0.01–70.62)	0.004
CRP, mg/L	82.65 (0.43–320.04)	50.14 (0.01–314.69)	0.001
ESR, mm/h	63.49 (2–120)	54.73 (2–120)	0.081
Ca^{2+}, mmol/L	2.04 (0.99–2.49)	2.15 (1.15–3.34)	0.001
Albumin, g/L	30.0 (16.5–44.7)	32.5 (17.1–47.2)	0.001
DDD	116 (36–255)	109 (0–300)	0.013

mNGS, metagenomic next generation sequencing; NLR, neutrophil-to-lymphocyte ratio; Cre, creatinine; PLR, platelet-to-lymphocyte ratio; DDD, defined daily dose; PCT, procalcitonin; CRP, C-reactive protein; ESR, erythrocyte sedimentation rate.
Data are presented as means (range).

The positive rate of mNGS for pathogenic bacteria was almost twice than that of BALF culture (**Figure 4**). Except for *K. pneumoniae* and *Acinetobacter baumannii*, the positive rate for mNGS of other pathogens were relatively higher. Not only that, *Haemophilus parainfluenzae*, *Mycobacterium tuberculosis*, *Nocardia*, *Legionella*, *Streptococcus parasanguis*, and *Tropheryma whipplei* were only detected by mNGS, and the BALF cultures of these microorganism were all negative. The positive rate of mNGS for fungi was seven times than that of BALF culture, and *C. albicans* was one of the most detected fungi in BALF culture. For *Pneumocystis jirovecii*, *Aspergillus*, and *Cryptococcus*, the positive rate of mNGS was much higher than that of BALF culture. Viruses and some special pathogens can only be detected by mNGS. *Human herpesvirus 1, 4,* and *5* were only considered pathogenic when the reads and abundance was relatively high. mNGS can detect rare pathogens such as *Orientia tsutsugamushi* and *Leptospira interrogans*, which was of great guiding significance for antibiotic adjustment. In addition, we also counted other pathogens in the mNGS report of 173 patients that we thought were not pathogenic (**Figure 5**). Among the non-pathogenic pathogens, *C. albicans* was the most common. But the *A. baumannii*, *K. pneumoniae*, etc. were also included which were "usually" considered to cause pneumonia. As there was no detailed uniform criteria or authoritative guide for the interpretation of mNGS reports, we always determined whether the pathogens were pathogenic, colonized, or contaminated based on clinical experience, patient's imaging findings and inflammation indicators.

The Influence of mNGS on Treatment and Prognosis

The correct use of antibiotics was extremely important for the treatment of CAP. Among the 116 patients with pathogen-positive pneumonia, 46 (40%) cases were completely covered by antibiotics before the pathogens were detected. These 46 cases were not adjusted for antibiotics after the pathogens were detected. Forty (34%) cases were partially covered by antibiotics before the pathogens were detected. After the pathogens were detected, 37 cases adjusted their antibiotics, and three cases did not adjust, of which one case were transferred to specialist hospitals for further treatment, and two cases died. Thirty (26%) cases were not covered by antibiotics at all, of which 25 cases were adjusted after the pathogens were detected, and the remaining five cases were transferred to other hospitals or death (**Figure 6**). All the pathogens detected by mNGS and culture, and the details of antibiotics therapy had been listed in **Supplementary Table 2**. As for pathogens were not detected or pathogens that were colonized and contaminated, we could only rely on laboratory test results, imaging findings, and empirical treatment to adjust antibiotics.

DISCUSSION

We retrospectively reviewed 346 CAP cases. Based on the patients' clinical characteristics and inflammatory indices, the patients in the mNGS group were relatively severer in our study, including a higher incidence of ARDS, WBC, PCT, neutrophils, ESR elevation, and peripheral blood calcium concentration decrease. We suggested that mNGS would be recommended to

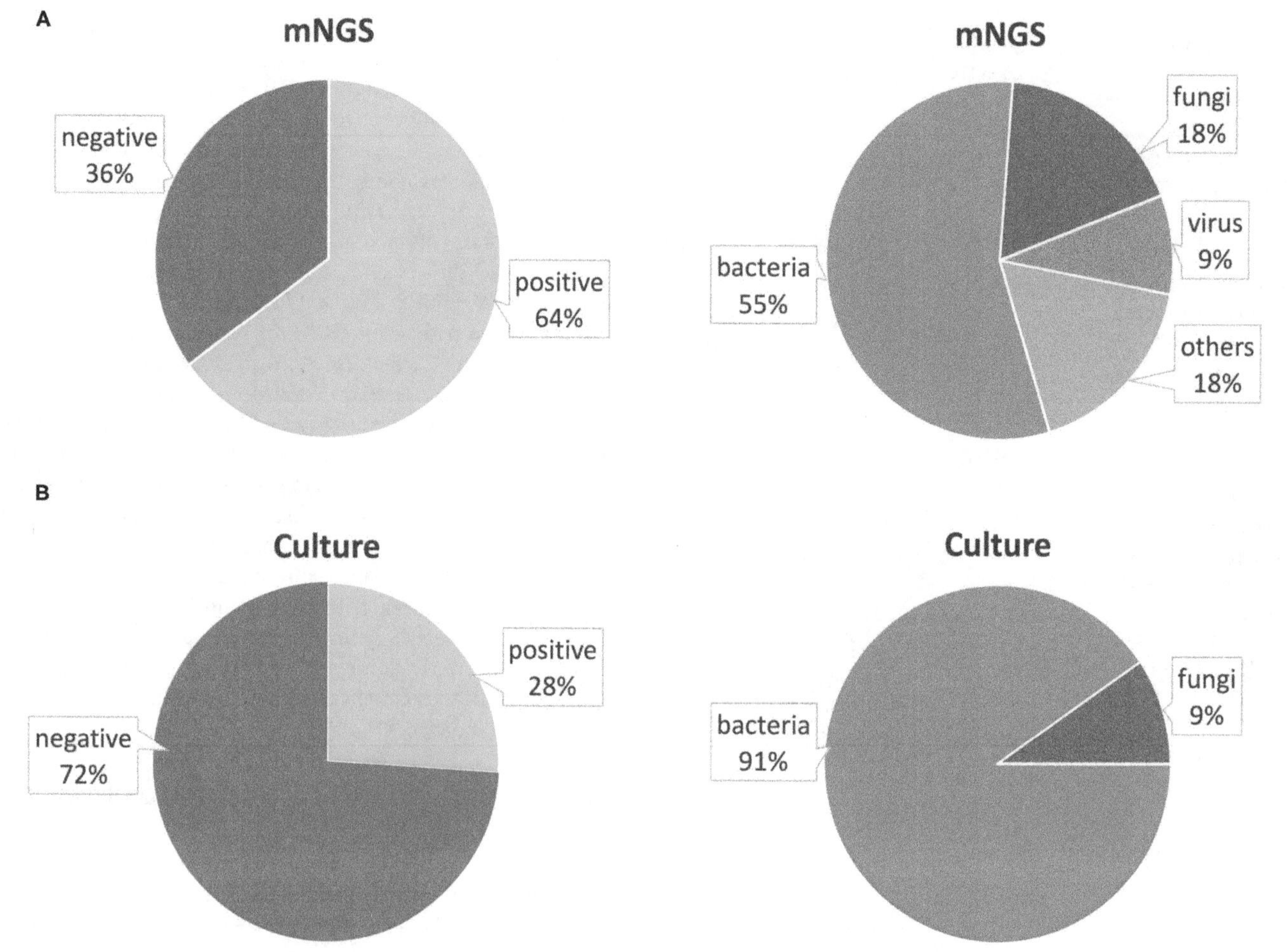

FIGURE 3 | Comparison of positive rate of pathogens by BALF mNGS and culture. **(A)** The positive rate of mNGS and the types of pathogens detected. **(B)** The positive rate of BALF culture and the types of pathogens detected. BALF, bronchoalveolar lavage fluid; mNGS, metagenomic next-generation sequencing.

patients with more complex and severer conditions to accurately identify the pathogens and timely adjust antibiotics. The DDD reflects the density of antibiotic application. The patients in the mNGS group treated more antibiotics because their conditions were more serious and complicated. However, we have also controlled it at a relatively low level which was benefited from the timely detection of pathogens by mNGS. The patients received timely targeted anti-infection treatment, and most of them had better prognosis. In addition, although patients in the mNGS group were with severer conditions, the 30-day mortality rate was basically the same as that in the control group, which indicated that the early diagnosis and promptly treatment of patients through mNGS could reduce the mortality. Moreover, mNGS can detect many pathogens that cannot be detected by traditional microbiological culture. During the incipient stage of the COVID-19 pandemic, mNGS supplied a quick and accurate identification for pathogenic virus (20).

In the past, we thought that *C. psittaci* was relatively rare. However, we detected 24 patients infected with *C. psittaci* through mNGS. Most of the cases were also accompanied by the infection of other pathogens (*C. albicans* was the top one), but many of the pathogens were the microbiota in oropharynx and colonized bacteria in respiratory tracts. Meanwhile, we found that after mNGS had been fully applied in our clinical practice from the year 2018, the incidence of *C. psittaci* pneumonia had been greatly increased, which meant that *C. psittaci* was widespread in the past, but it was difficult to be detected. Although miost patients infected with *C. psittaci* have severe pneumonia, clinicians can adjust the dosage and classes of antibiotics in time according to mNGS reports, and the overall outcome of the patients is better. Previous studies also confirmed that mNGS could improve the outcome of patients with severe pneumonia of *C. psittaci* and played a positive role in diagnosis and treatment of CAP, as well as adjustment of antibiotics (21).

Traditionally, the detection of tuberculosis could only be based on methods such as acid-fast staining of sputum smears, culture of *M. tuberculosis*, and interferon gamma release assay (IGRA), etc. These methods have disadvantages such as low sensitivity, low positive rate, time-consuming, and not direct enough. However, mNGS can detect as low as 1–2 reads of *M.*

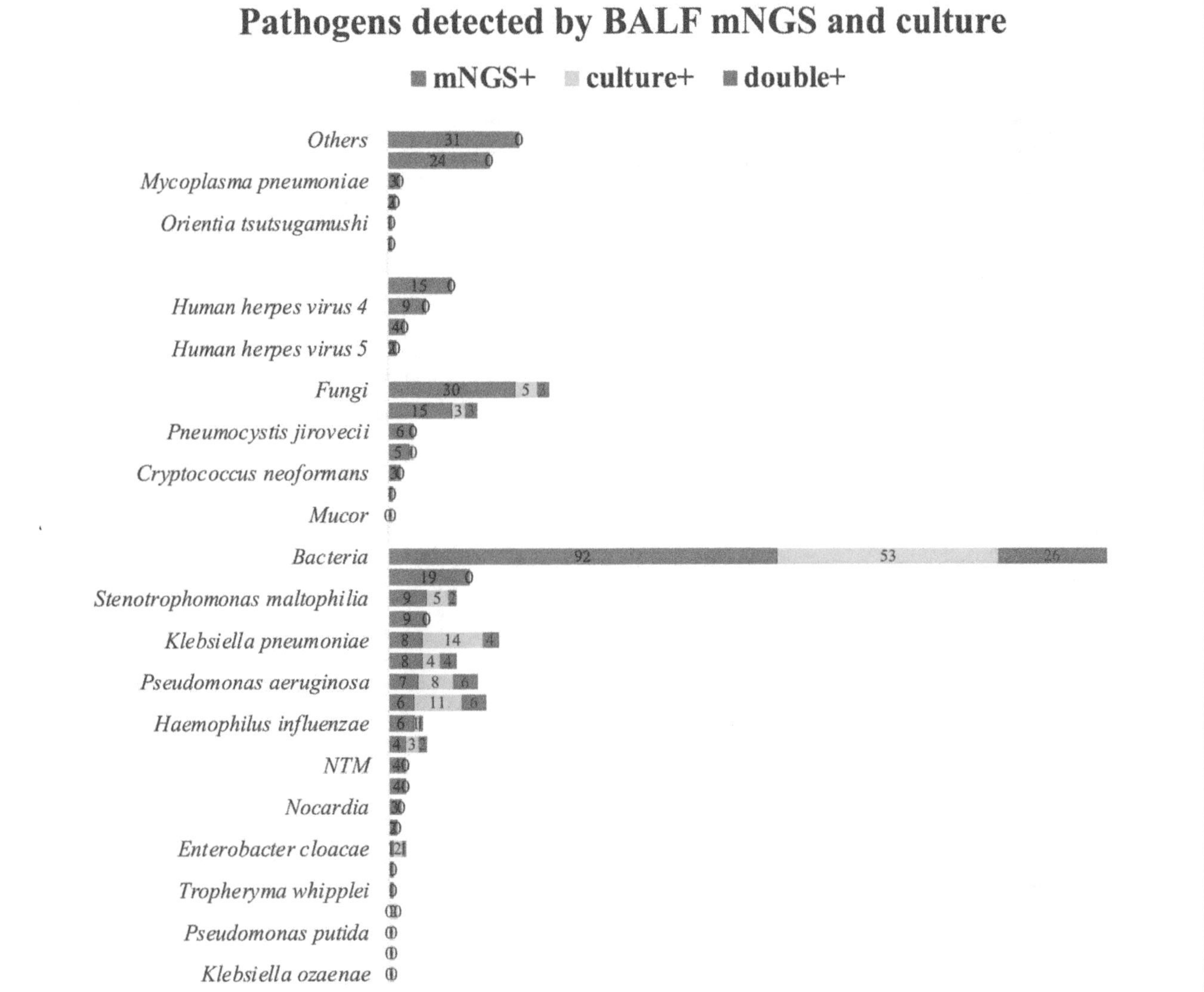

FIGURE 4 | The overlap of positivity between BALF mNGS and BALF culture. Bacteria were the most detected, followed by fungi, special pathogens, and viruses. The positive rate of BALF culture in detecting *Klebsiella pneumoniae* and *Acinetobacter baumannii* was higher than that of mNGS. *Chlamydia psittaci* was the most detected by mNGS, followed by *Haemophilus parainfluenzae* and *Candida albicans*. All viruses, special pathogens, MTB and NTM were only detected by mNGS, and the BALF culture of these pathogens were negative. BALF, bronchoalveolar lavage fluid; mNGS, metagenomic next generation sequencing; MTB, *Mycobacterium tuberculosis*; NTM, *nontuberculous mycobacteria*.

tuberculosis which provides an opportunity for patients to be transferred to specialist hospitals for tuberculosis therapy in time. In the past few decades, the detection of *O. tsutsugamushi* and *L. interrogans* could only rely on microscopic examination, but mNGS can currently detect these special pathogens sensitively, which provides a good guidance for clinicians to adjust treatment protocols. Among the 116 pathogen-positive cases, the positive rate of mNGS for bacteria and fungi were significantly higher than that of BALF culture, additionally mNGS can detect viruses and special pathogens sensitively.

Due to regional differences, the pathogens of our CAP cases were quite different from those in northern China. Chen et al. (22) reported that the bacteria such *as Citrobacter freundii*, *Salmonella enterica*, and *Aeromonas hydrophila* detected by mNGS are common pathogens in CAP. But those bacteria were not detected in any of our cases, which was possibly because the patients in Peking University People's Hospital was more complicated since the difficult and complicated patients around the country would like to go there for further treatment, so the pathogenic pathogens could have a multiple source.

Among the non-pathogenic pathogens detected by mNGS, *Human herpesvirus 4, 1,* and *5* were the most common viruses. These viruses can be latent in the host when the patient is immunocompetent (23). Most studies believed that they had no pathogenic significance when detected in BALF. But when the patient's immune function was low or suppressed, these viruses will be pathogenic (24). *C. albicans* was also detected relatively frequently, but pneumonia with *C. albicans* was relatively

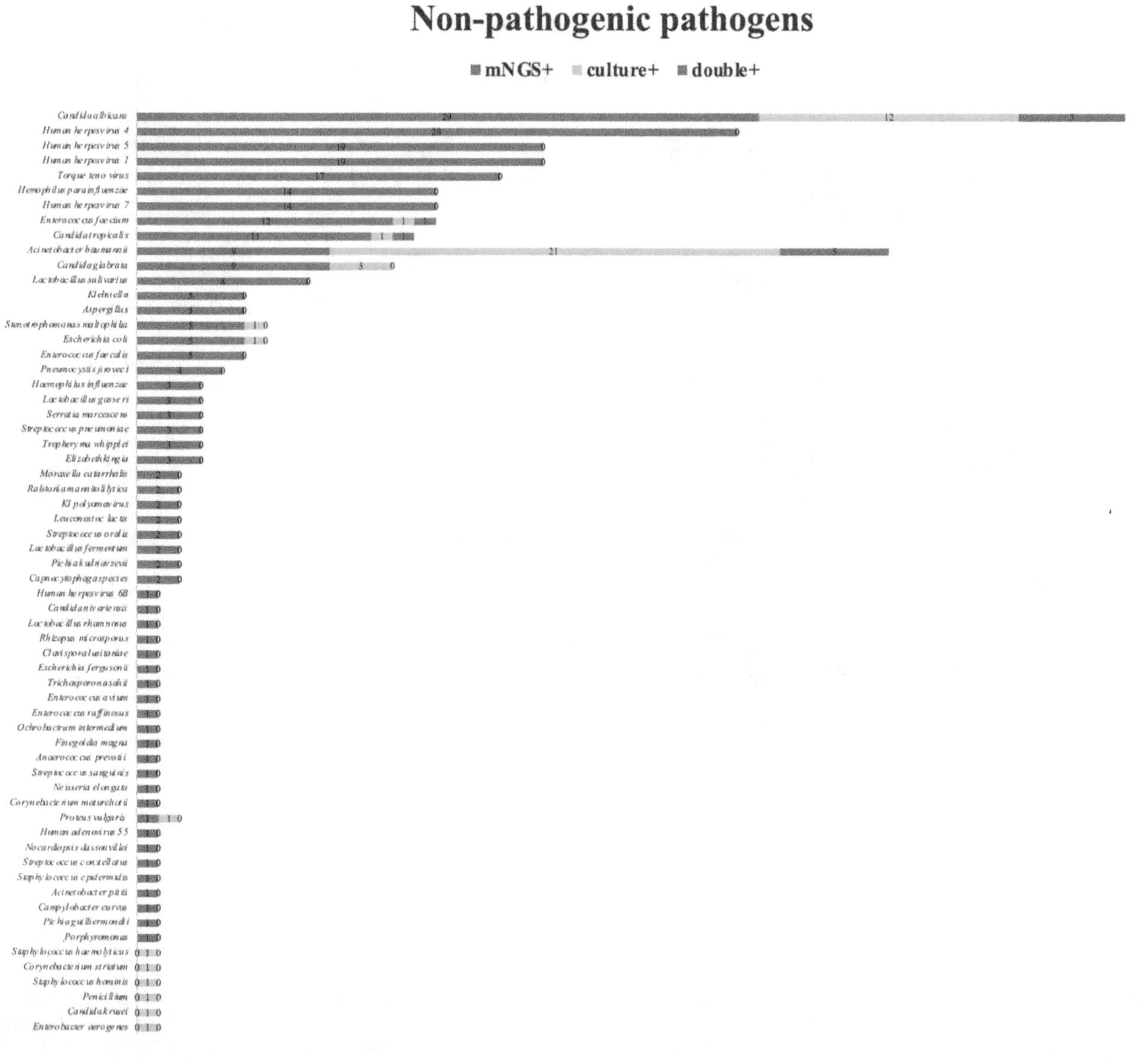

FIGURE 5 | Non-pathogenic pathogens detected by mNGS. A total of 64 different non-pathogenic pathogens were detected in the mNGS group. *Human herpesvirus 5*, *Candida albicans*, *Human herpesvirus 4* are the most common non-pathogenic pathogens detected by mNGS. *Acinetobacter baumannii*, *Candida albicans*, *Candida glabrata* are the most common non-pathogenic pathogens detected by sputum culture. mNGS, metagenomic next-generation sequencing.

rare (25), and most of it were hematogenous dissemination. Additionally, *Enterococcus faecium* and *Enterococcus faecalis* pneumonia were also very rare (26). When interpreting the mNGS reports, some clinicians thought that *C. albicans* was pathogenic. We believed that anti-*C. albicans* treatment must be determined based on the patient's imaging findings and inflammatory indicators. *Torque teno virus* is widely present in the human body, animals, air, and solid surfaces (27), which caused pneumonia only when patients were under immunosuppression condition (28). Therefore, the positive report of *Torque teno virus* may be sample contamination or in immunosuppression condition. When the reads of *H. parainfluenzae* are not high, it is necessary to comprehensively determine whether it is pathogenic based on clinical features, infection sites, inflammation indicators, and lung imaging findings. Some cases of *A. baumannii* and *K. pneumoniae* are in-hospital infection (29, 30). Patients with long-term use of antibiotics and longer hospital stays are prone to in-hospital infection. The impaired intestinal barrier, long-term use of acid inhibitors, long-term bed rest, and nasogastric reflux will cause bacterial translocation (31). The primary lesions of these patients are not in the lungs. Therefore, *A. baumannii* and *K. pneumoniae* detected in the BALF of these patients cannot be regarded as the pathogenic bacteria for pneumonia. The use of mNGS in patients with immunosuppression not only identifies pathogens, but also reflects the patient's immune status and microbiota

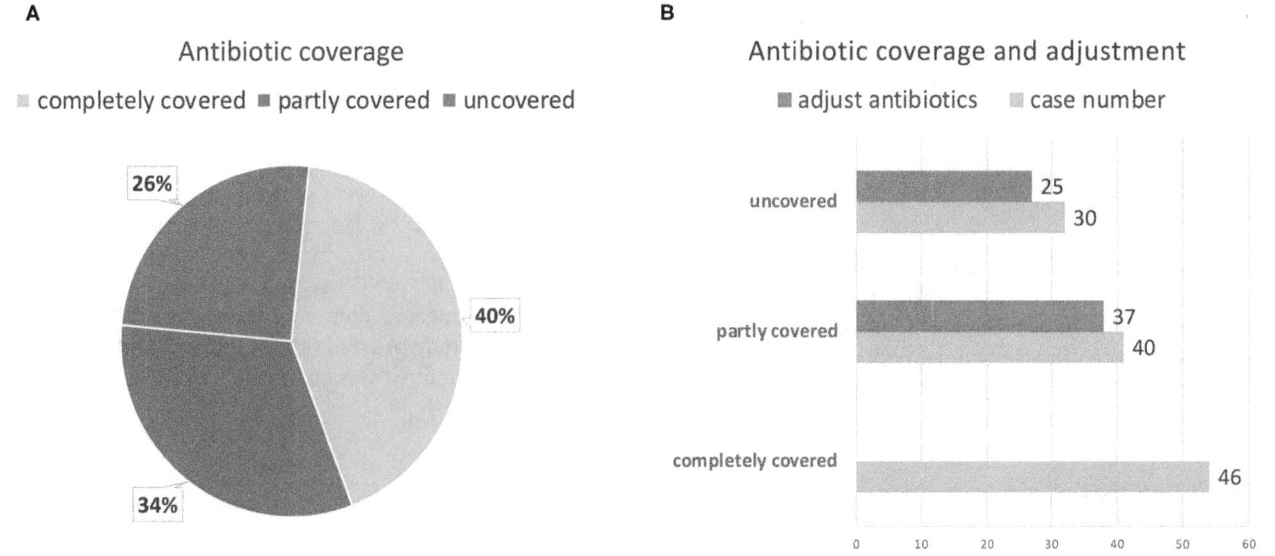

FIGURE 6 | The coverage and adjustment of antibiotics in the mNGS group. **(A)** Among patients in the mNGS group, complete antibiotic coverage was 54 (43%); partial coverage was 41 (32%); and no coverage was 32 (25%). **(B)** Antibiotics were adjusted for 38 partially covered patients, and for 27 uncovered patients. mNGS, metagenomic next-generation sequencing.

distribution. A small number of cases in which the detection was negative with mNGS, but the BALF culture was positive, which was possibly because: (1) the specimen may have been contaminated. For example, the positive *Aspergillus* BALF culture may be caused by contamination. (2) The low pathogens load in the specimen. Under suitable culture conditions, active micro bacteria or fungi could also be cultured, but micro pathogens could not reach the minimum threshold of mNGS detection. (3) Detection of some fungi requires breaking the cell wall to obtain DNA, but conventional sputum culture does not. Therefore, if this process was badly handled, negative results of mNGS may occur. Nevertheless, mNGS showed significant advantages for detecting fastidious bacteria.

Normal sputum culture takes 5–7 days. *M. tuberculosis* culture even takes about 6 weeks. But mNGS can detect pathogens within 48 h and even shorter, which greatly improves the timeliness of treatment. In the use of antibiotics, mNGS can be used to determine whether the current antibiotic therapy covered the pathogens and the reads of pathogens detected by mNGS will guide clinicians to adjust the dosage of antibiotics. Moxifloxacin was the common choice for the severe CAP regularly. However, after the *C. psittaci* was detected by mNGS, we adjusted the moxifloxacin to the doxycycline. Additionally, after the rare pathogens such as *L. interrogans* detected, adjusted to penicillin G was essential for the initial treatment stage. After the fungi detected by mNGS, we should take a comprehensive consideration between the specific reads and abundance of the pathogens to determine whether use the antifungal agents such as fluconazole or voriconazole.

However, there are still some disadvantages of mNGS. Due to the high sensitivity of mNGS, some colonized and contaminated pathogens will also be detected. Because of the differences in the ability of clinicians to interpret the mNGS reports, it may lead to the abuse of antibiotics. The mNGS performed during the early stage of hospitalization could clarify what the main pathogen is. After a period of hospitalization, patients with underlying diseases or immunocompromised patients may have in-hospital infections or colonization of some special bacteria, which will affect the interpretation of mNGS results. Besides, some clinicians are not strict enough on the indications for mNGS, which leads to a waste of medical resources. Otherwise, some laboratories will delete background bacteria, but occasionally the main pathogenic bacteria may be deleted. mNGS has some shortcomings, and it is not a routine pathogen detection method in the guideline. However, due to the large population and a vast extent of land, medical resources are not evenly distributed to a certain extent. The technology of pathogen detection in some remote areas is poor, and even the PCR technology for single pathogens is lacking. Therefore, it is necessary to use mNGS to detect pathogens in an appropriate and timely manner.

Therefore, we suggest that mNGS would be mainly used: (1) the infection is complicated and severe; (2) pathogens which are hard to detected by traditional microorganism test or culture, such as *M. tuberculosis* and *Cryptococcus*. We need to improve clinicians' ability of interpretation of mNGS reports to prevent the abuse of antibiotics caused by mNGS.

The limitation in our study is that this is a single-center retrospective study with a relatively small sample size, thus there was selection bias. Since we tended to compare the positive rate of mNGS and BALF culture, as well as the characteristics of the detected pathogens, the 173 control patients who only underwent BALF or sputum culture were not used for subsequent analysis of pathogen characteristics.

As the antibiotic coverage of pneumonia patients was close to 100%, the positive rate of BALF or sputum culture would be affected by antibiotics, possibly resulting in a relative higher positive rate of mNGS. All mNGS reports were interpreted by a senior clinician, so the consistency was ensured.

CONCLUSION

The positive rate of mNGS for pathogens in patients with CAP was higher than that of traditional BALF culture. mNGS can detect pathogens in a more timely and accurate manner and assist clinicians to adjust antibiotics in time. With available indications, we recommend mNGS for the complementary diagnosis of severe or complicated pneumonia.

from the individual(s) for the publication of any potentially identifiable images or data included in this article.

AUTHOR CONTRIBUTIONS

The study was conceived, designed, and supervised by CL and QZ. Statistical analyses were performed by YZ. Clinical data collection was done by HL. Sample collection was done by SS. Manuscript was written by HL and YZ. Figures and tables were drawn by GC. mNGS testing data was uploaded by FC. Manuscript editing was done by JW, HL, and YZ contributed equally to this study. All authors contributed to the article and approved the submitted version.

REFERENCES

1. Wunderink RG, Waterer G. Advances in the causes and management of community acquired pneumonia in adults. *BMJ.* (2017) 358:j2471. doi: 10.1136/bmj.j2471
2. Glaser CA, Honarmand S, Anderson LJ, Schnurr DP, Forghani B, Cossen CK, et al. Beyond viruses: clinical profiles and etiologies associated with encephalitis. *Clin Infect Dis.* (2006) 43:1565–77. doi: 10.1086/509330
3. Schlaberg R, Chiu CY, Miller S, Procop GW, Weinstock G, Professional Practice C, et al. Validation of metagenomic next-generation sequencing tests for universal pathogen detection. *Arch Pathol Lab Med.* (2017) 141:776–86. doi: 10.5858/arpa.2016-0539-RA
4. Kolditz M, Ewig S. Community-acquired pneumonia in adults. *Dtsch Arztebl Int.* (2017) 114:838–48. doi: 10.3238/arztebl.2017.0838
5. Wu X, Li Y, Zhang M, Li M, Zhang R, Lu X, et al. Etiology of severe community-acquired pneumonia in adults based on metagenomic next-generation sequencing: a prospective multicenter study. *Infect Dis Ther.* (2020) 9:1003–15. doi: 10.1007/s40121-020-00353-y
6. Musher DM, Roig IL, Cazares G, Stager CE, Logan N, Safar H. Can an etiologic agent be identified in adults who are hospitalized for community-acquired pneumonia: results of a one-year study. *J Infect.* (2013) 67:11–8. doi: 10.1016/j.jinf.2013.03.003
7. Jain S, Self WH, Wunderink RG, Fakhran S, Balk R, Bramley AM, et al. Community-Acquired Pneumonia Requiring Hospitalization among U.S. Adults. *N Engl J Med.* (2015) 373:415–27. doi: 10.1056/NEJMoa1500245
8. Simner PJ, Miller S, Carroll KC. Understanding the promises and hurdles of metagenomic next-generation sequencing as a diagnostic tool for infectious diseases. *Clin Infect Dis.* (2018) 66:778–88. doi: 10.1093/cid/cix881
9. Chiu CY, Miller SA. Clinical metagenomics. *Nat Rev Genet.* (2019) 20:341–55. doi: 10.1038/s41576-019-0113-7
10. Wang J, Han Y, Feng J. Metagenomic next-generation sequencing for mixed pulmonary infection diagnosis. *BMC Pulm Med.* (2019) 19:252. doi: 10.1186/s12890-019-1022-4
11. Duan H, Li X, Mei A, Li P, Liu Y, Li X, et al. The diagnostic value of metagenomic next rectanglegeneration sequencing in infectious diseases. *BMC Infect Dis.* (2021) 21:62. doi: 10.1186/s12879-020-05746-5
12. Gu W, Deng X, Lee M, Sucu YD, Arevalo S, Stryke D, et al. Rapid pathogen detection by metagenomic next-generation sequencing of infected body fluids. *Nat Med.* (2021) 27:115–24. doi: 10.1038/s41591-020-1105-z
13. Li H, Gao H, Meng H, Wang Q, Li S, Chen H, et al. Detection of pulmonary infectious pathogens from lung biopsy tissues by metagenomic next-generation sequencing. *Front Cell Infect Microbiol.* (2018) 8:205. doi: 10.3389/fcimb.2018.00205
14. Goldberg B, Sichtig H, Geyer C, Ledeboer N, Weinstock GM. Making the leap from research laboratory to clinic: challenges and opportunities for next-generation sequencing in infectious disease diagnostics. *MBio.* (2015) 6:e01888–e01815. doi: 10.1128/mBio.01888-15
15. Dickson RP, Erb-Downward JR, Martinez FJ, Huffnagle GB. The microbiome and the respiratory tract. *Annu Rev Physiol.* (2016) 78:481–504. doi: 10.1146/annurev-physiol-021115-105238
16. Amar Y, Lagkouvardos I, Silva RL, Ishola OA, Foesel BU, Kublik S, et al. Pre-digest of unprotected DNA by Benzonase improves the representation of living skin bacteria and efficiently depletes host DNA. *Microbiome.* (2021) 9:123. doi: 10.1186/s40168-021-01067-0
17. Miller S, Naccache SN, Samayoa E, Messacar K, Arevalo S, Federman S, et al. Laboratory validation of a clinical metagenomic sequencing assay for pathogen detection in cerebrospinal fluid. *Genome Res.* (2019) 29:831–42. doi: 10.1101/gr.238170.118
18. Bolger AM, Lohse M, Usadel B. Trimmomatic: a flexible trimmer for Illumina sequence data. *Bioinformatics.* (2014) 30:2114–20. doi: 10.1093/bioinformatics/btu170
19. Li H, Durbin R. Fast and accurate short read alignment with Burrows-Wheeler transform. *Bioinformatics.* (2009) 25:1754–60. doi: 10.1093/bioinformatics/btp324
20. Chen L, Liu W, Zhang Q, Xu K, Ye G, Wu W, et al. RNA based mNGS approach identifies a novel human coronavirus from two individual pneumonia cases in 2019 Wuhan outbreak. *Emerg Microbes Infect.* (2020) 9:313–9. doi: 10.1080/22221751.2020.1725399
21. Chen X, Cao K, Wei Y, Qian Y, Liang J, Dong D, et al. Metagenomic next-generation sequencing in the diagnosis of severe pneumonias caused by *Chlamydia psittaci. Infection.* (2020) 48:535–42. doi: 10.1007/s15010-020-01429-0
22. Chen H, Yin Y, Gao H, Guo Y, Dong Z, Wang X, et al. Clinical utility of in-house metagenomic next-generation sequencing for the diagnosis of lower respiratory tract infections and analysis of the host immune response. *Clin Infect Dis.* (2020) 71:S416–26. doi: 10.1093/cid/ciaa1516
23. Ho DY, Enriquez K, Multani A. Herpesvirus infections potentiated by biologics. *Infect Dis Clin North Am.* (2020) 34:311–39. doi: 10.1016/j.idc.2020.02.006
24. Clementi N, Cappelletti F, Criscuolo E, Castelli M, Mancini N, Burioni R, et al. Role and potential therapeutic use of antibodies against herpetic infections. *Clin Microbiol Infect.* (2017) 23:381–6. doi: 10.1016/j.cmi.2016.12.023
25. Ricard JD, Roux D. Candida pneumonia in the ICU: myth or reality? *Intensive Care Med.* (2009) 35:1500–2. doi: 10.1007/s00134-009-1563-8
26. Bonten MJ, Van Tiel FH, Van Der Geest S, Stobberingh EE, Gaillard CA. Enterococcus faecalis pneumonia complicating topical antimicrobial prophylaxis. *N Engl J Med.* (1993) 328:209–10. doi: 10.1056/NEJM199301213280311
27. Hino S, Miyata H. Torque teno virus (TTV): current status. *Rev Med Virol.* (2007) 17:45–57. doi: 10.1002/rmv.524
28. Fernandez-Ruiz M. Torque Teno virus load as a surrogate marker for the net state of immunosuppression: the beneficial side of the virome. *Am J Transplant.* (2020) 20:1963–4. doi: 10.1111/ajt.15872
29. Lee CR, Lee JH, Park M, Park KS, Bae IK, Kim YB, et al. Biology of *Acinetobacter baumannii*: pathogenesis, antibiotic resistance mechanisms,

and prospective treatment options. *Front Cell Infect Microbiol.* (2017) 7:55. doi: 10.3389/fcimb.2017.00055

30. Basso M, Zago D, Pozzetto I, De Canale E, Scaggiante R, Biasolo MA, et al. Intra-hospital acquisition of colonization and infection by *Klebsiella pneumoniae* strains producing carbapenemases and carriage evolution: a longitudinal analysis in an Italian teaching hospital from January 2017 to August 2019. *Int J Infect Dis.* (2020) 92:81–8. doi: 10.1016/j.ijid.2019.12.035
31. Balzan S, De Almeida Quadros C, De Cleva R, Zilberstein B, Cecconello I. Bacterial translocation: overview of mechanisms and clinical impact. *J Gastroenterol Hepatol.* (2007) 22:464–71. doi: 10.1111/j.1440-1746.2007.04933.x

6

Association of COVID-19 Case-Fatality Rate with State Health Disparity in the United States

Yu-Che Lee [1†], *Ko-Yun Chang* [2†] *and Mehdi Mirsaeidi* [3*]

[1] *Department of Medicine, University at Buffalo-Catholic Health System, Buffalo, NY, United States,* [2] *Division of Chest Medicine, Taichung Veterans General Hospital, Taichung, Taiwan,* [3] *Division of Pulmonary and Critical Care and Sleep Medicine, University of Florida College of Medicine, Jacksonville, FL, United States*

Correspondence:
Mehdi Mirsaeidi
m.mirsaeidi@ufl.edu

† These authors have contributed equally to this work and share first authorship

Background: The disproportionate burden of COVID-19 pandemic has become a major concern in the United States (US), but the association between COVID-19 case-fatality rate (CFR) and factors influencing health outcomes at a state level has not been evaluated.

Methods: We calculated COVID-19 CFR for three different waves using COVID Data Tracker from the Centers for Disease Control and Prevention. America's Health Rankings assesses the factors that influence health outcomes to determine state's health rankings. The association between COVID-19 CFR and state health disparities was analyzed by linear regression.

Results: States with better rankings of Physical Environment were associated with lower CFR for the 1st wave ($\beta = 0.06\%$, $R^2 = 0.170$, $P = 0.003$). There was a paradoxical association between the 2nd wave CFR and Clinical Care ($\beta = -0.04\%$, $R^2 = 0.112$, $P = 0.017$) and Overall health rankings ($\beta = -0.03\%$, $R^2 = 0.096$, $P = 0.029$). For the 3rd wave, states with better rankings of Overall health factors ($\beta = 0.01\%$, $R^2 = 0.179$, $P = 0.002$), Social & Economic Factors ($\beta = 0.01\%$, $R^2 = 0.176$, $P = 0.002$), Behaviors ($\beta = 0.01\%$, $R^2 = 0.204$, $P < 0.001$), and Health Outcomes ($\beta = 0.01\%$, $R^2 = 0.163$, $P = 0.004$) were associated with lower CFR. COVID-19 vaccination coverage was also associated with state health rankings (at least one dose: $\beta = -0.13\%$, $R^2 = 0.305$, $P < 0.001$; fully vaccinated: $\beta = -0.06\%$, $R^2 = 0.120$, $P = 0.014$).

Conclusions: These findings suggested targeted public health interventions and mitigation strategies addressing health disparities are essential to improve inequitable outcomes of COVID-19 in the US.

Keywords: COVID-19, case-fatality rate, health disparity, COVID-19 vaccination, USA

INTRODUCTION

The novel Coronavirus Disease 2019 (COVID-19), which is caused by the severe acute respiratory syndrome coronavirus 2 (SARS-CoV-2) and first discovered in Wuhan, China, on December 31, 2019, has continued to spread in the United States (US) and overwhelm healthcare systems all over the world (1–4). As of May 1, 2022, there are more than 510 million confirmed cases and 6 million deaths from COVID-19 worldwide (5). In the US, the impact of racial/ethnic and socioeconomic

TABLE 1 | Summary of COVID-19 case-fatality rate, state health rankings, and COVID vaccination rate of 50 states, as of April 1, 2021.

State	COVID-19 case-fatality rate (%)			2020 America's health rankings (AHR)						COVID-19 vaccination rate (%)	
	1st wave (March 25–June 3, 2020)	2nd wave (Jun 4–September 2, 2020)	3rd wave (September 3, 2020–April 1, 2021)	Overall	Behaviors	Social and economic factors	Physical environment	Clinical care	Health outcomes	At least one dose	Fully vaccinated
Alabama	3.50	1.43	2.19	46	46	43	23	43	48	24.2	13.7
Alaska	1.94	0.60	0.49	29	32	36	40	34	11	34.2	22.6
Arizona	4.64	2.26	1.86	32	24	35	26	39	29	30.1	17.4
Arkansas	1.81	1.29	1.85	48	45	48	11	42	47	26.6	14.3
California	3.75	1.48	1.55	20	14	27	49	23	5	31.3	16.4
Colorado	5.68	1.51	1.03	9	7	13	5	17	9	30.5	17.9
Connecticut	9.36	4.77	1.32	4	3	15	33	5	3	36.0	20.9
Delaware	4.00	2.69	1.23	23	30	16	18	16	35	31.8	16.8
Florida	4.47	1.57	1.57	33	31	29	36	41	27	28.5	16.3
Georgia	4.49	1.55	1.78	38	39	30	10	47	37	24.3	12.5
Hawaii	3.12	0.68	1.96	7	13	11	28	4	1	32.2	19.5
Idaho	2.88	1.04	1.08	22	17	23	30	37	14	26.3	16.8
Illinois	4.71	2.30	1.52	26	23	24	32	24	28	31.8	16.9
Indiana	6.21	1.86	1.39	36	36	32	27	38	36	25.8	17.0
Iowa	2.87	1.20	1.62	11	22	5	15	9	15	31.3	19.7
Kansas	2.19	0.70	1.74	24	26	21	35	28	26	30.5	17.2
Kentucky	4.35	1.30	1.17	44	48	34	19	31	46	31.5	17.9
Louisiana	7.21	1.94	1.75	50	50	50	48	40	50	26.6	16.8
Maine	4.13	1.72	1.32	14	20	12	13	7	23	35.2	20.2
Maryland	4.80	2.05	1.49	10	14	18	8	10	8	31.8	17.8
Massachusetts	7.10	7.43	1.67	2	9	7	29	1	2	34.9	19.5
Michigan	9.86	2.15	1.60	34	35	44	41	15	40	29.2	17.4
Minnesota	4.31	1.54	1.11	5	4	6	4	12	7	31.9	19.3
Mississippi	4.90	2.55	2.04	49	49	47	47	49	49	24.7	15.2
Missouri	5.75	1.03	1.42	39	43	26	25	35	38	25.9	15.6
Montana	3.65	1.28	1.37	28	8	25	22	32	41	31.3	19.7
Nebraska	1.27	1.10	1.07	17	18	17	21	13	20	31.6	19.3
Nevada	6.06	1.68	1.68	37	38	31	14	48	30	28.3	16.3
New Hampshire	5.63	6.64	1.05	1	5	1	24	6	17	36.8	18.2
New Jersey	7.45	7.08	1.21	13	11	3	50	26	4	34.1	19.5
New Mexico	4.66	2.38	1.89	42	34	49	31	29	31	38.7	24.0
New York	7.30	3.88	1.21	21	19	37	34	19	10	31.4	17.3
North Carolina	3.09	1.29	1.25	30	36	22	9	27	31	29.3	16.9

(Continued)

TABLE 1 | Continued

State	COVID-19 case-fatality rate (%)			2020 America's health rankings (AHR)						COVID-19 vaccination rate (%)	
	1st wave (March 25–June 3, 2020)	2nd wave (Jun 4–September 2, 2020)	3rd wave (September 3, 2020–April 1, 2021)	Overall	Behaviors	Social and economic factors	Physical environment	Clinical care	Health outcomes	At least one dose	Fully vaccinated
North Dakota	2.47	1.10	1.45	16	28	10	1	18	16	32.8	20.6
Ohio	6.32	2.11	1.21	41	41	42	39	29	39	29.6	17.2
Oklahoma	5.12	0.88	1.11	47	46	45	45	46	43	31.4	18.5
Oregon	3.60	1.35	1.38	19	12	20	42	22	19	28.7	17.1
Pennsylvania	8.70	3.08	1.95	27	33	27	46	8	34	32.4	17.2
Rhode Island	4.92	4.49	1.36	12	16	18	38	2	18	33.2	21.5
South Carolina	4.14	2.15	1.46	40	40	41	7	36	42	27.7	15.4
South Dakota	1.19	1.21	1.70	25	27	39	6	21	24	35.4	22.9
Tennessee	1.67	1.05	1.54	43	42	40	17	44	44	25.6	14.2
Texas	2.55	2.01	1.60	35	29	33	43	50	22	26.4	14.3
Utah	1.12	0.71	0.52	6	2	2	12	25	6	26.5	11.9
Vermont	5.35	0.47	0.94	3	1	9	20	3	12	34.0	19.2
Virginia	3.03	1.59	1.55	15	21	8	2	20	21	31.9	17.5
Washington	4.90	1.60	1.21	8	6	4	16	14	13	30.3	18.4
West Virginia	3.83	1.77	1.74	45	44	46	44	33	45	30.6	19.4
Wisconsin	3.23	0.86	1.11	18	10	14	37	11	33	32.5	19.0
Wyoming	1.72	0.80	1.26	31	25	38	3	45	25	27.8	18.8

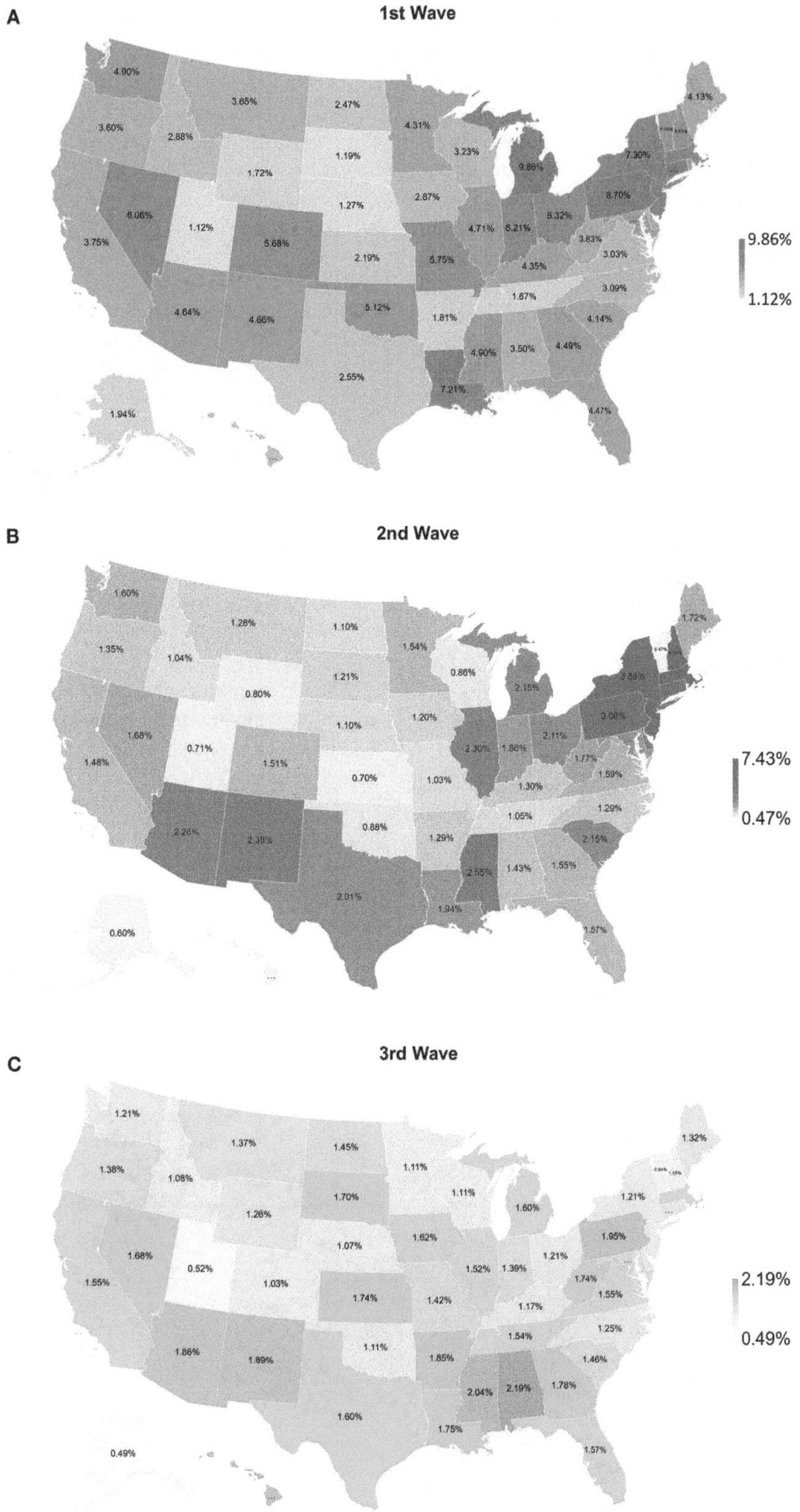

FIGURE 1 | Map of COVID-19 case-fatality rate for **(A)** 1st wave (March 25–June 3, 2020), **(B)** 2nd wave (June 4–September 2, 2020), and **(C)** 3rd wave (September 3, 2020–April 1, 2021) for 50 states of the US.

disparities on COVID-19 incidence, mortality and outcomes has been well established, with racial/ethnic minority groups consistently having higher incidence, mortality rates and adverse outcomes driven by sociodemographic disadvantage (6–10). The disproportionate and inequitable burden of the COVID-19 pandemic has become a major concern and emerging evidence on COVID-19 disparities is vitally important for guiding public health policy and healthcare resource allocation in the US (11).

Case-fatality rate (CFR), defined as the proportion of deaths among incident cases of a disease, has been used to investigate and compare the severity and outcomes of COVID-19, as well as the efficacy of treatment and healthcare capacity in response to the pandemic between countries (12–15). Prior literature also indicated that COVID-19 CFR was significantly higher in minority groups and rural counties and associated with socioeconomic status in the US (16, 17).

America's Health Rankings (AHR), a partnership of the United Health Foundation and the American Public Health Association, is an annual comprehensive assessment of the nation's health on a state-by-state basis since 1990. AHR assesses the factors that influence health outcomes and uses different measures to determine the state's health rankings, with "1" being the healthiest state and "50" the most unhealthy state.

Despite several studies focusing on the variation of impact on COVID-19 pandemic across the US, little is known about the role of the state-level health disparity in COVID-19 outcomes. In this study, we hypothesized that COVID-19 CFR correlated with state health rankings and COVID-19 vaccination coverage, which reflect the healthcare and socioeconomic disparities between states. We aimed to examine the association of COVID-19 CFR, state health rankings, and COVID-19 vaccination rates to provide another perspective of the impact between COVID-19 and health disparities in the US.

Abbreviations: AHR, America's Health Rankings; CDC, Centers for Disease Control and Prevention; CFR, Case-Fatality Rate; COVID-19, Coronavirus Disease 2019.

MATERIALS AND METHODS

Data Resources

COVID-19 confirmed cases and deaths from March 25, 2020 to April 1, 2021 were obtained from the COVID Data Tracker provided by the Centers for Disease Control and Prevention (CDC). CFR calculations were performed by dividing the number of confirmed deaths by the confirmed cases at the same time-period expressed as a percentage, where values approaching 0% represent an excellent disease outcome (lower severity) and those approaching 100% represent a poor outcome (higher severity). With these data, we calculated three specific CFR in different time-period for all 50 states: March 25 to June 3, 2020 as the "1st wave", June 4 to September 2, 2020 as the "2nd wave", and September 3, 2020 to April 1, 2021 as the "3rd wave" of COVID-19.

The state health rankings were calculated by a formula using different weighted measures in five main categories: 20% for Behaviors (Insufficient Sleep, Nutrition and Physical Activity, Sexual Health, Tobacco Use), 30% for Social and Economic Factors (Community and Family Safety, Economic Resources, Education, Social Support and Engagement), 10% for Physical

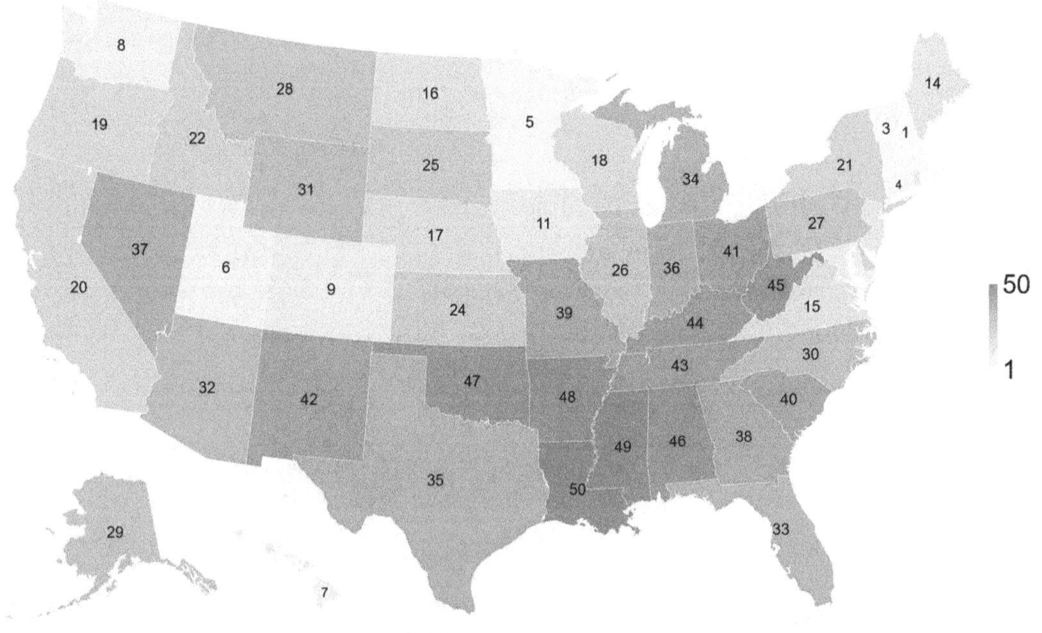

FIGURE 2 | Map of state overall health rankings for 50 states of the US, 2020.

Environment (Air and Water Quality, Housing and Transit), 15% for Clinical Care (Assess to Care, Preventive Clinical Services, Quality of Care), and 25% for Health Outcomes (Behavioral Health, Mortality, Physical Health). The Overall health rankings in 2020 and each category of rankings for Behaviors, Social and Economic Factors, Physical Environment, Clinical Care, and Health Outcomes were examined in the current study as we previously described (18, 19).

In addition, the percentages of people who received at least one dose of COVID-19 vaccine and fully vaccinated by state until April 1, 2021 were obtained from the CDC.

Statistical Analyses

Scatterplots of Overall health rankings, five core measures of health factor rankings by state, and the percentages of COVID-19 vaccinations vs. CFR were generated, respectively. Linear regression analyses were performed with the following formulas to calculate the association between state health rankings, COVID-19 vaccinations, and CFR: CFR = Overall Health Rankings * $\beta + \alpha$; CFR = Behaviors rankings * $\beta + \alpha$; CFR = Social & Economic Factors rankings * $\beta + \alpha$; CFR = Physical Environment rankings * $\beta + \alpha$; CFR = Clinical Care rankings * $\beta + \alpha$; CFR = Health Outcomes rankings * $\beta + \alpha$; CFR = COVID-19 vaccinations * $\beta + \alpha$. Separate regression models were used to avoid potential collinearity issues. Data management and statistical analyses were performed using Microsoft Excel and Statistics Software SAS. ® *P*-values < 0.05 using two-sided *T*-tests indicated statistical significance.

RESULTS

COVID-19 Case Fatality Rate by State

From the beginning of COVID-19 pandemic to April 1, 2021, a total of 30,481,267 people were diagnosed with COVID-19 and

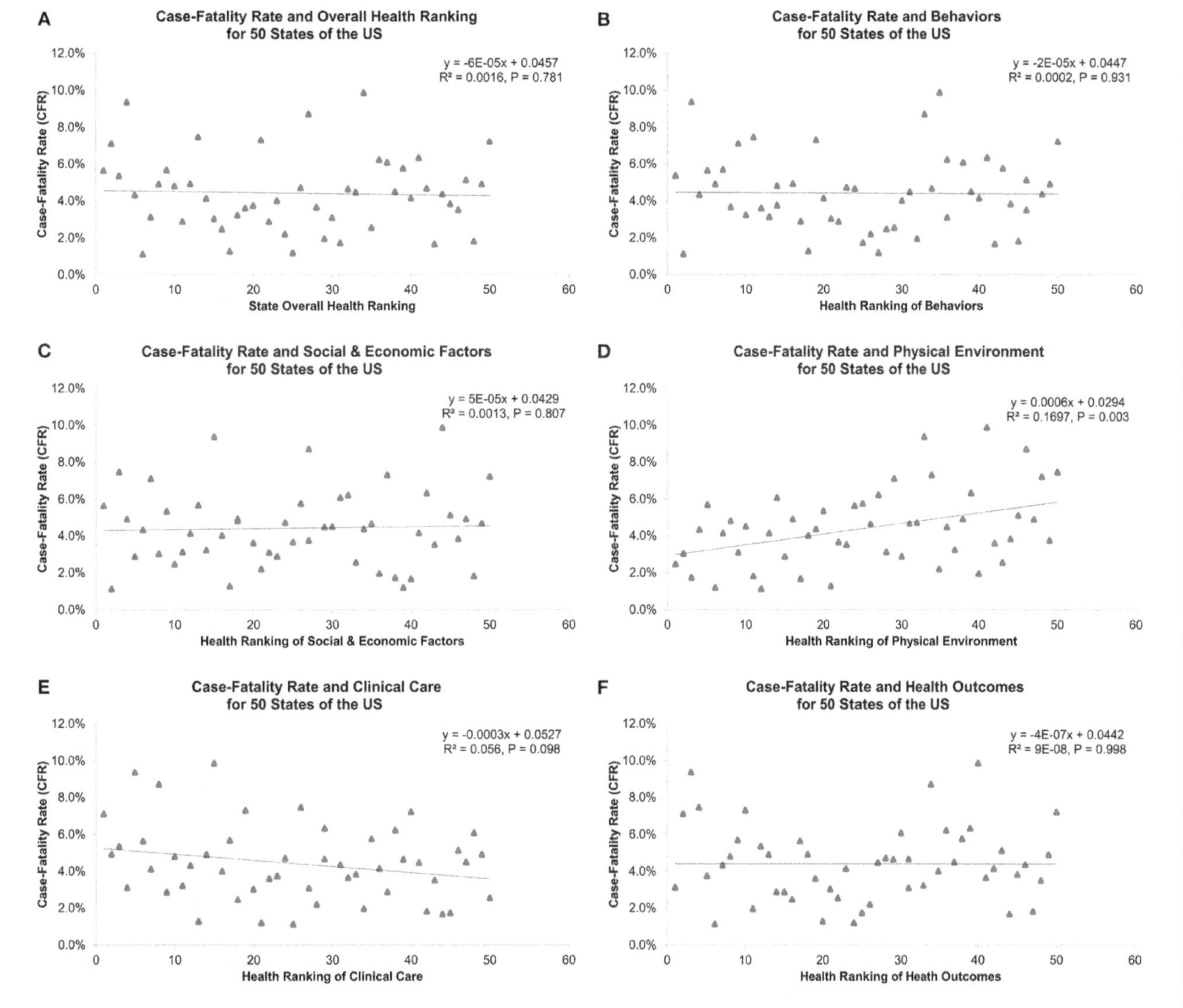

FIGURE 3 | Association of 1st wave COVID-19 case-fatality rate with **(A)** overall health ranking, **(B)** behaviors, **(C)** social and economic factors, **(D)** physical environment, **(E)** clinical care, and **(F)** health outcomes for 50 states of the US.

558,761 people died from COVID-19 in the US. The incidence, mortality, and CFR were 9,172 per 100,000 population, 168 per 100,000, and 1.8%, respectively. The confirmed cases, deaths, and CFRs in three different time-period were 1,923,996, 110,479, and 5.7% (1st wave), 4,335,732, 81,265, and 1.9% (2nd wave), and 24,221,539, 367,017, and 1.5% (3rd wave). There was a remarkable geographic difference in CFRs by state. During the 1st wave, Michigan had the highest CFR (9.9%) whereas Utah had the lowest CFR (1.1%). The highest CFR for the 2nd wave was recorded in Massachusetts (7.4%) and the lowest in Vermont (0.5%). Regarding the 3rd wave, the lowest CFR was reported in Alaska (0.5%) and the highest in Alabama (2.2%). The results are summarized in **Table 1** and shown in **Figure 1**.

Association Between State Health Rankings and COVID-19 CFR

Table 1 and **Figure 2** show overall health rankings and five main health factors rankings in 2020 for 50 states. Among 50 states, New Hampshire had the highest ranking for Overall health factors and Social and Economic Factors, whereas Louisiana had the lowest ranking for Overall health factors, Social and Economic Factors, Behaviors, and Health Outcomes. During the 1st wave, states with better health rankings of Physical Environment were associated with lower CFR ($\beta = 0.06\%$, $R^2 = 0.170$, $P = 0.003$, **Figure 3**). For the 2nd wave, states with better health rankings of Physical Environment were also associated with lower CFR ($\beta = 0.03\%$, $R^2 = 0.081$, $P = 0.045$), whereas an opposite association was found in Clinical Care ($\beta = -0.04\%$,

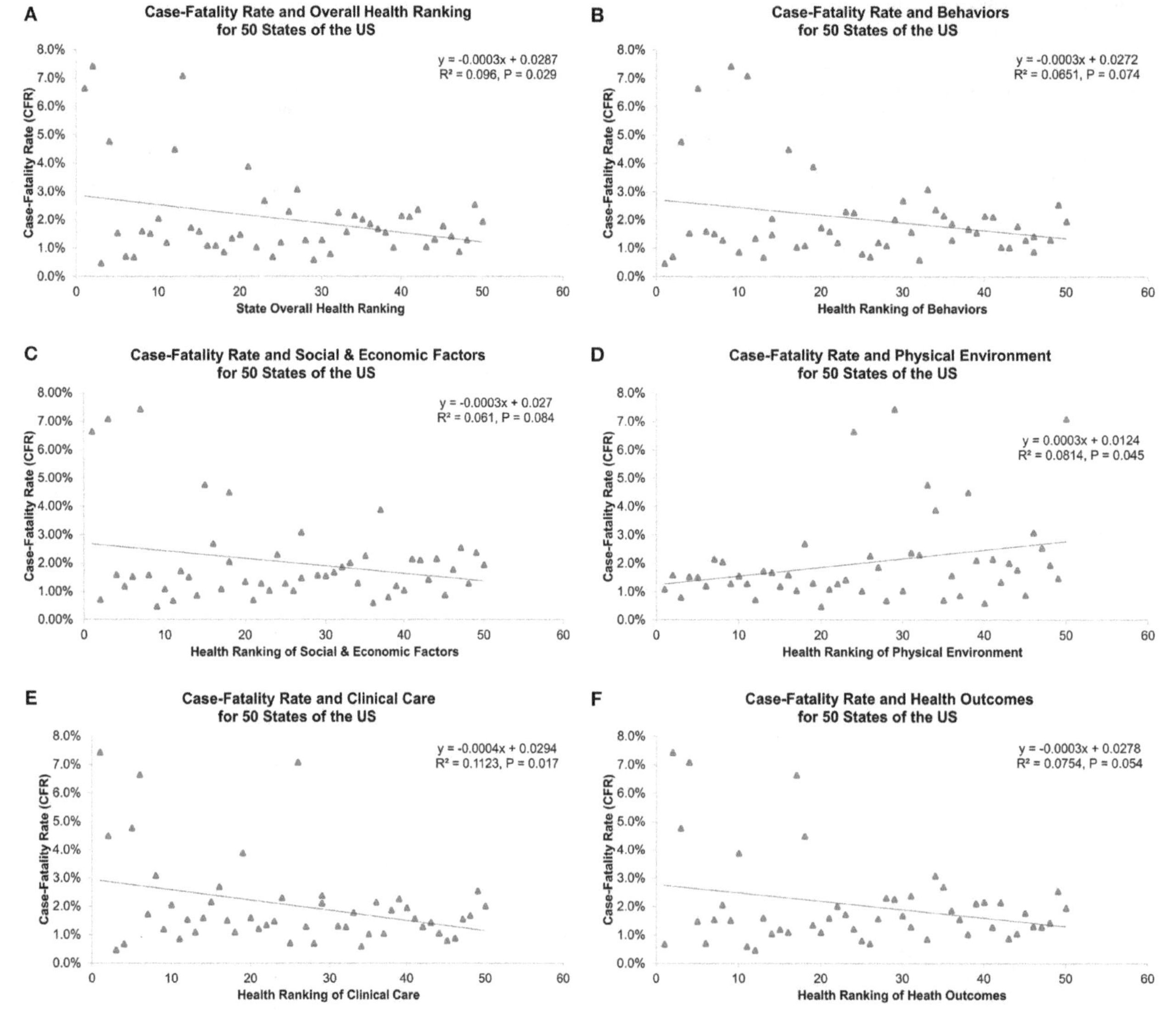

FIGURE 4 | Association of 2nd wave COVID-19 case-fatality rate with **(A)** overall health ranking, **(B)** behaviors, **(C)** social and economic factors, **(D)** physical environment, **(E)** clinical care, and **(F)** health outcomes for 50 states of the US.

$R^2 = 0.112$, $P = 0.017$) and Overall health rankings ($\beta = -0.03\%$, $R^2 = 0.096$, $P = 0.029$, **Figure 4**). Regarding the 3rd wave, states with better health rankings of Overall health factors ($\beta = 0.01\%$, $R^2 = 0.179$, $P = 0.002$, **Figure 5**), Social and Economic Factors ($\beta = 0.01\%$, $R^2 = 0.176$, $P = 0.002$), Behaviors ($\beta = 0.01\%$, $R^2 = 0.204$, $P < 0.001$), and Health Outcomes ($\beta = 0.01\%$, $R^2 = 0.163$, $P = 0.004$) were all associated with lower CFR. This is the most important finding of our study result which showed state health rankings of different health indicators were significantly associated with COVID-19 CFR during these three different waves of pandemic.

Association Between COVID-19 Vaccinations and COVID-19 CFR

Table 1 and **Figure 6** show COVID-19 vaccination rates for 50 states. The highest rates for at least one dose of vaccination and fully vaccinated were both in New Mexico (38.7 and 24.0%), but the lowest rates for at least one vaccination and fully vaccinated were in Alabama (24.2%) and Utah (11.9%), respectively. There was no association between COVID-19 vaccinations and the 3rd wave CFR (at least one dose: $R^2 = 0.049$, $P = 0.122$; fully vaccinated: $R^2 = 0.025$, $P = 0.274$, **Figure 7**).

DISCUSSION

To our knowledge, this is the first study to investigate the association between COVID-19 CFR and state health factors in the US. This study clearly shows geographic differences in COVID-19 outcomes between states and its significant association with state-level health disparities. During different pandemic waves, state-level COVID-19 CFRs were significantly associated with different health indicators, including

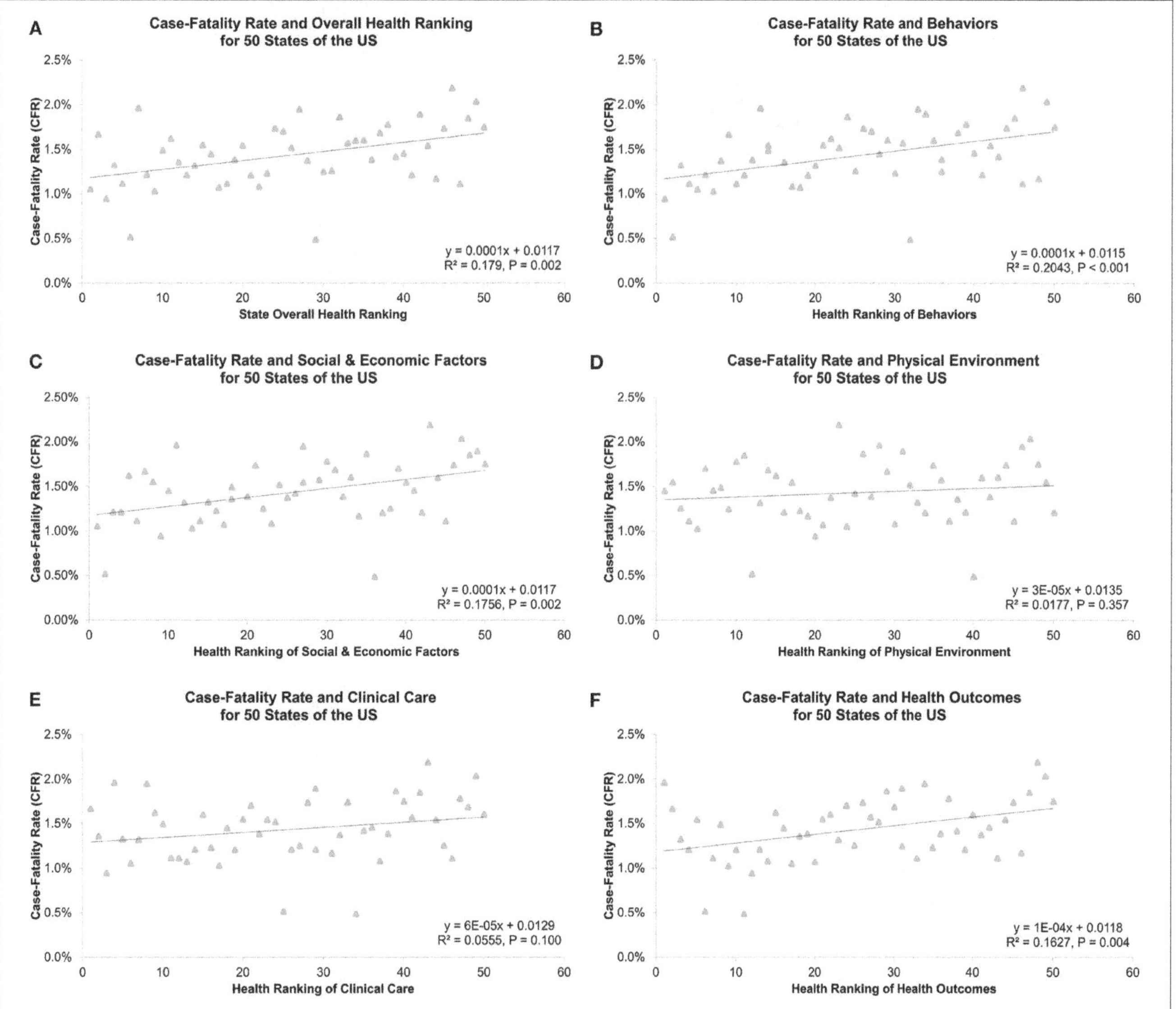

FIGURE 5 | Association of 3rd wave COVID-19 case-fatality rate with **(A)** overall health ranking, **(B)** behaviors, **(C)** social and economic factors, **(D)** physical environment, **(E)** clinical care, and **(F)** health outcomes for 50 states of the US.

Overall health factors, Social and Economic Factors, Behaviors, and Health Outcomes. The mapping of COVID-19 CFR demonstrates distinct distributions for the three waves. The highest CFRs for the 1st and 2nd waves were found in some Northeastern states (New York, New Jersey, Massachusetts, Connecticut, and Pennsylvania), Michigan and Louisiana, whereas the lowest in Utah, South Dakota and Nebraska. For the 3rd wave, the highest CFRs were seen in some Southern states (Alabama, Mississippi, Arkansas, Georgia, and Louisiana), Hawaii and Pennsylvania, but the lowest in Alaska, Utah and Vermont. These geographic findings align with the official COVID-19 reports from CDC and Johns Hopkins University Center for Systems Science and Engineering (20), indicating COVID-19 confirmed cases and deaths in the early

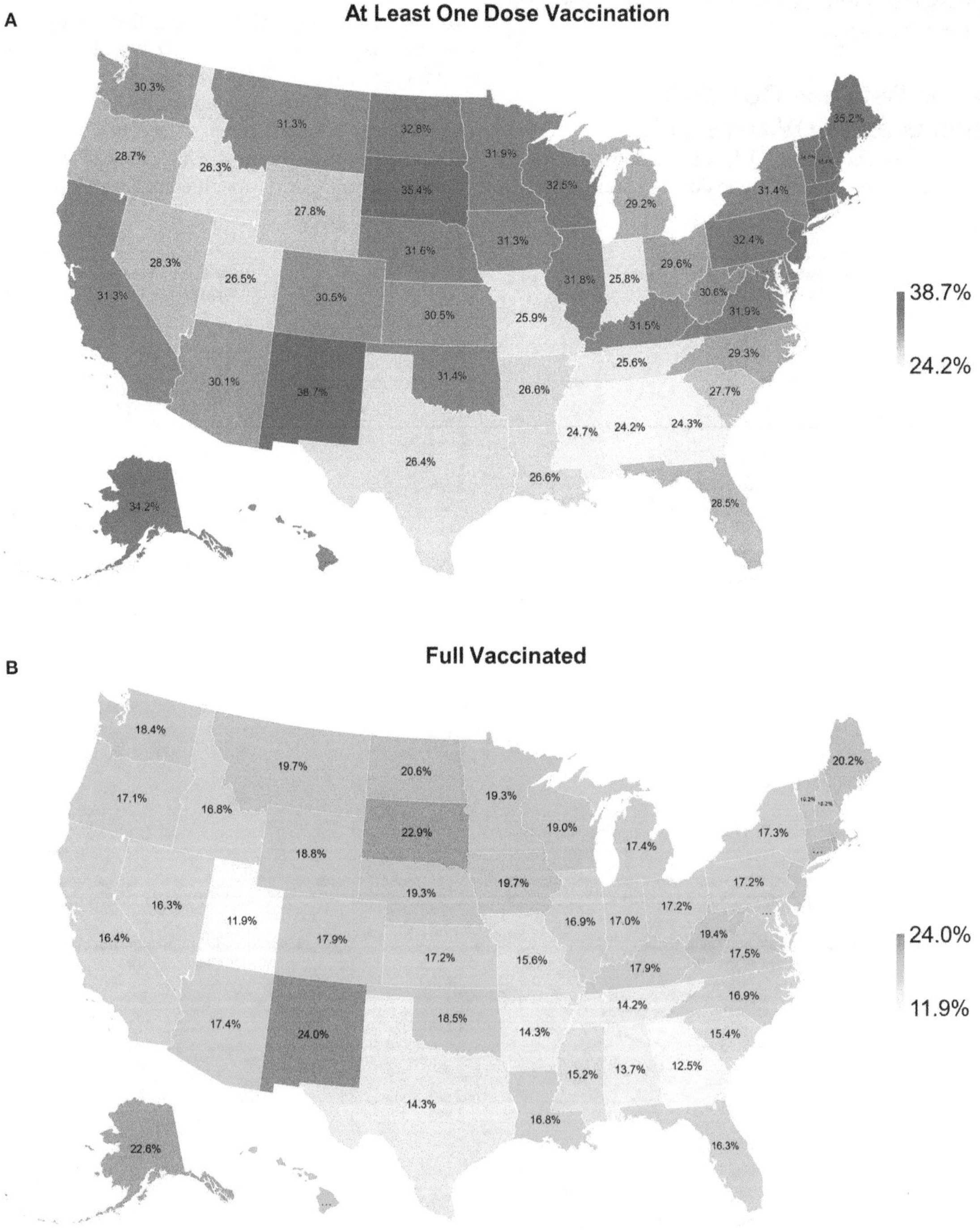

FIGURE 6 | Map of COVID-19 vaccination rate for **(A)** as least one dose vaccination and **(B)** fully vaccinated for 50 states of the US, as of April 1, 2021.

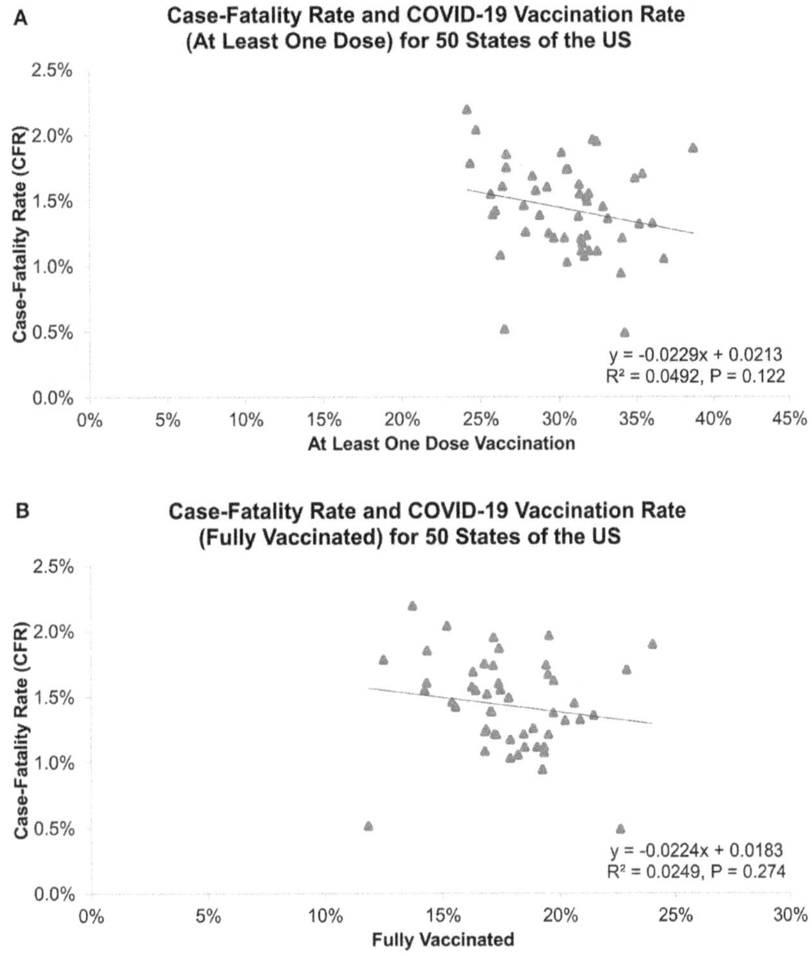

FIGURE 7 | Association of 3rd wave COVID-19 case-fatality rate with vaccination rate for **(A)** as least one dose vaccination and **(B)** fully vaccinated, as of April 1, 2021.

months of the pandemic were mostly concentrated in the metropolitan areas of New York (New York City), Louisiana (New Orleans), Massachusetts (Boston) and Michigan (Detroit), and the geography has shifted as COVID-19 spread across the US over time (21).

Geographic difference in COVID-19 cases, deaths and CFRs likely reflects variations in epidemiologic factors, clinical practices, and public health interventions. During the 1st and 2nd wave, we found a positive association between health rankings of Physical Environment and COVID-19 CFRs, suggesting unfavorable COVID-19 outcomes in states with worse physical environments. Since COVID-19 is primarily transmitted by exposure to infectious respiratory droplets and there were no effective treatments identified during these two waves, population density and mitigation strategies to reduce transmission might contribute to observed variation in COVID-19 infection rates and disease outcomes (21, 22). In our study, air quality and severe housing problems with overcrowding occupants and inadequate ventilation are the main measures of Physical Environment indicator. These factors can be the possible explanation for our study result as greater household crowding and poor indoor ventilation with outside air have shown to increase indoor airborne contaminants, the risk of COVID-19 infection and associated outcomes (16, 23, 24). In contrast, a surprising and interesting finding was the paradoxical relationship between COVID-19 CFRs and Clinical Care indicator and Overall health rankings during the 2nd wave. The negative association in this wave could be attributed to differences in COVID-19 testing availabilities and capacities across the US (25). This suggested that states with better Clinical Care and Overall health rankings may have greater access and abilities to test and identify cases, leading to higher testing volume, more precise calculation for incidence and mortality, and different outcomes of COVID-19.

During the 3rd wave, better understanding of the disease, more clear treatment guidelines, expanded medical resources and workforce, higher implementation of mitigation strategies, and vaccine development and administration have resulted in reduced disease severity and improved outcomes of COVID-19 (26). In this wave, our study demonstrated a positive association between state health rankings of Overall health factors, Social

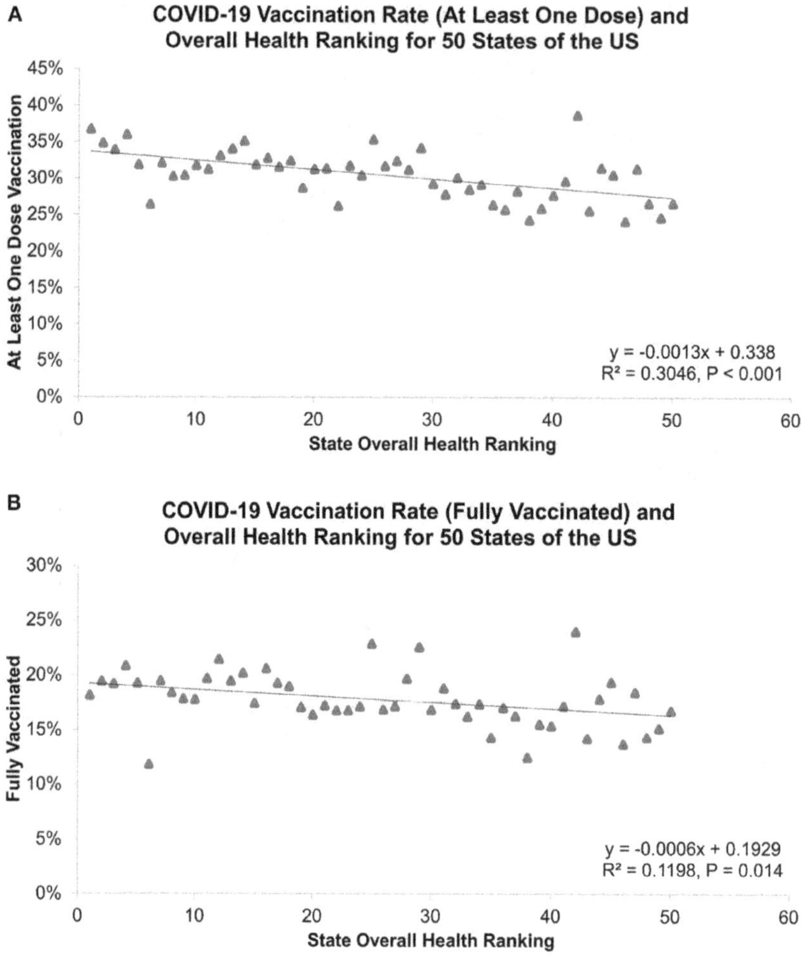

FIGURE 8 | Association of state overall health ranking with COVID-19 vaccination rate for **(A)** as least one dose vaccination and **(B)** fully vaccinated, as of April 1, 2021.

& Economic Factors, Behaviors, Health Outcomes and COVID-19 CFRs. Previous studies have identified that racial/ethnic health disparities and socioeconomic status, including poverty, unemployment, income inequality, education, occupation and uninsured rate have significant impacts on incidence, mortality and clinical outcomes of COVID-19 (27–34). Specifically, Dasgupta et al., Nayak et al., Karaye et al., Khazanchi et al., and Karmakar et al. all found that higher Social Vulnerability Index (SVI, a validated measure using four domains: Socioeconomic Status, Household Composition and Disability, Racial/Ethnic Minority and Language, and Housing and Transportation) was associated with greater COVID-19 incidence, mortality and adverse outcomes (16, 24, 35–37). Interestingly, some studies also indicated that limited English proficiency and socioeconomic disadvantage in social distancing are the important factors resulting in wide-ranging differences in the impact of COVID-19 pandemic across the US (24, 38). Taken together, all these findings are generally consistent with our study result as states with better overall health and socioeconomic status may have superior health care system, public health infrastructures and policies, contributing to favorable COVID-19 outcomes in the US.

COVID-19 vaccines, with the declaration of Emergency Use Authorization (EUA) by the US Food and Drug Administration (FDA) in December of 2020, have proven to reduce the risk of COVID-19 infection and its potentially severe complications and deaths (39–43). In contrast to the currently available evidence, our study showed no association between COVID-19 vaccination coverage and disease outcomes (the 3rd wave CFR). This result could be explained by the different distribution of time lag between reporting of infections and deaths among states, which affects the estimation of COVID-19 CFRs in the US. According to the CDC, ensuring equitable COVID-19 vaccine access is a priority for the US COVID-19 vaccination program. A recent study by Hughes et al. from CDC COVID-19 Response Team indicated that COVID-19 vaccination coverage was lower in high vulnerability counties than in low vulnerability counties (44). We thus performed a linear regression analysis to examine the relationship between COVID-19 vaccination rates and state health rankings, which showed states with better Overall health rankings were significant associated with higher COVID-19 vaccination coverage (at least one dose: $\beta = -0.13\%$, $R^2 = 0.305$, $P < 0.001$; fully vaccinated: $\beta = -0.06\%$, $R^2 = 0.120$, $P = 0.014$; **Figure 8**). This finding suggested that COVID-19 vaccination coverage was largely driven by socioeconomic and health disparities and tailored vaccine administration and outreach efforts should be developed to reduce COVID-19 vaccination inequities among states.

The current study is subject to some limitations. First, the CFR analyzed here was based on the reported COVID-19 cases and deaths by states, which is likely to be influenced by the time lags in report dates resulting in a challenge with accurate calculation of the CFR. Second, this cross-sectional, state-level study evaluates population-level risk, but no causal, individual-level inferences can be made, including age, comorbidities, socioeconomic and medical risks. Third, using health factor rankings from AHR to represent the health disparities among states may not be specific. We focused our analysis at the state-level using health indicators of Behaviors, Social and Economic Factors, Physical Environment, Clinical Care, and Health Outcomes, but important variation in socioeconomic and health disparities exists within states and some crucial parameters may not be included. Therefore, the results of this study should be interpreted cautiously, and future research is suggested to strengthen our findings.

In conclusion, this study provided the first state-level assessment and demonstrated substantial geographic differences in COVID-19 CFR in the US. State health rankings, including a wide range of health indicators, were significantly associated with COVID-19 outcomes and vaccination coverage among states. These findings suggested that targeted public health interventions (e.g., bans on public gatherings, stay-at-home policies, and telemedicine), mitigation strategies (e.g., mask use and social distancing) and policies (e.g., COVID-19 vaccination program) addressing health disparities are essential to improve inequitable outcomes of COVID-19 in the US.

AUTHOR CONTRIBUTIONS

Y-CL had full access to all the data in the study and takes responsibility for the integrity of the data and the accuracy of the data analysis. Y-CL, K-YC, and MM contributed to the literature review, study concept and design, data analysis and interpretation, and writing and revision of the manuscript. All authors contributed to the article and approved the submitted version.

ACKNOWLEDGMENTS

The authors would like to thank the Centers for Disease Control and Prevention, World Health Organization, and America's Health Rankings for providing the dataset.

REFERENCES

1. Zhu N, Zhang D, Wang W, Li X, Yang B, Song J, et al. A novel coronavirus from patients with pneumonia in China, 2019. *New Engl J Med.* (2020) 382:727–33. doi: 10.1056/NEJMoa2001017
2. Zhou P, Yang XL, Wang XG, Hu B, Zhang L, Zhang W, et al. A pneumonia outbreak associated with a new coronavirus of probable bat origin. *Nature.* (2020) 579:270–3. doi: 10.1038/s41586-020-2951-z
3. Cocconcelli E, Bernardinello N, Giraudo C, Castelli G, Giorgino A, Leoni D, et al. Characteristics and prognostic factors of pulmonary fibrosis after COVID-19 pneumonia. *Front Med.* (2021) 8:823600. doi: 10.3389/fmed.2021.823600
4. Pelosi P, Tonelli R, Torregiani C, Baratella E, Confalonieri M, Battaglini D, et al. Different methods to improve the monitoring of noninvasive respiratory support of patients with severe pneumonia/ARDS due to COVID-19: an update. *J Clin Med.* (2022) 11:1704. doi: 10.3390/jcm11061704
5. *WHO COVID-19 Dashboard.* Geneva: World Health Organization (2020). Available online at: https://covid19.who.int (accessed May 01, 2022).
6. Dyer O. Covid-19: black people and other minorities are hardest hit in US. *BMJ.* (2020) 369:m1483. doi: 10.1136/bmj.m1483
7. Gross CP, Essien UR, Pasha S, Gross JR, Wang S-y, Nunez-Smith M. Racial and ethnic disparities in population-level Covid-19 mortality. *J Gen Intern Med.* (2020) 35:3097–9. doi: 10.1007/s11606-020-06081-w
8. Hooper MW, Nápoles AM, Pérez-Stable EJ. COVID-19 and racial/ethnic disparities. *JAMA.* (2020) 323:2466–7. doi: 10.1001/jama.2020.8598
9. Price-Haywood EG, Burton J, Fort D, Seoane L. Hospitalization and mortality among black patients and white patients with Covid-19. *New Engl J Med.* (2020) 382:2534–43. doi: 10.1056/NEJMsa2011686
10. Yancy CW. COVID-19 and African Americans. *JAMA.* (2020) 323:1891–2. doi: 10.1001/jama.2020.6548
11. Alberti PM, Lantz PM, Wilkins CH. Equitable pandemic preparedness and rapid response: lessons from COVID-19 for pandemic health equity. *J Health Polit Policy Law.* (2020) 45:921–35. doi: 10.1215/03616878-8641469
12. Cao Y, Hiyoshi A, Montgomery S. COVID-19 case-fatality rate and demographic and socioeconomic influencers: worldwide spatial regression analysis based on country-level data. *BMJ Open.* (2020) 10:e043560. doi: 10.1136/bmjopen-2020-043560
13. Khafaie MA, Rahim F. Cross-country comparison of case fatality rates of COVID-19/SARS-CoV-2. *Osong Public Health Res Perspect.* (2020) 11:74–80. doi: 10.24171/j.phrp.2020.11.2.03
14. Kim D-H, Choe YJ, Jeong J-Y. Understanding and interpretation of case fatality rate of coronavirus disease 2019. *J Korean Med Sci.* (2020) 35:e137. doi: 10.3346/jkms.2020.35.e137
15. Sorci G, Faivre B, Morand S. Explaining among-country variation in COVID-19 case fatality rate. *Sci Rep.* (2020) 10:18909. doi: 10.1038/s41598-020-75848-2
16. Nayak A, Islam SJ, Mehta A, Ko YA, Patel SA, Goyal A, et al. Impact of social vulnerability on COVID-19 incidence and outcomes in the United States. *medRxiv.* (2020). doi: 10.1101/2020.04.10.20060962
17. Iyanda AE, Boakye KA, Lu Y, Oppong JR. Racial/ethnic heterogeneity and rural-urban disparity of COVID-19 case fatality ratio in the USA: a negative binomial and GIS-based analysis. *J Racial Ethn Health Disparities.* (2021) 9:708–21. doi: 10.1007/s40615-021-01006-7
18. Lee YC, Chang KY, Mirsaeidi M. State-level health disparity is associated with sarcoidosis mortality. *J Clin Med.* (2021) 10:2366. doi: 10.3390/jcm10112366
19. Lee YC, Calderon-Candelario RA, Holt GE, Campos MA, Mirsaeidi M. State-level disparity in lung cancer survival in the United States. *Front Oncol.* (2020) 10:1449. doi: 10.3389/fonc.2020.01449
20. Dong E, Du H, Gardner L. An interactive web-based dashboard to track COVID-19 in real time. *Lancet Infect Dis.* (2020) 20:533–4. doi: 10.1016/S1473-3099(20)30120-1
21. Bialek S, Bowen V, Chow N, Curns A, Gierke R, Hall AJ, et al. Geographic differences in COVID-19 cases, deaths, and incidence—United States, February 12–April 7, 2020. *Morb Mort Wkly Rep.* (2020) 69:465. doi: 10.15585/mmwr.mm6915e4

22. Stadnytskyi V, Bax CE, Bax A, Anfinrud P. The airborne lifetime of small speech droplets and their potential importance in SARS-CoV-2 transmission. *Proc Natl Acad Sci.* (2020) 117:11875–7. doi: 10.1073/pnas.2006874117
23. Morawska L, Tang JW, Bahnfleth W, Bluyssen PM, Boerstra A, Buonanno G, et al. How can airborne transmission of COVID-19 indoors be minimised? *Environ Int.* (2020) 142:105832. doi: 10.1016/j.envint.2020.105832
24. Karmakar M, Lantz PM, Tipirneni R. Association of social and demographic factors with COVID-19 incidence and death rates in the US. *JAMA Network Open.* (2021) 4:e2036462. doi: 10.1001/jamanetworkopen.2020.36462
25. Rader B, Astley CM, Sy KTL, Sewalk K, Hswen Y, Brownstein JS, et al. Geographic access to United States SARS-CoV-2 testing sites highlights healthcare disparities and may bias transmission estimates. *J Travel Med.* (2020) 27:taaa076. doi: 10.1093/jtm/taaa076
26. CDC COVID-19. *Centers for Disease Control and Prevention.* Available online at: https://www.cdc.gov/coronavirus/2019-ncov/index.html (accessed May 01, 2022).
27. Sy KTL, Martinez ME, Rader B, White LF. Socioeconomic disparities in subway use and COVID-19 outcomes in New York City. *Am J Epidemiol.* (2020) 190:1234–42. doi: 10.1093/aje/kwaa277
28. Quan D, Luna Wong L, Shallal A, Madan R, Hamdan A, Ahdi H, et al. Impact of race and socioeconomic status on outcomes in patients hospitalized with COVID-19. *J Gen Intern Med.* (2021) 36:1302–9. doi: 10.1007/s11606-020-06527-1
29. Paul A, Englert P, Varga M. Socio-economic disparities and COVID-19 in the USA. *J Phys Complex.* (2021) 2:035017. doi: 10.1088/2632-072X/ac0fc7
30. Abedi V, Olulana O, Avula V, Chaudhary D, Khan A, Shahjouei S, et al. Racial, economic, and health inequality and COVID-19 infection in the United States. *J Racial Ethn Health Disparities.* (2021) 8:732–42. doi: 10.1007/s40615-020-00833-4
31. Khanijahani A. Racial, ethnic, and socioeconomic disparities in confirmed COVID-19 cases and deaths in the United States: a county-level analysis as of November 2020. *Ethn Health.* (2021) 26:22–35. doi: 10.1080/13557858.2020.1853067
32. Liao TF, De Maio F. Association of social and economic inequality with coronavirus disease 2019 incidence and mortality across US counties. *JAMA Network Open.* (2021) 4:e2034578. doi: 10.1001/jamanetworkopen.2020.34578
33. Oronce CIA, Scannell CA, Kawachi I, Tsugawa Y. Association between state-level income inequality and COVID-19 cases and mortality in the USA. *J Gen Intern Med.* (2020) 35:2791–3. doi: 10.1007/s11606-020-05971-3
34. Little C, Alsen M, Barlow J, Naymagon L, Tremblay D, Genden E, et al. The impact of socioeconomic status on the clinical outcomes of COVID-19; a retrospective cohort study. *J Commun Health.* (2021) 46:794–802. doi: 10.1007/s10900-020-00944-3
35. Dasgupta S, Bowen VB, Leidner A, Fletcher K, Musial T, Rose C, et al. Association between social vulnerability and a county's risk for becoming a COVID-19 hotspot - United States, June 1-July 25, 2020. *Morb Mort Wkly Rep.* (2020) 69:1535–41. doi: 10.15585/mmwr.mm6942a3
36. Karaye IM, Horney JA. the impact of social vulnerability on COVID-19 in the U.S.: an analysis of spatially varying relationships. *Am J Prevent Med.* (2020) 59:317–25. doi: 10.1016/j.amepre.2020.06.006
37. Khazanchi R, Beiter ER, Gondi S, Beckman AL, Bilinski A, Ganguli I. County-level association of social vulnerability with COVID-19 cases and deaths in the USA. *J Gen Intern Med.* (2020) 35:2784–7. doi: 10.1007/s11606-020-05882-3
38. Garnier R, Benetka JR, Kraemer J, Bansal S. Socioeconomic disparities in social distancing during the COVID-19 pandemic in the United States: observational study. *J Med Internet Res.* (2021) 23:e24591. doi: 10.2196/24591
39. Baden LR, El Sahly HM, Essink B, Kotloff K, Frey S, Novak R, et al. Efficacy and safety of the mRNA-1273 SARS-CoV-2 vaccine. *New Engl J Med.* (2021) 384:403–16. doi: 10.1056/NEJMoa2035389
40. Food and Drug Administration. *Pfizer-BioNTech COVID-19 Vaccine.* Vaccines and Related Biological Products Advisory Committee Briefing Document – Sponsor. Available online at: https://www.fda.gov/media/144246/download (accessed January 01, 2019).
41. Food and Drug Administration. *Moderna COVID-19 Vaccine.* Vaccines and Related Biological Products Advisory Committee December 17, 2020 Meeting Briefing Document- Sponsor. Available online at: https://www.fda.gov/media/144452/download (accessed January 01, 2019).
42. Food and Drug Administration. *Janssen COVID-19 Vaccine.* Vaccines and Related Biological Products Advisory Committee February 26, 2021 Meeting Briefing Document – Sponsor. Available online at: https://www.fda.gov/media/146219/download (accessed January 01, 2019).
43. Polack FP, Thomas SJ, Kitchin N, Absalon J, Gurtman A, Lockhart S, et al. Safety and efficacy of the BNT162b2 mRNA Covid-19 vaccine. *New Engl J Med.* (2020) 383:2603–15. doi: 10.1056/NEJMoa2034577
44. Hughes MM, Wang A, Grossman MK, Pun E, Whiteman A, Deng L, et al. County-level COVID-19 vaccination coverage and social vulnerability—United States, December 14, 2020–March 1, 2021. *Morb Mort Wkly Rep.* (2021) 70:431. doi: 10.15585/mmwr.mm7012e1

7

The Association Between the Baseline and the Change in Neutrophil-to-Lymphocyte Ratio and Short-Term Mortality in Patients with Acute Respiratory Distress Syndrome

Wei Zhang[1*]*, Yadan Wang*[2]*, Weijie Li*[1] *and Guizuo Wang*[1]

[1] Department of Respiratory and Critical Care Medicine, Shaanxi Provincial People's Hospital, Xi'an, China, *[2] Ruibiao (Wuhan) Biotechnology Co. Ltd., Wuhan, China*

Correspondence:
Wei Zhang
zhangwei2384@126.com

Background: Two previous studies have shown that increased neutrophil to lymphocyte ratio (NLR) is associated with short-term prognosis in patients with acute respiratory distress syndrome (ARDS), but it is usually assessed as a single threshold value at baseline. We investigated the relationship between the baseline and the early change in NLR and 30-day mortality in patients with ARDS to evaluate the prognostic value of NLR baseline and NLR changes during the first 7 days after ICU admission.

Methods: This is a retrospective cohort study, with all ARDS patients diagnosed according to the Berlin definition from the Medical Information Mart for Intensive Care III (MIMIC-III) database. We calculated the NLR by dividing the neutrophil count by the lymphocyte count. The multivariable logistic regression analysis was used to investigate the relationship between the baseline NLR and short-term mortality. Then the generalized additive mixed model was used to compare trends in NLR over time among survivors and non-survivors after adjusting for potential confounders.

Results: A total of 1164 patients were enrolled in our study. Multivariable logistic regression analysis showed that after adjusting for confounders, elevated baseline NLR was a significant risk factor predicting 30-day mortality (OR 1.02, 95%CI 1.01, 1.03, $P = 0.0046$) and hospital mortality (OR 1.02, 95%CI 1.01, 1.03, $P = 0.0003$). The result of the generalized additive mixed model showed that the NLR decreased in the survival group and increased in the non-survival group gradually within 7 days after ICU admission. The difference between the two groups showed a trend of increase gradually and the difference increased by an average of 0.67 daily after adjusting for confounders.

Conclusions: We confirmed that there was a positive correlation between baseline NLR and short-term mortality, and we found significant differences in NLR changes over time between the non-survival group and the survival group. The early increase in NLR was associated with short-term mortality in ARDS patients.

Keywords: change, neutrophil to lymphocyte ratio, NLR, ARDS, 30-day mortality, intensive care unit

INTRODUCTION

Acute respiratory distress syndrome (ARDS) is a fatal form of acute respiratory failure requiring mechanical ventilation, which is caused by direct (pneumonia or aspiration) or indirect lung injury (sepsis or trauma) (1). It is a type of acute diffuse inflammatory lung injury that results in damage to the pulmonary endothelium, increased capillary permeability, pulmonary edema formation, and thus leads to decreased effective pulmonary ventilation area (2). Despite the efforts in early diagnosis and treatment, to our knowledge, there is no available treatment which can aim directly at the pathological mechanism of ARDS, and mechanical ventilation and supportive care are still the main approaches (1, 3). Approximately 35–46% of patients died consequently during hospitalization, making it one of the most common causes of death in intensive care units (ICU) (4). Therefore, it is urgent to find specific biological markers to accurately identify high-risk patients and adjust clinical treatment and nursing intervention to ultimately improve the prognosis of patients with ARDS.

Inflammatory response plays an important role in the development of ARDS, and is also an important factor affecting the prognosis of ARDS patients (2, 5). *In vivo* and *in vitro* studies have shown that inflammatory response can cause increased permeability of alveolar endothelium and epithelial cells, leading to the occurrence of pulmonary edema (5, 6). Neutrophil lymphocyte ratio (NLR) as a marker of systemic inflammation has been shown to be associated with the prognosis of a variety of diseases, including sepsis (7), COVID-19 pneumonia (8, 9), chronic obstructive pulmonary disease (COPD) (10), acute coronary syndrome (11), and several solid tumors (12–14). Two previous studies have shown that elevated baseline NLR was associated with short-term prognosis in ARDS patients (15, 16). However, these two studies only revealed the relationship between static NLR at baseline and short-term patient prognosis, which may not reflect the overall dynamics of the patient's condition. In this study, we investigated the relationship between baseline and early changes within the first week after ICU admission in NLR and short-term prognosis among ARDS patients.

PATIENTS AND METHODS

Data Sources

This is a retrospective cohort study of 1164 patients with ARDS according to the Berlin definition. We obtained all the data from the Medical Information Mart for Intensive Care III (MIMIC-III), which is a single-center and freely accessible database and contains more than 60,000 health-related hospitalizations from 2001 to 2012 in the ICU of Beth Israel Deaconess Medical Center in Boston. We have completed the online course and passed the online exams (no. 6182750) to gain access to the database. The establishment of the MIMIC III database was approved by the institutional review board of Beth Israel deacons Medical Center and Massachusetts Institute of Technology. Because hospitalization information is anonymous, the informed consent was not required.

Patients

We screened all the patients in the database. Our inclusion criteria were as follows: at least 16 years, ICU stay more than 72 h, ARDS diagnosis meeting Berlin standard at the time of ICU admission, had lymphocyte and neutrophil count within 24 h after ICU admission. We excluded patients with chronic hematologic disorders, lacked the baseline of lymphocyte and neutrophil records. If a patient was admitted repeatedly during the study period, we used only the record of his first ICU admission.

The Berlin standard included: acute onset, arterial oxygen partial pressure (PaO_2)/fraction of inspired oxygen (FiO_2) <300 mmHg and positive end-expiratory pressure (PEEP) $\geq$5 cm H_2O on the first day of ICU admission, bilateral infiltrates on chest radiograph, absence of heart failure. According to the Berlin standard, ARDS were classified into mild (>200 mmHg, $\leq$300 mmHg), moderate (>100 mmHg, $\leq$ 200 mmHg), and severe (<100 mmHg) based on the PaO_2/FiO_2 ratio.

Data Extraction

We used the Structured Query Language to extract the data. We extracted or calculated the following variables, including the baseline characteristics (age, gender, ethnicity, admission type), the patients' comorbidity, the Elixhauser Comorbidity Index (SID30), the risk factors leading to ARDS, the vital signs within 24 h after ICU admission (heart rate, temperature, mean arterial pressure, Spo2), the severity of organ dysfunction (Simplified Acute Physiology Score, SAPS II; Oxford Acute Severity of Illness Score, OASIS; Sequential Organ Failure Assessment, SOFA), PaO_2/FiO_2 at diagnosis, PEEP at diagnosis and the treatment received (ventilation received; vasopressor therapy; renal replacement therapy; corticosteroids therapy; antibiotic therapy). The serious score of organ dysfunction was estimated for all patients within 24 h of ICU admission.

The baseline of NLR was determined by the absolute neutrophil count divided by the absolute lymphocyte count based on the first laboratory parameters after ICU admission. Repeated measurements of NLR were performed during the first 7 days after ICU admission. The repeated measurements of NLR were irregularly spaced over time.

Statistical Analysis

We processed and analyzed all the data by EmpowerStats software (www.empowerstats.com version R.3.4.3) and statistical software package R. We presented the continuous variables as the mean (SD) and compared them by Student's *t*-test (normal distribution) or Mann-Whitney test (non-normal distribution); we presented the categorical variables as percentages and compared them by chi-square test. A two-tailed $P < 0.05$ was considered statistically significant.

We first analyzed the relationship between the baseline NLR and short-term clinical outcomes in ARDS patients. We divided the patients into three groups according to the tertile of the baseline NLR values. We used multivariable logistic regression analysis and smooth curve fitting to test the independent effects of the baseline NLR and in-hospital and 30-day mortality with crude and full models. The adjusted variables included age,

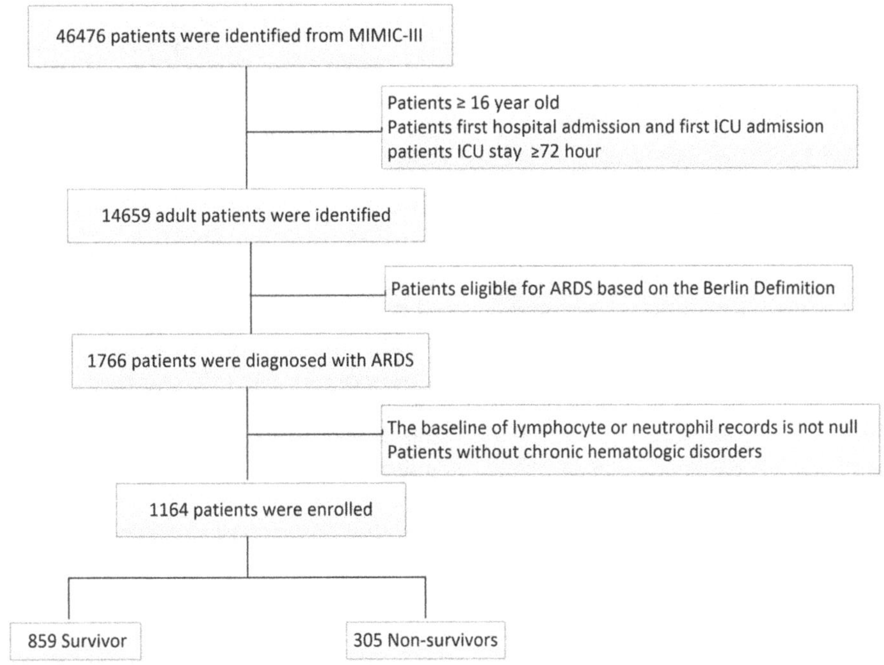

FIGURE 1 | Flow chart of the current study.

gender, ethnicity, smoking, admission type, COPD, hypertension, tumor, diabetes mellitus, renal failure, SID30, pneumonia, sepsis, aspiration, trauma/surgery, other non-pulmonary, PaO_2/FiO_2, SAPS II, OASIS, SOFA, corticosteroids therapy, antibiotic therapy, vasopressor therapy, ventilation received and renal replacement therapy. We selected those confounders based on their associations with the outcomes of interest or a change in effect estimate of more than 10%.

Then we analyzed the relationship between the early change of NLR and 30-day mortality. We showed the difference in NLR between survivors and non-survivors within the first 7 days after ICU admission. We used the generalized additive mixed model (GAMM) to investigate the early changes of NLR over time between survivors and non-survivors, with crude and full models. The GAMM is commonly used to analyze the results of repeated measurements, especially when the interval between repeated measurements is irregular and some data is missing (17, 18).

RESULTS

Characteristics of Patients

A total of 1164 patients with ARDS were included in this study, which contained 859 survivors and 305 non-survivors who were stratified on 30-day mortality. The flowchart of study cohort selection was shown in **Figure 1**. The characteristics of the study participants were displayed in **Table 1**.

The average age of the study participants was 60.27 ± 17.74 years and 40.87% of participants were female. The main risk factors of ARDS were non-pulmonary sepsis ($N = 549$ 47.12%) and pneumonia ($N = 345$ 29.64%). There were 208 (17.87%), 534 (45.88%), and 422 (36.25%) patients with mild, moderate and severe ARDS, respectively, upon ICU admission. The median values of NLR at baseline were 13.14 ± 10.66 in survivors and 16.78 ± 13.38 in non-survivors, respectively. We found that there was a significant difference between the two groups in terms of age, ethnicity, smoking and admission type; The SAPS II, OASIS, and SOFA scores within 24 h of ICU admission were significantly higher in non-survivors than that in survivors. There were also significant differences in vital signs (temperature, mean arterial pressure, Spo2, and PaO_2/FiO_2 at diagnosis) and treatment received (mechanical ventilation and antibiotic therapy).

Association Between Baseline NLR and Mortality

We divided all the patients into three groups according to the tertiles of baseline NLR and **Table 2** displayed the clinical outcomes of the subjects across the tertile of baseline NLR. Patients with high NLR (NLR $\geq$14.8) had shorter days free of mechanical ventilation, higher in-hospital, and 30-day mortality.

We used the smooth curve fitting to show the association between baseline NLR levels and risk of in-hospital and 30-day mortality which was presented in **Figure 2**. Taking NLR on admission as a continuous variable, there was a significant positive association with the short-term mortality in the adjusted model.

We further evaluated this finding by the multivariable logistic regression analysis, which was shown in **Table 3**. As a continuous variable, after adjusting for the clinical confounders listed, an SD increase in baseline NLR levels was associated with a 2% higher

TABLE 1 | Baseline characteristics of total cohort, 30-day survivors, and 30-day non-survivors.

Variables	Total cohort $N = 1164$	30-day survivor $N = 859$	30-day non-survivors $N = 305$	*P*-value
Age (years)	60.27 ± 17.74	58.23 ± 17.53	66.03 ± 17.06	<0.001
Female	479 (40.87%)	346 (40.28%)	129 (42.30%)	0.538
Ethnicity				<0.001
Caucasian	782 (67.18%)	606 (70.55%)	176 (57.70%)	
Black	64 (5.50%)	48 (5.59%)	16 (5.25%)	
Hispanic	30 (2.58%)	26 (3.03%)	4 (1.31%)	
Others	288 (24.74%)	179 (20.84%)	109 (35.74%)	
Smoking, *n* (%)	595 (51.12%)	452 (52.62%)	143 (46.89%)	<0.001
Admission type				0.033
Emergency	1021 (87.71%)	744 (86.61%)	277 (90.82%)	
Urgent	94 (8.08%)	80 (9.31%)	14 (4.59%)	
Elective	49 (4.21%)	35 (4.07%)	14 (4.59%)	
Risk factor, *n* (%)				
Pneumonia	345 (29.64%)	235 (27.36%)	110 (36.07%)	0.004
Non-pulmonary sepsis	549 (47.12%)	390 (45.40%)	159 (52.13%)	0.043
Aspiration	77 (6.62%)	56 (6.52%)	21 (6.89%)	0.825
Trauma/surgery	293 (25.17%)	250 (29.10%)	43 (14.10%)	<0.001
Other non-pulmonary	328 (28.18%)	236 (27.47%)	92 (30.16%)	0.370
Comorbidity				
COPD	61 (5.24%)	43 (5.01%)	18 (5.90%)	0.546
Tumor	78 (6.70%)	39 (4.54%)	39 (12.79%)	0.001
Renal failure	140 (12.03%)	98 (11.41%)	42 (13.77%)	0.276
Hypertension	121 (10.40%)	92 (10.71%)	29 (9.51%)	0.555
Diabetes mellitus	272 (23.37%)	204 (23.75%)	68 (22.30%)	0.606
SID30	8.51 ± 7.58	7.73 ± 7.40	10.70 ± 7.63	<0.001
Severity scale				
SAPSII	44.36 ± 15.02	41.89 ± 13.79	51.30 ± 16.16	<0.001
OASIS	38.86 ± 8.08	37.92 ± 7.81	41.50 ± 8.25	<0.001
SOFA	7.20 ± 3.65	6.81 ± 3.35	8.30 ± 4.22	<0.001
Baseline vital data				
Temperature, °C	37.12 ± 0.79	37.20 ± 0.76	36.89 ± 0.81	<0.001
HR, beats/min	91.40 ± 17.28	91.66 ± 17.21	90.64 ± 17.49	0.375
MAP mmHg	76.52 ± 9.63	77.42 ± 9.58	73.98 ± 9.33	<0.001
Spo2	96.82 ± 2.95	97.01 ± 2.84	96.30 ± 3.18	<0.001
PaO_2/FiO_2 at diagnosis	136.57 ± 64.37	140.08 ± 63.98	126.69 ± 64.54	<0.001
PEEP at diagnosis	8.33 ± 13.57	7.91 ± 3.96	9.51 ± 25.65	0.076
NLR at diagnosis	14.10 ± 11.54	13.14 ± 10.66	16.78 ± 13.38	<0.001
Berlin classification, *n* (%)				0.007
Mild	208 (17.87%)	162 (18.86%)	46 (15.08%)	
Moderate	534 (45.88%)	408 (47.50%)	126 (41.31%)	
Severe	422 (36.25%)	289 (33.64%)	133 (43.61%)	
Treatment received				
Ventilation received	1032 (88.66%)	776 (90.34%)	256 (83.93%)	0.002
Vasopressor therapy	586 (50.34%)	426 (49.59%)	160 (52.46%)	0.390
Renal replacement therapy	74 (6.36%)	57 (6.64%)	17 (5.57%)	0.514
Corticosteroids therapy	87 (7.47%)	62 (7.22%)	25 (8.20%)	0.576
Antibiotic therapy	549 (47.16%)	444 (51.69%)	105 (34.43%)	<0.001

Data were mean ± SD, n (%). p-values comparing groups were from Student's t-test or Mann-Whitney test for continuous data and chi-squared test for categorical variables. COPD, chronic obstructive pulmonary disease; SID30, elixhauser comorbidity score; MAP, mean arterial pressure; HR, heart rate; PaO_2/FiO_2, arterial oxygen partial pressure/fraction of inspired oxygen; SAPSII, Simplified Acute Physiology Score; OASIS, Oxford Acute Severity of Illness Score; SOFA, Sequential Organ Failure Assessment; PEEP, positive end-expiratory pressure.

TABLE 2 | Outcomes of the patients with ARDS across tertile of the baseline NLR.

Variables	All patients	NLR			*P*-value
		<7.5	≥7.5, <14.8	≥14.8	
n	1,164	388	388	388	
Time in ICU (days)	15.53 ± 13.13	15.13 ± 12.20	15.81 ± 12.80	15.63 ± 14.33	0.757
Time in hospital (days)	22.34 ± 16.68	22.56 ± 17.67	22.25 ± 14.94	22.21 ± 17.34	0.950
Days free of MV at day 30	15.37 ± 11.07	16.39 ± 10.62	16.54 ± 10.69	13.19 ± 11.57	<0.001
In-hospital mortality	336 (28.87%)	91 (23.45%)	103 (26.55%)	142 (36.60%)	<0.001
30-day mortality	305 (26.20%)	82 (21.13%)	91 (23.45%)	132 (34.02%)	<0.001

Data were mean ± SD, n (%). p-values comparing groups were from Student's t-test for continuous data and chi-squared test for categorical variables.

risk of 30-day mortality (OR 1.02, 95% CI, 1.01, 1.03, $P = 0.0046$), and there was a similar trend for in-hospital mortality (OR 1.02, 95% CI, 1.01, 1.03, $P = 0.0004$). When RDW was assessed as tertiles, we found that patients in high baseline NLR (NLR ≥14.8) also had significantly higher risks of in-hospital (OR 1.48, 95% CI 1.03–2.12, $P = 0.0319$) and 30-day (OR 1.48, 95% CI 1.02–2.16, $P = 0.0409$) mortality than patients in low group (NLR <7.5) in the adjusted model.

The subgroup analyses for the relationship between baseline NLR and mortality were presented in **Supplementary Table 1**, which were performed according to age, gender, race, smoking, type of admission, risk factor, comorbidity, Berlin classification, and treatment received. The results showed that in different subgroups the relationship between baseline NLR and the risk of mortality stably existed except for patients of other race.

Association Between Early Change in NLR and Mortality

We compared the difference in NLR between 30-day survivors and 30-day non-survivors on admission, on the 2–3th, the 4–5th, and the 6–7th day. We found that there were significant differences in NLR between the survival and the non-survival at the time points mentioned above. The result was shown in **Table 4**.

We used GAMM to show the changes in NLR over time (the first week after ICU admission) between 30-day survivors and 30-day non-survivors after adjusted for clinical confounders listed. The result was presented in **Figure 3**. We found that, as time went on, NLR increased in the non-survival group. While the trend was reversed and it decreased in the survival group gradually within 1 week after ICU admission. And the difference between the two groups increased over time.

Furthermore, we revealed the association between early changes in NLR and 30-day mortality in ARDS patients which was presented in **Table 5**. The results indicated that NLR in the non-survival group was significantly higher than that in the survival group, and more importantly the difference between the two groups showed an increasing trend within 1 week after ICU admission. This difference increased by an average of 0.69 per day, and the results were consistent in the adjusted model ($\beta = 0.67$, 95% CI 0.23 1.11, $P = 0.0030$). These trends were also observed for in-hospital mortality.

DISCUSSION

In this retrospective cohort study, we confirmed that there was a significant positive correlation between baseline NLR and short-term mortality of patients with ARDS. High NLR at ICU admission was associated with higher 30-day and in-hospital mortality. Moreover, the NLR dynamic during the first 7-days after ICU admission also appears to be a good prognostic factor in patients with ARDS. We found that NLR increased gradually within 7 days after ICU admission in the non-survival group, but decreased gradually in the survival group. Furthermore, this difference between the two groups increased significantly over time. The relationship remained stable after adjusting for clinical confounders. This might suggest that an early increase in NLR is associated with poor short-term prognosis in ARDS patients.

Previous studies have shown that increased NLR was associated with short-term prognosis in a variety of diseases, including tumors, cardiovascular disease, and inflammatory diseases (7, 8, 10–12, 14, 19, 20). To our knowledge, there are only two previous studies on the relationship between baseline NLR and clinical outcomes of ARDS. The results of these two studies both showed that increased NLR on admission was associated with poor outcomes of ARDS patients. Wang et al. suggested that NLR >14 can be used as the cut-off threshold for predicting the 28-day mortality in patients with ARDS (16). Li et al. found that combining NLR could improve the prognostic value of APACHE II score and Berlin classification than using any of them alone (15). Our results for the relationship between baseline NLR and short-term prognosis in ARDS patients were consistent with previous studies. However, there is no study to explore the association between an early change of NLR and mortality in ARDS patients, which may reflect the comprehensive dynamic changes of the patient's condition and the evolution of the disease.

Therefore, we first used the GAMM model to explore the temporal variation of NLR in ARDS patients and its relationship with short-term outcomes. First, our study showed that NLR changed over time in ARDS patients within the first 7 days after ICU admission. Second, we compared the different trends of NLR over time between survival and death groups. Finally, the GAMM model was used to investigate the relationship between early changes in NLR and short-term prognosis in ARDS patients. We found that the difference between the two groups showed an

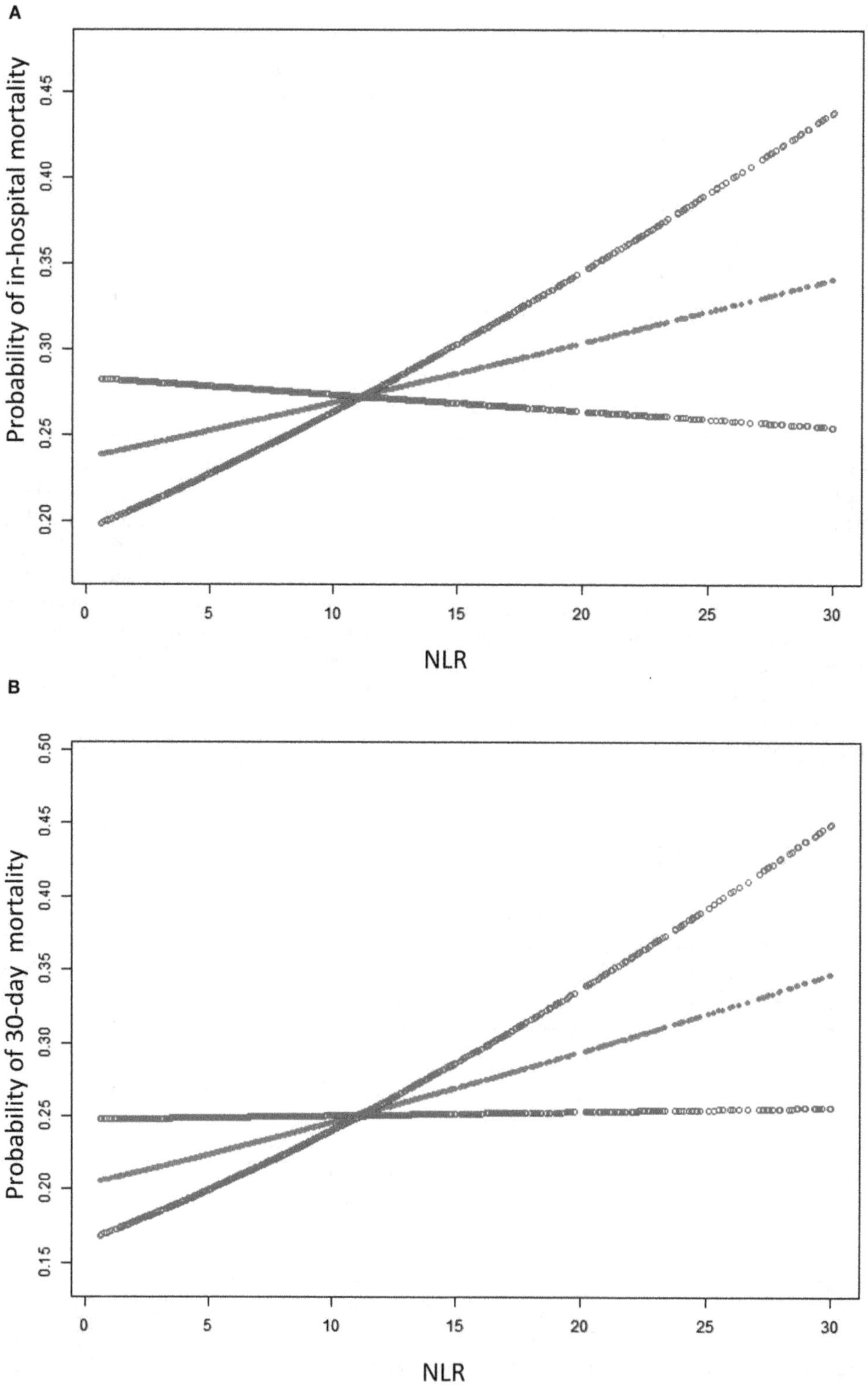

FIGURE 2 | A smooth curve fitting for the relationship between the baseline NLR and the risk of in-hospital mortality **(A)** and 30-day mortality **(B)**. The resulting figures show the risk of mortality in the y-axis and the NLR (continuous variable) in the x-axis. The red line shows the dose-response curve between NLR and probability of short-term mortality, the two blue lines refer to 95% CIs. A positive relationship between NLR and the risk of short-term mortality was observed after adjusting for age, gender, ethnicity, smoking, admission type, COPD, hypertension, tumor, diabetes mellitus, renal failure, SID30, pneumonia, sepsis, aspiration, trauma/surgery, other non-pulmonary, PaO_2/FiO_2, SAPS II, OASIS, SOFA, corticosteroids therapy, antibiotic therapy, vasopressor therapy, ventilation received, and renal replacement therapy by spline smoothing plot.

TABLE 3 | Multivariable logistic regression analysis of baseline NLR for mortality.

Exposure	Non-adjusted			Adjust I			Adjust II		
30-day mortality	**OR**	**95% CI**	***p*-value**	**OR**	**95% CI**	***p*-value**	**OR**	**95% CI**	***p*-value**
NLR Per 1 sd	1.03	(1.01, 1.04)	<0.0001	1.02	(1.01, 1.03)	0.0003	1.02	(1.01, 1.03)	0.0046
NLR tertile									
T1	1.0	(Reference)		1.0	(Reference)		1.0	(Reference)	
T2	1.14	(0.82, 1.60)	0.4378	1.07	(0.75, 1.53)	0.6921	1.09	(0.74, 1.60)	0.6643
T3	1.92	(1.39, 2.65)	<0.0001	1.74	(1.24, 2.45)	0.0015	1.48	(1.02, 2.16)	0.0409
In-hospital mortality	**OR**	**95% CI**	***p*-value**	**OR**	**95% CI**	***p*-value**	**OR**	**95% CI**	***p*-value**
NLR Per 1 sd	1.03	(1.02, 1.04)	<0.0001	1.02	(1.01, 1.04)	<0.0001	1.02	(1.01, 1.03)	0.0004
NLR tertile									
T1	1.0	(Reference)		1.0	(Reference)		1.0	(Reference)	
T2	1.18	(0.85, 1.63)	0.3201	1.11	(0.78, 1.54)	0.5510	1.15	(0.80, 1.66)	0.4544
T3	1.88	(1.38, 2.58)	<0.0001	1.71	(1.23, 2.39)	0.0014	1.48	(1.03, 2.12)	0.0319

OR, odds ratio; CI, confidence interval.
Adjusted I for age, gender, ethnicity, smoking, admission type.
Adjusted II for age, gender, ethnicity, smoking, admission type, COPD, hypertension, tumor, diabetes mellitus, renal failure, SID30, pneumonia, sepsis, aspiration, trauma/surgery, other non-pulmonary, PaO_2/FiO_2, SAPSII, OASIS, SOFA, corticosteroids therapy, antibiotic therapy, vasopressor therapy, ventilation received, and renal replacement therapy.

TABLE 4 | The evolution of NLR after ICU admission between 30-day survivors and 30-day non survivors.

Time	NLR, mean (SD) median (25th–75th percentile)		
	Survivors	**Non-survivors**	***P*-value**
On admission	13.14 (10.66), 9.89 (5.97–16.40)	16.78 (13.38), 12.67 (6.96–22.32)	<0.001
On 2–3th day	11.97 (9.16), 9.08 (6.15–15.48)	17.39 (15.09), 13.33 (6.87–20.74)	<0.001
On 4-5th day	12.52 (9.31), 9.66 (5.86–15.70)	18.68 (19.04), 12.09 (8.06–20.53)	<0.001
On 6–7th day	11.73 (9.89), 9.25 (5.90–14.11)	21.25 (22.87), 13.56 (8.21–21.83)	<0.001

p-value: as for the difference between survivors and non-survivors; Mann-Whitney test was applied for the variables with a skewed distribution.

increasing trend (an average of 0.69 per day) within 1 week after ICU admission.

The systemic inflammatory response is closely related to the occurrence and development of ARDS (2, 5). Elevated levels of inflammatory markers were associated with poor clinical outcomes of ARDS patients (21). Previous studies have shown that increased NLR including neutrophils rising and lymphocytes apoptosis, can be used as a marker of systemic inflammation to reflect the relative degree of inflammation and host immune status (22). In the latest study, the increased NLR can be used as an indicator to predict the development of ARDS in patients with COVID-19 (8). However, the physiologic mechanism behind the association between elevated NLR and poor clinical outcomes in ARDS remains unclear. We can give some possible reasons.

The literature showed that neutrophil counts are positively correlated with the degree of inflammation in ARDS (23). It has been reported that neutrophils and neutrophil-derived particles are significantly increased in bronchoalveolar lavage fluid of ARDS patients (24, 25). Several studies have shown that during the occurrence of acute lung injury (ALI), neutrophils are the first immune cells to be recruited to inflammatory sites, after being stimulated by chemokines released from damaged lung tissue. Activated neutrophils can trigger oxidative stress, release proteases, and form neutrophils extracellular traps (NETs), which induce positive feedback and further enhance the inflammatory response to lung damage (5, 23, 26). Recent studies also showed that increased neutrophils and neutrophil extracellular traps are key pathological drivers of progressive lung injury in COVID-19 patients (27). Targeting neutrophil therapy may improve the clinical outcomes of ARDS caused by SARS-COV-2 infection (19). Previous studies have shown that lymphopenia was associated with high mortality in patients with systemic inflammatory response syndrome and ARDS caused by COVID-19 (28, 29). Lymphocytes play an important role in regulating appropriate inflammatory responses, and lymphopenia may perpetuate harmful inflammation (15). Moreover, *in vitro* experiments, when lymphocytes were cultured with neutrophils, their cytolytic activity was inhibited, and the degree of inhibition increased with the addition of neutrophils (30). NLR reflects the balance between lymphocytes and neutrophils and may reflect the immune status more comprehensively. Therefore, we speculated that the dynamic elevation of NLR may reflect the severity of inflammatory response in ARDS patients, which can be an important indicator for monitoring the clinical prognosis of ARDS.

Although many studies have assessed the prognosis of ARDS patients, none of the biomarkers is perfect (31). NLR is the ratio of neutrophil count to lymphocyte count that can be obtained through routine blood tests without any additional cost, which may make it more convenient for clinical use. Early changes in

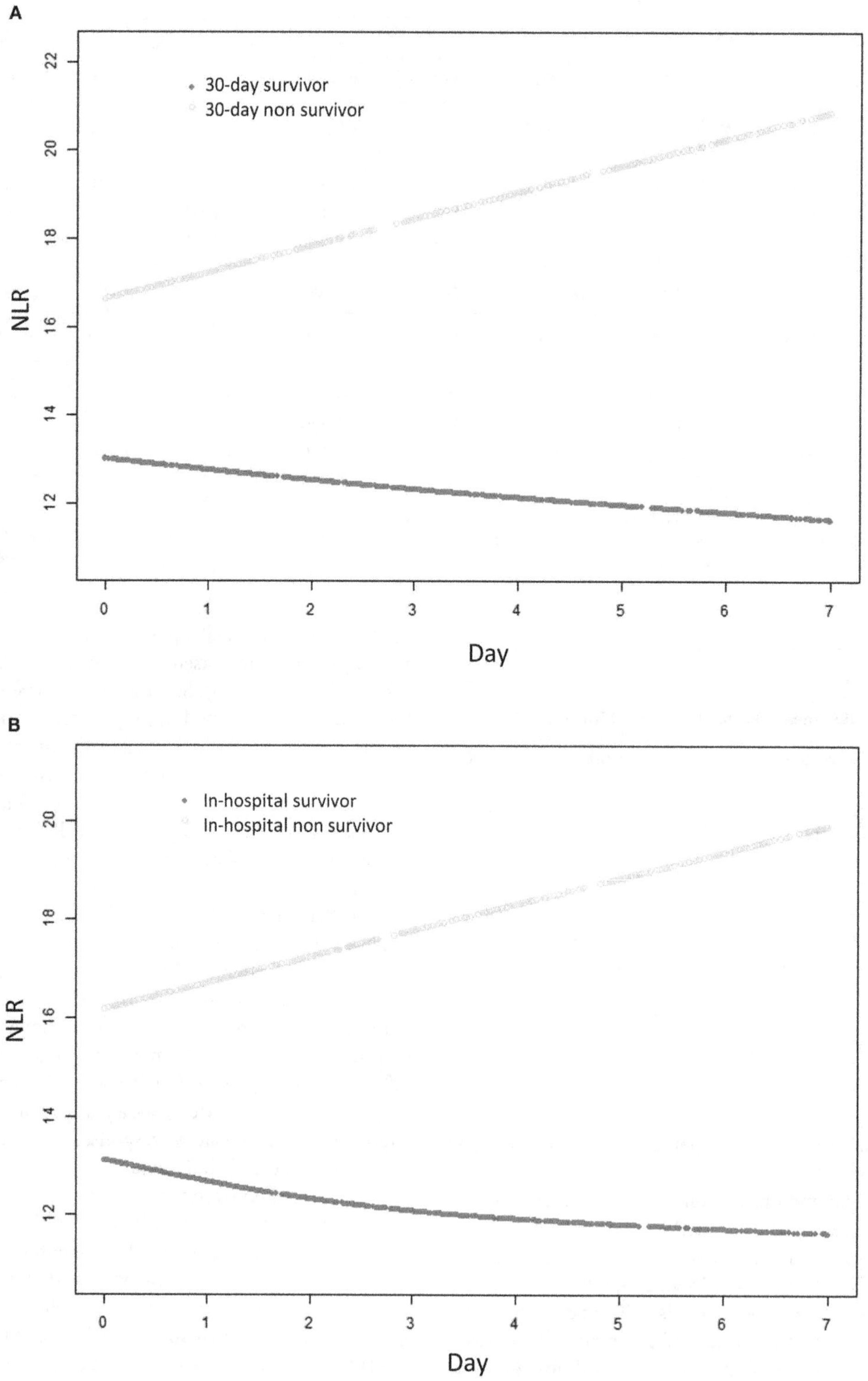

FIGURE 3 | Association between changes in NRL and 30-day mortality **(A)** and in-hospital mortality **(B)**. A linear association between changes in NLR and mortality was found in a generalized additive mix model (GAMM). Smooth curve fitting graph illustrated the NLR in 1164 ARDS patients based on the days after admission to ICU. The red line represented the survivors. The blue line represented the non-survivors. All adjusted for age, gender, ethnicity, smoking, admission type, COPD, hypertension, tumor, diabetes mellitus, renal failure, SID30, pneumonia, sepsis, aspiration, trauma/surgery, other non-pulmonary, PaO_2/FiO_2, SAPS II, OASIS, SOFA, corticosteroids therapy, antibiotic therapy, vasopressor therapy, ventilation received, and renal replacement therapy.

TABLE 5 | Relationship between changes (0–7 days) NLR and short-term mortality in patients with ARDS derived from a generalized additive mixed model (GAMM).

	Unadjusted		Adjusted I		Adjusted II	
30-day mortality	**β (95%CI)**	***P*-value**	**β (95%CI)**	***P*-value**	**β (95%CI)**	***P*-value**
Day	−0.23 (−0.46, −0.001)	0.0496	−0.23 (−0.46, 0.01)	0.0562	−0.25 (−0.48, −0.02)	0.0358
Death	3.86 (2.43, 5.28)	<0.0001	3.43 (1.97, 4.88)	<0.0001	2.64 (1.09, 4.19)	0.0009
Day × death	0.69 (0.25, 1.13)	0.0022	0.68 (0.24, 1.12)	0.0026	0.67 (0.23, 1.11)	0.0030
In-hospital mortality	**β (95%CI)**	***P*-value**	**β (95%CI)**	***P*-value**	**β (95%CI)**	***P*-value**
Day	−0.30 (−0.54, −0.06)	0.0132	−0.29 (−0.53, −0.06)	0.0159	−0.31 (−0.55, −0.07)	0.0103
Death	3.38 (2.00, 4.77)	<0.0001	2.98 (1.56, 4.39)	<0.0001	2.22 (0.76, 3.73)	0.0032
Day × death	0.75 (0.33, 1.18)	0.0005	0.74 (0.32, 1.16)	0.0006	0.73 (0.31, 1.15)	0.0007

CI, confidence interval; Day, the mean of the increasing of NLR at death = 0 over time (daily); Death, the difference of NLR at day = 0 between the group of death = 1 and the group of death = 0; Day × death, the average increasing in NLR daily under the condition of the group of death = 1 compared with the group of death = 0.
Adjusted I for age, gender, ethnicity, smoking, admission type.
Adjusted II for age, gender, ethnicity, smoking, admission type, COPD, hypertension, tumor, diabetes mellitus, renal failure, SID30, pneumonia, sepsis, aspiration, trauma/surgery, other non-pulmonary, PaO_2/FiO_2, SAPSII, OASIS, SOFA, corticosteroids therapy, antibiotic therapy, vasopressor therapy, ventilation received, and renal replacement therapy.

NLR can be a sensitive indicator of disease severity. Therefore, we believe that dynamic monitoring of NLR after ICU admission is helpful for the early detection of patients with poor prognosis and early adoption of different treatments and nursing measures.

There were some limitations in our study. First, this was a single-center retrospective cohort study, so there was the possibility of selection bias; Second, although we have shown that the increased baseline NLR and an increasing trend over time after ICU admission were related to the poor prognosis of patients with ARDS, the causal relationship between baseline elevated NLR, early change in NLR and mortality cannot be established. So further basic research is needed. Third, the accuracy of the results may be affected due to the lack of information on the active infection (bacterial infection or viral infection) and the medication which can alter NLR levels. Fourth, as a single-center study, the results should be interpreted with caution when implicating in other populations and areas.

CONCLUSION

In our study, there was a positive correlation between baseline NLR and short-term prognosis in ARDS patients. Furthermore, we found that there was a significant difference in the changes of NLR over time between non-survival and survival groups. The early increase in NLR was associated with higher short-term mortality in ARDS patients. These results suggest the potential benefit of monitoring early change in NLR for patients with ARDS. However, prospective studies are needed for further validation.

AUTHOR CONTRIBUTIONS

WZ designed the study, collected and analyzed data, and contributed to writing this manuscript. YW collected and analyzed data. GW and WL designed and supervised the study and drafted the manuscript. All authors have read and approved the final manuscript.

ACKNOWLEDGMENTS

The authors thank all the researchers who created and managed the MIMIC III database.

REFERENCES

1. Fan E, Brodie D, Slutsky AS. Acute respiratory distress syndrome: advances in diagnosis and treatment. *JAMA.* (2018) 319:698–710. doi: 10.1001/jama.2017.21907
2. Huppert LA, Matthay MA, Ware LB. Pathogenesis of acute respiratory distress syndrome. *Semin Resp Crit Care.* (2019) 40:31–9. doi: 10.1055/s-0039-1683996
3. Ben Salem C. Acute respiratory distress syndrome. *N Engl J Med.* (2017) 377:1903–5. doi: 10.1056/NEJMc1711824
4. Bellani G, Laffey JG, Pham T, Fan E, Brochard L, Esteban A, et al. Epidemiology, patterns of care, and mortality for patients with acute respiratory distress syndrome in intensive care units in 50 countries. *JAMA.* (2016) 315:788–800. doi: 10.1001/jama.2016.0291
5. Yang S, Tsai Y, Pan Y, Hwang T. Understanding the role of neutrophils in acute respiratory distress syndrome. *Biomed J.* (2020) 9:10. doi: 10.1016/j.bj.2020.09.001
6. Wang M, Zhang T, Li L, Xie Q, Wang Y, Li Y, et al. Protective effects of HY1702 on lipopolysaccharide-induced mild acute respiratory distress syndrome in mice. *Eur J Pharmacol.* (2020) 887:173563. doi: 10.1016/j.ejphar.2020.173563
7. Ni J, Wang H, Li Y, Shu Y, Liu Y. Neutrophil to lymphocyte ratio (NLR) as a prognostic marker for in-hospital mortality of patients with sepsis: a secondary analysis based on a single-center, retrospective, cohort study. *Medicine.* (2019) 98:e18029. doi: 10.1097/MD.0000000000018029
8. Ma A, Cheng J, Yang J, Dong M, Liao X, Kang Y. Neutrophil-to-lymphocyte ratio as a predictive biomarker for moderate-severe ARDS in severe COVID-19 patients. *Crit Care.* (2020) 24:288. doi: 10.1186/s13054-020-03007-0
9. Liu Y, Li G, He J, Liu Y, Li M, Zhang R, et al. Combined use of the neutrophil-to-lymphocyte ratio and CRP to predict 7-day disease severity in 84 hospitalized patients with COVID-19 pneumonia: a retrospective cohort study. *Ann Transl Med.* (2020) 8:635. doi: 10.21037/atm-20-2372
10. Guo R, Li J, Ma X, Pan L. The predictive value of neutrophil-to-lymphocyte ratio for chronic obstructive pulmonary disease: a systematic

review and meta-analysis. *Expert Rev Resp Med.* (2020) 14:929–36. doi: 10.1080/17476348.2020.1776613
11. Dong C, Wang Z, Chen S. Neutrophil to lymphocyte ratio predict mortality and major adverse cardiac events in acute coronary syndrome: a systematic review and meta-analysis. *Clin Biochem.* (2018) 52:131–6. doi: 10.1016/j.clinbiochem.2017.11.008
12. McLellan P, Henriques J, Ksontini F, Doat S, Hammel P, Desrame J, et al. Prognostic value of the early change in neutrophil-to-lymphocyte ratio in metastatic pancreatic adenocarcinoma. *Clin Res Hepatol Gas.* (2020) 11:101541. doi: 10.1016/j.clinre.2020.08.016
13. Li M, Spakowicz D, Burkart J, Patel S, Husain M, He K, et al. Change in neutrophil to lymphocyte ratio during immunotherapy treatment is a non-linear predictor of patient outcomes in advanced cancers. *J Cancer Res Clin.* (2019) 145:2541–6. doi: 10.1007/s00432-019-02982-4
14. Kim HS, Ku JH. Systemic inflammatory response based on neutrophil-to-lymphocyte ratio as a prognostic marker in bladder cancer. *Dis Markers.* (2016) 2016:8345286. doi: 10.1155/2016/8345286
15. Li W, Ai X, Ni Y, Ye Z, Liang Z. The association between the neutrophil-to-lymphocyte ratio and mortality in patients with acute respiratory distress syndrome: a retrospective cohort study. *Shock.* (2019) 51:161–7. doi: 10.1097/SHK.0000000000001136
16. Wang Y, Ju M, Chen C, Yang D, Hou D, Tang X, et al. Neutrophil-to-lymphocyte ratio as a prognostic marker in acute respiratory distress syndrome patients: a retrospective study. *J Thor Dis.* (2018) 10:273–82. doi: 10.21037/jtd.2017.12.131
17. Najjar SS, Scuteri A, Shetty V, Wright JG, Muller DC, Fleg JL, et al. Pulse wave velocity is an independent predictor of the longitudinal increase in systolic blood pressure and of incident hypertension in the Baltimore Longitudinal Study of Aging. *J Am Coll Cardiol.* (2008) 51:1377–83. doi: 10.1016/j.jacc.2007.10.065
18. Zhao X, Wang K, Zuo P, Liu Y, Zhang M, Xie S, et al. Early decrease in blood platelet count is associated with poor prognosis in COVID-19 patients-indications for predictive, preventive, and personalized medical approach. *EPMA J.* (2020) 11:1–7. doi: 10.1007/s13167-020-00208-z
19. Chiang C, Korinek M, Cheng W, Hwang T. Targeting neutrophils to treat acute respiratory distress syndrome in coronavirus disease. *Front Pharmacol.* (2020) 11:572009. doi: 10.3389/fphar.2020.572009
20. Guo Z, Yu S, Xiao L, Chen X, Ye R, Zheng P, et al. Dynamic change of neutrophil to lymphocyte ratio and hemorrhagic transformation after thrombolysis in stroke. *J Neuroinflamm.* (2016) 13:199. doi: 10.1186/s12974-016-0680-x
21. Calfee CS, Delucchi K, Parsons PE, Thompson BT, Ware LB, Matthay MA. Subphenotypes in acute respiratory distress syndrome: latent class analysis of data from two randomised controlled trials. *Lancet Respir Med.* (2014) 2:611–20 doi: 10.1016/S2213-2600(14)70097-9
22. Faria SS, Fernandes PCJ, Silva MJB, Lima VC, Fontes W, Freitas-Junior R, et al. The neutrophil-to-lymphocyte ratio: a narrative review. *Ecancermedicalscience.* (2016) 10:702. doi: 10.3332/ecancer.2016.702
23. Grommes J, Soehnlein O. Contribution of neutrophils to acute lung injury. *Mol Med.* (2011) 17:293–307. doi: 10.2119/molmed.2010.00138
24. Zhao J, Zhang G, Cui W, Tian B. [Progress of neutrophil extracellular traps in airway inflammation of acute lung injury/acute respiratory distress syndrome: Review]. *Xi Bao Yu Fen Zi Mian Yi Xue Za Zhi.* (2020) 36:664–70.
25. Ojima M, Yamamoto N, Hirose T, Hamaguchi S, Tasaki O, Kojima T, et al. Serial change of neutrophil extracellular traps in tracheal aspirate of patients with acute respiratory distress syndrome: report of three cases. *J Intensive Care.* (2020) 8:25. doi: 10.1186/s40560-020-00444-5
26. Vassallo A, Wood AJ, Subburayalu J, Summers C, Chilvers ER. The counter-intuitive role of the neutrophil in the acute respiratory distress syndrome. *Brit. Med Bull.* (2019) 131:43–55. doi: 10.1093/bmb/ldz024
27. Narasaraju T, Tang BM, Herrmann M, Muller S, Chow VTK, Radic M. Neutrophilia and NETopathy as key pathologic drivers of progressive lung impairment in patients with COVID-19. *Front Pharmacol.* (2020) 11:870. doi: 10.3389/fphar.2020.00870
28. Riff R, Cohen Y, Eini-Rider H, Naamani O, Mazar J, Haviv YS, et al. Systemic inflammatory response syndrome-related lymphopenia is associated with adenosine A(1) receptor dysfunction. *J Leukocyte Biol.* (2017) 102:95–103. doi: 10.1189/jlb.3A0816-345RR
29. Wang A, Gao G, Wang S, Chen M, Qian F, Tang W, et al. Clinical characteristics and risk factors of Acute Respiratory Distress Syndrome (ARDS) in COVID-19 patients in Beijing, China: a retrospective study. *Med Sci Monitor.* (2020) 26:e925974. doi: 10.12659/MSM.925974
30. Chen Y, Yan H, Wang Y, Shi Y, Dai G. Significance of baseline and change in neutrophil-to-lymphocyte ratio in predicting prognosis: a retrospective analysis in advanced pancreatic ductal adenocarcinoma. *Sci Rep.* (2017) 7:753. doi: 10.1038/s41598-017-00859-5
31. Bime C, Camp SM, Casanova N, Oita RC, Ndukum J, Lynn H, et al. The acute respiratory distress syndrome biomarker pipeline: crippling gaps between discovery and clinical utility. *Transl Res.* (2020) 226:105–15. doi: 10.1016/j.trsl.2020.06.010

8

Healthcare Utilization and Medical Cost of Gastrointestinal Reflux Disease in Non-Tuberculous Mycobacterial Pulmonary Disease: A Population-Based Study, South Korea, 2009–2017

Taehee Kim [1†], Jai Hoon Yoon [2†], Bumhee Yang [3†], Jiin Ryu [4], Chang Ki Yoon [5], Youlim Kim [6], Jang Won Sohn [7], Hyun Lee [7] and Hayoung Choi [1*]*

[1] Division of Pulmonary, Allergy, and Critical Care Medicine, Department of Internal Medicine, Hallym University Kangnam Sacred Heart Hospital, Hallym University College of Medicine, Seoul, South Korea, [2] Department of Gastroenterology, Hanyang University Hospital, Seoul, South Korea, [3] Division of Pulmonary and Critical Care Medicine, Department of Internal Medicine, Chungbuk National University Hospital, Chungbuk National University College of Medicine, Cheongju, South Korea, [4] Biostatistical Consulting and Research Lab, Medical Research Collaborating Center, Hanyang University, Seoul, South Korea, [5] Department of Ophthalmology, Seoul National University Hospital, Seoul, South Korea, [6] Division of Pulmonary and Allergy, Department of Internal Medicine, Konkuk University Hospital, School of Medicine, Konkuk University, Seoul, South Korea, [7] Division of Pulmonary Medicine and Allergy, Department of Internal Medicine, Hanyang University College of Medicine, Seoul, South Korea

***Correspondence:**
Hyun Lee
namuhanayeyo@hanynang.ac.kr
Hayoung Choi
hychoimd@gmail.com

† These authors have contributed equally to this work

Gastroesophageal reflux disease (GERD) is a common non-respiratory comorbidity in patients with non-tuberculous mycobacterial pulmonary disease (NTM-PD). However, little is known about the association between GERD and healthcare utilization and medical costs of NTM-PD. Thus, we evaluated this association using the Health Insurance Review and Assessment Service National Patient Sample. NTM-PD patients with GERD had significantly higher healthcare use and spent a higher total on medical costs (5,098 vs. 2,675 USD/person/year) than those without GERD ($P < 0.001$ for all). Therefore, an appropriate management of GERD in NTM-PD patients can be an important factor to reduce the disease burden.

Keywords: NTM, non-tuberculous mycobacteria, GERD (gastroesophageal reflux disease), population base study, medical cost, disease burden

INTRODUCTION

The prevalence and incidence of non-tuberculous mycobacterial pulmonary disease (NTM-PD) has been increasing worldwide (1). Furthermore, both the attributable mortality and financial burden associated with this disease are high (2). Thus, clinical studies that identify preventable or treatable factors to address the high disease burden of NTM-PD are urgently needed to determine strategies for reducing the burden. Gastroesophageal reflux disease (GERD) is a common non-respiratory comorbidity in NTM-PD patients, with a prevalence of 26–44% (3, 4). GERD is associated with an increased number of aspiration symptoms, higher bacterial burden, and more severe radiologic findings (3, 4). Although these results indicate that the disease burden in NTM-PD patients with GERD can be more substantial than in those without GERD, there is limited information on this issue. Thus, we aimed to evaluate whether GERD is associated with a higher disease burden, specifically healthcare use, medical costs, and in-hospital mortality, in patients with NTM-PD.

METHODS

Data Source

We used the 2009–2017 Health Insurance Review and Assessment Service, National Patient Sample (HIRA-NPS), which includes ~1,400,000 individuals each year drawn by 3% stratified random sampling by age and sex from the entire population with claims records during the year. The dataset included patient diagnosis, treatment, procedures, surgical history, and prescription drugs. Diagnosis was coded according to the 10th edition of the International Classification of Diseases (ICD-10). Generic drugs were coded according to the Korean National Code System (5).

Study Population

NTM-PD was defined by ICD-10 diagnosis codes of A31.0, A31.8, and A31.9; GERD was defined by ≥2 claims under the ICD-10 code K21 and proton pump inhibitors prescribed for ≥2 weeks (6). We included 6,589 patients with NTM-PD from January 2009 to December 2017 using the ICD-10 code, of which 1,407 patients had GERD. The Institutional Review Board of Chungbuk National University Hospital approved the study and waived the requirement for informed consent because the HIRA-NPS data were deidentified (application no. CBNUH 2021-03-020).

Outcomes

Respiratory-related healthcare use was defined as healthcare use under the ICD-10 codes of respiratory diseases (J00–J99). We compared healthcare use (outpatient department [OPD] visits, emergency room [ER] visits, or hospitalizations), medical costs, and in-hospital mortality in NTM-PD patients with GERD to those in patients without GERD. The medical cost consists of expenses related to diagnostic tests, procedures, and treatments covered by the National Health Insurance (7).

Covariables

Comorbidities were also defined using ICD-10 codes. Pulmonary comorbidities were defined as chronic obstructive pulmonary disease (COPD; J42–J44, except J43.0 [unilateral emphysema]), asthma (J45–J46), bronchiectasis (J47, excluding E84 [cystic

TABLE 1 | Characteristics of study population.

	Total (N = 6,589)	NTM-PD with GERD (n = 1,407)	NTM-PD without GERD (n = 5,182)	P-value
Age, years				<0.001
20–29	499 (7.6)	25 (1.8)	474 (9.2)	
30–39	877 (13.3)	96 (6.8)	781 (15.1)	
40–49	789 (12.0)	125 (8.9)	664 (12.8)	
50–59	1,360 (20.5)	311 (22.1)	1,049 (20.1)	
60–69	1,407 (21.4)	403 (28.6)	1,004 (19.4)	
≥70	1,657 (25.2)	447 (31.8)	1,210 (23.4)	
Sex				0.614
Male	2,458 (37.3)	533 (37.9)	1,925 (37.2)	
Female	4,131 (62.7)	874 (62.1)	3,257 (62.8)	
Type of insurance				<0.001
Health insurance	6,283 (95.3)	1,302 (92.5)	4,981 (96.2)	
Medical aid	301 (4.6)	102 (7.3)	199 (3.8)	
Veteran status	5 (0.1)	3 (0.2)	2 (0.0)	
Comorbidities				
COPD	1,720 (26.1)	528 (37.5)	1,192 (23.0)	<0.001
Asthma	1,909 (29.0)	575 (40.9)	1,334 (25.7)	<0.001
Bronchiectasis	1,653 (25.1)	406 (28.9)	1,247 (24.1)	<0.001
Cerebrovascular disease	626 (9.5)	221 (15.7)	405 (7.8)	<0.001
Hypertension	2,051 (31.1)	620 (44.1)	1,431 (27.6)	<0.001
Diabetes mellitus	1,464 (22.2)	478 (34.0)	986 (19.0)	<0.001
Connective tissue disease	405 (6.2)	173 (12.3)	232 (4.5)	<0.001
Charlson comorbidity index				<0.001
0–1	2,952 (44.8)	307 (21.8)	2,645 (51.0)	
≥2	3,637 (55.2)	1,100 (78.2)	2,537 (49.0)	

Data are presented as numbers (percentages).
NTM-PD, non-tuberculous mycobacterial pulmonary disease; GERD, gastroesophageal reflux disease; COPD, chronic obstructive pulmonary disease.

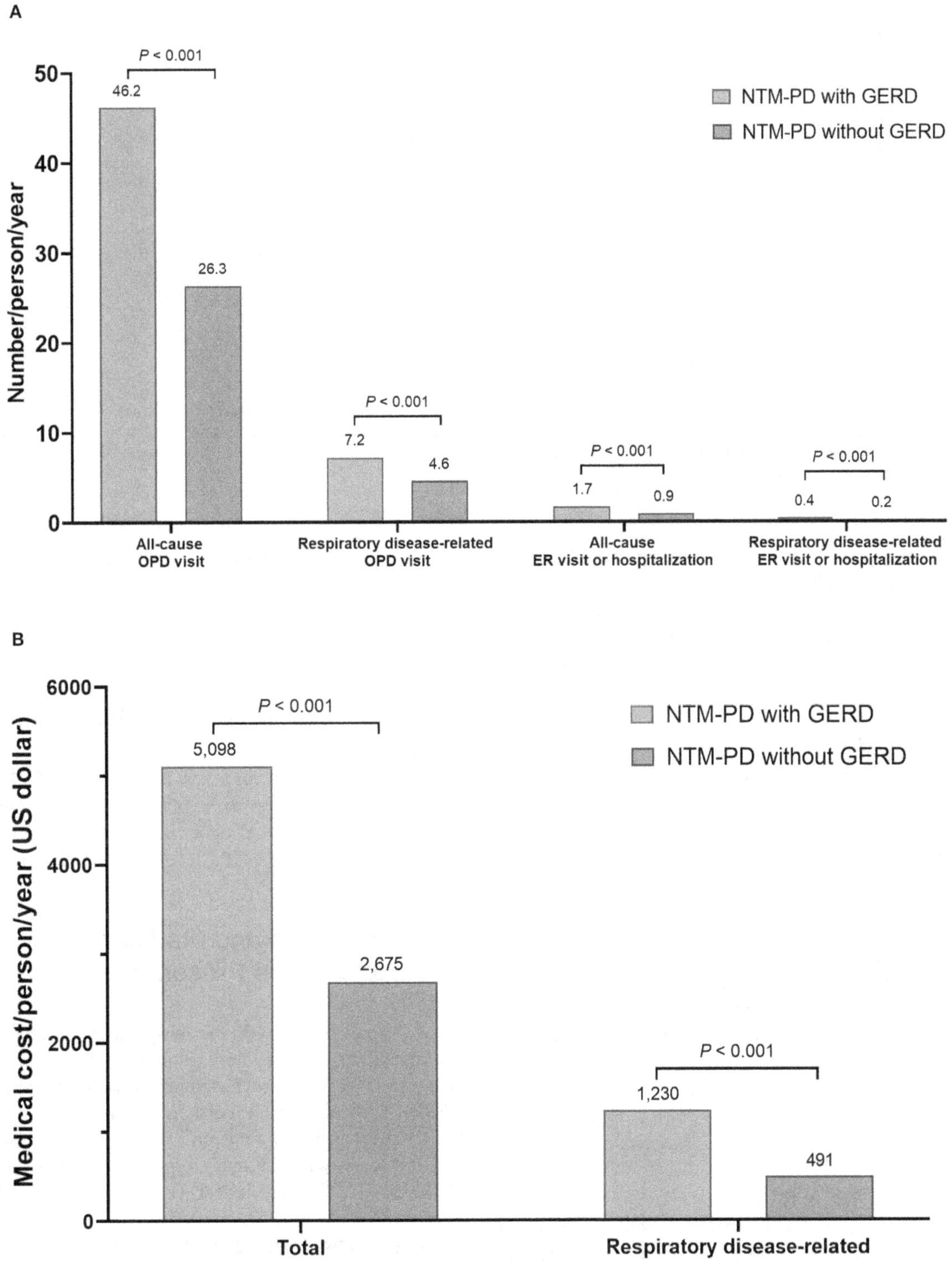

FIGURE 1 | Disease burden of GERD in patients with NTM-PD: **(A)** healthcare use of patients with NTM-PD according to presence or absence of GERD (number of events/person/year), and **(B)** medical costs of patients with NTM-PD according to presence or absence of GERD (medical cost/person/year, unit US dollar). NTM-PD, non-tuberculous mycobacterial pulmonary disease; GERD, gastroesophageal reflux disease; OPD, outpatient department; ER, emergency room.

fibrosis] or Q33.4, Q89.3 [congenital bronchiectasis]), pulmonary tuberculosis (TB; A15–19), and lung cancer (C33–C34). Extrapulmonary comorbidities were defined as cerebrovascular disease (G45–G46, I60–I69, and H34.0), hypertension (I10–I15), angina or myocardial infarction (MI; I20, I21, I22, and I25.2), congestive heart failure (I43, I50, I09.9, I11.0, I25.5, I13.0, I13.2,

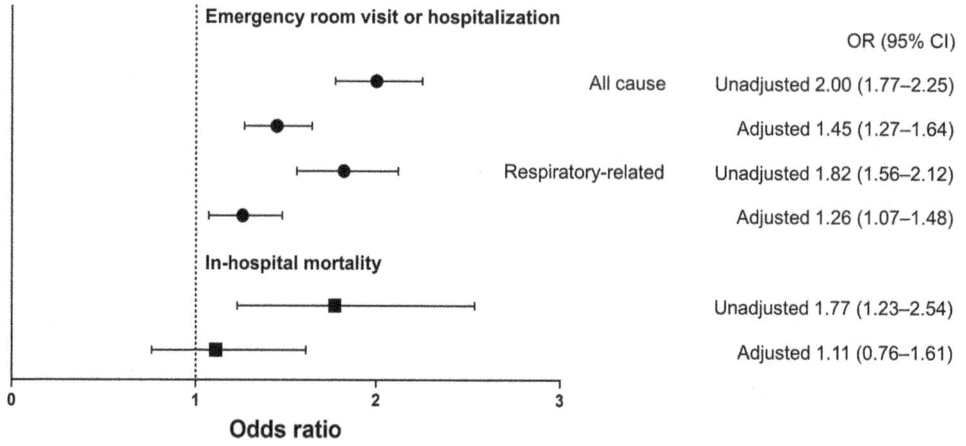

FIGURE 2 | Odds ratio and 95% confidence interval for emergency room visits, hospitalization, and in-hospital mortality in NTM-PD patients with GERD relative to those without GERD. The multivariable model was adjusted for age, sex, type of insurance (health insurance, medical aid, and veteran status), bronchiectasis, and Charlson comorbidity index (0–1 and 2). NTM-PD, non-tuberculous mycobacterial pulmonary disease; GERD, gastroesophageal reflux disease; ER, emergency room; OR, odds ratio; CI, confidence interval.

I42.0, I42.5–I42.9, and P29.0), inflammatory bowel disease (K50–K51), diabetes mellitus (E10–E14), chronic kidney disease (N18), and connective tissue disease (M05, M06, M315, M32, M33, M34, M351, M353, and M360) (5, 8). The Charlson comorbidity index (CCI) was calculated using a modified version consisting of 17 comorbidities (9).

Statistical Analysis

We calculated the age-adjusted prevalence of GERD among patients with NTM-PD by dividing the number of events by 1,000 person-years. All categorized variables were compared using Pearson's chi-squared test. To compare the medical use of NTM-PD patients with and without GERD, logistic regression analysis was used to determine the odds ratio (OR) for healthcare use (ER visits or hospitalizations) and in-hospital mortality in NTM-PD patients with GERD relative to those without GERD. A multivariable model was adjusted for age, sex, type of insurance (health insurance, medical aid, and veteran status), bronchiectasis, and CCI (0–1 and ≥2). All statistical analyses were performed with SAS 9.4 (SAS Institute, Cary, NC, USA). Statistical significance was set at $P < 0.05$.

RESULTS

Baseline Characteristics

The baseline characteristics of the patients are summarized in **Table 1**. The prevalence of NTM-PD in patients with GERD was significantly higher in older age groups (≥60 years [60.4 vs. 42.8%], $P < 0.001$). However, there was no difference in the sex ratio (~62% of the cases were female). The proportion of patients who received medical aid was higher in the NTM-PD with GERD group than in those without GERD (7.3 vs. 3.8%, $P < 0.001$). Analysis of comorbidities indicated that the rates of asthma (40.9 vs. 25.7%), chronic obstructive pulmonary disease (37.5 vs. 23.0%), bronchiectasis (28.9 vs. 24.1%), hypertension (44.1 vs. 27.6%), diabetes mellitus (34.0 vs. 19.0%), cerebrovascular disease (15.7 vs. 7.8%), connective tissue disease (12.3 vs. 4.5%), and CCI ≥ 2 (78.2 vs. 49.0%) were significantly higher in NTM-PD patients with GERD than in those without GERD ($P < 0.001$ for all).

Prevalence of GERD in Patients With NTM-PD

Of the 6,589 patients with NTM-PD, 1,407 had GERD. During the study period, the prevalence of GERD in patients with NTM-PD was 21.4%, which was higher than that in patients aged ≥20 years (7.4%) in the HIRA-NPS database. The prevalence of GERD in patients with NTM-PD increased with age.

Healthcare Use and Medical Costs According to the Presence or Absence of GERD

NTM-PD patients with GERD had significantly higher healthcare use, including all-cause and respiratory disease-specific OPD visits and ER visits or hospitalizations, than those without GERD ($P < 0.001$ for all). Furthermore, NTM-PD patients with GERD spent a higher total on medical costs (5,098 vs. 2,675 USD/person/year), including respiratory disease-related costs (1,230 vs. 491 USD/person/year) ($P < 0.001$ for both) (**Figure 1**).

Association Between GERD and Increased Healthcare Use

GERD was independently associated with more ER visits or hospitalizations in patients with NTM-PD: all-cause (adjusted OR, 1.45; 95% confidence interval [CI], 1.27–1.64) and respiratory disease-related (adjusted OR, 1.26; 95% CI, 1.07–1.48). However, GERD was not significantly associated with in-hospital mortality (adjusted OR 1.11, 95% CI, 0.76–1.61) (**Figure 2**).

DISCUSSION

To our knowledge, this study is the first to evaluate the impact of GERD on the estimated disease burden based on healthcare use, medical costs, and in-hospital mortality in patients with NTM-PD. NTM-PD patients with GERD had significantly higher healthcare use and medical costs than those without GERD; however, there were no significant intergroup differences in in-hospital mortality.

GERD is prevalent in patients with NTM-PD, affecting up to 44% of patients (3, 4). In agreement with previous reports, 21% of patients with NTM-PD had GERD, which was significantly higher than the prevalence of GERD (7%) in the overall population aged ≥20 years during the study period. GERD has been recognized not only as an underlying disease for the occurrence of NTM-PD (10) but also as an important comorbidity that can influence the symptoms and severity of the disease (3, 10). In this regard, this study revealed NTM-PD patients with GERD are hampered by greater healthcare use and higher medical costs, which denote a significant disease burden, compared to those without GERD.

Gastro-esophageal refluxate can aggravate respiratory disease by either stimulating the sensitized esophageal-bronchial neuronal pathway or by microaspiration, which involves aspiration into the airway (11). Conversely, it has been suggested that progression of chronic lung disease can lead to deterioration of GERD (12). Consequently, it can be postulated that the interaction between the two diseases may further deteriorate the health of patients with NTM-PD and GERD. Considering the potential bidirectional process between reflux disease and chronic respiratory disease (13), appropriate treatment of GERD may lead to decreased disease burden and improvement in overall treatment outcomes in patients with NTM-PD. However, since acid reduction cannot reduce refluxate other than acid, there is a possibility that non-acid refluxate can still cause lung damage. Thus, it should be acknowledged that it is challenging to reduce reflux itself.

Our study has several strengths that support our hypothesis and was based on a large, nationally representative database. However, there are some limitations to this study. First, we used a cross-sectional study design; thus, long-term mortality was not fully evaluated based on the presence or absence of GERD. Second, there is a possibility of misclassification because we used the ICD-10 codes to define NTM-PD and GERD. Therefore, a large prospective cohort study is needed to clarify the role of GERD in NTM-PD.

In conclusion, GERD significantly increased healthcare use and medical costs in patients with NTM-PD. Thus, appropriate diagnostic and management plans to reduce the GERD-associated disease burden would bring significant improvements to patients with NTM-PD.

AUTHOR CONTRIBUTIONS

HL and HC were responsible for the conception and design of the study. TK, JHY, BY, JR, CKY, YK, JWS, HL, and HC undertook the analysis and interpretation of the data. TK, JHY, BY, HL, and HC drafted the manuscript. All authors made a critical revision of the manuscript, and read and approved the final manuscript.

REFERENCES

1. Prevots DR, Marras TK. Epidemiology of human pulmonary infection with non-tuberculous mycobacteria: a review. *Clin Chest Med.* (2015) 36:13–34. doi: 10.1016/j.ccm.2014.10.002
2. Diel R, Jacob J, Lampenius N, Loebinger M, Nienhaus A, Rabe KF, et al. Burden of non-tuberculous mycobacterial pulmonary disease in Germany. *Eur Respir J.* (2017) 49:2016. doi: 10.1183/13993003.02109-2016
3. Koh WJ, Lee JH, Kwon YS, Lee KS, Suh GY, Chung MP, et al. Prevalence of gastroesophageal reflux disease in patients with non-tuberculous mycobacterial lung disease. *Chest.* (2007) 131:1825–30. doi: 10.1378/chest.06-2280
4. Thomson RM, Armstrong JG, Looke DF. Gastroesophageal reflux disease, acid suppression, and Mycobacterium avium complex pulmonary disease. *Chest.* (2007) 131:1166–72. doi: 10.1378/chest.06-1906
5. Choi H, Yang B, Nam H, Kyoung DS, Sim YS, Park HY, et al. Population-based prevalence of bronchiectasis and associated comorbidities in South Korea. *Eur Respir J.* (2019) 54:1900194. doi: 10.1183/13993003.00194-2019
6. Kim SY, Min C, Oh DJ, Choi HG. Bidirectional association between GERD and asthma: two longitudinal follow-up studies using a national sample cohort. *J Allergy Clin Immunol Pract.* (2020) 8:1005–13. doi: 10.1016/j.jaip.2019.10.043
7. Kim JA, Yoon S, Kim LY, Kim DS. Towards Actualizing the value potential of Korea health insurance review and assessment (HIRA) data as a resource for health research: strengths, limitations, applications, and strategies for optimal use of HIRA data. *J Korean Med Sci.* (2017) 32:718–28. doi: 10.3346/jkms.2017.32.5.718
8. Choi H, Han K, Yang B, Shin DW, Sohn JW, Lee H. Female reproductive factors and incidence of non-tuberculous mycobacterial pulmonary disease among postmenopausal women in Korea. *Clin Infect Dis.* (2022). doi: 10.1093/cid/ciac134
9. Brusselaers N, Lagergren J. The charlson comorbidity index in registry-based research. *Methods Inf Med.* (2017) 56:401–6. doi: 10.3414/ME17-01-0051
10. Griffith DE, Girard WM, Wallace RJ Jr. Clinical features of pulmonary disease caused by rapidly growing mycobacteria An analysis of 154 patients. *Am Rev Respir Dis.* (1993) 147:1271–8. doi: 10.1164/ajrccm/147.5.1271
11. Houghton LA, Lee AS, Badri H, DeVault KR, Smith JA. Respiratory disease and the oesophagus: reflux, reflexes, and microaspiration. *Nat Rev Gastroenterol Hepatol.* (2016) 13:445–60. doi: 10.1038/nrgastro.2016.91
12. Morehead RS. Gastro-oesophageal reflux disease and non-asthma lung disease. *Eur Respir Rev.* (2009) 18:233–43. doi: 10.1183/09059180.00002509
13. McDonnell MJ, Hunt EB, Ward C, Pearson JP, O'Toole D, Laffey JG, et al. Current therapies for gastro-esophageal reflux in the setting of chronic lung disease: state of the art review. *ERJ Open Res.* (2020) 6:190. doi: 10.1183/23120541.00190-2019

9

PEP-sNASP Peptide Alleviates LPS-Induced Acute Lung Injury Through the TLR4/TRAF6 Axis

Yu-Chih Wu [1†], Sung-Po Hsu [2,3†], Meng-Chun Hu [4], Yu-Ting Lan [4], Edward T. H. Yeh [5,6] and Feng-Ming Yang [1]*

[1] School of Respiratory Therapy, College of Medicine, Taipei Medical University, Taipei, Taiwan, [2] Department of Physiology, School of Medicine, College of Medicine, Taipei Medical University, Taipei, Taiwan, [3] Graduate Institute of Medical Sciences, College of Medicine, Taipei Medical University, Taipei, Taiwan, [4] Graduate Institute of Physiology, National Taiwan University College of Medicine, Taipei, Taiwan, [5] Department of Internal Medicine, University of Arkansas for Medical Sciences, Little Rock, AK, United States, [6] Winthrop P. Rockefeller Cancer Institute, University of Arkansas for Medical Sciences, Little Rock, AK, United States

***Correspondence:**
Feng-Ming Yang
fmyang1229@tmu.edu.tw

† These authors have contributed equally to this work and share first authorship

Specialty section:

Acute lung injury (ALI) is a severe inflammatory lung disease associated with macrophages. Somatic nuclear autoantigenic sperm protein (sNASP) is a negative regulator of Toll-like receptor (TLR) signaling that targets tumor necrosis factor (TNF) receptor-associated factor 6 (TRAF6) in macrophages, which is required to maintain homeostasis of the innate immune response. In the present study, we generated a cell permeable PEP-sNASP peptide using the sNASP protein N-terminal domain, and examined its potential therapeutic effect in a mouse model of ALI induced by the intranasal administration of lipopolysaccharide (LPS) and elucidated the underlying molecular mechanisms in RAW 264.7 cells. *In vivo*, PEP-sNASP peptide treatment markedly ameliorated pathological injury, reduced the wet/dry (W/D) weight ratio of the lungs and the production of proinflammatory cytokines (interleukin (IL)-1β, IL-6, and TNF-α). *In vitro*, we demonstrated that when the PEP-sNASP peptide was transduced into RAW 264.7 cells, it bound to TRAF6, which markedly decreased LPS-induced proinflammatory cytokines by inhibiting TRAF6 autoubiquitination, nuclear factor (NF)-κB activation, reactive oxygen species (ROS) and cellular nitric oxide (NO) levels. Furthermore, the PEP-sNASP peptide also inhibited NLR family pyrin domain containing 3 (NLRP3) inflammasome activation. Our results therefore suggest that the PEP-sNASP may provide a potential protein therapy against oxidative stress and pulmonary inflammation *via* selective TRAF6 signaling.

Keywords: TLR4, TRAF6, inflammation, acute lung injury, NASP

INTRODUCTION

Acute lung injury (ALI) and its severe form of acute respiratory distress syndrome (ARDS) were first described in 1967 (1) and are both known to be common causes of respiratory failure in critically ill patients (2). Pathologically, ALI is often characterized by an uncontrolled acute pulmonary inflammatory response, decreased lung compliance, and impaired gas exchange, ultimately leading to various clinical disorders, such as pneumonia, pulmonary edema, and sepsis (3–5). Despite advances in understanding of the pathogenesis and treatment of this disease, the morbidity and mortality from ALI/ARDS remain high. It was estimated that the overall mortality rate of ALI/ARDS range 38.5~41.1%, which significantly depends on various comorbidities (5–7). A study conducted in Taiwan found that the in-hospital mortality rate increasing from 33.5 to 68.2% was correlated with patients' ages (8). Currently, the treatments of ALI/ARDS available in clinical practice are still limited, which emphasizes the urgent need for the development of novel therapeutic strategies to improve clinical outcomes.

Various inflammation are transmitted through a family of receptors of the innate immune system, known as Toll-like receptors (TLRs), which are known to play essential roles in the pathogenesis of pulmonary inflammation (9–12). TLR4 is the dominant mammalian receptor for the microbial product, lipopolysaccharide (LPS), a major biologically active component of gram-negative bacterial cell walls, and which is widely used to induce ALI models that are similar to pathological features of ALI in humans by triggering excessive inflammatory mediators (13–15). Our previous work showed that the somatic nuclear autoantigenic sperm protein (sNASP) is a negative regulator of the TLR4-mediated innate immune response (16, 17). In unstimulated cells, it binds tumor necrosis factor (TNF) receptor-associated factor 6 (TRAF6) to avoid excessive inflammation and maintain homeostasis of the innate immune response. Once TLR4 binds to its ligands, sNASP is phosphorylated and released from TRAF6, which ultimately stimulates expressions of proinflammatory cytokines, such as interleukin (IL)-6 and TNF-α. In addition, using a cecal ligation and puncture (CLP)-induced sepsis model with dominant-negative sNASP mutant mice, these mutant mice were more susceptible to bacterial infection due to ineffective clearance of bacteria in the lungs after CLP, indicating that the sNASP may be involved in pathological changes in lung inflammation. Those results suggested that sNASP functions as a negative regulator of innate immunity and may contribute to its protective effects against ALI and underling mechanisms.

PEP-1 is a 21-residue peptide carrier that can efficiently transduce proteins into various cells and tissues (18, 19). It consists of three domains: (1) a hydrophobic tryptophan-rich motif (KETWWETWWTEW) for targeting cell membranes, (2) a spacer (SQP), and (3) a hydrophilic lysine-rich domain (KKKRKV) for intracellular delivery and peptide solubility. Recently, it was shown that PEP fusion proteins successfully protected against various diseases including lung inflammation and neuronal diseases (20–22). In this study, we designed a PEP-NASP fusion protein to investigate whether the transduced PEP-NASP protects cells against LPS-induced inflammation. We found that PEP-NASP was efficiently transduced into RAW 264.7 cells through a membrane barrier, and that the transduced PEP-NASP reduced LPS-induced proinflammatory cytokines and nitric oxide (NO) production as well as NLR family pyrin domain containing 3 (NLRP3) inflammasome activation. *In vivo*, administration of the PEP-NASP markedly attenuated LPS-induced lung injury, with significant reductions in neutrophil infiltration, myeloperoxidase (MPO) activity, and bronchoalveolar lavage fluid (BALF) protein content. Therefore, we suggest that the PEP-NASP fusion protein might be useful as a potential therapeutic agent against ALI.

MATERIALS AND METHODS

Mice and LPS-Induced ALI Model

Pathogen-free, 8-week-old male C57BL/6 mice were purchased from the National Laboratory Animal Center (Taipei, Taiwan). Mice were housed in a pathogen-free animal facility at Taipei Medical University (Taipei, Taiwan). Animal protocols described in this study were approved by the animal and ethics review committee of the Laboratory Animal Center at Taipei Medical University.

ALI was induced by intranasal (i.n.) instillation of LPS [5 mg/kg body weight (BW)] as described previously (23, 24). LPS was obtained from Sigma-Aldrich (St. Louis, MO, USA). Forty mice were randomly divided into four groups: sham+NASP, sham+PEP-NASP, LPS+NASP, and LPS+PEP-NASP groups. Mice in the sham and LPS groups received i.n. instillation of phosphate-buffered saline (PBS) and LPS (5 mg/kg), respectively, while mice in the LPS+NASP and LPS+PEP-NASP groups received an i.n. injection of NASP or PEP-NASP (0.1 mg/kg) at 1 h before LPS inhalation. The experiment was terminated at 24 h after LPS inhalation, after which lung tissues and BALF were harvested and collected.

Preparation of the PEP-NASP

The His-PEP-NASP (HHHHHHKETWWETWWTEWSQP KKKRKVMAMESTATAAVAAELVSADKIEDVPAPSTSA) and control His-NASP (HHHHHHMAMESTATAAVAAELVSADKI EDVPAPSTSA) fusion proteins were synthesized by Biotools (Taipei, Taiwan). All peptides were dissolved in 0.1% DMSO and stored at −80°C.

Cell Culture and Transduction of the PEP-NASP

The mouse macrophage RAW 264.7 cell line (ATCC TIB-71, American Type Culture Collection, Manassas, VA, USA) and embryonic kidney epithelial HEK293 cell line (ATCC CRL-1573) were both cultured in Dulbecco's modified Eagle medium (DMEM) supplemented with 10% fetal bovine serum (FBS), and 1% penicillin and streptomycin at 37°C and 5% CO_2 in air as previously described (16).

To determine the dose-dependent transduction ability of the PEP-NASP, cells were grown to 75% confluency for 24 h, and then various concentrations (0.1 ~ 0.4 μM) of the PEP-NASP were added to the culture medium for 1 h at 37 °C. For time-dependent transduction, cells were treated with 0.4 μM of the PEP-NASP for 10 ~6 0 min. To determine the intracellular stability of the transduced PEP-NASP, cells were treated with 0.4 μM PEP-NASP for 1 h and washed with fresh medium to remove fusion proteins that had not been transduced into cells. Cells were further incubated for 60 h.

Plasmids and Transfection

Plasmids encoding Flag-TRAF6 and green fluorescent protein (GFP)-sNASP were previously described (16). After the pGFP-sNASP plasmid had been digested with SbfI/ApaI or EcoNI/ApaI, the ends were blunted with Klenow and then self-ligated to generate pGFP-sNASP 1-233 (dTRP3) and pGFP-sNASP 1-348 (sNLS). The pGFP-sNASP 1-31 (dTRP1/2/3), 1-93 (dTRP2/3), and 94-449 (dTRP1) plasmids were constructed by polymerase chain reaction (PCR) amplification using relevant primers incorporating a KpnI site and an ApaI site, and the resulting fragment was inserted into the KpnI/ApaI-digested pGFP-sNASP. Transfection of HEK293 and RAW 264.7 cells was performed using Lipofectamine 3000 (L3000015, Invitrogen, USA) according to the manufacturer's protocol.

Immunoprecipitation (IP) and Western Blotting

Harvested cells were subjected to IP, lysates were resolved on sodium dodecylsulfate polyacrylamide gel electrophoresis (SDS-PAGE), and a Western blot analysis was performed as previously described (16, 25). Signals were detected using the Trident femto Western horseradish peroxidase (HRP) substrate (GTX14698, GeneTex, Taiwan). Images were captured and the density of the bands was measured using the UVP BioSpectrum 815 (Jena, Germany). The detected bands were quantitated using ImageJ image analytical software. Antibodies used for the immunoblot analysis were mouse anti-NASP (SC-161915, Santa Cruz Biotechnology, Santa Cruz, CA, USA), mouse anti-TRAF6 (SC-7221, Santa Cruz), mouse anti-ubiquitin (SC-8017, Santa Cruz), mouse anti-β-actin (A1544, Sigma-Aldrich, St. Louis, MO, USA), mouse anti-phospho-TAK1 (4531, Cell Signaling, USA), mouse anti-TAK1 (4505, Cell Signaling), mouse anti-phospho-p38 mitogen-activated protein kinase (MAPK) (9211, Cell Signaling), anti-p38 MAPK (9212, Cell Signaling), mouse anti-phospho-c-Jun N-terminal kinase (JNK) (4671, Cell Signaling), mouse anti-JNK (9252, Cell Signaling), mouse anti-GFP (632281, Clontech, USA), mouse anti-COS-2 (SC-19999, Santa Cruz), mouse anti-His (SC-8036, Santa Cruz), mouse anti-Flag (F1804, Sigma-Aldrich), rabbit anti-inducible NO synthase (iNOS) (2982, Cell Signaling), rabbit anti-NLRP3 (15101, Cell Signaling), rabbit anti-capase-1 (GTX11701, GeneTex), and rabbit anti-ASC (67824, Cell Signaling). Antibodies were diluted according to the manufacturers' instructions.

RNA Isolation and Real-Time Quantitative (q)PCR

RNA was extracted from cells using the Toolsmart RNA extractor (TB-DPT-BD24, Biotools), and then reverse-transcribed into complementary (c)DNA with a magic RT cDNA synthesis kit (Bio-Genesis Technologies, Taipei, Taiwan) according to the manufacturer's instructions. qPCRs were performed using TaqMan Gene Expression Master Mix (4369016, Thermo Fisher Scientific, Waltham, MA, USA) in an StepOnePlusTM machine (Thermo Fisher Scientific, Waltham, MA, USA). The TaqMan Gene Expression Assay used as follows: *IL-6* (Mm00446190_m1), *TNF-α* (Mm00443260_g1), and *IL-1β* (Mm00434228_m1, was all from Thermo Fisher Scientific, Waltham, MA, USA). Results were normalized to the expression of the gene encoding 18s and were quantified by the change-in-threshold method (ΔΔCT).

Enzyme-Linked Immunosorbent Assay (ELISA)

Concentrations of cytokines in bronchoalveolar lavage fluid (BALF) and cell culture supernatants were measured using Mouse Ready-Set-Go ELISA for IL-6 (88-7064), TNF-α (88-7324), and IL-1β (88-7013) purchased from BioLegend (San Diego, CA, USA), according to the manufacturer's protocol.

Luciferase Assays

Luciferase reporter assays were conducted according to our previous publication (26). RAW 264.7 cells were subcultured in 24-well tissue culture plates and transfected with NF-κB luciferase and pRL-TK Renilla luciferase. After 24 h, cells were transduced with the NASP or PEP-NASP 1 h before LPS stimulation, and then cells were lysed with lysis buffer, and firefly luciferase, and Renilla luciferase activities were determined using the Dual-Glo Luciferase Assay System (E2920, Promega, Madison, WI, USA).

Immunofluorescence (IF) Staining

IF staining was conducted as described previously (27). Cells were maintained on 12-mm glass slides for 24 h and then were stimulated with 1 μg/mL LPS for 30 min in the presence of the NASP or PEP-NASP (0.4 μM) added 1 h before stimulation. Then cells were fixed with 4% paraformaldehyde for 10 min and blocked with Blocking One Histo (06349-64, Nacalai Tesque, Kyoto, Japan) for 1 h, followed by incubation with rabbit anti-NF-κB p65 Alexa Fluor 594 (SC-8008 AF594, Santa Cruz) and mouse anti-His antibodies (34650, Qiagen, USA) overnight at 4 °C. After being washed, cells were incubated with an FITC-labeled goat anti-mouse immunoglobulin G (IgG) antibody for 1 h. Nuclear DNA was stained with DAPI for 10 min. Images were captured using confocal microscopy on a Leica TCS SP5 (Wetzlar, Germany).

Histological Analysis

Hematoxylin and eosin (H&E) staining of paraffin-embedded lung tissue sections was performed to determine cellular infiltration. Lung tissues were fixed with 10% buffered formalin for 24 h, embedded in paraffin, and sectioned at 4-μm thickness. After deparaffinization and dehydration, sections were stained with H&E and were observed with an Echo Revolve Fluorescence Microscope (San Diego, CA, USA).

Lung Wet/Dry (W/D) Ratio

The left lung was harvested and weighed to obtain the wet weight. The lung was then placed into a drying oven at 80°C for 48 h to obtain the dry weight. The W/D weight ratio was calculated to evaluate the degree of lung edema.

Myeloperoxidase (MPO) Activity Assay

Lung tissues were homogenized with MPO assay buffer after collection and then centrifuged at 13,000 g for 10 min at 4°C. The supernatant was assayed for MPO activity according to the manufacturer's instructions (K744-100, Biovision, USA). MPO activity was One unit of MPO activity was defined as the quantity of enzyme that converted 1 μmol hydrogen peroxide to water each minute at 37°C. MPO activity is expressed as units per gram (U/g) wet weight.

Bronchoalveolar Lavage Fluid (BALF) Collection and Analysis

BALF was harvested according to a previous description (28). Briefly, mice were euthanized, and a catheter was installed in the open trachea. Then, 0.8 ml of ice-cold PBS was instilled into the lungs three times, and the recovered BALF was centrifuged at 450 ×*g* for 10 min. The cell pellet was used to count numbers of total cells, macrophages, and neutrophils counted with a hemocytometer and Wright-Giemsa staining (K1438-30, Biovision, USA).

Measurement of Reactive Oxygen Species (ROS) and Glutathione (GSH) Level

ROS and GSH level were estimated by using Fluorometric Intracellular ROS Kit (MAK144, Sigma-Aldrich, St. Louis, MO, USA) and Reduced Glutathione (GSH) Assay Kit (MAK364, Sigma-Aldrich, St. Louis, MO, USA), respectively, according to the manufacturer's instructions. Fluorescence intensity was measured using a SpectraMax® i3x microplate reader (Molecular Devices, San Jose, CA, USA).

Cell Viability Determination

The Cell Proliferation Kit I (MTT) (11465007001, Merck, USA) was used to detect cell viability. According to the manufacturer's instructions, cells were cultured onto a 96-well plate under the indicated conditions. At the indicated time, 10 μl of MTT labeling reagent were added into each well and incubated at 37°C for 4 h. Then 100 μl of Solubilization solution was added to dissolve the purple formazan crystals. Absorbance at wavelength 570 nm was detected with a SpectraMax® i3x microplate reader (Molecular Devices, San Jose, CA, USA).

Statistical Analysis

GraphPad Prism 6 software was used for all statistical analyses by Student's *t*-test for two groups or a one-way analysis of variance (ANOVA) for three or more groups. Values of $p < 0.05$ were considered statistically significant.

RESULTS

N-Terminal Region of sNASP Physically Interacts With TRAF6

In our previous publication, sNASP was identified as a TRAF6-binding protein (16). The sNASP protein has three tetratricopeptide repeat (TPR) motifs (amino acids 43 ~ 76, 203 ~ 236, and 245 ~ 278), a region of coiled-coil domains (CCDs), and a nuclear localization sequence (NLS; amino acids 379 ~ 397) (29). To identify specific regions of the sNASP that interacts with TRAF6, various sNASP deletion mutants were generated with GFP-tagged fusion proteins (**Figure 1A**). Reciprocal IP and Western blot analyses confirmed that sNASP binds to TRAF6 (**Figures 1B,C** and **Supplementary Figure 1**). The N-terminal region (amino acids 1 ~ 31) of sNASP, which contains the ring and zinc fingers, was able to bind to TRAF6. Deletion of the N-terminal sNASP abolished the association with TRAF6 (**Figures 1B,C** and **Supplementary Figure 1**). Among sNASP deletion mutants, TRAF6 bound to the dTRP1/2/3 (amino acids 1 ~ 31), dTRP2/3 (amino acids 1 ~ 93), dTRP3 (amino acids 1 ~ 233), and dNLS (amino acids 1 ~ 348) mutants but not to dTRP1 (amino acids 94 ~ 449), indicating that the minimal N-terminal of sNASP containing residues 1 ~ 31 is required for TRAF6 interactions.

Transduction of the PEP-NASP Into RAW 264.7 Cells

TRAF6 is a crucial mediator that transmits intracellular signals through TLRs to a wide range of immunostimulatory cytokines and chemokines against invading microorganisms (9, 30, 31). In this study, sNASP residues 1 ~ 31 fused with PEP-1 (PEP-NASP) were synthesized to determine whether the increase in sNASP by protein transduction had a negative regulatory effect on the LPS-induced inflammatory response in the mouse macrophage RAW 264.7 cell line.

To evaluate the transduction ability of the PEP-NASP, RAW 264.7 cells were incubated with various concentrations (0.1 ~ 0.4 μM, 1 h) of the PEP-NASP and for various times (10 ~ 60 min, 0.4 μM). Then protein transduction was analyzed by Western blotting with an anti-His antibody. As shown in **Figures 2A,B**, the PEP-NASP was successfully transduced into RAW 264.7 cells in dose- and time-dependent manners, whereas the control NASP lacking the PEP-1 domain was not transduced into cells. The intracellular concentration of the transduced PEP-NASP in cells was detected within 10 min and had gradually increased by 60 min (**Figure 2B**). Since stability is an important factor in protein therapy, we examined the stability of the transduced PEP-NASP at various time periods. Western blotting revealed that the transduced PEP-NASP in RAW 264.7 remained stable until 36 h after treatment, subsequently decomposing over time (**Figure 2C**). The viability of RAW 264.7 cells wasn't affected when treated with PEP-NASP, suggesting that PEP-NASP did not cause cytotoxicity in cells (**Supplementary Figure 2**). In addition, cellular localization of the transduced PEP-NASP in cells was determined by IF staining. PEP-1-NASP fluorescence was distributed in both the nucleus and cytoplasm, but no fluorescent signal was observed in control NASP-transduced cells (**Figure 2D**). These results demonstrated that the PEP-NASP was efficiently transduced into cells and persisted for 36 h after transduction.

Transduced PEP-NASP Inhibits the LPS-Induced Inflammatory Response Through TRAF6

Our previous report showed that sNASP binds to TRAF6 and inhibits TRAF6 autoubiquitination and its downstream signaling (16); we wanted to evaluate whether the transduced PEP-NASP would affect TRAF6 autoubiquitination following LPS stimulation. Results indicated that transduction of the PEP-NASP, but not the control NASP, diminished LPS-induced TRAF6 autoubiquitination in RAW 264.7 cells (**Figure 3A**). Next, we investigated whether the PEP-NASP could interact

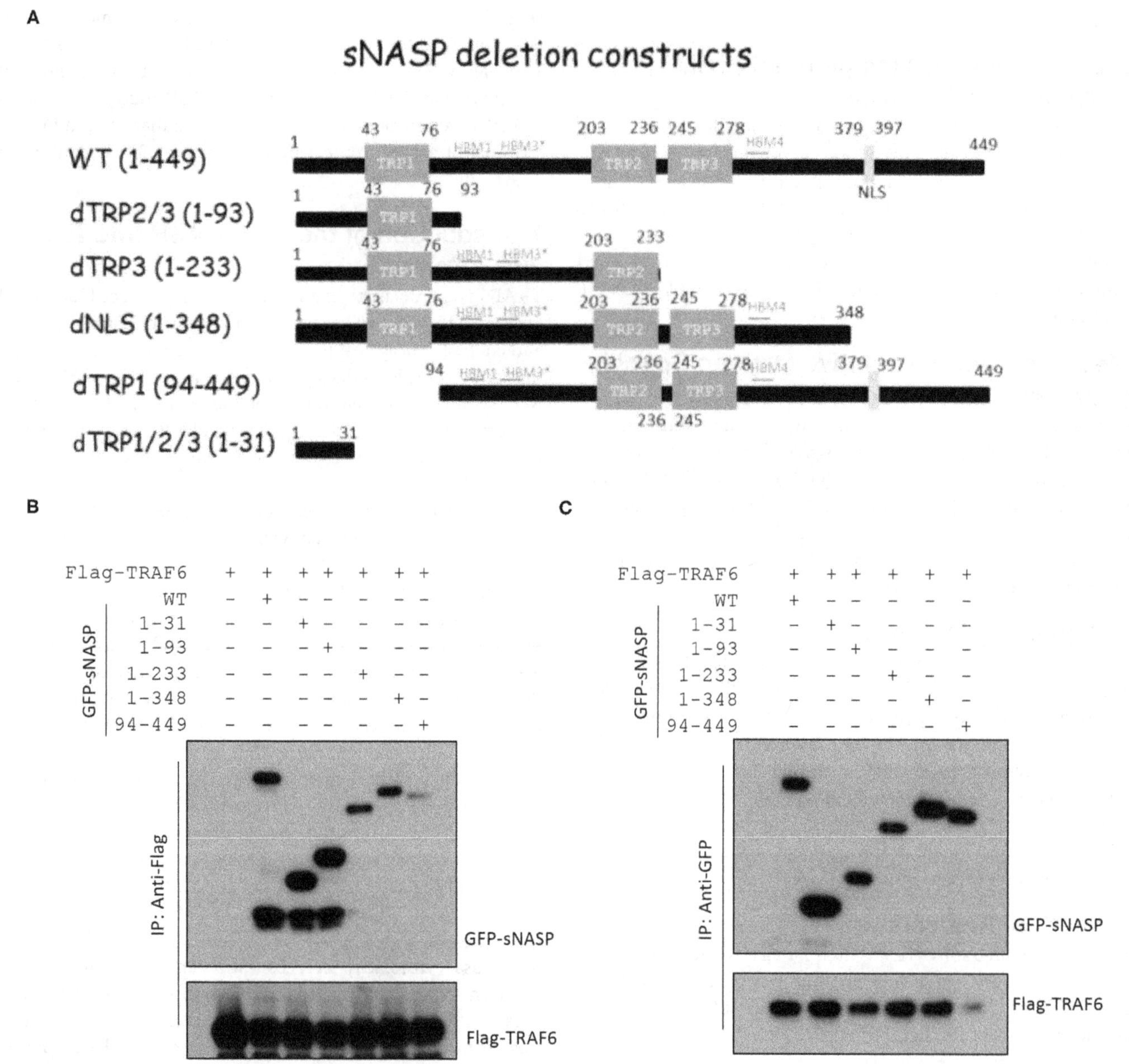

FIGURE 1 | The N-terminal 1∼31 domain of the somatic nuclear autoantigenic sperm protein (sNASP) is essential for interaction with tumor necrosis factor receptor-associated factor 6 (TRAF6). **(A)** Schematic representation of sNASP deletion constructs fused to the C-terminal enhanced green fluorescent protein (EGFP) tag. **(B,C)** Immunoprecipitation (IP) of Flag-TRAF6 **(B)** (with anti-Flag agarose) or GFP-sNASP **(C)** (with GFP-Trap) from HEK293 cells transiently transfected with GFP-sNASP wild-type or deletion mutants plus Flag-TRAF6, followed by immunoblotting (IB) with an antibody against Flag or GFP. Data represent a minimum of three independent experiments.

with endogenous TRAF6 during regulation of TLR4 signaling. There was a clear interaction between endogenous TRAF6 and the PEP-NASP, but not the control NASP (**Figures 3B,C**). IP assays also showed that transduction of the PEP-NASP led to reduced interactions between endogenous sNASP and TRAF6 (**Figure 3B**). Following LPS stimulation, transduction of the PEP-NASP accelerated the dissociation of the sNASP from TRAF6 (**Figure 3C**), indicating that the PEP-NASP had a much higher affinity for endogenous TRAF6 than endogenous sNASP. These results suggested that transduction of the PEP-NASP may compete with endogenous sNASP for the TRAF6-binding motif.

Since NF-κB activation is crucial for the LPS/TLR4 signaling-induced inflammatory response in RAW 264.7 cells, we examined the effect of the PEP-NASP against LPS-induced TRAF6 downstream signaling and the nuclear translocation of p65 in RAW 264.7 cells following LPS stimulation. As shown in **Figure 4A**, LPS-induced phosphorylation of transforming

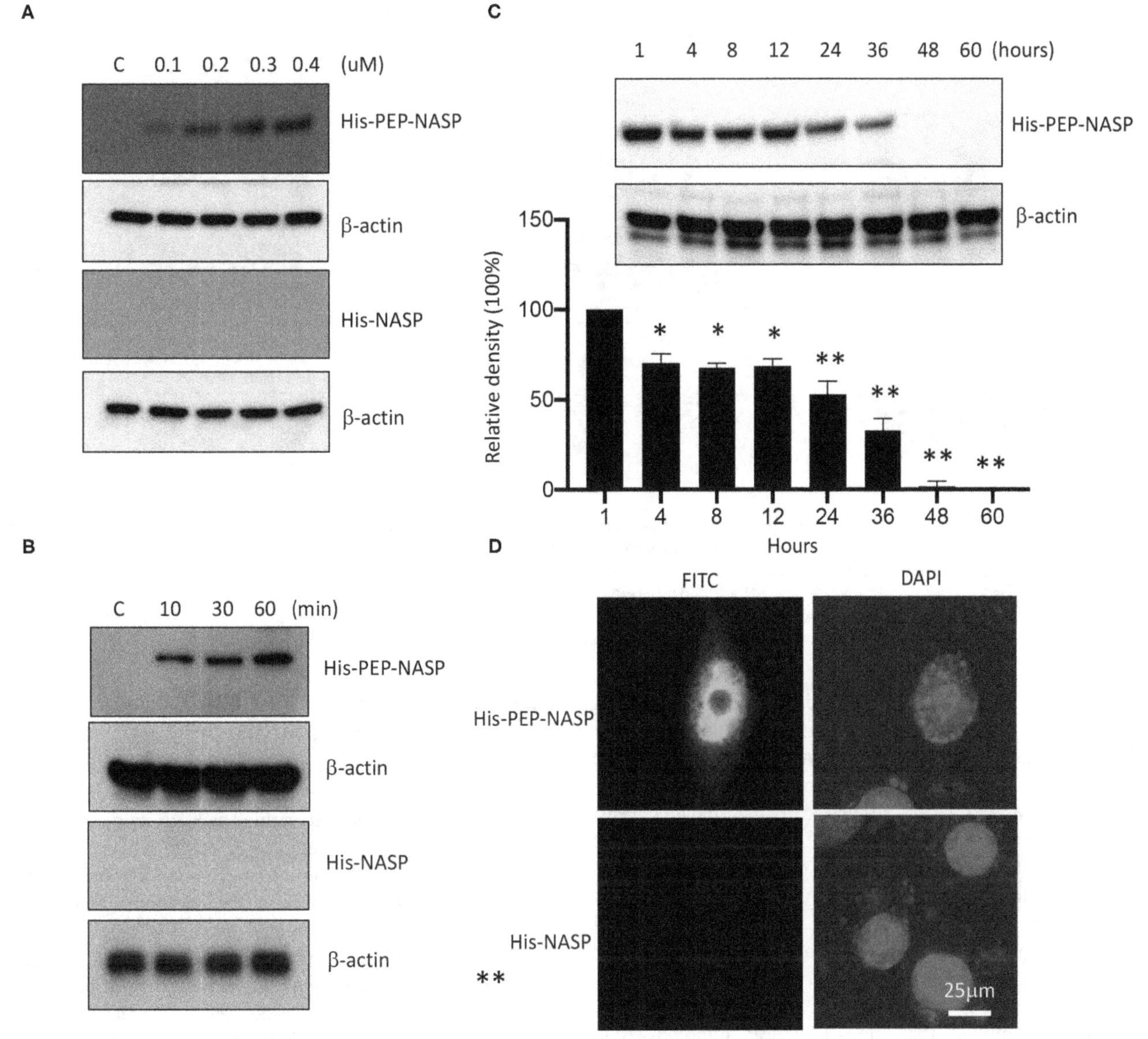

FIGURE 2 | Transduction of the PEP-NASP into RAW 264.7 cells. Cells were cultured in 60-mm culture dishes. Then, PEP-NASP (0.1 ~ 0.4 μM) and control NASP were added to the culture media for 1 h **(A)**, and PEP-NASP (0.4 μM) and control NASP were added to the culture media for 10 ~ 60 min **(B)**, and analyzed by immunoblotting (IB) with an antibody against His or β-actin. Transduction of PEP-NASP stability was assessed after various time periods (1 ~ 60 h). Cells pretreated with 0.4 μM PEP-NASP for 1 h and analyzed by IB with an antibody against His or β-actin **(C)**. The intracellular distribution of the transduced PEP-NASP and NASP was observed by confocal microscopy **(D)**. Scale bar = 25 μm. Data represent a minimum of three independent experiments.

growth factor (TGF)-β activated kinase 1 (TAK1), p38 MAPK, and JNK decreased when the PEP-NASP was transduced into RAW 264.7 cells. Furthermore, the amount of NF-κB p65 in the nucleus markedly increased upon exposure to LPS alone, but the PEP-NASP suppressed the LPS-mediated nuclear translocation of NF-κB p65 (**Figure 4B**). Transduced PEP-NASP, but not control NASP, was also found to inhibit LPS-mediated NF-κB activation (**Figure 4C**). In additional, the PEP-NASP significantly decreased the production of the proinflammatory cytokines: TNF-α, IL-6, and IL-1β (**Figure 4D**). These results suggested that the transduced PEP-NASP negatively regulates activation of the LPS-triggered TLR4 pathway by regulating TRAF6 autoubiquitination.

PEP-NASP Suppresses LPS-Induced ROS/NO Production and NLRP3 Inflammasome Activation

The production of excessive ROS and NO after LPS challenge is an important reflection of the inflammatory process involved in local immune responses. Since iNOS and cyclooxygenase (COX)-2 proteins are associated with NO production, we

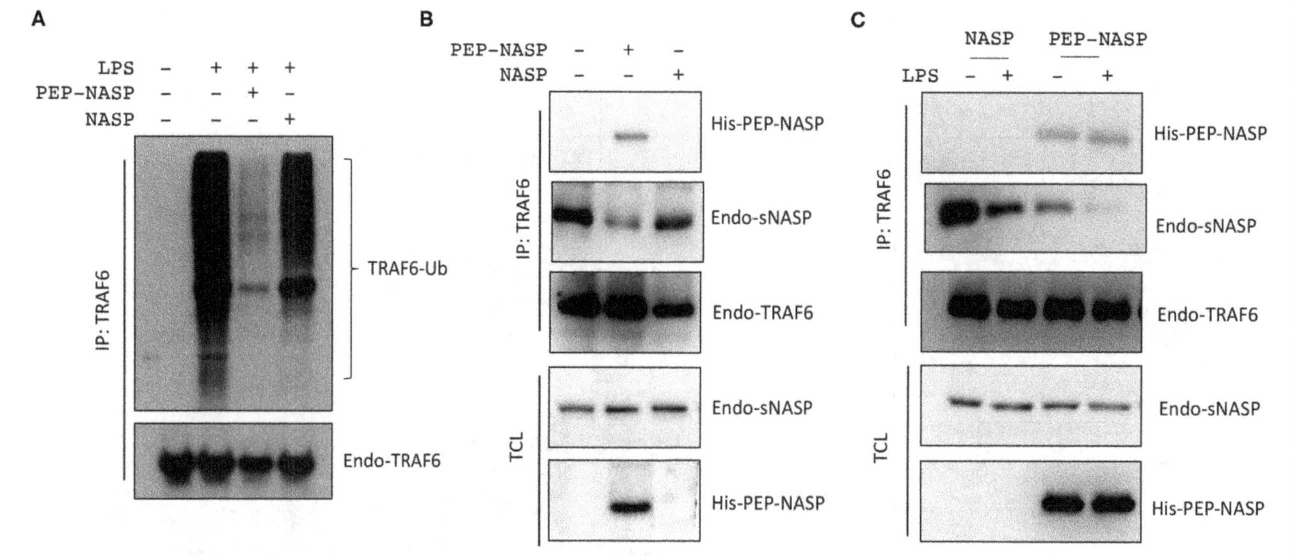

FIGURE 3 | The PEP-NASP significantly inhibits tumor necrosis factor receptor-associated factor 6 (TRAF6) polyubiquitination in LPS-stimulated RAW 264.7 cells. **(A)** Cells were pretreated with or without the PEP-NASP or NASP (0.4 μM) for 1 h before the addition of LPS (1 μg/mL) for 30 min. Cell lysates were immunoprecipitated with an anti-TRAF6 followed by immunoblotting (IB) with an antibody against Ub or TRAF6. **(B)** Immunoprecipitation (IP) of endogenous TRAF6 (with anti-TRAF6) from RAW 264.7 cells transduced with the PEP-NASP or NASP, followed by IB with an antibody against His, NASP, or TRAF6. Total cell lysate (TCL) IB was done with anti-NASP and anti-His. **(C)** Cells were transduced with the PEP-NASP or NASP, stimulated with LPS, and assessed by IB with an antibody against His, NASP, or TRAF6 after IP with anti-TRAF6 or by IB with anti-NASP and anti-His in TCL. Data represent a minimum of three independent experiments.

assessed whether the LPS-induced production of NO mediated by iNOS and COX-2 was regulated by the transduced PEP-NASP. As shown in **Figure 5A**, expressions of the iNOS and COX-2 proteins significantly increased in LPS-stimulated RAW 264.7 cells compared to unstimulated cells. However, the transduced PEP-NASP dose-dependently (0.2 and 0.4 μM) inhibited expressions of iNOS and COX-2 in the presence of LPS (**Figure 5A**). Similar result was found in ROS production. As shown in **Figures 5B,C**, ROS production significantly decreased, and GSH, as the major free radical scavenger, level significantly increased in PEP-NASP transduced group compared with the LPS group. These results implied that the PEP-NASP inhibited ROS and NO production by downregulating iNOS and COX-2 expressions.

Our study showed that the PEP-NASP could reduce IL-1β production in LPS-induced RAW 264.7 cells (**Figure 4D**), and the NLRP3 inflammasome was reported to be essential to turn the inactive precursor (pro-IL-1β) into the active form (IL-1β). Consequently, to elucidate whether its anti-inflammatory effect was related to the NLRP3 inflammasome, we further explored the effect of the PEP-NASP on activating the NLRP3 inflammasome. As shown in **Figure 5D**, LPS challenge significantly enhanced expressions of NLRP3, ASC, and caspase-1 proteins, indicating that the NLRP3 inflammasome was activated by LPS in macrophages. PEP-NASP transduction dramatically blocked the LPS-induced upregulation of NLRP3, ASC, and caspase-1 compared to treatment with LPS alone (**Figure 5D**). These results indicated that the PEP-NASP might reduce promotion of the NLRP3 inflammasome to inhibit inflammation.

PEP-NASP Transduction Attenuates LPS-Induced Lung Injury in Mice

Next, we investigated the protective effects of the PEP-NASP in a mouse model of ALI induced by the i.n. administration of LPS. Lung histopathology was determined by H&E staining. We found that LPS administration resulted in obvious histopathological lung injury, including pulmonary edema, inflammatory cell infiltration, and alveolar damage, whereas transduction of the PEP-NASP markedly ameliorated these pathological changes (**Figure 6A**). There were no obvious pathological changes in the control group (**Figure 6A**). Edema is a typical pathological characteristic of ALI lungs. The elevated lung W/D weight indicated edema in LPS-challenged mice (**Figure 6B**). In contrast, the transduced PEP-NASP markedly decreased the W/D ratio compared to that in the ALI group (**Figure 6B**). These data suggested that the PEP-NASP alleviated the pulmonary pathological injury observed in LPS-treated mice.

PEP-NASP Negatively Regulates LPS-Induced Production of Inflammatory Cytokines in the Lungs

Expressions of inflammatory cytokines (TNF-α, IL-6, and IL-1β) in lung tissues were determined using a qPCR and ELISA. We found that mRNA expressions in lung tissues and protein expressions of TNF-α, IL-6, and IL-1β in BALF had dramatically increased in the LPS group (**Figures 7A,B**). By contrast, transduction of the PEP-NASP resulted in significant decreases in expressions of these cytokines (**Figures 7A,B**). These data indicated that the PEP-NASP negatively regulated expressions of inflammatory cytokines in LPS-induced lung injury.

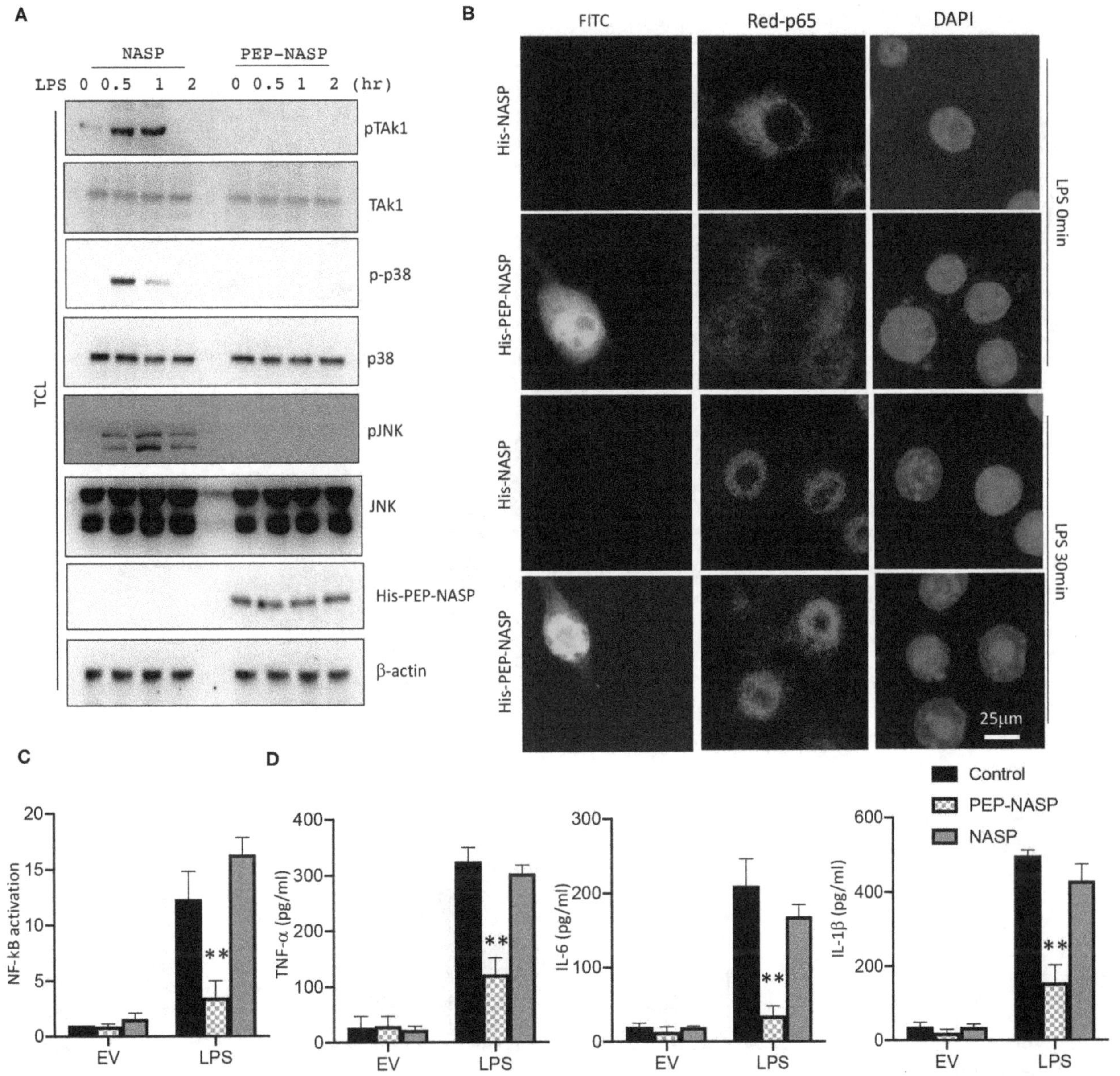

FIGURE 4 | The PEP-NASP inhibited LPS-induced activation of NF-κB and expression of proinflammatory cytokine production in macrophages. **(A)** RAW 264.7 cells pretreated with the PEP-NASP or NASP were stimulated with LPS for different time points and assessed by an immunoblotting (IB) analysis with the indicated antibodies. **(B)** FITC-labeled PEP-NASP or NASP was transduced into RAW 264.7 cells. After 48 h, cells were fixed and immunostained with an anti-p65 (Red) antibody. Nuclei were counterstained with DAPI. Images were visualized by confocal microscopy. Scale bar = 25 μm. **(C)** Luciferase activity in RAW 264.7 cells transfected with a luciferase reporter vector driven by an NF-κB-responsive promoter, plus the control, PEP-NASP, or NASP. Results were standardized to an empty vector (EV; set to 1). Data are the mean ± standard error (SE) for each group. **(D)** Production of TNF-α, IL-6, and IL-1β by RAW 264.7 cells transduced with the PEP-NASP or NASP and stimulated with LPS. Data are the mean ± SE for each group. $^{**}p < 0.01$ (by a one-way ANOVA). Data represent a minimum of three independent experiments.

PEP-NASP Reduces Neutrophil Recruitment in the Lungs and Ameliorates Lung Tissue Damage During LPS-Induced ALI

Next, the infiltration of proinflammatory cells, including macrophages and neutrophils, was evaluated. Numbers of total cells in BALF had increased at 24 h after the LPS challenge, and numbers of total cells in mice with PEP-NASP pretreatment were significantly reduced (**Figure 8A**). Next, lung MPO activity was measured, as a specific marker for neutrophil infiltration and ALI severity, and LPS-challenged animals showed a significant increase in lung tissue MPO activity, while administration of the PEP-NASP dramatically reduced MPO activity (**Figure 8B**).

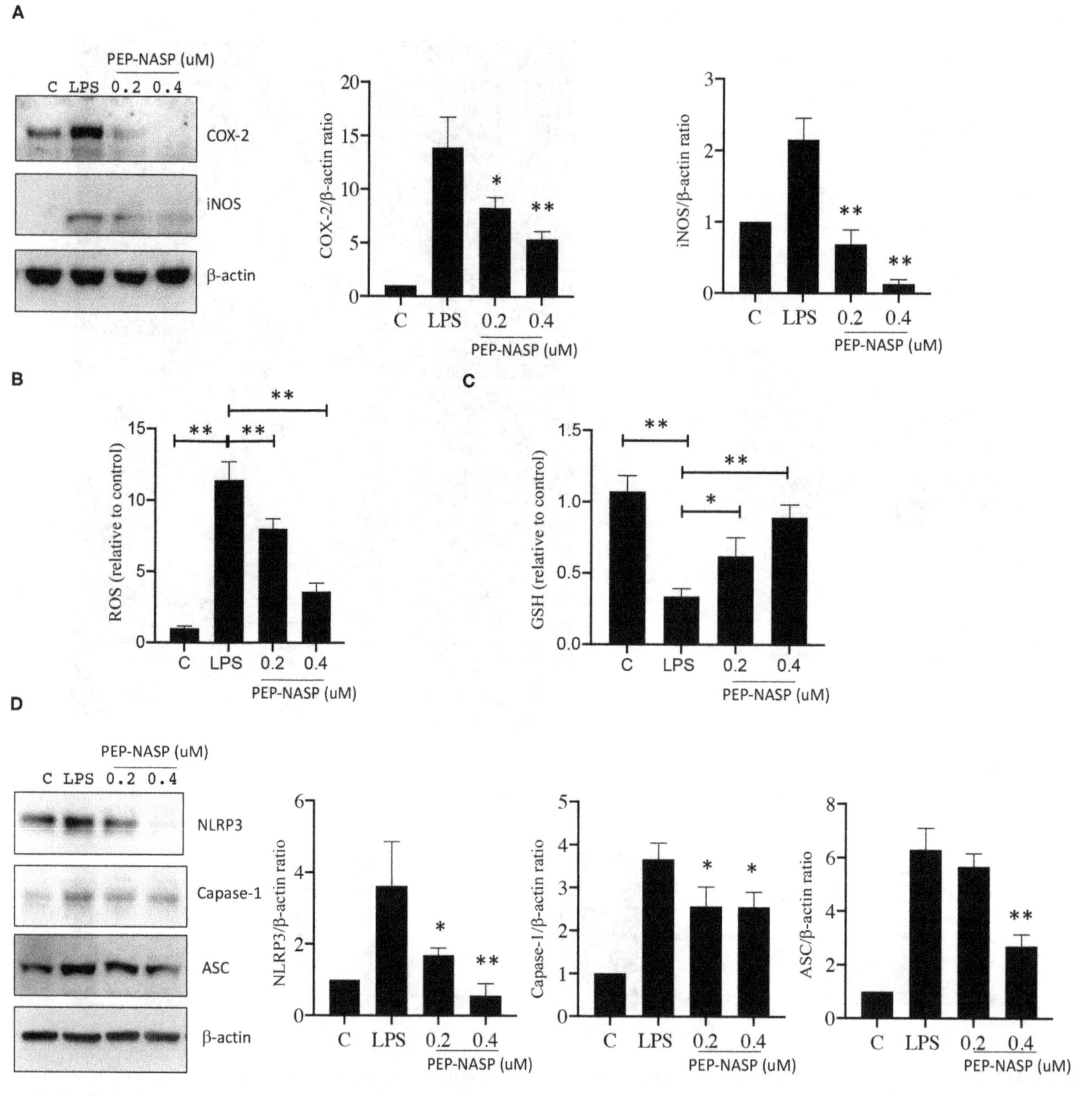

FIGURE 5 | LPS-induced NLRP3 inflammasome and NO production were inhibited by the PEP-NASP. **(A)** Protein expression levels of COX-2, iNOS, and β-actin in RAW 264.7 cells pretreated with the PEP-NASP and stimulated with LPS as detected by a Western blot analysis. **(B)** Production of ROS, **(C)** GSH level and **(D)** Protein expression levels of NLRP3, caspase-1, ASC, and β-actin in RAW 264.7 cells transduced as in A and stimulated with LPS. Western blots were quantified by normalizing densitometric values to those of β-actin. Data are expressed as mean ± standard error for each group. Signal values were compared to unstimulated conditions. $^{*}p < 0.05$, $^{**}p < 0.01$ (by a one-way ANOVA). Data represent at least three independent experiments.

We next explored the neutrophil and macrophage percentage changes in total cells by Wright-Giemsa staining. As shown in **Figures 8C,D**, percentages of neutrophils and macrophages had both significantly increased at 24 h after LPS challenge, while pretreatment with the PEP-NASP fusion protein reduced the percentage of neutrophils by 70% and macrophages by 28% compared to the LPS group. In addition, we also found that PEP-NASP fusion protein decreased the ROS production and increased the levels of GSH in mice of ALI (**Figures 8E,F**). These findings indicated that the transduced PEP-NASP suppressed ROS production and the infiltration of inflammatory cells into the lungs induced by LPS.

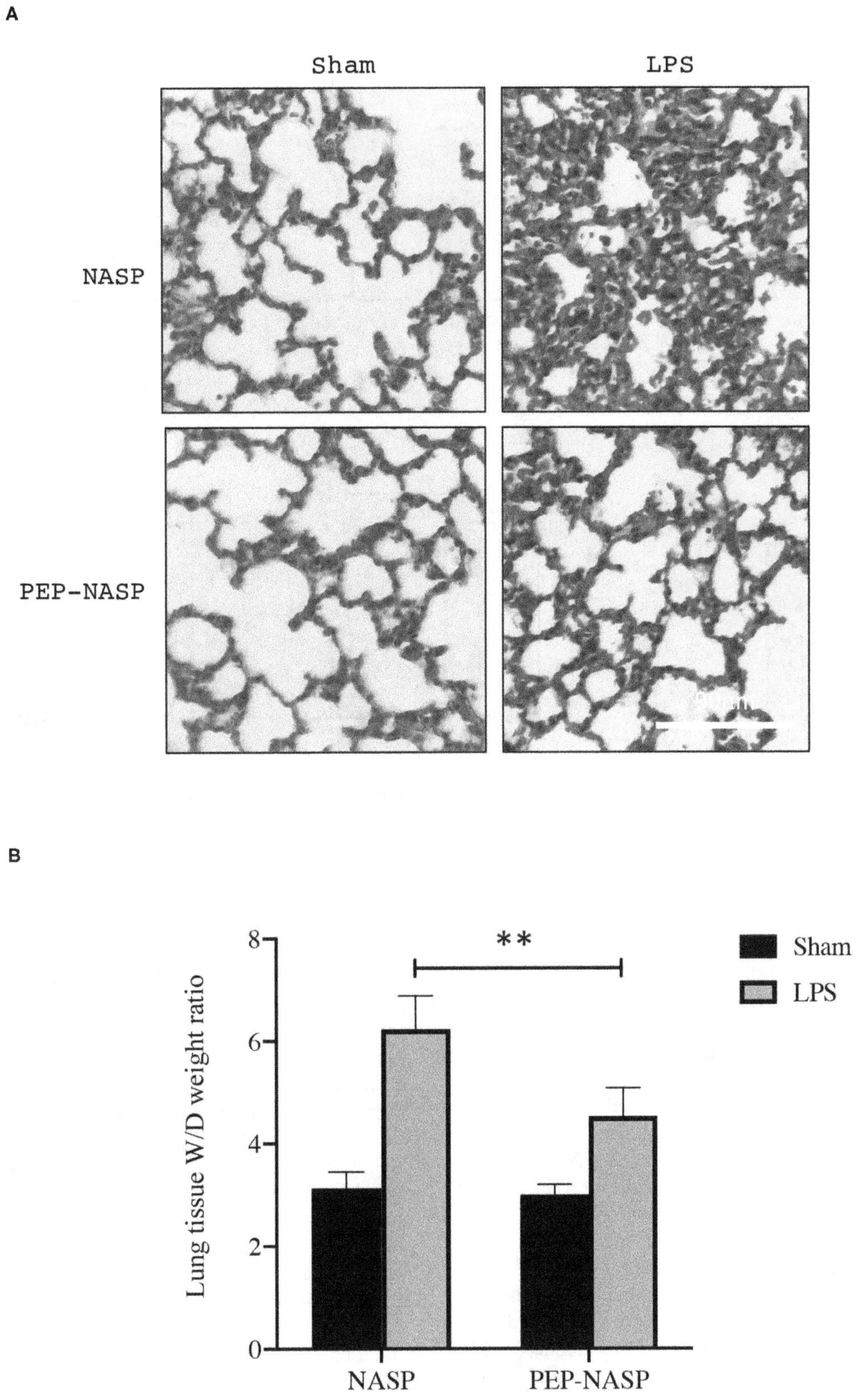

FIGURE 6 | The PEP-NASP significantly suppresses LPS-induced acute lung injury. Pathological changes in lung tissues stained with H&E. Scale bar = 90 μm **(A)**, and the lung wet/dry (W/D) ratio **(B)** was detected in all groups. **$p < 0.01$ (by a one-way ANOVA). ($n = 10$ per group per experiment).

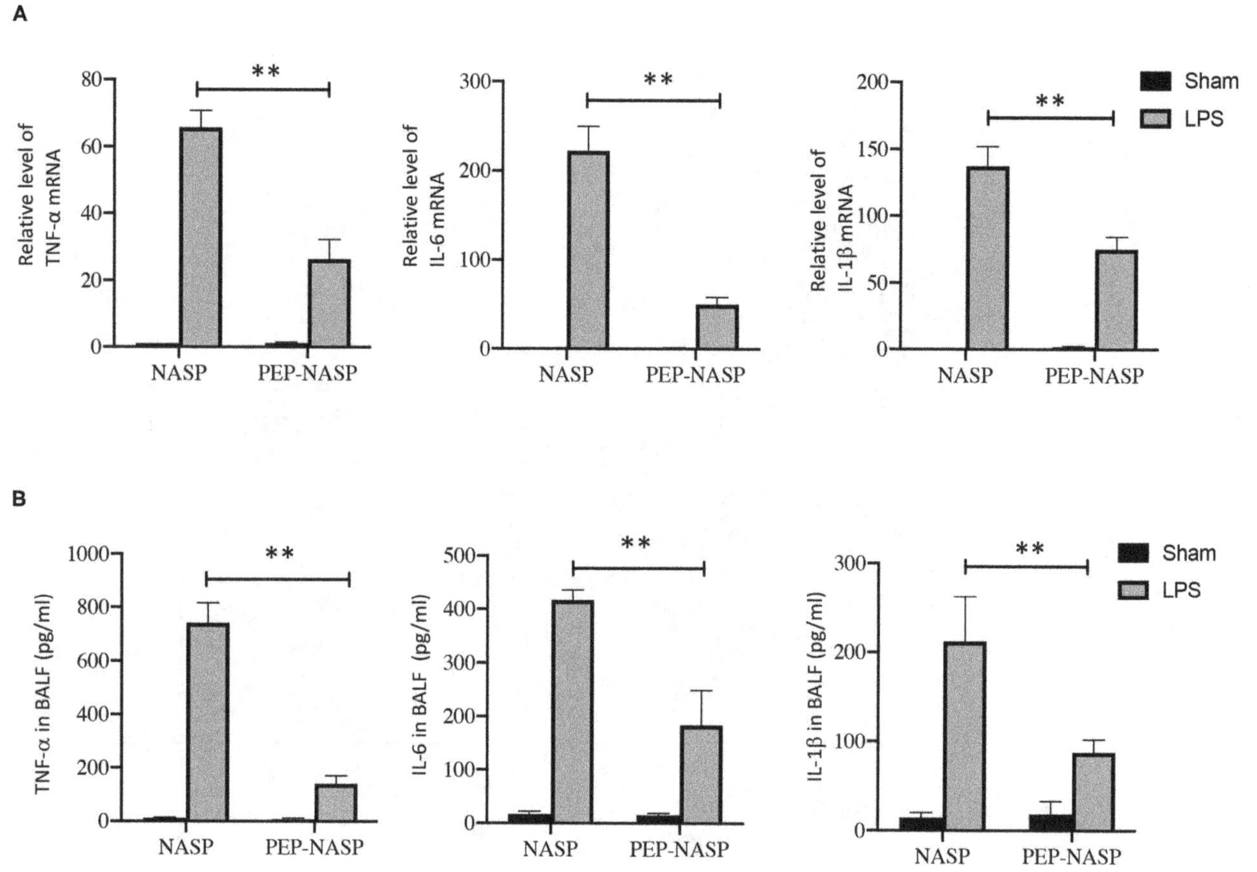

FIGURE 7 | The PEP-NASP reduced expressions of TNF-α, IL-6, and IL-1β in mice treated with LPS. **(A)** RNA expressions of TNF-α, IL-6 and IL-1β in lung tissues were determined by an RT-qPCR. **(B)** Levels of proinflammatory factors (TNF-α, IL-6, and IL-1β) in bronchoalveolar lavage fluid (BALF) were detected by an ELISA. $N = 10$, $^{**}p < 0.01$ (by a one-way ANOVA).

DISCUSSION

ALI, which is mainly characterized by pulmonary inflammation, is a common clinical disease in humans, and the mortality remains high at 30% ~ 40% in most studies (32, 33). Our previous study suggested that the sNASP had the ability to negatively regulate TLR signaling through targeting TRAF6 (16, 17). In a polymicrobial sepsis model, sNASP-mutant mice had defective bacterial clearance from the lungs due to marked reductions in IL-1β, TNF-α, and IFN-γ production associated with poor adhesion molecule expression and leukocyte recruitment, and defective phagolysosome formation. In this study, we demonstrated, for the first time, that administration of the PEP-NASP fusion protein effectively protected mice against LPS-induced ALI, with significantly attenuated pulmonary polymorphonuclear (PMN) infiltration, decreased lung MPO activity, suppressed inflammation, reduced BALF protein content, and ameliorated lung pathological changes. Moreover, we showed that the PEP-NASP alleviated the LPS-induced inflammatory response by inhibiting activation of the TLR/TRAF6 signaling pathway in macrophages *in vitro*. Thus, our data indicated that the PEP-NASP fusion protein conferred protection against lung injury induced by LPS.

Inflammation is a defense mechanism against exogenous pathogens, and it has been implicated in various aggressive and excessive inflammatory responses leading to serious tissue damage (34–36). Development of ALI is due to uncontrolled inflammation, which is connected to the overproduction of various inflammatory mediators released by diverse immune cells, such as endothelial cells, neutrophils, and macrophages. LPS, a major constituent of gram-negative bacterial cells, is a ligand of TLR4 that induces inflammatory syndromes, such as multiple organ injury and sepsis, and is generally recognized as a key factor in inducing ALI (35–37). Challenge of macrophages with LPS can produce high levels of NO, subsequently leading to proinflammatory and destructive effects mainly caused by iNOS (38, 39). In this study, we found that the PEP-NASP inhibited expressions of iNOS and COX-2 in LPS-stimulated macrophages. As is known, overproduction of inflammatory cytokines drives both COX-2 and iNOS gene expressions in macrophages, causing NO release (40). NO is a highly reactive free radical that participates in many inflammatory processes (41). Studies showed that *iNOS* and *COX-2* gene expressions

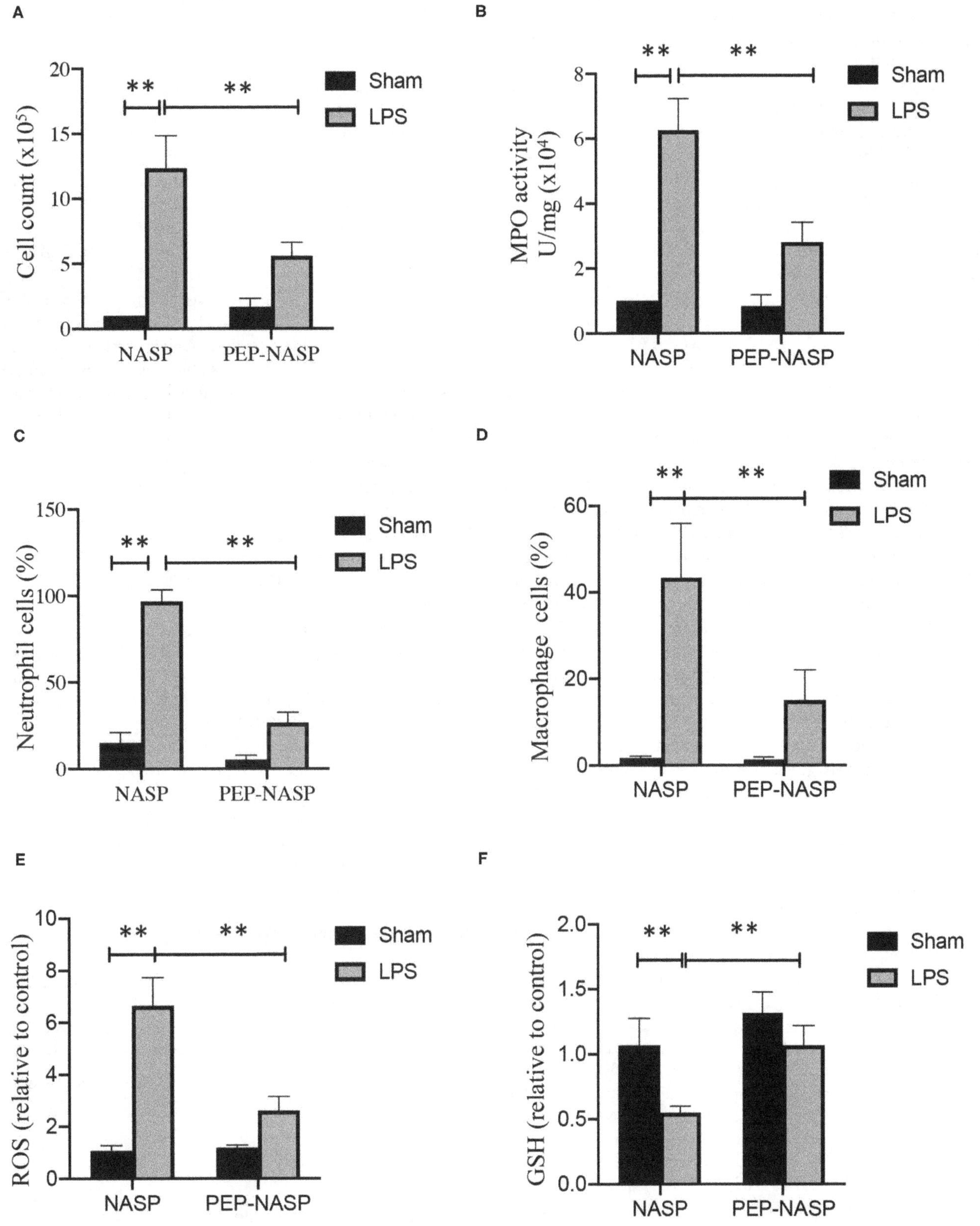

FIGURE 8 | The PEP-NASP inhibited the infiltration of inflammatory cells in LPS-induced acute lung injury. **(A)** Total infiltrated cells in bronchoalveolar lavage fluid (BALF) were counted using a counting chamber. **(B)** Effect of the PEP-NASP on myeloperoxidase (MPO) activity in lung tissue homogenates. **(C,D)** Statistical analysis of percentages of neutrophils and macrophages in BALF by hemocytometer and Wright-Giemsa staining. **(E)** Production of ROS and **(F)** GSH level were measured in BALF. Values represent the mean ± standard error of the mean (SEM), $n = 10$, $^{**}p < 0.01$ (by a one-way ANOVA).

markedly increased during ALI induced by LPS (42). These potential effects of the PEP-NASP on reducing NO suggest an anti-reactive oxygen species (ROS) role of the PEP-NASP in bacterium-induced inflammation.

TRAF6 is a key adaptor for TLR4/NF-κB signaling in regulating innate and adaptive immunity (43, 44). Increasing evidence indicates that the TLR4/TRAF6 pathway is considered to be involved in the process of inflammation-related ALI (45–47). For example, Ding et al. and Liu et al. both demonstrated that the inhibition of TRAF6 alleviated the severity of inflammation and lung injury in an ALI mouse model (45, 47). Inhibition of TRAF6 ubiquitination can attenuate TRAF6-mediated NF-κB activation and proinflammatory cytokine expressions (45, 46, 48). In recent years, many bioactive ingredients extracted from herbs have been reported to effectively ameliorate ALI *via* different mechanisms. For example, glycyrrhizic acid attenuates LPS-induced ALI *via* modulation of the PI3K/AKT/mTOR pathway (49); picrasma quassiodes attenuates LPS-induced pulmonary inflammation and pulmonary edema by regulating the iNOS, HO-1, NF-κB and MAPK signaling (50); and magnoflorine exerts anti-inflammatory effects against LPS-induced ALI through regulation of TLR4-mediated MAPK and NF-κB signaling pathways (51). Moreover, isoalantolactone, a traditional Chinese herbal medicine, was reported to improve pulmonary inflammation and permeability through inhibiting TRAF6 ubiquitination (45). Our findings indicated that the PEP-NASP prevented TRAF6 ubiquitination by directly interacting with TRAF6 in RAW 264.7 cells. Transduction of the PEP-NASP also negatively regulates TRAF6-downstream TAK1/p38/JNK and NF-κB activation. LPS-induced proinflammatory cytokines also decreased by the PEP-NASP in lung tissue *in vivo* and in macrophages *in vitro*. We also showed that the PEP-NASP inhibited activation of the NLRP3 inflammasome in RAW 264.7 cells. These results suggested that the PEP-NASP exerts its anti-inflammatory effects through suppressing TRAF6. Whether PEP-NASP regulate multiple levels of cellular process in response to LPS-induced inflammation is needed to be investigated in future studies.

Macrophages as important inflammatory cells were reported to attract neutrophil infiltration into the lungs and induce lung tissue damage (52). Meanwhile, clinical studies indicated that augmentation of the proinflammatory cytokines TNF-α, IL-1β, and IL-6 has a major role in the development of inflammatory diseases, including ALI (53). These cytokines amplify lung inflammation in ALI patients and were correlated with severity and poor outcomes, such as high protein pulmonary edema and respiratory failure (54, 55). The lung W/D ratio is an indicator of pulmonary edema. We found that LPS induced a higher lung W/D ratio than that of control mice, and administration of the PEP-NASP ameliorated the degree of pulmonary edema due to LPS. Higher levels of total proteins induced by LPS in BALF were also inhibited by the PEP-NASP. In addition, due to cytokines, neutrophils infiltrated into lung tissues, leading to the production of proinflammatory cytokines, which are secreted by activated macrophages in ALI patients and influence pulmonary gas exchange (56, 57). Inhibition of these proinflammatory cytokines provides important guidance for treating ALI. Our *in vivo* analysis performed in the ALI mouse model showed that the PEP-NASP suppressed the release of proinflammatory cytokines, including TNF-α, IL-1β, and IL-6, in lung tissues and BALF. These effects of the PEP-NASP on macrophages also revealed that the PEP-NASP might attenuate LPS-induced ALI *via* inhibiting cytokine production in macrophages. MPO is an enzyme stored in cytoplasmic granules of neutrophils, and its activity reflects the infiltration of neutrophils into lung tissues (58). We found that the PEP-NASP significantly decreased the activity of MPO induced by LPS and attenuated neutrophil infiltration into the lungs in LPS-induced ALI, indicating that the PEP-NASP can suppress neutrophil recruitment into lung tissues.

Studies have also found that the expression of TRAR6 was increased in lung tissues in mice with ALI (59–61). Clinically, TRAF6 variant (rs4755453) was significantly associated with susceptibility to sepsis-induced ALI in Chinese Han population (59). Therefore, it suggests that genetic variants in TRAF6 could influence TRAF6 mRNA stability and subsequently the production of inflammatory cytokines, which directly impacted lung tissue injury. The results of this study indicated the potent therapeutic effects of the novel peptide PEP-NASP against oxidative stress and pulmonary inflammation *via* selective TRAF6 signaling. Thus, PEP-NASP may exert potent therapeutic effects targeting genetic variants in TLR signaling, especially focused on high expression of TRAF6 population. We are planning to investigate the mechanism of PEP-NASP beyond genetic variants (rs4755453) in TRAF6 to further explore the clinical application.

In summary, we demonstrated for the first time that the human NASP, a negative inflammatory mediator, with its N-terminal fused to the PEP-1 peptide (PEP-NASP), can be efficiently transduced *in vivo* and *in vitro*. We also revealed that the transduced PEP-NASP has anti-inflammatory and antioxidant effects which ameliorated lung injury by regulating inflammatory responses and oxidative stress. The mechanisms for the protective role of the PEP-NASP are associated with the inhibition of TLR4-mediated TRAF6/NF-κB signaling pathways. Thus, our success in the protein transduction of PEP-NASP may provide a new therapeutic agent for protecting against inflammation-associated lung diseases, like ALI.

AUTHOR CONTRIBUTIONS

F-MY, Y-CW, and S-PH developed the concepts. F-MY, Y-CW, and Y-TL designed and performed the experiments and analyzed the data. M-CH provided resource support. Y-CW contributed to the ALI animal model. M-CH, EY, Y-CW, and S-PH assisted in interpreting the data and writing, review, and editing. All authors contributed to the article and approved the submitted version.

FUNDING

This work was financially supported of the Higher Education Sprout Project by the Ministry of Education (MOE) in Taiwan. F-MY was also supported by grants (TMU 108-AE1-B14, DP2-109-21121-01-T-04-02, and DP2-110-21121-01-T-04-02) from Taipei Medical University and (MOST 108-2320-B-038-069-MY2 and MOST 110-2320-B-038-065-MY3) from the Ministry of Science and Technology of Taiwan. Y-CW was also supported by grants (TMU 105-AE1-B53) from Taipei Medical University.

REFERENCES

1. Ashbaugh DG, Bigelow DB, Petty TL, Levine BE. Acute respiratory distress in adults. *Lancet.* (1967) 2:319–23. doi: 10.1016/S0140-6736(67)90168-7
2. Mowery NT, Terzian WTH, Nelson AC. Acute lung injury. *Curr Probl Surg.* (2020) 57:100777. doi: 10.1016/j.cpsurg.2020.100777
3. Matthay MA, Ware LB, Zimmerman GA. The acute respiratory distress syndrome. *J Clin Invest.* (2012) 122:2731–40. doi: 10.1172/JCI60331
4. Wheeler AP, Bernard GR. Acute lung injury and the acute respiratory distress syndrome: a clinical review. *Lancet.* (2007) 369:1553–64. doi: 10.1016/S0140-6736(07)60604-7
5. Rubenfeld GD, Caldwell E, Peabody E, Weaver J, Martin DP, Neff M, et al. Incidence and outcomes of acute lung injury. *N Engl J Med.* (2005) 353:1685–93. doi: 10.1056/NEJMoa050333
6. Goss CH, Brower RG, Hudson LD, Rubenfeld GD, Network A. Incidence of acute lung injury in the United States. *Crit Care Med.* (2003) 31:1607–11. doi: 10.1097/01.CCM.0000063475.65751.1D
7. Suresh R, Kupfer Y, Tessler S. Acute respiratory distress syndrome. *N Engl J Med.* (2000) 343:660–1. doi: 10.1056/NEJM200008313430914
8. Chen W, Chen YY, Tsai CF, Chen SC, Lin MS, Ware LB, et al. Incidence and outcomes of acute respiratory distress syndrome: a Nationwide Registry-Based Study in Taiwan, 1997 to (2011). *Medicine.* (2015) 94:e1849. doi: 10.1097/MD.0000000000001849
9. O'Shea JJ, Murray PJ. Cytokine signaling modules in inflammatory responses. *Immunity.* (2008) 28:477–87. doi: 10.1016/j.immuni.2008.03.002
10. Duggan JM, You D, Cleaver JO, Larson DT, Garza RJ, Guzman Pruneda FA, et al. Synergistic interactions of TLR2/6 and TLR9 induce a high level of resistance to lung infection in mice. *J Immunol.* (2011) 186:5916–26. doi: 10.4049/jimmunol.1002122
11. Ware HH, Kulkarni VV, Wang Y, Pantaleon Garcia J, Leiva Juarez M, Kirkpatrick CT, et al. Inducible lung epithelial resistance requires multisource reactive oxygen species generation to protect against bacterial infections. *PLoS ONE.* (2019) 14:e0208216. doi: 10.1371/journal.pone.0208216
12. Kumar V. Pulmonary innate immune response determines the outcome of inflammation during pneumonia and sepsis-associated acute lung injury. *Front Immunol.* (2020) 11:1722. doi: 10.3389/fimmu.2020.01722
13. Chen JQ, Szodoray P, Zeher M. Toll-like receptor pathways in autoimmune diseases. *Clin Rev Allergy Immunol.* (2016) 50:1–17. doi: 10.1007/s12016-015-8473-z
14. Kawasaki T, Kawai T. Toll-like receptor signaling pathways. *Front Immunol.* (2014) 5:461. doi: 10.3389/fimmu.2014.00461
15. Lee WL, Downey GP. Neutrophil activation and acute lung injury. *Curr Opin Crit Care.* (2001) 7:1–7. doi: 10.1097/00075198-200102000-00001
16. Yang FM, Zuo Y, Zhou W, Xia C, Hahm B, Sullivan M, et al. sNASP inhibits TLR signaling to regulate immune response in sepsis. *J Clin Invest.* (2018) 128:2459–72. doi: 10.1172/JCI95720
17. Yang FM, Chang HM, Yeh ETH. Regulation of TLR4 signaling through the TRAF6/sNASP axis by reversible phosphorylation mediated by CK2 and PP4. *Proc Natl Acad Sci USA.* (2021) 118:e2107044118. doi: 10.1073/pnas.2107044118
18. Kurzawa L, Pellerano M, Morris MC. PEP and CADY-mediated delivery of fluorescent peptides and proteins into living cells. *Biochim Biophys Acta.* (2010) 1798:2274–85. doi: 10.1016/j.bbamem.2010.02.027
19. Morris MC, Depollier J, Mery J, Heitz F, Divita G. A peptide carrier for the delivery of biologically active proteins into mammalian cells. *Nat Biotechnol.* (2001) 19:1173–6. doi: 10.1038/nbt1201-1173
20. Yan XT, He XH, Wang YL, Zhang ZZ, Tang JJ. Transduced PEP-1-Heme Oxygenase-1 fusion protein attenuates lung injury in septic shock rats. *Oxid Med Cell Longev.* (2018) 2018:6403861. doi: 10.1155/2018/6403861
21. Kim MJ, Jeong HJ, Kim DW, Sohn EJ, Jo HS, Kim DS, et al. PEP-1-PON1 protein regulates inflammatory response in raw 264.7 macrophages and ameliorates inflammation in a TPA-induced animal model. *PLoS ONE.* (2014) 9:e86034. doi: 10.1371/journal.pone.0086034
22. Kim DS, Sohn EJ, Kim DW, Kim YN, Eom SA, Yoon GH, et al. PEP-1-p18 prevents neuronal cell death by inhibiting oxidative stress and Bax expression. *BMB Rep.* (2012) 45:532–7. doi: 10.5483/BMBRep.2012.45.9.083
23. Khadangi F, Forgues AS, Tremblay-Pitre S, Dufour-Mailhot A, Henry C, Boucher M, et al. Intranasal versus intratracheal exposure to lipopolysaccharides in a murine model of acute respiratory distress syndrome. *Sci Rep.* (2021) 11:7777. doi: 10.1038/s41598-021-87462-x
24. Man F, Nadkarni S, Kanabar V, RR EL, Gomes Ferreira S, Federici Canova D, et al. A peptide derived from chaperonin 60.1, IRL201104, inhibits LPS-induced acute lung inflammation. *Am J Physiol Lung Cell Mol Physiol.* (2021) 321:L803–13. doi: 10.1152/ajplung.00155.2021
25. Yang FM, Pan CT, Tsai HM, Chiu TW, Wu ML, Hu MC. Liver receptor homolog-1 localization in the nuclear body is regulated by sumoylation and cAMP signaling in rat granulosa cells. *FEBS J.* (2009) 276:425–36. doi: 10.1111/j.1742-4658.2008.06785.x
26. Hsieh HT, Wang CH, Wu ML, Yang FM, Tai YC, Hu MC. PIASy inhibits LRH-1-dependent CYP11A1 expression by competing for SRC-1 binding. *Biochem J.* (2009) 419:201–9. doi: 10.1042/BJ20081402
27. Yang FM, Lin YC, Hu MC. Identification of two functional nuclear localization signals mediating nuclear import of liver receptor homologue-1. *Cell Mol Life Sci.* (2011) 68:1241–53. doi: 10.1007/s00018-010-0521-5
28. Zhang D, Li X, Hu Y, Jiang H, Wu Y, Ding Y, et al. Tabersonine attenuates lipopolysaccharide-induced acute lung injury via suppressing TRAF6 ubiquitination. *Biochem Pharmacol.* (2018) 154:183–92. doi: 10.1016/j.bcp.2018.05.004
29. Finn RM, Ellard K, Eirin-Lopez JM, Ausio J. Vertebrate nucleoplasmin and NASP: egg histone storage proteins with multiple chaperone activities. *FASEB J.* (2012) 26:4788–804. doi: 10.1096/fj.12-216663
30. Aderem A, Ulevitch RJ. Toll-like receptors in the induction of the innate immune response. *Nature.* (2000) 406:782–7. doi: 10.1038/35021228
31. Cook DN, Pisetsky DS, Schwartz DA. Toll-like receptors in the pathogenesis of human disease. *Nat Immunol.* (2004) 5:975–9. doi: 10.1038/ni1116
32. Lin S, Wu H, Wang C, Xiao Z, Xu F. Regulatory T cells and acute lung injury: cytokines, uncontrolled inflammation, and therapeutic implications. *Front Immunol.* (2018) 9:1545. doi: 10.3389/fimmu.2018.01545
33. Matthay MA, Zemans RL, Zimmerman GA, Arabi YM, Beitler JR, Mercat A, et al. Acute respiratory distress syndrome. *Nat Rev Dis Primers.* (2019) 5:18. doi: 10.1038/s41572-019-0069-0
34. Medzhitov R. Origin and physiological roles of inflammation. *Nature.* (2008) 454:428–35. doi: 10.1038/nature07201
35. Jin C, Chen J, Gu J, Zhang W. Gut-lymph-lung pathway mediates sepsis-induced acute lung injury. *Chin Med J.* (2020) 133:2212–8. doi: 10.1097/CM9.0000000000000928
36. Shih HJ, Chang CY, Chiang M, Le VL, Hsu HJ, Huang CJ. Simultaneous inhibition of three major cytokines and its therapeutic effects: a peptide-based novel therapy against endotoxemia in mice. *J Pers Med.* (2021) 11:436. doi: 10.3390/jpm11050436
37. Chang CY, Hsu HJ, Foo J, Shih HJ, Huang CJ. Peptide-based TNF-alpha-binding decoy therapy mitigates lipopolysaccharide-induced liver injury in mice. *Pharmaceuticals.* (2020) 13:280. doi: 10.3390/ph13100280
38. Korhonen R, Lahti A, Kankaanranta H, Moilanen E. Nitric oxide production and signaling in inflammation. *Curr Drug Targets Inflamm Allergy.* (2005) 4:471–9. doi: 10.2174/1568010054526359
39. Lee JH, Ko HJ, Woo ER, Lee SK, Moon BS, Lee CW, et al. Moracin M inhibits airway inflammation by interrupting the JNK/c-Jun and NF-kappaB pathways *in vitro* and *in vivo*. *Eur J Pharmacol.* (2016) 783:64–72. doi: 10.1016/j.ejphar.2016.04.055
40. Hori M, Kita M, Torihashi S, Miyamoto S, Won KJ, Sato K, et al. Upregulation of iNOS by COX-2 in muscularis resident macrophage of rat intestine stimulated with LPS. *Am J Physiol Gastrointest Liver Physiol.* (2001) 280:G930–8. doi: 10.1152/ajpgi.2001.280.5.G930
41. Chen L, Deng H, Cui H, Fang J, Zuo Z, Deng J, et al. Inflammatory responses and inflammation-associated diseases in organs. *Oncotarget.* (2018) 9:7204–18. doi: 10.18632/oncotarget.23208

42. Singh G, Kaur J, Kaur M, Singh P, Bhatti R. Anti-nociceptive and anti-inflammatory effect of imperatorin: evidences for involvement of COX-2, iNOS, NFkappaB and inflammatory cytokines. *Int J Neurosci.* (2020) 130:176–85. doi: 10.1080/00207454.2019.1667789
43. Shi JH, Sun SC. Tumor necrosis factor receptor-associated factor regulation of nuclear factor kappaB and mitogen-activated protein kinase pathways. *Front Immunol.* (2018) 9:1849. doi: 10.3389/fimmu.2018.01849
44. Dainichi T, Matsumoto R, Mostafa A, Kabashima K. Immune control by TRAF6-mediated pathways of epithelial cells in the EIME (Epithelial Immune Microenvironment). *Front Immunol.* (2019) 10:1107. doi: 10.3389/fimmu.2019.01107
45. Ding YH, Song YD, Wu YX, He HQ, Yu TH, Hu YD, et al. Isoalantolactone suppresses LPS-induced inflammation by inhibiting TRAF6 ubiquitination and alleviates acute lung injury. *Acta Pharmacol Sin.* (2019) 40:64–74. doi: 10.1038/s41401-018-0061-3
46. Tian F, Lu Q, Lei J, Ni Y, Xie N, Zhong D, et al. Negative Effects of SIGIRR on TRAF6 ubiquitination in acute lung injury *in vitro*. *J Immunol Res.* (2020) 2020:5097920. doi: 10.1155/2020/5097920
47. Liu X, Lin Z, Xu Y. Pellino1 promoted inflammation in lung injury model of sepsis by TRAF6/ NF-kappaB signal pathway. *J Inflamm.* (2021) 18:11. doi: 10.1186/s12950-021-00276-6
48. Lv Y, Kim K, Sheng Y, Cho J, Qian Z, Zhao YY, et al. YAP controls endothelial activation and vascular inflammation through TRAF6. *Circ Res.* (2018) 123:43–56. doi: 10.1161/CIRCRESAHA.118.313143
49. Qu L, Chen C, He W, Chen Y, Li Y, Wen Y, et al. Glycyrrhizic acid ameliorates LPS-induced acute lung injury by regulating autophagy through the PI3K/AKT/mTOR pathway. *Am J Transl Res.* (2019) 11:2042–55.
50. Lee JW, Park JW, Shin NR, Park SY, Kwon OK, Park HA, et al. Picrasma quassiodes (D. Don) Benn. attenuates lipopolysaccharide (LPS)-induced acute lung injury. *Int J Mol Med.* (2016) 38:834–44. doi: 10.3892/ijmm.2016.2669
51. Guo S, Jiang K, Wu H, Yang C, Yang Y, Yang J, et al. Magnoflorine ameliorates lipopolysaccharide-induced acute lung injury via suppressing NF-kappaB and MAPK activation. *Front Pharmacol.* (2018) 9:982. doi: 10.3389/fphar.2018.00982
52. Gauna AE, Cha S. Akt2 deficiency as a therapeutic strategy protects against acute lung injury. *Immunotherapy.* (2014) 6:377–80. doi: 10.2217/imt.14.5
53. Goodman RB, Pugin J, Lee JS, Matthay MA. Cytokine-mediated inflammation in acute lung injury. *Cytokine Growth Factor Rev.* (2003) 14:523–35. doi: 10.1016/S1359-6101(03)00059-5
54. Ganter MT, Roux J, Miyazawa B, Howard M, Frank JA, Su G, et al. Interleukin-1beta causes acute lung injury via alphavbeta5 and alphavbeta6 integrin-dependent mechanisms. *Circ Res.* (2008) 102:804–12. doi: 10.1161/CIRCRESAHA.107.161067
55. Ware LB. Pathophysiology of acute lung injury and the acute respiratory distress syndrome. *Semin Respir Crit Care Med.* (2006) 27:337–49. doi: 10.1055/s-2006-948288
56. Parsey MV, Tuder RM, Abraham E. Neutrophils are major contributors to intraparenchymal lung IL-1 beta expression after hemorrhage and endotoxemia. *J Immunol.* (1998) 160:1007–13.
57. Ubags ND, Vernooy JH, Burg E, Hayes C, Bement J, Dilli E, et al. The role of leptin in the development of pulmonary neutrophilia in infection and acute lung injury. *Crit Care Med.* (2014) 42:e143–51. doi: 10.1097/CCM.0000000000000048
58. Klebanoff SJ. Myeloperoxidase: friend and foe. *J Leukoc Biol.* (2005) 77:598–625. doi: 10.1189/jlb.1204697
59. Song Z, Yao C, Yin J, Tong C, Zhu D, Sun Z, et al. Genetic variation in the TNF receptor-associated factor 6 gene is associated with susceptibility to sepsis-induced acute lung injury. *J Transl Med.* (2012) 10:166. doi: 10.1186/1479-5876-10-166
60. Shen CH, Lin JY, Chang YL, Wu SY, Peng CK, Wu CP, et al. Inhibition of NKCC1 modulates alveolar fluid clearance and inflammation in ischemia-reperfusion lung injury via TRAF6-mediated pathways. *Front Immunol.* (2018) 9:2049. doi: 10.3389/fimmu.2018.02049
61. Zhou X, Li Y, Ding J, Wang L, Wang R, Zhou B, et al. Down-regulation of tumor necrosis factor-associated factor 6 is associated with progression of acute pancreatitis complicating lung injury in mice. *Tohoku J Exp Med.* (2009) 217:279–85. doi: 10.1620/tjem.217.279

10

Molecular Analysis of IL-5 Receptor Subunit Alpha as a Possible Pharmacogenetic Biomarker in Asthma

Sandra Elena-Pérez [1], David Hansoe Heredero-Jung [1], Asunción García-Sánchez [2,3,4], Miguel Estravís [2,3,4], Maria J. Martin [2,4], Jacinto Ramos-González [5], Juan Carlos Triviño [6], María Isidoro-García [1,2,4,7], Catalina Sanz [2,4,8] and Ignacio Dávila [2,3,4,9]*

[1] Department of Clinical Biochemistry, University Hospital of Salamanca, Salamanca, Spain, [2] Allergic Disease Research Group IIMD-01, Institute for Biomedical Research of Salamanca, Salamanca, Spain, [3] Department of Biomedical Sciences and Diagnostics, University of Salamanca, Salamanca, Spain, [4] Network for Cooperative Research in Health - RETICS ARADyAL, Carlos III Health Institute, Madrid, Spain, [5] Department of Pneumology, University Hospital of Salamanca, Salamanca, Spain, [6] Sistemas Genómicos, Paterna, Spain, [7] Department of Medicine, University of Salamanca, Salamanca, Spain, [8] Department of Microbiology and Genetics, University of Salamanca, Salamanca, Spain, [9] Department of Allergy, University Hospital of Salamanca, Salamanca, Spain

***Correspondence:**
Catalina Sanz
catsof@usal.es

Background: Asthma is a heterogeneous syndrome with a broad clinical spectrum and high drug response variability. The inflammatory response in asthma involves multiple effector cells and mediator molecules. Based on asthma immunopathogenesis, precision medicine can be a promising strategy for identifying biomarkers. Biologic therapies acting on the IL-5/IL-5 receptor axis have been developed. IL-5 promotes proliferation, differentiation and activation of eosinophils by binding to the IL-5 receptor, located on the surface of eosinophils and basophils. This study aimed to investigate the expression of *IL5RA* in patients with several types of asthma and its expression after treatment with benralizumab, a biologic directed against IL-5 receptor subunit alpha.

Methods: Sixty peripheral blood samples, 30 from healthy controls and 30 from asthmatic patients, were selected for a transcriptomic RNAseq study. Differential expression analysis was performed by statistical assessment of fold changes and *P*-values. A validation study of *IL5RA* expression was developed using qPCR in 100 controls and 187 asthmatic patients. The effect of benralizumab on *IL5RA* expression was evaluated in five patients by comparing expression levels between pretreatment and after 3 months of treatment. The *IL5RA* mRNA levels were normalized to *GAPDH* and *TBP* expression values for each sample. Calculations were made by the comparative $\Delta\Delta$Ct method. All procedures followed the MIQE guidelines.

Results: *IL5RA* was one of the most differentially overexpressed coding transcripts in the peripheral blood of asthmatic patients ($P = 8.63E\text{-}08$ and fold change of 2.22). In the qPCR validation study, *IL5RA* expression levels were significantly higher in asthmatic patients than in controls ($P < 0.001$). Significant expression differences were present in different asthmatic types. In the biological drug study, patients treated with benralizumab showed a significant decrease in *IL5RA* expression and blood eosinophil counts. A notable improvement in ACT and lung function was also observed in these patients.

Conclusions: These results indicate that *IL5RA* is overexpressed in patients with different types of asthma. It could help identify which asthmatic patients will respond more efficiently to benralizumab, moving toward a more personalized asthma management. Although further studies are required, *IL5RA* could play a role as a biomarker and pharmacogenetic factor in asthma.

Keywords: asthma, pharmacogenetic biomarker, transcriptomic, *IL5RA*, benralizumab, precision medicine

INTRODUCTION

Asthma is a chronic inflammatory disease of the airways affecting more than 300 million people worldwide, and its prevalence is increasing, becoming a health and economic problem (1). It is defined by variable expiratory airflow limitation and respiratory symptoms such as wheeze, cough and shortness of breath, which vary in frequency and intensity (2). Asthma is recognized as a heterogeneous syndrome with different underlying disease processes, determined by complex interactions between genetic and environmental factors. This variety of interactions results in different clinical presentations, phenotypes and response to treatment (3).

Despite the broad clinical spectrum of asthma, the presence of inflammation of the airway is a common pathologic feature and the primary treatment target. Nevertheless, the relationship between the intensity of inflammation and the severity of asthma has not been consistently established (4). The characteristic inflammatory pattern in most asthmatic patients includes an increase in type 2 helper T (Th2) lymphocytes, eosinophils, basophils, mast cells and type 2 innate lymphoid cells (ILC2). These effector cells release numerous mediating molecules that cause disease symptoms (5). Type 2 inflammation is characterized by an increase in type 2 cytokines, particularly IL-4, IL-5, IL-9, and IL-13, involved in eosinophil activation and immunoglobulin E production (6).

Asthma comprises different phenotypes with similar clinical manifestations but probably involving different underlying mechanisms (7). These phenotypes have been characterized based on the age of onset of disease, clinical presentation, severity and presence of other disorders such as atopy and eosinophilia (8–10). Eosinophilic asthma is the best-studied inflammatory phenotype and is characterized by elevated eosinophils in peripheral blood and sputum. Patients in whom eosinophilic inflammation persists despite treatment with high doses of corticosteroids are often associated with more severe asthma and a higher risk of exacerbations (11, 12). Therefore, phenotype characterization in patients with severe uncontrolled or poorly controlled asthma could help in guiding specific treatments (13).

Asthma management aims to achieve and maintain control of the disease and reduce the risk of exacerbations. Understanding the underlying pathophysiologic mechanisms is necessary for stratifying patients toward individualized therapy. The implementation of precision medicine requires identifying specific biomarkers easily measurable in biological fluids, which can help in evaluating treatment effectiveness (14, 15). In this context, new biologic therapies are being developed targeting cytokines and their receptors. IL-5 plays a crucial role in eosinophilic asthma pathophysiology and has been proposed as a novel therapeutic target. This cytokine is involved in the proliferation, differentiation, survival and activation of eosinophils by binding to the IL-5 receptor, located on the surface of eosinophils and basophils (16, 17). The IL-5 receptor is a heterodimer comprising one alpha subunit (IL-5RA) and one beta subunit, also found in both IL-3 and GM-CSF receptors (18).

In recent years, new drugs based on monoclonal antibodies have been developed against the action of IL-5 in eosinophilic-mediated inflammation. Benralizumab is a humanized IgG1κ monoclonal antibody that binds to IL-5RA via its Fab domain with high affinity and specificity, blocking IL-5 signaling (19). Besides, this antibody can bind through its afucosylated Fc domain to the Fcγ receptor IIIa, expressed on the surface of natural killer cells, macrophages and neutrophils, thus inducing antibody-directed cell-mediated cytotoxicity of eosinophils and basophils. As a result, the administration of benralizumab results in a dramatic depletion of eosinophils counts in blood, sputum, airway mucosa and bone marrow (20). In this context, benralizumab has proved effectivity in treating patients with severe eosinophilic asthma, improving lung function and asthma control and reducing the rate of exacerbations (21).

The present study aims to investigate the expression of *IL5RA* in patients with different types of asthma and its role as a possible biomarker of response to treatment with benralizumab.

MATERIALS AND METHODS

Study Population

The study involved 347 unrelated Caucasian individuals, 130 controls and 217 asthmatic patients, from the Allergy Department of the University Hospital of Salamanca. The study was approved by the Clinical Research Ethics Committee of the Institute for Biomedical Research of Salamanca (IBSAL) (PI 2020-02-433) and all participants signed a written informed consent. Controls had to fulfill the following criteria: (i) no symptoms or history of asthma, rhinitis or other pulmonary diseases; (ii) no symptoms or history of allergic diseases; (iii) negative skin prick tests with a battery of locally adapted common aeroallergens; (iv) absence of family history of asthma, rhinitis or atopy; and (v) age >16 years old. Asthmatic patients were recruited if they met all the following criteria: (i) at least two symptoms consistent with asthma (cough, wheeze and dyspnea); (ii) either a positive bronchodilator or methacholine test; and (iii) absence of other pulmonary disorders; and (iv) age >16 years old.

Lung function was measured by spirometry according to the American Thoracic Society (ATS) criteria (22). Asthma severity was established following the Spanish Guide for the Management of Asthma (GEMA) guidelines (7) and severe asthma was diagnosed according to the ERS/ATS criteria (23). Skin prick tests were performed with a battery of common aeroallergens (24), according to The European Academy of Allergy and Clinical Immunology (EAACI) recommendations (25). Skin tests were considered positive if there was at least one wheal reaction of >3 mm of diameter. Patients were considered atopic if they had a positive skin prick test to at least one allergen. Patients were considered monosensitized if they had a positive skin prick test result to only one group of aeroallergens (pollens, mites, molds or animal dander) and polysensitized if they had positive skin tests for two or more groups. Early-onset asthma was defined as the presence of asthma symptoms that appeared before 18 years, and late-onset asthma was defined as the presence after the age of 18 years (26). Asthmatic patients were classified into two subgroups, eosinophilic and non-eosinophilic asthma, according to the number of eosinophils (cut-off point of 150 cells per µl) (2). Blood cell counts were determined on the XN-1000 hematology analyzer (Sysmex Corporation, Kobe, Japan) and total serum IgE levels were measured using a fluoroenzyme immunoassay (Thermo Fisher Scientific, Waltham, MA, USA).

Transcriptomic RNAseq Study

A total of 60 peripheral blood samples, 30 from healthy controls and 30 from patients with pollen allergic asthma, were selected for a transcriptomic RNAseq study. Total RNA extraction was performed using the Ambion RiboPure^{TM}-Blood kit (Thermo Fisher Scientific, Waltham, MA, USA). After Ambion DNAse I treatment (Thermo Fisher Scientific, Waltham, MA, USA), RNA was purified and concentrated with the RNeasy MinElute Cleanup Kit (Qiagen, Hilden, Germany). All purification protocols were performed with the modifications indicated by the manufacturers. RNA was quantified by Nanodrop 1000 spectrophotometer (Thermo Fisher Scientific, Waltham, MA, USA). The RNA integrity number (RIN) algorithm was used to determine RNA quality on the Agilent 2100 Bioanalyzer using the Eukaryote Total RNA Nano kit (Agilent Technologies, Waldbronn, Germany). RNA samples with a RIN value above 8 were used. Globin transcripts and ribosomal RNA were removed, and RNA was cleaved to prepare RNA strand-specific libraries. Finally, the generated libraries were sequenced on the Illumina HiSeq 2500 platform (Illumina, San Diego, CA, USA).

Bioinformatic Analysis

In the bioinformatic analysis of the transcriptomic data, the FastQC software (27) was used to analyze the quality of raw reads. Sequencing reads were mapped on the human reference genome (GRCh38) using the TopHat2 software (28). The low-quality readings were removed with Picard Tools (29) and the unmapped and non-properly paired reads were re-mapped using the BWA-MEM algorithm (30). Gene and isoform prediction were estimated using the Cufflinks method (31). The HTSeq software (v.0.6.0) (32) was used to calculate gene expression levels. Differential expression analysis was performed by DESeq2 package (33) and only the transcripts with a fold change value $\geq$1.5 or ≤ -1.5 and a FDR-adjusted P-value <0.05 were considered as differentially expressed genes. Potential interactions between selected proteins were examined by cluster analysis using the STRING software (34), a database which include functional and physical associations between known and predicted proteins.

qPCR Validation Assays

For the validation of the transcriptomic gene expression data, 287 peripheral blood samples were selected including 100 samples from controls and 187 from asthmatic patients. Total RNA was isolated using the RiboPure-Blood kit (Ambion, Thermo Fisher Scientific, Waltham, MA, USA). DNAse treatment was performed using Ambion DNAse I (Thermo Fisher Scientific, Waltham, MA, USA). Concentrations and RNA quality ratios were determined in a Nanodrop 1000 spectrophotometer (Thermo Fisher Scientific, Waltham, MA, USA). cDNA was generated from 500 ng of total RNA using Superscript III First-Strand Synthesis System for RT-PCR (Invitrogen, Thermo Fisher Scientific, Waltham, MA, USA), in a final volume of 20 µl. Conditions for PCR included a single cycle and incubation periods of 65°C for 5 min, 25°C for 10 min, 50°C for 50 min, 85°C for 5 min, and 37°C for 20 min.

qPCR reactions were performed in a LightCycler480 system (Roche Applied Science, Indianapolis, IN, USA). *IL5RA* primers were designed using Primer 3.0 (35) and the Beacon Designer (36) software. *GAPDH* and *TBP* reference gene primers were chosen from The Real Time ready Human Reference GenePanel (Roche Applied Science, Indianapolis, IN, USA). The sequence of the primers used are shown in **Table 1**. Primers efficacies were analyzed by amplifying serial dilutions of cDNA sample of known concentration and according to the following equation: $E = (10^{-1/\text{slope}} - 1) \times 100$. All efficiencies ranged from 90 to 110%. The reaction mixture in each well-contained a final volume of 15 µl based on 7.5 µl of Master Mix SYBR Green I (Roche Applied Science, Indianapolis, IN, USA), 10 µM of each primers and 20 ng of cDNA. All reactions were performed in triplicate. In each experiment, non-template controls and calibrator were included. The PCR conditions included 10 min at 95°C followed by 45 cycles of 10 s at 95°C for denaturation, 10 s at 60°C for annealing and 10 s at 72°C for polymerization. Finally, melting curve analyses were carried out to verify the specificity of the qPCR products. *IL5RA* mRNA levels were normalized to *GAPDH* and *TBP* expression levels

TABLE 1 | Sequences of primers used in the qPCR assay.

	Primer	Sequence 5′ → 3′
IL5RA	Forward	TGAAAGAGTGAAGAACCGCC
	Reverse	CCTGGCCTGAGAAATGCG
GAPDH	Forward	CTCTGCTCCTCCTGTTCGAC
	Reverse	ACGACCAAATCCGTTGACTC
TBP	Forward	GAACATCATGGATCAGAACAACA
	Reverse	ATAGGGATTCCGGGAGTCAT

TABLE 2 | Characteristics of the study population in the RNAseq study and the validation analyses.

	N	Sex (% Female)	Age (Mean ± SD)	FeNO, ppb (Mean ± SD)	IgE, kU/l (Median ± IQR)
RNAseq study					
Controls	30	46.7	57 ± 17	-	46.7 ± 87.8
Asthmatic patients	30	56.7	30 ± 13	-	179.0 ± 239.0
Validation analysis					
Controls	100	66.0	57 ± 17	-	28.8 ± 57.7
Asthmatic patients	187	55.1	45 ± 19	44.8 ± 48.3	174.0 ± 398.2
Non-allergic asthma (NAA)	76	60.5	58 ± 15	38.1 ± 40.6	77.0 ± 118.8
NAA without NP	33	72.7	56 ± 16	24.8 ± 19.3	37.9 ± 103.5
NAA with NP	43	51.2	61 ± 14	52.2 ± 51.7	83.0 ± 258.7
Allergic asthma (AA)	111	51.4	35 ± 16	49.8 ± 53.0	312.5 ± 472.3
AA without NP	82	57.3	31 ± 14	39.8 ± 29.5	312.5 ± 445.5
AA with NP	29	34.5	46 ± 17	79.6 ± 88.7	307.0 ± 747.0
Early-onset asthma	76	61.8	31 ± 17	42.5 ± 43.1	271.0 ± 402.1
Late-onset asthma	111	50.5	54 ± 16	46.5 ± 51.9	126.0 ± 406.5
Non-eosinophilic asthma	32[a]	59.4	44 ± 17	26.4 ± 18.2	109.0 ± 260.5
Eosinophilic asthma	120[a]	53.3	46 ± 20	49.7 ± 54.5	196.0 ± 405.4

SD, standard deviation; IQR, interquartile range.
[a]Blood eosinophil counts were not available for all non-eosinophilic and eosinophilic asthma patients.

using the formula $2^{-\Delta\Delta Ct}$ by the comparative $\Delta\Delta$Ct method (37). All procedures followed the Minimum Information for Publication of Quantitative Real-Time PCR Experiment (MIQE) guidelines (38).

Pharmacogenetic Study

A proof-of-concept study of the *IL5RA* expression in peripheral blood before and after 3 months of treatment with benralizumab was performed in five severe eosinophilic asthmatic patients. Benralizumab was administered at a dose of 30 mg by subcutaneous injection once every 4 weeks. Asthma control test (ACT), fractional exhaled nitric oxide (FeNO) and lung function parameters were performed before and after 3 months of treatment. Patients were considered responders in the ACT score if they achieved a score of 25 or an increase of 3 or more points after 3 months of treatment. Also, they were considered FEV1 responders if they achieved a FEV1.0 $\geq$ 200 ml or FEV1.0 $\geq$ 12% after 3 months of treatment. As only three doses were evaluated, exacerbations were not considered. Blood samples were collected and lung function tests were performed at each time point. All patients provided their informed consent to receive benralizumab therapy.

Statistical Analysis

Descriptive analysis was carried out using central (mean and median) and dispersion tendency (standard deviation and interquartile range) measurements, followed by bivariate and multivariate analysis. The normality distribution was assessed by Kolmogorov-Smirnov test and the homoscedasticity was also tested before applying statistical tests. Continuous variables were evaluated using either ANOVA or Kruskal-Wallis test. Statistical significance was assessed by Wilcoxon's test for changes before

TABLE 3 | The 26 protein-coding transcripts most differentially expressed ($P < 0.025$) between the group of controls and patients with allergic asthma, listed by their fold change value.

Ensemble ID	External ID gene	Fold change	*P*-value
Up-regulated expression			
ENSG00000161905	*ALOX15*	2.45	3.91E-05
ENSG00000091181	*IL5RA*	2.22	8.63E-08
ENSG00000103056	*SMPD3*	2.16	1.44E-07
ENSG00000105205	*CLC*	2.04	4.63E-06
ENSG00000183134	*PTGDR2*	1.99	2.64E-06
ENSG00000134489	*HRH4*	1.93	7.21E-07
ENSG00000152207	*CYSLTR2*	1.84	1.15E-09
ENSG00000171659	*GPR34*	1.83	1.27E-08
ENSG00000143297	*FCRL5*	1.75	3.18E-05
ENSG00000255587	*RAB44*	1.74	8.10E-06
ENSG00000132465	*JCHAIN*	1.70	0.007
ENSG00000276231	*PIK3R6*	1.67	9.12E-06
ENSG00000131203	*IDO1*	1.67	0.014
Down-regulated expression			
ENSG00000118113	*MMP8*	−2.75	3.17E-04
ENSG00000012223	*LTF*	−2.35	4.79E-04
ENSG00000124469	*CEACAM8*	−2.19	2.47E-03
ENSG00000123689	*G0S2*	−2.02	4.95E-03
ENSG00000118520	*ARG1*	−2.00	4.51E-05
ENSG00000168209	*DDIT4*	−1.91	4.11E-04
ENSG00000179094	*PER1*	−1.86	6.80E-04
ENSG00000096006	*CRISP3*	−1.78	0.002
ENSG00000005961	*ITGA2B*	−1.75	6.90E-04
ENSG00000179869	*ABCA13*	−1.73	0.001
ENSG00000100985	*MMP9*	−1.69	0.001
ENSG00000124102	*PI3*	−1.65	7.32E-04
ENSG00000122025	*FLT3*	−1.64	3.66E-05

and after treatment. A *P*-value <0.05 was considered statistically significant. All statistical analyses were performed using SPSS Statistics version 21 (IBM, Armonk, NY, USA). Graphs were plot using GraphPad Prism version 6 (San Diego, CA, USA).

RESULTS

Study Population

The phenotypic characteristics of the studied subjects of the RNAseq study and the validation analysis are shown in **Table 2.** In both assays, control individuals were older to permit a more extended period for asthma to have appeared. Thus, age was significantly higher in the control group than in patients ($P <$ 0.001), except in the case of non-allergic and late-onset asthma groups, in which the disease had begun at older ages. According to the inclusion criteria, total IgE levels were significantly higher in all patient groups than in controls ($P \leq 0.001$). Moderate persistent asthma was the most common type in both the RNAseq study and the validation analysis (43.3 and 45.7%, respectively), followed by intermittent asthma (33.3 and 26.3%, respectively). The most common aeroallergen sensitization in the validation analysis patients was pollen, followed by animal dander. No patient was receiving oral corticosteroids.

Transcriptomic RNAseq Study

Significant differences between control and asthmatic patients were observed in the transcriptomic assay ($P < 0.05$). **Table 3** shows the top 26 most differentially expressed transcripts between controls and patients with allergic asthma, according to *P*-value and fold change. The main biological roles of these

TABLE 4 | Gene Ontology term enrichment analysis of the more differentially expressed genes.

Term ID	Biological process	FDR	Genes
Immune system			
GO:0002376	Immune system process	1.74E-07	*ABCA13, ARG1, CEACAM8, CRISP3, CYSLTR2, DDIT4, FLT3, IDO1, IL5RA, LTF, MMP8, MMP9, PI3, PTGDR2, RAB44, SMPD3.*
GO:0006955	Immune response	5.94E-06	*ABCA13, ARG1, CEACAM8, CRISP3, CYSLTR2, IL5RA, LTF, MMP8, MMP9, PI3, PTGDR2, RAB44.*
GO:0043312	Neutrophil degranulation	7.28E-05	*ABCA13, ARG1, CEACAM8, CRISP3, LTF, MMP8, MMP9, RAB44.*
Cellular process			
GO:0001775	Cell activation	1.32E-06	*ABCA13, ARG1, CEACAM8, CRISP3, FLT3, ITGA2B, LTF, MMP8, MMP9, PIK3R6, RAB44.*
GO:0019221	Cytokine-mediated signaling pathway	8.10E-03	*ALOX15, FLT3, IL5RA, MMP9.*
GO:0007166	Cell surface receptor signaling pathway	0.017	*ALOX15, DDIT4, FLT3, G0S2, GPR34, IL5RA, MMP9.*
GO:0007165	Signal transduction	0.012	*ALOX15, CYSLTR2, DDIT4, FLT3, G0S2, GPR34, HRH4, IL5RA, MMP9, PIK3R6, PTGDR2.*
Cellular response			
GO:0050896	Response to stimulus	2.52E-06	*ABCA13, ALOX15, ARG1, CEACAM8, CRISP3, CYSLTR2, DDIT4, FLT3, G0S2, GPR34, HRH4, IDO1, IL5RA, ITGA2B, LTF, MMP8, MMP9, PER1, PI3, PIK3R6, PTGDR2, RAB44.*
GO:0006952	Defense response	9.28E-05	*ALOX15, ARG1, CRISP3, DDIT4, HRH4, IDO1, IL5RA, LTF.*
GO:0006950	Response to stress	3.00E-04	*ALOX15, ARG1, CRISP3, DDIT4, HRH4, IDO1, IL5RA, ITGA2B, LTF, MMP9, PIK3R6.*
GO:0006954	Inflammatory response	2.50E-03	*ALOX15, HRH4, IDO1, IL5RA.*
GO:0071345	Cellular response to cytokine stimulus	9.30E-03	*ALOX15, ARG1, FLT3, IL5RA, MMP9.*
Biological regulation			
GO:0048583	Regulation of response to stimulus	6.84E-05	*ALOX15, ARG1, CLC, CYSLTR2, DDIT4, FLT3, G0S2, HRH4, IDO1, LTF, MMP9, PER1, PIK3R6, PTGDR2.*
GO:0009966	Regulation of signal transduction	6.84E-05	*ALOX15, ARG1, CYSLTR2, DDIT4, FLT3, G0S2, HRH4, LTF, MMP9, PER1, PIK3R6 PTGDR2.*
GO:0051239	Regulation of multicellular organismal process	2.30E-04	*ARG1, CLC, CYSLTR2, IDO1, IL5RA, ITGA2B, LTF, MMP9, PER1, PIK3R6, PTGDR2.*
GO:0001817	Regulation of cytokine production	6.20E-03	*ARG1, CLC, IDO1, IL5RA, LTF, PER1.*
GO:0050794	Regulation of cellular process	0.018	*ALOX15, ARG1, CLC, CRY2, CYSLTR2, DDIT4, FLT3, G0S2, GPR34, HRH4, IDO1, IL5RA, ITGA2B, LTF, MMP9, PER1, PI3, PIK3R6, PTGDR2, SMPD3.*

FDR, false discovery rate.

genes are described in **Table 4**, which highlights the biological processes related to the immune system. Among these genes, *IL5RA* attracted our attention as a putative asthma biomarker because it was the best positioned when considering both fold change and *P*-value data, and because of its role in different immune processes.

A protein-protein interaction network analysis was performed with the selected transcripts to analyze the interactions among them. Four main clusters were obtained, referred to as clusters A, B, C, and D (**Figure 1**). *IL5RA* was found in cluster A, which included seven genes: *IL5RA, IL5, FLT3* (receptor-type tyrosine-protein kinase), *PTGDR2* (prostaglandin D2 receptor 2), *HRH4* (histamine H4 receptor), *TIMP1* (metalloproteinase inhibitor 1) and *IDO1* (indoleamine 2,3-dioxygenase 1). Regarding the role of *IL5RA* in biological processes, the most significant terms were "immune system process" (FDR 1.74E-07) and "response to stimulus" (FDR 2.52E-06) (**Table 4**), as well as in Reactome pathways, such as "signaling by interleukins" and "RAF/MAP kinase cascade."

qPCR Validation Assays

A validation qPCR analysis was performed to confirm the differences observed in the RNAseq study. Patients were classified according to the presence of atopy and nasal polyposis (NP), the severity of asthma and the age of onset of asthma. As summarized in **Table 5**, asthmatic patients had significantly higher levels of peripheral blood eosinophil counts and *IL5RA* expression than controls ($P < 0.001$). That also occurred in all subgroups except for non-eosinophilic asthma ($P = 0.707$). Interestingly, the lower increase in *IL5RA* expression levels was observed in patients with non-allergic asthma (NAA) without NP (10.3 ± 11.2; $P = 0.037$). Significant differences were observed when comparing these patients with the subgroup of patients who had NAA with NP ($P = 0.047$). These significant differences were not observed among the other subgroups, although *IL5RA* expression levels were significantly higher in eosinophilic asthma than in non-eosinophilic asthma ($P < 0.001$). Also, *IL5RA* expression levels were slightly higher in monosensitized patients to pollens.

In general, there was an association between asthma severity and increased levels of *IL5RA* expression (**Table 5**). Patients with intermittent asthma had the lowest expression levels of *IL5RA* (12.0 ± 13.7), while patients with severe asthma had the highest levels (19.9 ± 20.3; $P = 0.056$). In addition, there was a statistically significant association between asthma severity and the number of eosinophils ($P = 0.015$).

To discard a possible influence of anti-inflammatory treatments on the expression of *IL5RA*, patients receiving inhaled corticosteroids or allergen immunotherapy were compared with patients not receiving these treatments. One hundred thirty-nine patients were receiving therapy with inhaled corticosteroids; 54 patients were receiving allergen immunotherapy. No statistically significant differences in the *IL5RA* expression levels were observed between patients receiving corticosteroid treatment or allergen immunotherapy and patients not receiving these treatments.

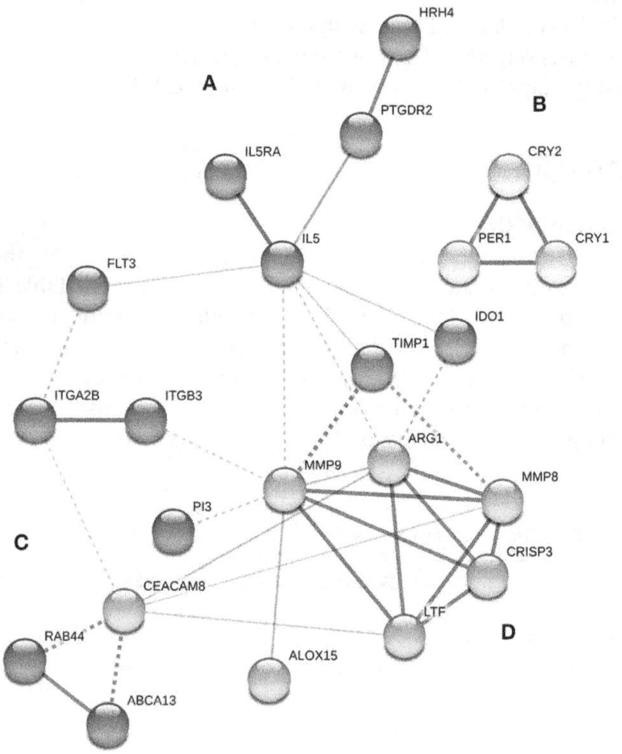

FIGURE 1 | Protein interaction network of proteins encoded by differentially expressed genes between controls and asthmatic patients using STRING software. The strength of data support is indicated by line thickness. The four main clusters are shown in blue **(A)**, yellow **(B)**, red **(C)**, and green **(D)**.

The relationship between *IL5RA* expression levels and peripheral blood eosinophil counts was also analyzed, observing some correlation with a Pearson's correlation coefficient of 0.520 ($P < 0.001$). Remarkably, as shown in **Figure 2A**, there were patients with the same eosinophil counts and very different expression levels of *IL5RA*. In addition, an eosinophil count-dependent increase in both *IL5RA* expression levels and dispersion was observed when the eosinophil counts were divided into quartiles (**Figure 2B**). This fact was also observed according to asthma severity. The more severe the asthma was, the greater the *IL5RA* levels were (**Figure 3**).

Pharmacogenetic Study

The clinical parameters of the patients included in the proof-of-concept study are shown in **Table 6**. Three of the patients had NP, and three were sensitized to pollens, without present clinical relevance. All patients were in treatment with high dose inhaled corticosteroids and tiotropium bromide at entry, although no patient was treated with oral corticosteroids. Before treatment with benralizumab, *IL5RA* expression levels and eosinophil counts were high in two patients, intermediate in two, and lower in another one. After 3 months of treatment, a dramatic reduction (90–100%) of peripheral eosinophil count was observed in all patients ($P = 0.042$) (**Figure 4A**). *IL5RA*

TABLE 5 | Blood eosinophil counts and *IL5RA* expression levels according to asthma diagnosis, sensitization and severity.

	N	Eosinophils/μl[a] (Mean ± SD)	*IL5RA*, relative expression (Mean ± SD)	*P*-value[b]	*P*-value[c]
Controls	100	127.8 ± 89.4	7.1 ± 6.3		
Asthmatic patients	187	380.4 ± 331.0	15.5 ± 15.4	<0.001	
Non-allergic asthma (NAA)	76	373.4 ± 367.1	13.9 ± 13.7	<0.001	
NAA without NP	33	223.7 ± 169.4	10.3 ± 11.2	0.037	0.047
NAA with NP	43	510.0 ± 441.6	16.6 ± 14.9	<0.001	
Allergic asthma (AA)	111	385.6 ± 303.3	16.6 ± 16.4	<0.001	
AA without NP	82	308.4 ± 222.9	16.5 ± 17.0	<0.001	0.982
AA with NP	29	577.1 ± 386.9	16.6 ± 15.0	<0.001	
Monosensitized to pollens	22	478.7 ± 301.6	20.2 ± 17.3	<0.001	
Monosensitized to animal dander	6	300.0 ± 205.2	21.4 ± 29.2	0.050	
Monosensitized to mites	10	411.1 ± 513.4	14.5 ± 14.5	0.064	
Polysensitized	73	358.8 ± 266.4	15.2 ± 14.7	<0.001	
Intermittent asthma	49	290.8 ± 199.3	12.0 ± 13.7	0.003	0.056
Mild persistent asthma	29	337.4 ± 192.7	17.7 ± 18.4	<0.001	
Moderate persistent asthma	85	380.5 ± 340.9	15.4 ± 13.4	<0.001	
Severe persistent asthma	23	574.0 ± 494.3	19.9 ± 20.3	<0.001	
Early-onset asthma	76	364.0 ± 307.4	14.5 ± 14.4	<0.001	
Late-onset asthma	111	391.1 ± 346.7	16.1 ± 16.0	<0.001	
Non-eosinophilic asthma	32	98.5 ± 66.1	6.6 ± 5.8	0.707	<0.001
Eosinophilic asthma	120	455.6 ± 332.9	18.2 ± 15.4	<0.001	

SD, standard deviation.

[a]All P-value results for blood eosinophil counts were significant ($P < 0.05$) among each patient group vs. controls, except for non-eosinophilic asthma ($P = 0.082$).

[b]P-value obtained for the comparison of IL5RA expression levels from each patient group vs. controls.

[c]P-value obtained for comparison of IL5RA expression levels from NAA without NP vs. NAA with NP; AA without NP vs. AA with NP; intermittent asthma vs. severe persistent asthma; and non-eosinophilic asthma vs. eosinophilic asthma, respectively.

expression levels were reduced between 70–96% after treatment ($P = 0.043$) (**Figure 4B**). A strong correlation was found between *IL5RA* levels and peripheral blood eosinophil counts at pretreatment (**Figure 4C**) with a Pearson's correlation coefficient of 0.940 ($P = 0.017$). In addition, all patients achieved an ACT score >20 and a mean increase of 30% in FEV1, except patient 4. This patient had the highest pretreatment levels of *IL5RA* expression, and the improvement of FEV1 reached 50% (**Figure 5**).

DISCUSSION

Novel biological therapies have increased clinical treatment options for asthma. The necessity of identifying biomarkers to achieve a proper selection of these expensive compounds has led to the application of transcriptomic methods as a starting point for discovering new genes involved in the disease. In a previous transcriptomic study, increased expression of interleukin-4 receptor (IL-4R) on B cells was observed in allergic asthma patients (39). In the present study, we have focused on another type 2 cytokine, IL-5, which is also involved in asthma pathophysiology. Thus, IL-5RA has been analyzed due to its implication with eosinophilic-mediated immunity.

In the RNAseq study, significant gene expression differences were observed between the peripheral blood samples of controls and allergic asthmatic patients, with a top 26 differentially expressed genes, as shown in **Table 3**. Interestingly, most of these genes are involved in biological processes related to the immune system, suggesting their potential implication in the pathophysiology of asthma. *IL5RA* turned out to be one of the genes with the highest differential expression, which is also supported by its relevant role in asthma (16, 17) and its interactions with other immune response effector molecules that were detected in the protein-protein interaction network analysis. All proteins of the *IL5RA* cluster had already been reported to participate in functions related to inflammatory response, signal transduction and eosinophil mediated immunity, such as eosinophil chemotaxis, regulation of type 2 cytokine production or cell differentiation and proliferation (40–44). These functions are consistent with the biological processes obtained in our transcriptomic study, described in **Table 4**. Furthermore, differential *IL5RA* expression levels have also been described in the literature, both between asthmatic patients and controls (45, 46) and pre and post-benralizumab treatment samples (47).

Following the results obtained in the RNAseq study, we decided to carry out a qPCR validation study to evaluate

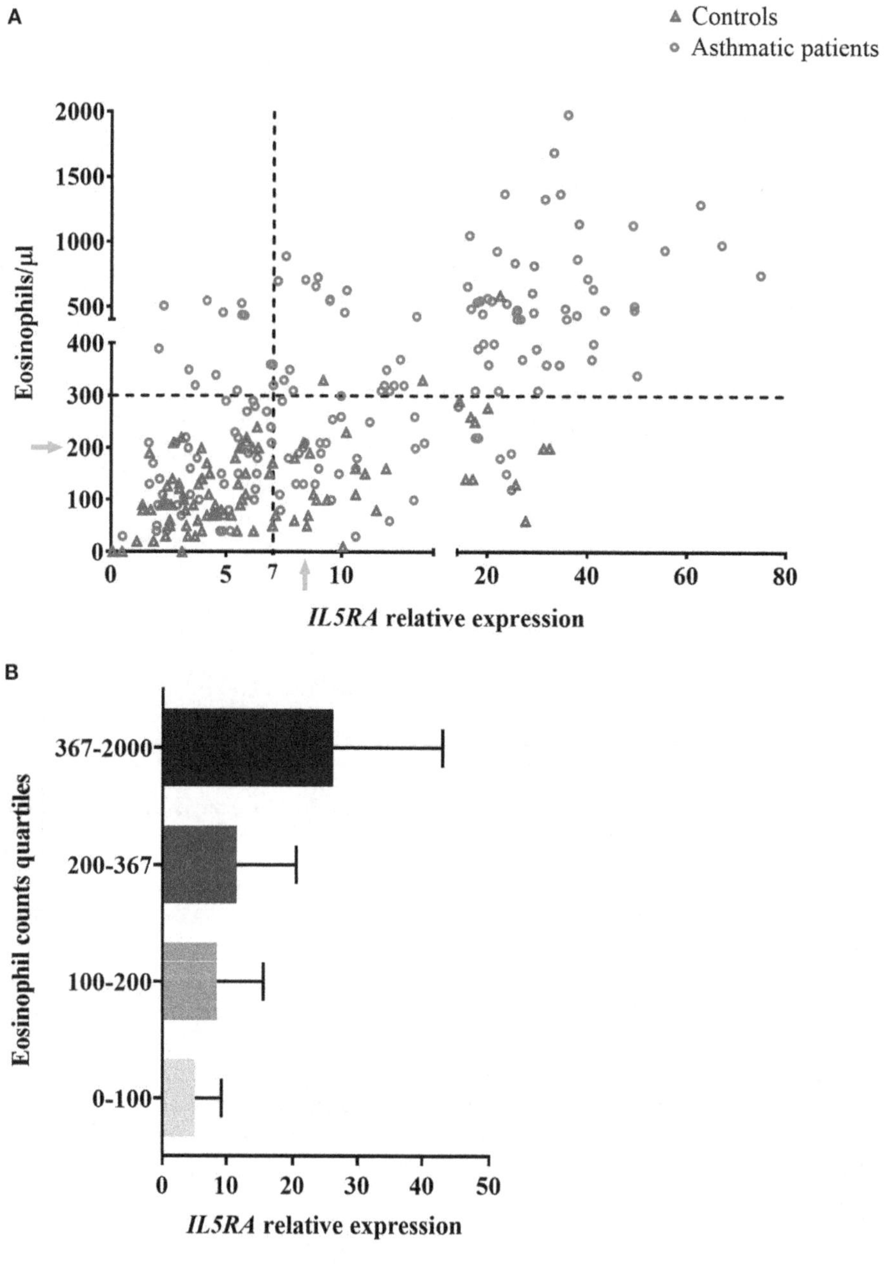

FIGURE 2 | (A) Correlation between *IL5RA* expression levels and peripheral blood eosinophil counts of controls and asthmatic patients from the validation analysis. Four quadrants were obtained by dividing according to the normality values for eosinophil counts (300/μl) and *IL5RA* expression (7-fold). The green arrows indicate a constant value of eosinophils at which a wide range of expressed *IL5RA* values is observed, and vice versa. **(B)** *IL5RA* expression levels (mean ± SD) in eosinophil count quartiles.

the performance of the peripheral blood *IL5RA* expression levels in the diagnosis of asthma. Levels were significantly higher in asthmatic patients than in controls, independently of the type of asthma (**Table 5**). This result suggests that it could be a potential marker in the diagnosis of asthma. One main limitation is its correlation with eosinophil counts, as a moderate correlation was observed ($r = 0.520$). Nevertheless, as shown by green arrows in **Figure 2A**, there was a notable dispersion of values, and some patients had high *IL5RA* expression levels compared to their eosinophil counts and vice versa. Also, we found that patients with the same eosinophil counts can show very different *IL5RA* expression levels. For example, *IL5RA* expression values ranging from 4 to 32 were observed for counts of 200 eosinophils/μl. This distribution was also found in controls, as variability in *IL5RA* expression levels was observed at low eosinophil counts. However, the dispersion was considerably more significant in patients with high eosinophil counts. This dispersion was also observed

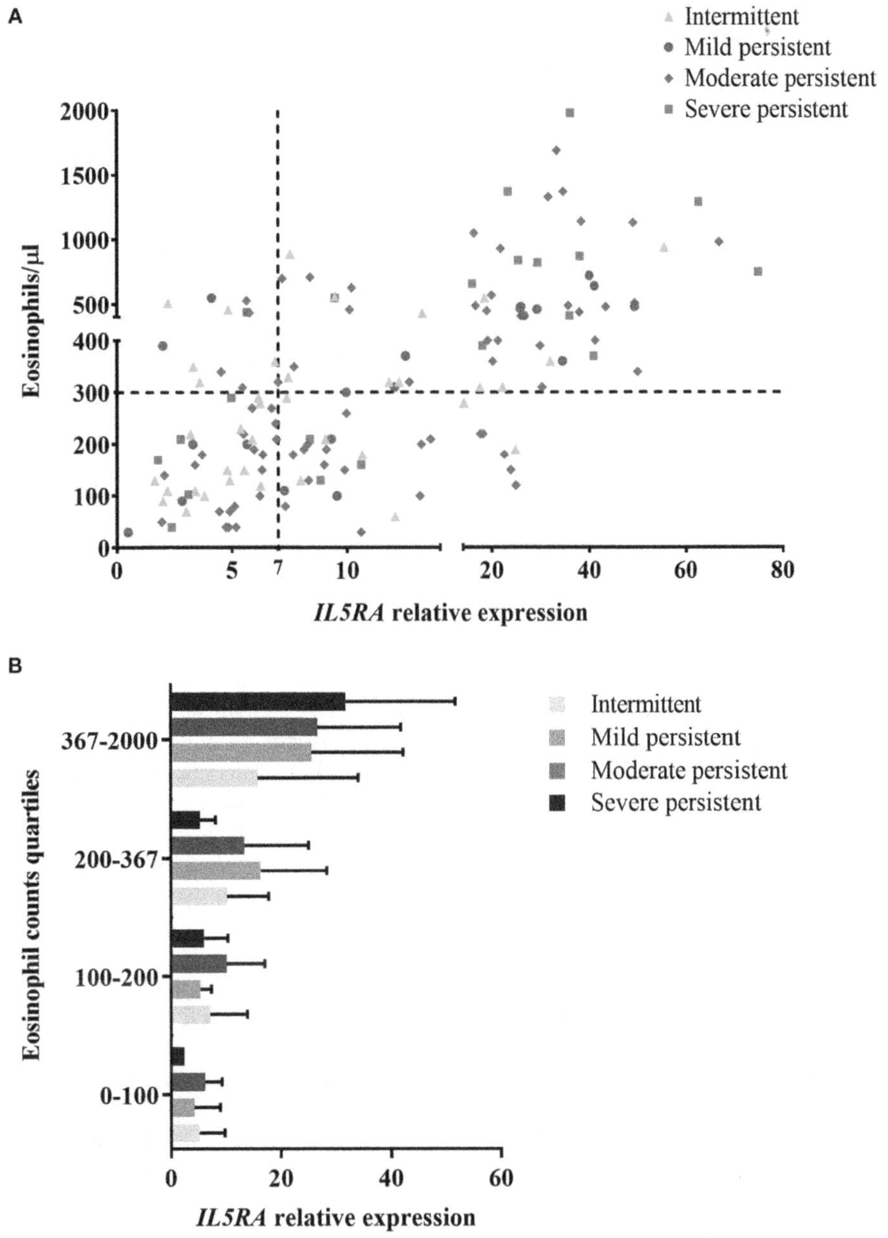

FIGURE 3 | (A) Correlation between *IL5RA* expression levels and peripheral blood eosinophil counts according to asthma severity of patients from the validation analysis. Four quadrants were obtained by dividing according to the normality values for eosinophil counts (300/µl) and *IL5RA* expression (7-fold). **(B)** *IL5RA* expression levels (mean ± SD) in eosinophil count quartiles according to asthma severity.

in all subgroups according to asthma severity. It can be speculated that differences could be due to different levels of expression of the *IL5RA* by eosinophils, caused by unknown elements, such as genetic or environmental factors driving the expression of the receptor. Besides, differences could reflect the expression by other cell types, such as basophils (20). In this sense, basophils have been involved in the immunology of eosinophilic asthma (48). Furthermore, this differential expression of *IL5RA* could be related to the different responses observed to biologics directed against *IL5RA*. In fact, in the proof-of-concept study, the patient with the highest levels of *IL5RA* expression was the best responder in terms of ACT and FEV1 (see below).

Concerning the different types of asthma, *IL5RA* expression levels were elevated in both allergic and non-allergic asthma. This finding is in agreement with the fact that responses to benralizumab are not influenced by the atopy status (49). In addition, we observed a progressive increase in the expression of *IL5RA* levels from intermittent to severe asthma, which could be related to the number of eosinophils to a great extent.

TABLE 6 | *IL5RA* expression levels and clinical parameters in pretreatment and after 3 months of benralizumab treatment.

	Eosinophils/μl	*IL5RA*, relative expression	FEV1, ml	FeNO, ppb	ACT
Patient 1					
Pretreatment	630	1.8	1,897	43	13
3 months	10	0.6	2,462	68	22
Patient 2					
Pretreatment	820	29.2	1,960	-	8
3 months	10	1.2	2,520	-	24
Patient 3[a]					
Pretreatment	437	10.9	2,310	154	12
3 months	0	1.0	3,100	113	22
Patient 4					
Pretreatment	1,290	62.5	1,890	66	19
3 months	0	4.7	2,840	198	25
Patient 5[a]					
Pretreatment	630	12.6	2,060	65	12
3 months	10	0.8	2,630	64	21

[a]Patients previously treated with other biological drugs, but no improvement was observed.

One streaking feature was that *IL5RA* expression levels were significantly higher in non-allergic asthma patients with NP respect to non-allergic asthma patients without NP. In this sense, it has been described that *IL5RA* expression is increased in patients with NP, particularly those with Aspirin-Exacerbated Respiratory Disease (50). Whether this could be related to response to the treatment with biologics in patients with chronic rhinosinusitis with NP remains speculative.

In the proof-of-concept pharmacogenetic study, we selected peripheral blood because it is easily accessible, a crucial characteristic of an ideal biomarker (51). In addition, as we were trying to check the *IL5RA* expression as a biomarker, we selected benralizumab treatment as it is directed against *IL5RA* (21). All patients were good responders, as demonstrated by the increase of ACT and FEV1. It is known that anti-IL-5 and anti-IL-5RA treatments do not significantly modify FeNO levels (52), as it happened in most of our patients. The increase observed in some of them could be due to acute exposure to allergens (53) because adherence to inhaled corticosteroids seemed to be appropriated. Due to the short follow-up period, exacerbations were not considered, although no patient had an exacerbation after treatment with benralizumab; even more, they almost did not require rescue bronchodilators. All patients showed a dramatic decrease in peripheral blood eosinophil counts with values between 0 and 10 eosinophils/μl, as observed in the phase III studies (21). The pretreatment levels of *IL5RA* were highly variable in patients, ranging from 1.8 to 62.5, and were strongly correlated with pretreatment peripheral blood eosinophil counts ($r = 0.940$). Thus, we believe that *IL5RA* expression level could add value to peripheral blood eosinophil counts. Accordingly, the patient with the highest *IL5RA* expression levels showed the best lung function response and reached an ACT of 25. In a very recent study, Nakajima et al. (54) described a group of super responder to benralizumab patients that had higher expression of genes related to eosinophils in peripheral blood, together with significant reductions in the expressions of genes associated with eosinophilic inflammatory responses after treatment with benralizumab, with *IL5RA* among them. So, the expression of *IL5RA* could be a useful biomarker of response, as it seems to be more discriminant than eosinophil counts.

This study is not without limitations since it is a unicentric study, and the number of patients is low. Nevertheless, this fact gives uniformity to the study. Additionally, we have mainly focused on *IL5RA*, and other genes may also be relevant in response to treatment. Nevertheless, we selected *IL5RA* by its crucial implication in the immunology of T2-asthma and because benralizumab is directed against this molecule. Finally, the proof-of-concept study has a limited number of patients and a short period of follow-up.

CONCLUSION

There is an urgent need for biomarkers of response to biologics in asthma. In this study, we have explored the peripheral blood *IL5RA* expression levels as a possible useful biomarker for several reasons. First, *IL5RA* is a plausible etiopathogenic target and a biologic target for the treatment of asthma. Second, peripheral blood is easily accessible. Third, its expression is easily measurable and reproducible. Fourth, it varies in different types of asthma. And, finally, although it has a moderate correlation with eosinophils, *IL5RA* expression levels probably do not reflect the same, as these levels vary for a particular count of peripheral blood eosinophils. Further studies are required for confirming the findings of the present study.

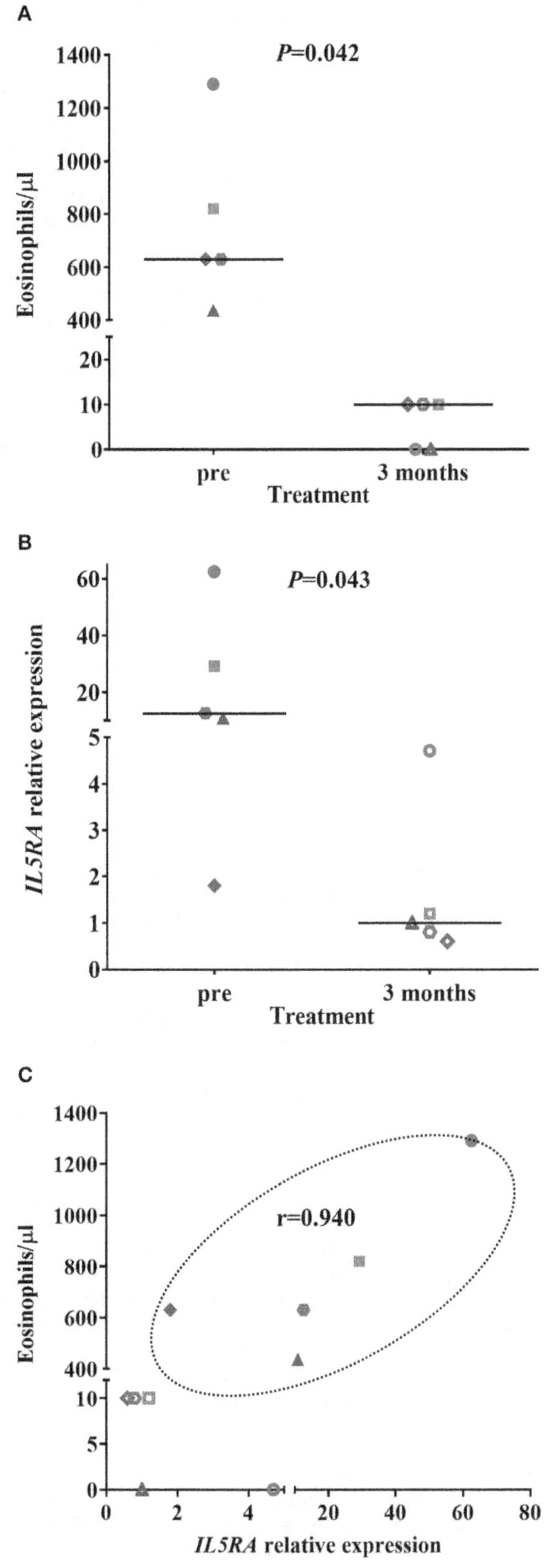

FIGURE 4 | **(A)** Peripheral blood eosinophil counts and **(B)** *IL5RA* expression levels in pretreatment and after 3 months of benralizumab treatment. The

(Continued)

FIGURE 4 | median of each group is also shown. **(C)** Correlation between *IL5RA* expression levels and peripheral blood eosinophil counts at pretreatment and after 3 months of benralizumab treatment. Pearson's correlation coefficient in the pretreatment is also shown. Each symbol represents a patient (◆ Patient 1; ■ Patient 2; ▲ Patient 3; ● Patient 4; ⬢ Patient 5). The filled symbols correspond to the pretreatment and the empty symbols to after 3 months of benralizumab treatment.

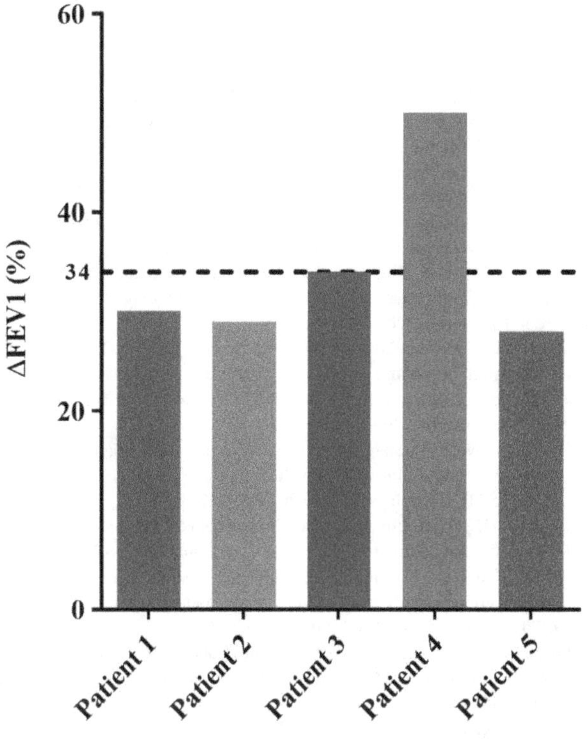

FIGURE 5 | Percentage of FEV1 value variation in each patient between pretreatment and after 3 months of treatment with benralizumab. The dotted line shows the mean of all patients.

AUTHOR CONTRIBUTIONS

SE-P, DH-J, AG-S, ME, MM, JR-G, JT, MI-G, CS, and ID have contributed in designing research studies, conducting experiments, acquiring data, analyzing data, and writing the manuscript. All authors read and approved the final manuscript.

FUNDING

This work was supported by the Instituto de Salud Carlos III and the European Regional Development Fund (Grant Nos. PI17/00818 and PI20/00268), by a grant of the Junta de Castilla y León and the European Regional Development Fund (IES161P20) and by a grant of the Instituto de Salud Carlos III to the Red temática de investigación en salud Asma, Reacciones Adversas y Alérgicas (ARADYAL) RD16/0006/0019.

REFERENCES

1. Vos T, Abajobir AA, Abbafati C, Abbas KM, Abate KH, Abd-Allah F, et al. Global, regional, and national incidence, prevalence, and years lived with disability for 328 diseases and injuries for 195 countries, 1990-2016: a systematic analysis for the global burden of disease study 2016. *Lancet.* (2017) 390:1211–59. doi: 10.1016/S0140-6736(17)32154-2
2. Global Initiative for Asthma. *Global Strategy for Asthma Management and Prevention.* (2020). Available online at: https://www.ginasthma.org/ (accessed April 25, 2020).
3. Wenzel SE. Asthma phenotypes: the evolution from clinical to molecular approaches. *Nat. Med.* (2012) 18:716–25. doi: 10.1038/nm.2678
4. Levine SJ, Wenzel SE. Narrative review: The role of Th2 immune pathway modulation in the treatment of severe asthma and its phenotypes. *Ann. Intern. Med.* (2010) 152:232–7. doi: 10.7326/0003-4819-152-4-201002160-00008
5. Lambrecht BN, Hammad H. The immunology of asthma. *Nat. Immunol.* (2015) 16:45–56. doi: 10.1038/ni.3049
6. Caminati M, Le Pham D, Bagnasco D, Canonica GW. Type 2 immunity in asthma. *World Allergy Organ. J.* (2018) 11:13. doi: 10.1186/s40413-018-0192-5
7. GEMA 4.4. *Guía española para el manejo del asma.* (2020). Available online at: https://www.gemasma.com/ (accessed May 1, 2020).
8. Kaur R, Chupp G. Phenotypes and endotypes of adult asthma: moving toward precision medicine. *J. Allergy Clin. Immunol.* (2019) 144:1–12. doi: 10.1016/j.jaci.2019.05.031
9. Moore WC, Meyers DA, Wenzel SE, Teague WG, Li H, Li X, et al. Identification of asthma phenotypes using cluster analysis in the severe asthma research program. *Am. J. Respir. Crit. Care Med.* (2010) 181:315–23. doi: 10.1164/rccm.200906-0896OC
10. Haldar P, Pavord ID, Shaw DE, Berry MA, Thomas M, Brightling CE, et al. Cluster analysis and clinical asthma phenotypes. *Am. J. Respir. Crit. Care Med.* (2008) 178:218–24. doi: 10.1164/rccm.200711-1754OC
11. Coumou H, Bel EH. Improving the diagnosis of eosinophilic asthma. *Expert Rev. Respir. Med.* (2016) 10:1093–103. doi: 10.1080/17476348.2017.1236688
12. Buhl R, Humbert M, Bjermer L, Chanez P, Heaney LG, Pavord I, et al. Severe eosinophilic asthma: a roadmap to consensus. *Eur. Respir. J.* (2017) 49:1700634. doi: 10.1183/13993003.00634-2017
13. Fitzpatrick AM, Moore WC. Severe asthma phenotypes—how should they guide evaluation and treatment? *J. Allergy Clin. Immunol. Pract.* (2017) 5:901–8. doi: 10.1016/j.jaip.2017.05.015
14. Isidoro-García M, Sánchez-Martín A, García-Sánchez A, Sanz C, García-Berrocal B, Dávila I. Pharmacogenetics and the treatment of asthma. *Pharmacogenomics.* (2017) 18:1271–80. doi: 10.2217/pgs-2017-0024
15. Canonica GW, Ferrando M, Baiardini I, Puggioni F, Racca F, Passalacqua G, et al. Asthma: personalized and precision medicine. *Curr. Opin. Allergy Clin. Immunol.* (2018) 18:51–8. doi: 10.1097/ACI.0000000000000416
16. Kouro T, Takatsu K. IL-5- and eosinophil-mediated inflammation: from discovery to therapy. *Int. Immunol.* (2009) 21:1303–9. doi: 10.1093/intimm/dxp102
17. Brussino L, Heffler E, Bucca C, Nicola S, Rolla G. Eosinophils target therapy for severe asthma: critical points. *Biomed. Res. Int.* (2018) 2018:7582057. doi: 10.1155/2018/7582057
18. Tavernier J, Devos R, Cornelis S, Tuypens T, Van der Heyden J, Fiers W, et al. A human high affinity interleukin-5 receptor (IL5R) is composed of an IL5-specific α chain and a β chain shared with the receptor for GM-CSF. *Cell.* (1991) 66:1175–84. doi: 10.1016/0092-8674(91)90040-6
19. Kupczyk M, Kuna P. Benralizumab: an anti-IL-5 receptor α monoclonal antibody in the treatment of asthma. *Immunotherapy.* (2018) 10:349–59. doi: 10.2217/imt-2017-0161
20. Kolbeck R, Kozhich A, Koike M, Peng L, Andersson CK, Damschroder MM, et al. MEDI-563, a humanized anti-IL-5 receptor α mAb with enhanced antibody-dependent cell-mediated cytotoxicity function. *J. Allergy Clin. Immunol.* (2010) 125:1344–53. doi: 10.1016/j.jaci.2010.04.004
21. Dávila González I, Moreno Benítez F, Quirce S. Benralizumab: a new approach for the treatment of severe eosinophilic asthma. *J. Investig. Allergol. Clin. Immunol.* (2019) 29:84–93. doi: 10.18176/jiaci.0385
22. American Thoracic Society. Standards for the diagnosis and care of patients with chronic obstructive pulmonary disease. *Am. J. Respir. Crit. Care Med.* (1995) 152:77–121.
23. Chung KF, Wenzel SE, Brozek JL, Bush A, Castro M, Sterk PJ, et al. International ERS/ATS guidelines on definition, evaluation and treatment of severe asthma. *Eur. Respir. J.* (2014) 43:343–73. doi: 10.1183/09031936.00202013
24. Sanz C, Isidoro-García M, Dávila I, Moreno E, Laffond E, Ávila C, et al. Promoter genetic variants of prostanoid DP receptor (PTGDR) gene in patients with asthma. *Allergy.* (2006) 61:543–8. doi: 10.1111/j.1398-9995.2006.01025.x
25. Sub-Committee on Skin Tests of the European Academy of Allergology and Clinical Immunology. Skin tests used in type I allergy testing Position paper. *Allergy.* (1989) 44 Suppl 10:1–59.
26. Sendín-Hernández MP, Ávila-Zarza C, Sanz C, García-Sánchez A, Marcos-Vadillo E, Muñoz-Bellido FJ, et al. Cluster analysis identifies 3 phenotypes within allergic asthma. *J. Allergy Clin. Immunol. Pract.* (2018) 6:955–61. doi: 10.1016/j.jaip.2017.10.006
27. Babraham Bioinformatics. *FastQC A Quality Control Tool for High Throughput Sequence Data.* (2020). Available online at: http://www.bioinformatics.babraham.ac.uk/projects/fastqc/ (accessed August 17, 2020).
28. Kim D, Pertea G, Trapnell C, Pimentel H, Kelley R, Salzberg SL. TopHat2: Accurate alignment of transcriptomes in the presence of insertions, deletions and gene fusions. *Genome Biol.* (2013) 14:R36. doi: 10.1186/gb-2013-14-4-r36
29. Picard Tools. By Broad Institute (2020). Available online at: http://broadinstitute.github.io/picard/ (accessed August 28, 2020).
30. Li H. Aligning sequence reads, clone sequences and assembly contigs with BWA-MEM. (2013) *arXiv[Preprint].* arXiv:1303.3997.
31. Trapnell C, Williams BA, Pertea G, Mortazavi A, Kwan G, Van Baren MJ, et al. Transcript assembly and quantification by RNA-Seq reveals unannotated transcripts and isoform switching during cell differentiation. *Nat. Biotechnol.* (2010) 28:511–5. doi: 10.1038/nbt.1621
32. Anders S, Pyl PT, Huber W. HTSeq-A Python framework to work with high-throughput sequencing data. *Bioinformatics.* (2015) 31:166–9. doi: 10.1093/bioinformatics/btu638
33. Love MI, Huber W, Anders S. Moderated estimation of fold change and dispersion for RNA-seq data with DESeq2. *Genome Biol.* (2014) 15:550. doi: 10.1186/s13059-014-0550-8
34. STRING. *Functional Protein Association Networks.* (2020). Available online at: https://string-db.org/ (accessed October 13, 2020).
35. Primer3.0. (2018). Available online at: http://bioinfo.ut.ee/primer3-0.4.0/ (accessed March 6, 2018).
36. Beacon Designer (2020). Available online at: http://www.premierbiosoft.com/qOligo/Oligo.jsp?PID=1 (accessed March 6, 2018).
37. Livak KJ, Schmittgen TD. Analysis of relative gene expression data using real-time quantitative PCR and the 2-ΔΔCT method. *Methods.* (2001) 25:402–8. doi: 10.1006/meth.2001.1262
38. Bustin SA, Benes V, Garson JA, Hellemans J, Huggett J, Kubista M, et al. The MIQE guidelines: minimum information for publication of quantitative real-time PCR experiments. *Clin. Chem.* (2009) 55:611–22. doi: 10.1373/clinchem.2008.112797
39. Pascual M, Roa S, García-Sánchez A, Sanz C, Hernandez-Hernandez L, Greally JM, et al. Genome-wide expression profiling of B lymphocytes reveals IL4R increase in allergic asthma. *J. Allergy Clin. Immunol.* (2014) 134:972–5. doi: 10.1016/j.jaci.2014.05.015
40. Agrawal DK, Hopfenspirger MT, Chavez J, Talmadge JE. Flt3 ligand: a novel cytokine prevents allergic asthma in a mouse model. *Int. Immunopharmacol.* (2001) 1:2081–9. doi: 10.1016/S1567-5769(01)00122-9
41. Domingo C, Palomares O, Sandham DA, Erpenbeck VJ, Altman P. The prostaglandin D2 receptor 2 pathway in asthma: a key player in airway inflammation 11 medical and health sciences 1107 immunology 11 medical and health sciences 1102 Cardiorespiratory Medicine and Haematology. *Respir. Res.* (2018) 19:189. doi: 10.1186/s12931-018-0893-x
42. Ling P, Ngo K, Nguyen S, Thurmond RL, Edwards JP, Karlsson L, et al. Histamine H4 receptor mediates eosinophil chemotaxis with cell shape change and adhesion molecule upregulation. *Br. J. Pharmacol.* (2004) 142:161–71. doi: 10.1038/sj.bjp.0705729
43. Hassan N, Mohamed-Hussein A, Mohamed E, Mohamed O, Mohamed H, Tammam M. Matrix metalloproteinase- 9 (MMP-9) and tissue inhibitor of metalloproteinase-1(TIMP-1) as non-invasive biomarkers of remodelling in asthma. *Eur. Respir. J.* (2015)

46(Suppl. 59):OA1467. doi: 10.1183/13993003.congress-2015.OA1467
44. Hayashi T, Beck L, Rossetto C, Gong X, Takikawa O, Takabayashi K, et al. Inhibition of experimental asthma by indoleamine 2,3-dioxygenase. *J. Clin. Invest.* (2004) 114:270–9. doi: 10.1172/JCI21275
45. Bigler J, Boedigheimer M, Schofield JPR, Skipp PJ, Corfield J, Rowe A, et al. A severe asthma disease signature from gene expression profiling of peripheral blood from U-BIOPRED cohorts. *Am. J. Respir. Crit. Care Med.* (2017) 195:1311–20. doi: 10.1164/rccm.201604-0866OC
46. Virkud Y V., Kelly RS, Croteau-Chonka DC, Celedón JC, Dahlin A, Avila L, et al. Novel eosinophilic gene expression networks associated with IgE in two distinct asthma populations. *Clin. Exp. Allergy.* (2018) 48:1654–64. doi: 10.1111/cea.13249
47. Sridhar S, Liu H, Pham TH, Damera G, Newbold P. Modulation of blood inflammatory markers by benralizumab in patients with eosinophilic airway diseases. *Respir. Res.* (2019) 20:14. doi: 10.1186/s12931-018-0968-8
48. Suzuki Y, Wakahara K, Nishio T, Ito S, Hasegawa Y. Airway basophils are increased and activated in eosinophilic asthma. *Allergy Eur. J. Allergy Clin. Immunol.* (2017) 72:1532–9. doi: 10.1111/all.13197
49. Chipps BE, Newbold P, Hirsch I, Trudo F, Goldman M. Benralizumab efficacy by atopy status and serum immunoglobulin E for patients with severe, uncontrolled asthma. *Ann. Allergy Asthma Immunol.* (2018) 120:504–11. doi: 10.1016/j.anai.2018.01.030
50. Buchheit KM, Dwyer DF, Ordovas-Montanes J, Katz HR, Lewis E, Vukovic M, et al. IL-5Rα marks nasal polyp IgG4- and IgE-expressing cells in aspirin-exacerbated respiratory disease. *J. Allergy Clin. Immunol.* (2020) 145:1574–84. doi: 10.1016/j.jaci.2020.02.035
51. Medrek SK, Parulekar AD, Hanania NA. Predictive biomarkers for asthma therapy. *Curr. Allergy Asthma Rep.* (2017) 17:69. doi: 10.1007/s11882-017-0739-5
52. Hoyte FCL, Gross LM, Katial RK. Exhaled nitric oxide: an update. *Immunol. Allergy Clin. North Am.* (2018) 38:573–85. doi: 10.1016/j.iac.2018.06.001
53. Sordillo JE, Webb T, Kwan D, Kamel J, Hoffman E, Milton DK, et al. Allergen exposure modifies the relation of sensitization to fraction of exhaled nitric oxide levels in children at risk for allergy and asthma. *J. Allergy Clin. Immunol.* (2011) 127:1165–72.e5. doi: 10.1016/j.jaci.2011.01.066
54. Nakajima M, Matsuyama M, Arai N, Yamada H, Hyodo K, Nonaka M, et al. Identification of whole blood gene expressions correlated with responsiveness to benralizumab. *J. Allergy Clin. Immunol.* (2020) S0091-6749:31110–6. doi: 10.1016/j.jaci.2020.08.004

11

Trends in Influenza Vaccination Rates in Participants with Airflow Limitation: The Korea National Health and Nutrition Examination Survey 2007–2018

Hyun Lee [1†]***, Hayoung Choi*** [2†] ***and Yong Suk Jo*** [3*]

[1] Division of Pulmonary Medicine and Allergy, Department of Internal Medicine, Hanyang University College of Medicine, Seoul, South Korea, [2] Division of Pulmonary, Allergy, and Critical Care Medicine, Department of Internal Medicine, Hallym University Kangnam Sacred Heart Hospital, Hallym University College of Medicine, Seoul, South Korea, [3] Division of Pulmonary and Critical Care Medicine, Department of Internal Medicine, Seoul St. Mary's Hospital, College of Medicine, The Catholic University of Korea, Seoul, South Korea

Correspondence:
Yong Suk Jo
lucidyonge@gmail.com

† These authors have contributed equally to this work

Background: Influenza vaccination is strongly recommended for people with chronic lung diseases, including chronic obstructive pulmonary disease, to reduce risk of exacerbation. We assess the influenza vaccination rate and its related factors in participants with airflow limitation (AFL) using nationally representative data in Korea.

Methods: We conducted a cross-sectional study from the Korea National Health and Nutrition Examination Survey from 2007 to 2018. Individuals $\geq$ 40 years who underwent spirometry and had identifiable information on influenza vaccination status were included.

Results: Overall influenza vaccination coverage was 61.2% in participants with AFL and 41.8% in participants without AFL. Age had a significant impact on the yearly vaccination rate in participants with AFL. Over the 10 years of study period, while the yearly vaccination rate steadily increased from 58.3 to 61.9% in elderly participants ($\geq$65 years) with AFL (*p* for trend = 0.117), the yearly vaccination rate decreased from 41.5% to 30.8% in younger participants (<65 years) (*p* for trend = 0.038). In multivariable analyses, younger age [adjusted odds ratio (OR) for unvaccinated = 0.88, 95% confidence interval (CI) = 0.87–0.90], male (adjusted OR = 1.64; 95% CI = 1.23–2.19), and current smokers (adjusted OR = 1.42, 95% CI = 1.01–2.00) were associated with increased odds of being unvaccinated.

Conclusions: The vaccination rate in participants with AFL affected by age. Younger age, male sex, and current smoking were associated with unvaccinated status. More attention and targeted interventions are required to improve the influenza vaccination rate in those with AFL.

Keywords: influenza, vaccination, airflow limitation, risk factor, National Health and Nutrition Examination Survey (NHANES)

INTRODUCTION

Chronic obstructive pulmonary disease (COPD), which is a representative disease with airflow limitation (AFL), is the leading causes of death worldwide, with a prevalence of 5.6% in 2015, which is expected to increase to 7.8% by 2030 (1, 2). COPD is a chronic inflammatory airway disease characterized by fixed airflow limitation and chronic respiratory symptoms, such as cough, sputum, and progressive dyspnea. Acute exacerbation of COPD (AECOPD) can occur during the natural course of disease (3). AECOPD not only affects an individual's physical health status but also decreases lung function and increases future risk of exacerbation and even mortality (4–6). AECOPD also increases medical expense and resource use, causing increased socioeconomic burden (7).

AECOPD is a heterogeneous event thought to be caused by complex interactions between the host, respiratory viruses or bacteria, and environmental pollution (8, 9). The most common causes of AECOPD are respiratory infections, most of which are viral. Although the most frequent viruses associated with exacerbation are human rhinoviruses (8), influenza is also important, accounting for up to 28% of COPD exacerbations (10). Influenza can lead to hospitalization, frequent exacerbation, and even death in patients with COPD (11, 12). The disease course of influenza is worse in patients with COPD compared with those without COPD.

Influenza vaccination is the main strategy for prevention and control of seasonal influenza (13). The influenza vaccination has been shown to reduce AECOPD, influenza-related hospitalization, and mortality (14, 15). Thus, seasonal influenza vaccination is recommended to stable COPD patients from groups A to D classified by combining exacerbation history and severity of dyspnea suggested by Global Initiative for Chronic Obstructive Lung Disease (GOLD) (16). Despite this recommendation, it is not known whether influenza vaccination coverage has increased among COPD patients because most studies evaluated vaccination rates for a certain year (17–20). Such information is even scarcer within the past 10 years (21).

In addition to COPD, influenza vaccination should be considered in relation to other respiratory diseases including asthma and bronchiectasis. A previous meta-analysis found that influenza vaccination reduced febrile illnesses and prevented asthma attacks requiring emergency visits and hospitalizations (22). Despite limited studies regarding the efficacy of influenza vaccination in bronchiectasis, international bronchiectasis guidelines strongly recommend influenza vaccination in patients with bronchiectasis (23, 24). Consequently, more studies are needed to evaluate the factors associated with influenza vaccination coverage among individuals with AFL to develop ways to encourage vaccination and improve their health outcomes.

In this study, we measure the influenza vaccination rate among participants with AFL in a nationally representative sample of Korea, and assess factors associated with influenza vaccination.

METHODS

Study Population

For this study, cross-sectional data were used from the Korea National Health and Nutrition Examination Survey (KNHANES), which provides nationwide statistical data on the Korean population's health and diet from January 2007 to December 2018. The questionnaire on the influenza vaccination was investigated for only 3 months in 2013 and was not disclosed to the public; thus, data from 2013 were not included in this study. The KNHANES uses a complex, stratified, multistage probability cluster sampling design with sampling units of households based on geographic region, age, and gender. A health-related interview, nutrition survey, and physical examination were performed for each participant selected throughout Korea by trained interviewers. All participants agreed to participate in this study. Since publicly available data were used, ethical approval was waived. The KNHANES surveys were approved by the relevant institutional review boards, and informed consent was provided by all participants.

Because spirometry is only performed in individuals older than 40 years, we only included participants ≥40 years in the analyses. Participants who did not undergo spirometry and those who had missing data for influenza vaccination were excluded from the study.

Of the total 38,247 participants, influenza vaccination data were available for 34,464, of whom 4,873 (14.1%) had AFL on spirometry and 29,591 (85.9%) did not. Finally, this study included 4,873 participants with AFL, comprising those without influenza vaccination (n = 1,890) and those with influenza vaccination (n = 2,983) (**Figure 1**).

Exposure

The main exposure variable was influenza vaccination, which was determined by the response to a question about influenza vaccination status during the previous 1 year: "Have you been vaccinated for influenza during the previous 1 year?"

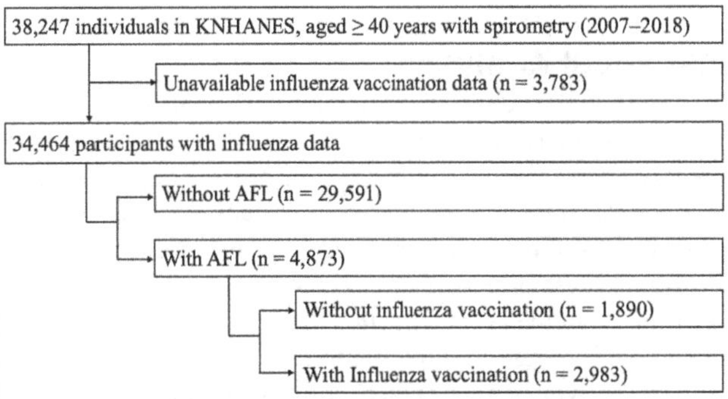

FIGURE 1 | Selection of study population. AFL, airflow limitation; KNHANES, Korea National Health and Nutrition Examination Survey.

Study Outcomes

The study outcomes were (1) influenza vaccination rate according to presence or absence of AFL during the study period; (2) influenza vaccination rate in participants with AFL stratified by age and AFL severity; and (3) factors associated with vaccination status in participants with AFL.

To reduce the disease burden of influenza, the Korean government instituted a national immunization program in 2005, which provides free influenza vaccination for people aged ≥ 65 years. Accordingly, we divided subjects into two age groups (65 years or older vs. under 65 years).

AFL was defined as spirometry revealing forced expiratory volume in 1 s (FEV_1)/forced vital capacity (FVC) <0.7. Severity of AFL was classified according to the percentage of the predicted FEV_1 (% pred): mild (FEV_1 %pred of >70), moderate (FEV_1 %pred of 60–69), moderately severe (FEV_1 %pred of 50–59), severe (FEV_1 %pred of 35–49), and very severe (FEV_1 %pred of <35) (25).

Covariates

The KNHANES provides various demographic data [age, sex, body mass index (BMI), education level, marital status, and self-perceived income status] and spirometry results. The Korean version of the EuroQol-5 dimensions questionnaire (EQ-5D), a simple health-related quality of life instrument consisting of 5 health dimensions (mobility, self-care, usual activities, pain/discomfort, and anxiety/depression), was used to measure QoL status (26, 27). Several comorbid conditions were also included in this study. The presence of hypertension was determined by high blood pressure (mean systolic blood pressure ≥140 mmHg or mean diastolic blood pressure ≥90 mmHg on examination or current intake of antihypertensive medications). Hypercholesterolemia was defined as total cholesterol >200 mg/dL or current intake of lipid-lowering medications (28). Diabetes was defined as fasting glucose >126 mg/dL or HbA1c >6.5% or current use of oral hypoglycemic agents or insulin for glycemic control (29). The presence of other comorbid conditions was determined by a positive response to the following two questions: "Have you been diagnosed with [disease] by a doctor?" or "Do you take medicine or treatment for [disease]?" (30).

Statistical Analyses

Data are presented as medians and interquartile ranges for continuous variables and as frequencies (percentages) for categorical variables. Data were compared using the Mann-Whitney U test for continuous variables because of non-normality. Continuous variables were compared using Pearson's chi-squared test or Fisher's exact test, as appropriate. For the analyses of influenza vaccination rate by AFL severity and multivariable logistic regression to evaluate factors associated with not receiving influenza vaccination, we classified the severity of AFL into four groups [mild (FEV_1 %pred of >70), moderate (FEV_1 %pred of 60–69), moderately severe (FEV_1 %pred of 50–59), and severe to very severe (FEV_1 %pred of <50)] because there only 1.3% of participants ($n = 64$) had severe to very severe AFL (FEV_1 %pred of <50) in the NHANES dataset. In the multivariable logistic regression model, we adjusted for age, sex, BMI, marital status, type of medical insurance, economic activity, education level, EQ-5D, chronic bronchitis, smoking history, the severity of AFL, comorbidities (hypertension, ischemic heart disease, diabetes mellitus, and asthma). All tests were two-sided, and a p-value ≤ 0.05 was considered statistically significant. Statistical analyses were performed using STATA software (ver. 16; StataCorp, College Station, TX, USA).

RESULTS

Influenza Vaccination Rate According to Presence of Airflow Limitation

Influenza vaccination trends from 2007 to 2018 are shown in **Figure 2**. Compared to 61.2% of participants with AFL (2,983/4,873) being vaccinated, 41.8% participants without AFL (12,357/29,591) were vaccinated.

Figure 3 shows the influenza vaccination trends according to AFL status based on age. While the overall vaccination rate in participants 65 years or older was ~80% (**Figure 3A**), the vaccination rate in participants younger than 65 years was <40% (**Figure 3B**). AFL had a significantly different impact on the age-stratified vaccination rate. In participants 65 years or older, the overall vaccination rate (80.2% with AFL vs. 80.3% without AFL; $p = 0.894$) was not different by AFL. Regardless of AFL, the yearly vaccination rate steadily increased during the study period [58.3% in 2007 to 61.9% in 2018 (p for trend = 0.117) in participants with AFL; 40.2% in 2007 to 44.7% in 2018 (p for trend <0.001) in participants without AFL; **Figure 3A**].

However, among individuals 65 years or less, the vaccination rate was higher in participants with AFL than in those without AFL (34.7% with AFL vs. 29.2% without AFL; $p < 0.001$). Additionally, while there was a decreasing trend in the yearly vaccination rate among participants with AFL, the vaccination rate in subjects without AFL fluctuated [41.5% in 2007 to 30.8% in 2018 (p for trend = 0.038) for participants with AFL; 28.6% in 2007 to 29.9% in 2018 (p for trend < 0.001) in participants without AFL; **Figure 3B**].

Comparison of Clinical Features in Participants With AFL According to Influenza Vaccination

Differences in clinical characteristics according to influenza vaccination status in participants with AFL are presented in **Table 1**. Vaccinated participants tended to be older and were less likely to be male and current smokers compared with unvaccinated participants ($p < 0.001$ for both). Regarding socioeconomics, vaccinated participants had lower economic activity and lower QoL compared with unvaccinated participants ($p < 0.001$ for both). Comorbid conditions including hypertension, ischemic heart disease, hypercholesterolemia, diabetes mellitus, cerebrovascular disease, asthma, and osteoporosis were more common among vaccinated participants than unvaccinated participants. Except for FEV_1

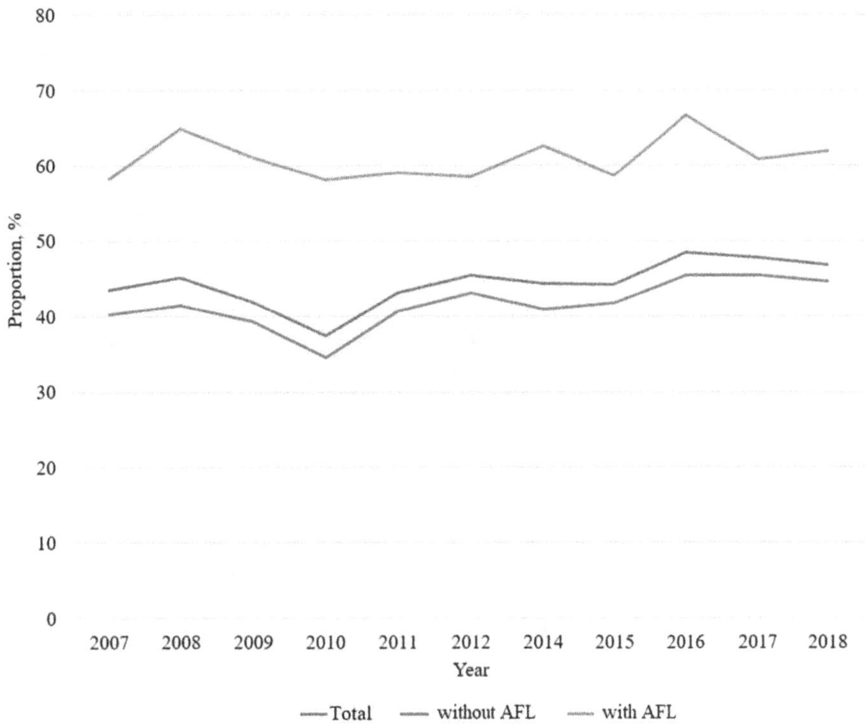

FIGURE 2 | Influenza vaccination trends in participants with AFL. AFL, airflow limitation.

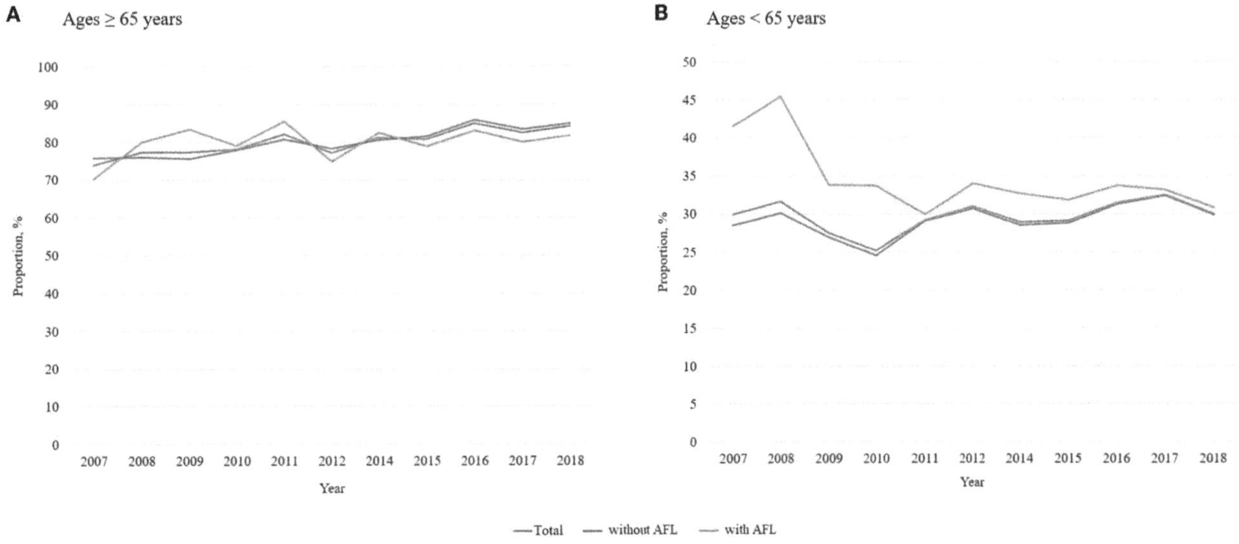

FIGURE 3 | Influenza vaccination trends according to age (≥65 vs. <65 years). AFL, airflow limitation. **(A)** Age ≥ 65 years, **(B)** Age < 65 years. AFL, airflow limitation.

% predicted, vaccinated participants had lower lung function parameters [FEV_1 (L), FVC (L), FVC % pred, and FEV_1/FVC] compared with unvaccinated participants ($p < 0.001$ for the latter four variables).

Influenza Vaccination Rate According to AFL Severity

Influenza vaccination rate was further analyzed according to AFL severity. The overall vaccination rates were 59.8% (2,027/3,392),

TABLE 1 | Comparison of clinical features in participants with airflow limitation according to influenza vaccination.

	Participants with airflow limitation (*N* = 4,873)		
	Without influenza vaccination (*n* = 1,890)	**With influenza vaccination (*n* = 2,983)**	***P*-value**
Age (years)	60 (53–66)	70 (65–75)	<0.001
Male sex	1,449 (76.7)	2,061 (69.1)	<0.001
Current smoker	883 (47.1)	1,009 (34.1)	<0.001
Smoking amount (pack-years) (*n*=3,182)	5 (0–26)	0 (0–24.5)	0.004
Body mass index, kg/m^2	23.5 (21.6–25.5)	23.5 (21.7–25.3)	0.782
Education beyond high school	1,107 (59.1)	1,149 (38.8)	<0.001
Marriage status (yes)	1,853 (98.2)	2,953 (99.2)	0.001
Economic activity status	1,257 (66.9)	1,352 (45.5)	<0.001
Health insurance	1,798 (95.8)	2,791 (94.4)	0.027
Symptoms (*n* = 3,558)			
Cough ≥3 months	45 (3.2)	88 (4.1)	0.207
Sputum ≥3 months	108 (7.8)	206 (9.5)	0.075
Chronic bronchitis	118 (8.5)	223 (10.3)	0.076
Quality of life, EQ-5D	1 (0.907–1)	1 (0.817–1)	<0.001
Comorbidities			
Hypertension (*n* = 3,576)	667 (51.5)	1,472 (64.5)	<0.001
Ischemic heart disease (*n* = 2,383)	53 (6.0)	152 (10.2)	<0.001
Hypercholesterolemia (*n* = 4,559)	298 (16.8)	571 (20.5)	0.002
Diabetes mellitus (*n* = 4,130)	853 (54.3)	1,512 (59.1)	0.003
Cerebrovascular disease (*n* = 2,354)	32 (3.6)	88 (6.0)	0.012
Asthma (*n* = 2,612)	63 (6.6)	200 (12.1)	<0.001
Osteoporosis (*n* = 1,958)	25 (3.5)	141 (11.4)	<0.001
Tuberculosis (*n* = 2,663)	49 (4.9)	87 (5.3)	0.633
Depression (*n* = 2,602)	26 (2.7)	61 (3.7)	0.151
Any cancer history* (*n* = 1,361)	33 (3.8)	52 (3.5)	0.757
Spirometry			
FEV_1, L	2.45 (1.96–2.90)	2.07 (1.60–2.49)	<0.001
FEV_1, % pred	78.2 (68.6–86.6)	77.6 (66.5–87.6)	0.287
FVC, L	3.81 (3.12–4.44)	3.32 (2.66–3.90)	<0.001
FVC, % pred	91.9 (82.3–100.6)	87.2 (76.9–96.9)	<0.001
FEV_1/FVC	66.0 (61.9–68.3)	65.0 (59.8–67.9)	<0.001

Data are presented as median (interquartile range) or number (percentage). The numbers in brackets for each comorbidity represent the number of participants who responded to the questions regarding each comorbidity.

**Includes gastric, liver, colon, breast, cervical, lung, or thyroid cancer.*

EQ-5D, EuroQol-5 dimensions questionnaire; FEV_1, forced expiratory volume in 1s; % pred, percentage of the predicted value; FVC, forced vital capacity.

61.7% (484/784), 66.6% (273/410), and 69.3% (199/287) in participants with mild, moderate, moderately severe, and severe to very severe AFL subjects, respectively (**Figure 4**; $p = 0.001$).

Factors Related to Non-vaccination in Participants With AFL

As shown in **Table 2**, in multivariable analyses, younger age [adjusted odds ratio (OR) for being unvaccinated = 0.88, 95% confidence interval (CI) = 0.87–0.90], male (adjusted OR = 1.70; 95% CI = 1.21–2.42), and current smoking (adjusted OR = 1.42, 95% CI = 1.01–2.00) were associated with increased odds for being unvaccinated. Although participants with more severe AFL were more likely to be vaccinated according to the univariable analysis, the severity of AFL was not related to vaccination status in multivariable analyses.

DISCUSSION

This study evaluated influenza vaccination trends from 2007 and 2018 among participants with AFL in Korea. During the study period, the overall influenza vaccination rate was higher in participants with AFL than in those without AFL. While the influenza vaccination rate in the elderly with AFL steadily increased similar to that of those without AFL, the rate in young participants with AFL decreased, while the rate among young participants without AFL fluctuated. In multivariable analyses,

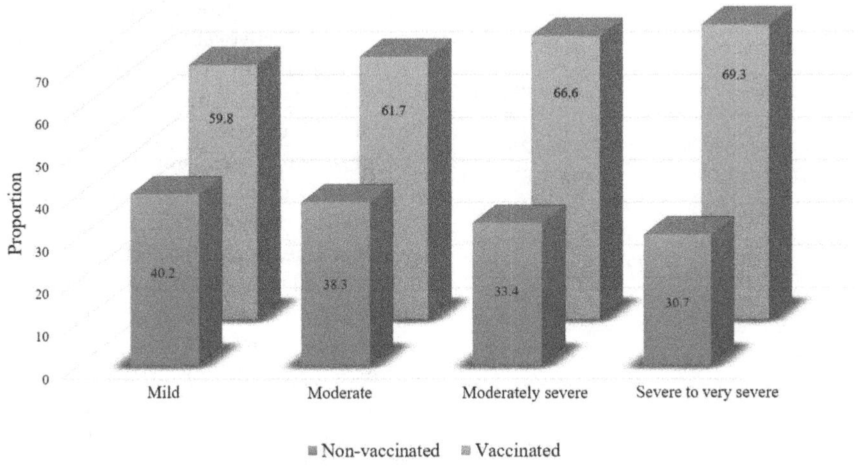

FIGURE 4 | Influenza vaccination rate according to AFL severity. AFL, airflow limitation.

younger age, male, and current smoking were associated with increased odds of unvaccinated status.

Influenza vaccination has been considered as important management in individuals with chronic airway diseases with AFL, such as COPD, asthma, and bronchiectasis. The current guidelines strongly recommend influenza vaccination in COPD. Influenza vaccination is known to reduce not only acute exacerbations but also serious lower respiratory infections in COPD participants. The benefits of influenza vaccination in participants with COPD extend beyond the prevention of respiratory illness. Studies have shown that influenza vaccination can reduce mortality and risk of ischemic heart disease, especially in the elderly (31). Furthermore, chronic comorbidities are highly prevalent in patients with COPD and are associated with frequent exacerbations and increased risk of exacerbation (32). Hence, influenza vaccination should be emphasized in patients with AFL and other comorbidities.

The vaccination rate in patients with COPD varies widely by country. While the rates of influenza vaccination in patients with COPD were relatively high in the US (~64%) (21), Spain (~60%) (17, 18), and Korea (~60% in this study), the vaccination rate was relatively low in Hungary (24%) (19), Taiwan (32%) (33), and Turkey (40%) (20). Unfortunately, few studies have evaluated influenza vaccination coverage within a specific country. In our study, the influenza vaccination rate was relatively stable, suggesting more effort is needed to increase coverage in patients with COPD in Korea. Because the current data suggest that vaccination rates can vary widely, we suggest that studies evaluating vaccination rates over time would be informative to set country-specific vaccination strategies for COPD patients.

Regarding asthma, a previous meta-analysis demonstrated influenza vaccination reduced febrile illness by 72% and prevented 59-78% of cases of acute exacerbation of asthma requiring emergency visits and/or hospitalizations (22), suggesting influenza vaccination could be a cost-effective strategy to reduce acute exacerbation of asthma. Although there is limited evidence directly showing the effectiveness of vaccination in patients with bronchiectasis, influenza virus may play a crucial role in triggering exacerbation of bronchiectasis (34), which supports providing influenza vaccination to this population (23, 24). However, to provide solid evidence for influenza vaccination in patients with bronchiectasis, future studies evaluating the role of influenza vaccination in bronchiectasis are needed.

Importantly, our study results suggested whom clinicians should persuade to receive influenza vaccination, which includes younger patients, males, and current smokers. As shown in previous studies, the vaccination rate was significantly lower in the younger population with AFL than in the older population with AFL (17, 20, 21, 33, 35). Additionally, younger age was independently associated with unvaccinated status in participants with AFL. Beyond this, we further performed a trend analysis for vaccination over 10 years according to age group, which has not been performed in previous studies. While the vaccination rate in elderly subjects with AFL had a steadily increasing trend, the rate showed a decreasing trend. The reasons for this phenomenon are not clear. For a possible reason, young participants with AFL are likely to have unhealthy lifestyles, while their symptoms are mild or absent in the early stage of AFL. Accordingly, the importance of influenza vaccination is likely to be neglected in this population. This information suggests the importance of age in predicting influenza vaccination in those with AFL. We need to pay more attention to increasing the vaccination rate in the young population with AFL.

Consistent with previous studies, our study revealed that males and current smokers are more likely to be unvaccinated among participants with AFL. Generally, males are more likely to be current smokers than females, especially in Asian countries, including Korea (30). Furthermore, being a male and a smoker increases the risk of severe disease presentation, including mortality (36–38). Thus, it is plausible that such male patients who also have AFL have a much higher risk of worse prognosis

TABLE 2 | Factors associated with non-vaccination against influenza in participants with airflow limitation.

Variables	Univariable	Multivariable*
	OR (95% CI)	OR (95% CI)
Male sex	1.47 (1.29–1.68)	1.70 (1.21–2.42)
Age, year	0.89 (0.88–0.90)	0.88 (0.87–0.90)
Married state	0.43 (0.26–0.73)	2.33 (0.85–6.40)
Medicaid	0.73 (0.56–0.97)	0.85 (0.47–1.52)
Economic activity	2.42 (2.15–2.73)	0.96 (0.75–1.22)
Education beyond high school	2.28 (2.01–2.57)	1.15 (0.91–1.45)
EQ-5D	8.47 (5.21–13.78)	0.57 (0.21–1.50)
Body mass index, kg/m^2	1.00 (0.98–1.02)	0.97 (0.93–1.01)
Chronic bronchitis	0.81 (0.64–1.02)	0.89 (0.57–1.37)
Current smoker	1.79 (1.55–2.05)	1.42 (1.01–2.00)
Severity of airflow limitation[†]		
Mild (FEV_1 %pred of >70)	Reference	Reference
Moderate (FEV_1 %pred of 60–69)	0.92 (0.78–1.08)	1.07 (0.78–1.49)
Moderately severe (FEV_1 %pred of 50–59)	0.75 (0.60–0.93)	1.14 (0.77–1.69)
Severe to very severe (FEV_1 %pred of <50)	0.66 (0.51–0.85)	1.22 (0.75–1.97)
Comorbidities		
Hypertension	0.58 (0.51–0.67)	0.91 (0.72–1.16)
Ischemic heart disease	0.56 (0.41–0.78)	0.80 (0.47–1.34)
Diabetes mellitus	0.82 (0.72–0.93)	0.92 (0.70–1.22)
Asthma	0.51 (0.78–0.68)	0.61 (0.33–1.13)

Data are presented as ratios (95% confidence intervals).

[†] *Severity of airflow limitation was graded according to ATS/ERS guideline (25), and severe and very severe were combined into one group due to the small number of participants with severe to very severe AFL (n = 64).*

[*] *Multivariate analysis was adjusted for age, sex, smoking PY, marriage status (married vs. unmarried or divorced), economic activity (active vs. inactive), education level (college or above vs. high school or less), EQ-5D, severity of airflow limitation, and comorbid conditions (hypertension, ischemic heart disease, diabetes mellitus, and asthma).*

OR, odds ratio; EQ-5D, EuroQol-5 dimensions questionnaire; FEV_1, forced expiratory volume in 1s; % pred; percentage of the predicted value.

than those without these risk factors. However, our study results alone cannot explain sex differences in vaccination rates. We believe that an unhealthy lifestyle in men may have influenced this observation. Additionally, there is a possibility that women might be more compliant with clinicians' recommendations for influenza vaccination than men, as shown by the sex difference in medication adherence in Korea (39).

There have been conflicting results on the relationship between AFL severity and influenza vaccination rate. While a lower rate of vaccination was observed in subjects with more severe AFL (17), other studies showed a positive association between AFL severity and influenza vaccination rate (18–20). Similarly, our study showed a positive association between AFL severity and vaccination rate, although it diminished after adjustment of covariables. Given that severe AFL can be associated with severe pneumonia in patients with AFL (40), and the protective effects of influenza vaccination seem to be correlated with AFL severity (13), strategies focusing on improving the vaccination rate in patients with severe AFL might be more cost-effective.

Our findings yield important insights that can be helpful to design targeted strategies to increase influenza vaccination coverage in patients with AFL. The identification of factors (younger age, male, and current smokers) associated with unvaccinated status can help design tailored strategies to increase influenza vaccination in patients with AFL. We also suggest a change in strategy of influenza vaccination policy for adults in Korea. Currently, the Korean government-led free influenza vaccination policy for adults is a one-size-fits-all strategy that is applied to all subjects aged 65 or older, and it does not consider risk factors other than age. Thus, a large number of young patients with AFL who are at a high risk of influenza have not been considered for the benefit of government-led free vaccination programs. However, given the broad benefits of influenza infection on respiratory diseases with AFL, a more advanced and personalized free vaccination strategy that estimates individual risk might be helpful, and it could include young patients with AFL.

There are limitations to our study that should be acknowledged. First, this study was performed in Korea, limiting the generalizability of our findings. Second, because KNHANES does not have data on post-bronchodilator spirometry, we defined AFL using pre-bronchodilator spirometry. However, prebronchodilator spirometry has been widely used to define AFL in many previous studies of COPD epidemiology (30, 41, 42). Third, this study could not evaluate the presence of bronchiectasis, which may be an important comorbidity to consider when interpreting the results of our study. This was because a questionnaire on bronchiectasis was only available in the 2007–2009 NHANES dataset. Fourth, we could not provide a reasonable explanation for our observation of the relationship between socioeconomic and influenza vaccination status in participants with AFL. Poor socioeconomic status, such as low education level, inactive economic status, and reduced QoL, showed increased odds of non-vaccination in the univariable analysis but no significant relationship in multivariable analyses. Although the reasons are not clear, it is possible that the Korean government-led free influenza vaccination program attenuated the influence of these factors on influenza vaccination. The free influenza vaccination program in Korea targets people receiving Medicaid and the elderly population whose socioeconomic status and QoL are poor, which leads to disproportionally higher influenza vaccination rates in these subjects despite their poor socioeconomic status. Thus, the simultaneous consideration of these factors (age, Medicaid, economic activity, educational level, and QoL) might have yielded the non-significance of socioeconomic variables. As socioeconomic status and government health policies might differ between countries, our study results should be interpreted with caution in other countries.

In conclusion, over the past 10 years, the influenza vaccination rate in elderly participants with AFL steadily increased, while the rate in younger participants with AFL decreased. Younger participants, males, and current smokers were most likely to have unvaccinated status among those with AFL. More attention and targeted interventions are required to improve the influenza vaccination rate in individuals with AFL.

AUTHOR CONTRIBUTIONS

HL and YJ take responsibility for the data, analysis, and wrote the first draft of the manuscript. HL, HC, and YJ designed the study. YJ performed statistical analysis of data. All authors provided critical review and approved the version for publication.

FUNDING

This work was supported by the National Research Foundation (NRF) of Korea Grant funded by the Ministry of Science, Information and Communications Technologies (MSIT) (NRF-2020R1F1A1070468), the Bio and Medical Technology Development Program of the National Research Foundation funded by the Korean Government (MSIT) (NRF-2021M3E5D1A01015176), and the Korea Medical Device Development Fund Grant funded by the Korea Government (the Ministry of Science and ICT, the Ministry of Trade, Industry and Energy, the Ministry of Health and Welfare, the Ministry of Food and Drug Safety) (Project Number: 1711138447, KMDF_PR_20200901_0214).

REFERENCES

1. Mathers CD, Loncar D. Projections of global mortality and burden of disease from 2002 to 2030. *PLoS Med.* (2006) 3:e442. doi: 10.1371/journal.pmed.0030442
2. Mannino DM, Braman S. The epidemiology and economics of chronic obstructive pulmonary disease. *Proc Am Thorac Soc.* (2007) 4:502–6. doi: 10.1513/pats.200701-001FM
3. Suissa S. Dell'Aniello S, Ernst P. Long-term natural history of chronic obstructive pulmonary disease: severe exacerbations and mortality. *Thorax.* (2012) 67:957–63. doi: 10.1136/thoraxjnl-2011-201518
4. McGhan R, Radcliff T, Fish R, Sutherland ER, Welsh C, Make B. Predictors of rehospitalization and death after a severe exacerbation of COPD. *Chest.* (2007) 132:1748–55. doi: 10.1378/chest.06-3018
5. Dransfield MT, Kunisaki KM, Strand MJ, Anzueto A, Bhatt SP, Bowler RP, et al. Acute exacerbations and lung function loss in smokers with and without chronic obstructive pulmonary disease. *Am J Respir Crit Care Med.* (2017) 195:324–30. doi: 10.1164/rccm.201605-1014OC
6. Garcia-Aymerich J, Serra Pons I, Mannino DM, Maas AK, Miller DP, Davis KJ. Lung function impairment, COPD hospitalisations and subsequent mortality. *Thorax.* (2011) 66:585–90. doi: 10.1136/thx.2010.152876
7. Press VG, Konetzka RT, White SR. Insights about the economic impact of chronic obstructive pulmonary disease readmissions post implementation of the hospital readmission reduction program. *Curr Opin Pulm Med.* (2018) 24:138–46. doi: 10.1097/MCP.0000000000000454
8. Wedzicha JA, Seemungal TA. COPD exacerbations: defining their cause and prevention. *Lancet.* (2007) 370:786–96. doi: 10.1016/S0140-6736(07)61382-8
9. Sapey E, Stockley RA. COPD exacerbations. 2: aetiology. *Thorax.* (2006) 61:250–8. doi: 10.1136/thx.2005.041822
10. Papi A, Luppi F, Franco F, Fabbri LM. Pathophysiology of exacerbations of chronic obstructive pulmonary disease. *Proc Am Thorac Soc.* (2006) 3:245–51. doi: 10.1513/pats.200512-125SF
11. Lall D, Cason E, Pasquel FJ, Ali MK, Narayan KM. Effectiveness of influenza vaccination for individuals with chronic obstructive pulmonary disease (COPD) in low- and middle-income countries. *COPD.* (2016) 13:93–9. doi: 10.3109/15412555.2015.1043518
12. Ouaalaya EH, Falque L, Dupis JM, Sabatini M, Bernady A, Nguyen L, et al. Susceptibility to frequent exacerbation in COPD patients: impact of the exacerbations history, vaccinations and comorbidities? *Respir Med.* (2020) 169:106018. doi: 10.1016/j.rmed.2020.106018
13. Chan TC, Fan-Ngai Hung I, Ka-Hay Luk J, Chu LW, Hon-Wai Chan F. Effectiveness of influenza vaccination in institutionalized older adults: a systematic review. *J Am Med Dir Assoc.* (2014) 15:226.e1–e6. doi: 10.1016/j.jamda.2013.10.008
14. Kopsaftis Z, Wood-Baker R, Poole P. Influenza vaccine for chronic obstructive pulmonary disease (COPD). *Cochrane Database Syst Rev.* (2018) 6:CD002733. doi: 10.1002/14651858.CD002733.pub3
15. Schembri S, Morant S, Winter JH, MacDonald TM. Influenza but not pneumococcal vaccination protects against all-cause mortality in patients with COPD. *Thorax.* (2009) 64:567–72. doi: 10.1136/thx.2008.106286
16. Global Initiative for Chronic Obstructive Lung Disease. *Global Strategy for the Diagnosis, Management, and Prevention of Chronic Obstructive Pulmonary Disease.* Global Initiative for Chronic Obstructive Lung Disease (2021). Available online at: http://www.goldcopd.org/ (accessed December 7, 2021).
17. Garrastazu R, Garcia-Rivero JL, Ruiz M, Helguera JM, Arenal S, Bonnardeux C, et al. Prevalence of influenza vaccination in chronic obstructive pulmonary disease patients and impact on the risk of severe exacerbations. *Arch Bronconeumol.* (2016) 52:88–95. doi: 10.1016/j.arbr.2015.09.022
18. Ruiz Azcona L, Roman-Rodriguez M, Llort Bove M, van Boven JF, Santibanez Marguello M. Prevalence of seasonal influenza vaccination in chronic obstructive pulmonary disease (COPD) patients in the Balearic Islands (Spain) and its effect on COPD exacerbations: a population-based retrospective cohort study. *Int J Environ Res Public Health.* (2020) 17:27. doi: 10.3390/ijerph17114027
19. Fekete M, Pako J, Nemeth AN, Tarantini S, Varga JT. Prevalence of influenza and pneumococcal vaccination in chronic obstructive pulmonary disease patients in association with the occurrence of acute exacerbations. *J Thorac Dis.* (2020) 12:4233–42. doi: 10.21037/jtd-20-814
20. Ozlu T, Bulbul Y, Aydin D, Tatar D, Kuyucu T, Erboy F, et al. Immunization status in chronic obstructive pulmonary disease: a multicenter study from Turkey. *Ann Thorac Med.* (2019) 14:75–82. doi: 10.4103/atm.ATM_145_18
21. Saeed GJ, Valero-Elizondo J, Mszar R, Grandhi GR, Cainzos-Achirica M, Omer SB, et al. Prevalence and disparities in influenza vaccination among patients with COPD in the United States. *Chest.* (2021) 159:1411–4. doi: 10.1016/j.chest.2020.10.058
22. Vasileiou E, Sheikh A, Butler C, El Ferkh K, von Wissmann B, McMenamin J, et al. Effectiveness of influenza vaccines in asthma: a systematic review and meta-analysis. *Clin Infect Dis.* (2017) 65:1388–95. doi: 10.1093/cid/cix524
23. Hill AT, Sullivan AL, Chalmers JD, De Soyza A, Elborn SJ, Floto AR, et al. British Thoracic Society Guideline for bronchiectasis in adults. *Thorax.* (2019) 74:1–69. doi: 10.1136/thoraxjnl-2018-212463
24. Polverino E, Goeminne PC, McDonnell MJ, Aliberti S, Marshall SE, Loebinger MR, et al. European Respiratory Society guidelines for the management of adult bronchiectasis. *Eur Respir J.* (2017) 50:1700629. doi: 10.1183/13993003.00629-2017
25. Pellegrino R, Viegi G, Brusasco V, Crapo RO, Burgos F, Casaburi R, et al. Interpretative strategies for lung function tests. *Eur Respir J.* (2005) 26:948–68. doi: 10.1183/09031936.05.00035205
26. EuroQol G. EuroQol-a new facility for the measurement of health-related quality of life. *Health Policy.* (1990) 16:199–208. doi: 10.1016/0168-8510(90)90421-9
27. Lee YK, Nam HS, Chuang LH, Kim KY, Yang HK, Kwon IS, et al. South Korean time trade-off values for EQ-5D health states: modeling

with observed values for 101 health states. *Value Health.* (2009) 12:1187–93. doi: 10.1111/j.1524-4733.2009.00579.x
28. National Cholesterol Education Program (NCEP) Expert Panel on Detection, Evaluation, and Treatment of High Blood Cholesterol in Adults (Adult Treatment Panel III). Third report of the national cholesterol education program (NCEP) expert panel on detection, evaluation, and treatment of high blood cholesterol in adults (Adult Treatment Panel III) final report. *Circulation.* (2002) 106:3143–421. doi: 10.1161/circ.106.25.3143
29. American Diabetes Association. Standards of medical care in diabetes—2013. *Diabetes Care.* (2013) 36(Suppl. 1):S11–66. doi: 10.2337/dc13-S011
30. Lee H, Shin SH, Gu S, Zhao D, Kang D, Joi YR, et al. Racial differences in comorbidity profile among patients with chronic obstructive pulmonary disease. *BMC Med.* (2018) 16:178. doi: 10.1186/s12916-018-1159-7
31. Huang CL, Nguyen PA, Kuo PL, Iqbal U, Hsu YH, Jian WS. Influenza vaccination and reduction in risk of ischemic heart disease among chronic obstructive pulmonary elderly. *Comput Methods Programs Biomed.* (2013) 111:507–11. doi: 10.1016/j.cmpb.2013.05.006
32. Westerik JA, Metting EI, van Boven JF, Tiersma W, Kocks JW, Schermer TR. Associations between chronic comorbidity and exacerbation risk in primary care patients with COPD. *Respir Res.* (2017) 18:31. doi: 10.1186/s12931-017-0512-2
33. Huang HH, Chen SJ, Chao TF, Liu CJ, Chen TJ, Chou P, et al. Influenza vaccination and risk of respiratory failure in patients with chronic obstructive pulmonary disease: a nationwide population-based case-cohort study. *J Microbiol Immunol Infect.* (2019) 52:22–9. doi: 10.1016/j.jmii.2017.08.014
34. Gao YH, Guan WJ, Xu G, Lin ZY, Tang Y, Lin ZM, et al. The role of viral infection in pulmonary exacerbations of bronchiectasis in adults: a prospective study. *Chest.* (2015) 147:1635–43. doi: 10.1378/chest.14-1961
35. Hsu DJ, North CM, Brode SK, Celli BR. Identification of barriers to influenza vaccination in patients with chronic obstructive pulmonary disease: analysis of the 2012 behavioral risk factors surveillance system. *Chronic Obstr Pulm Dis.* (2016) 3:620–7. doi: 10.15326/jcopdf.3.3.2015.0156
36. Martinez A, Soldevila N, Romero-Tamarit A, Torner N, Godoy P, Rius C, et al. Risk factors associated with severe outcomes in adult hospitalized patients according to influenza type and subtype. *PLoS ONE.* (2019) 14:e0210353. doi: 10.1371/journal.pone.0210353
37. Wong CM, Yang L, Chan KP, Chan WM, Song L, Lai HK, et al. Cigarette smoking as a risk factor for influenza-associated mortality: evidence from an elderly cohort. *Influenza Other Respir Viruses.* (2013) 7:531–9. doi: 10.1111/j.1750-2659.2012.00411.x
38. Godoy P, Castilla J, Soldevila N, Mayoral JM, Toledo D, Martin V, et al. Smoking may increase the risk of influenza hospitalization and reduce influenza vaccine effectiveness in the elderly. *Eur J Public Health.* (2018) 28:150–5. doi: 10.1093/eurpub/ckx130
39. Jeong H, Kim H, Lee K, Lee JH, Ahn HM, Shin SA, et al. Medical visits, antihypertensive prescriptions and medication adherence among newly diagnosed hypertensive patients in Korea. *Environ Health Prev Med.* (2017) 22:10. doi: 10.1186/s12199-017-0619-6
40. Eom JS, Song WJ, Yoo H, Jeong BH, Lee HY, Koh WJ, et al. Chronic obstructive pulmonary disease severity is associated with severe pneumonia. *Ann Thorac Med.* (2015) 10:105–11. doi: 10.4103/1817-1737.151441
41. Shin SH, Park J, Cho J, Sin DD, Lee H, Park HY. Severity of airflow obstruction and work loss in a nationwide population of working age. *Sci Rep.* (2018) 8:9674. doi: 10.1038/s41598-018-27999-6
42. Kim DS, Kim YS, Jung KS, Chang JH, Lim CM, Lee JH, et al. Prevalence of chronic obstructive pulmonary disease in Korea: a population-based spirometry survey. *Am J Respir Crit Care Med.* (2005) 172:842–7. doi: 10.1164/rccm.200502-259OC

12

Air Pollution Effects to the Subtype and Severity of Lung Cancers

Hung-Chi Lee[1,2], *Yueh-Hsun Lu*[1,2*], *Yen-Lin Huang*[1,2], *Shih Li Huang*[3] and *Hsiao-Chi Chuang*[4,5,6]

[1] *Department of Radiology, Shuang-Ho Hospital, Taipei Medical University, New Taipei City, Taiwan,* [2] *Department of Radiology, School of Medicine, College of Medicine, Taipei Medical University, Taipei, Taiwan,* [3] *Medical Department, Tai An Hospital Shuang Shi Branch, Taichung, Taiwan,* [4] *School of Respiratory Therapy, College of Medicine, Taipei Medical University, Taipei, Taiwan,* [5] *Division of Pulmonary Medicine, Department of Internal Medicine, Shuang Ho Hospital, Taipei Medical University, New Taipei City, Taiwan,* [6] *Cell Physiology and Molecular Image Research Center, Wan Fang Hospital, Taipei Medical University, Taipei, Taiwan*

Correspondence:
Yueh-Hsun Lu
s20001@s.tmu.edu.tw

The correlation between lung cancer incidence and air pollution has been established in previous research, but the other detail impact of air pollution to lung cancer is still under investigation. This study aimed to explore if air pollution affected the subtype and staging of lung cancer. At the same time, we investigated the effect of individual pollutant to subtypes and staging. Single center data were extracted from January 1, 2020 to June 30, 2020 using the search engine in the radiology reporting system of Shuang-Ho Hospital, New Taipei City, Taiwan. There were 169 patients finally included for analysis. The nationwide statistics data of lung cancer were extracted from the Taiwan Cancer Registry. The air quality data were extracted from the Taiwan air quality monitoring network. Comparison of the single center lung cancer characteristics with nationwide data was made using the chi-square test. Comparison of the air quality of the living space of the included cases with the average quality in Taiwan in 2020 was made using the *Z*-test. The result shows there was significant difference of cancer subtype and staging between the regional data and the nationwide data. The regional data demonstrated a tendency of higher incidence of adenocarcinoma and advanced stage disease. As for air quality, there was no significant difference. The regional PM10 level presented generally lower levels in regional data as compared to Taiwan in 2020 with near statistically significant *P*-value (0.052); the regional NO_2 level presented generally higher levels in regional data as compared to Taiwan in 2020 with near statistically significant *P*-value (0.060). The results indicate that air pollution might be related to increase in adenocarcinoma ratio and advanced stage of lung cancer at initial presentation. The NO_2 was probably the leading pollutant causing this trend.

Keywords: air pollution, lung cancer, staging, adenocarcinoma, squamous cell carcinoma, PM2.5, PM10, NO2

INTRODUCTION

Lung cancer remains one of the most commonly diagnosed cancer in recent years. With the high incidence, a large number of patients were diagnosed at the late stage of disease, making it the leading cause of overall cancer death (1). To cease the impact of lung cancer, much effort has been made to determine risk factors for prevention (2–11). To date, many risk factors of lung cancer have been identified, including cigarette smoking, radon, asbestos, family history of lung cancer, and air pollution (1). Cigarette smoking, as the leading cause for lung cancer and a modifiable risk factor, has attracted much attention in recent years (12, 13). Following the undertaken measures to prevent the population from smoking, the proportional number of smokers decreased significantly. Recently, air pollution was identified as a risk factor, when in 2013 the International Agency for Research on Cancer (IARC) declared air pollution as a category 1 for human carcinogens (14–24). Being a highly modifiable risk factor of lung cancer, the effect of air pollution on lung cancer gained more attention in recent years. Prior studies identified a correlation between air pollution and cases of lung cancer (25–28). However, there are other studies investigating the effect of air pollution on lung cancer in more detail. These include, for instance, survival rate, type, severity, and the effects of individual pollutants that are still being investigated. In this study we aimed to explore whether air pollution affected the subtype and staging of lung cancer. At the same time, we investigated the effect of individual pollutant to subtypes and staging of lung cancer.

MATERIALS AND METHODS

A search engine in the radiology reporting system of Shuang-Ho Hospital, New Taipei City, Taiwan was used for data extraction. The data from January 1, 2020 to June 30, 2020 were included, using the key word "lung cancer(s)" for searching. The search results present a total of 372 imaging studies belonging to 227 patients. The images and clinical history of the 227 patients were checked to exclude not truly diagnosed lung cancer, which appeared in the search machine due to the phrase "lung cancer(s)" that was present in the imaging cases for other reasons. The patients who were clinically diagnosed as having lung cancer, yet without pathologic proof, have also been excluded. A total of 169 patients that were diagnosed as having lung cancer with pathologic proof were considered in this study (**Table 1**). The staging, pathologic cell type, and living spaces of these patients were documented. As for staging, using pathologic staging as a priority, in case if there was no detected pathologic staging, for instance, a patient with stage IV cancer, the clinical staging was used as a substitute. For patients with recurrent or progression of the disease, or who received neoadjuvant therapy, the staging at initial presentation was used for statistical analysis.

As for data on air quality, the data were extracted from the Taiwan air quality monitoring network, an official website maintained by the Environmental Protection Administration, Executive Yuan, Taiwan (29). The website revealed the real-time data of monitoring stations all over Taiwan, also the yearly statistics data from 1993 to now (**Figures 1, 2**). The data of 2020 were used for analysis in this study.

The statistical data on lung cancer in Taiwan were accessed from the Taiwan Cancer Registry (30), which is a population-based cancer registry founded in 1979, and operated by the National Public Health Association. At the time of finalizing this study the most recent data were on 2018, which were used for the statistical analysis.

TABLE 1 | Demographic characteristics.

Total	169
Age, mean (SD)	66.5 (12)
Sex (%)	
M	74 (43.8)
F	95 (56.2)
Tumor location (%)	
Right	106 (62.7)
Left	63 (37.3)
Stage (%)	
0	4 (2.4)
1	35 (20.7)
2	8 (4.7)
3	25 (14.8)
4	97 (57.3)
Tumor type (%)	
Adenocarcinoma	136 (80.4)
Squamous cell carcinoma	23 (13.6)
Other	10 (5.9)

The comparison of the single center lung cancer characteristics with nationwide data was made using the chi-square test. The comparison of the air quality of the living spaces of the 169 included cases with the data of all of Taiwan in 2020 was made using the Z-test.

RESULTS

All 169 cases were sorted by living space of the included patients, into four major neighboring districts of Shuang-Ho Hospital, including Zhonghe/Yonghe (ZY), Banqiao (BQ), Tucheng (TC), and Xinzhuang (XZ). The data of corresponding air quality in the four districts were extracted from the Taiwan Air Quality Monitoring Network (**Tables 2–4**).

As for cell type of lung cancer, the data for all of Taiwan were 71.6% of adenocarcinoma, 12.0% of squamous cell carcinoma, and 16.3% of other cell types. The included 169 cases presented in total 80.4% of adenocarcinoma, 13.6% of squamous cell carcinoma, and 5.9% of other cell types. The ZY district presented 82.3% of adenocarcinoma, 14.6% of squamous cell carcinoma, and 3.1% of other cell types. The BQ district presented 84.2% of adenocarcinoma, 5.3% of squamous cell carcinoma, and 10.5% of other cell types. The TC district presented 71.4% of adenocarcinoma, 19.0% of squamous cell carcinoma, and 9.5% of other cell types. The XZ district presented 75.0% of adenocarcinoma, 25.0% of squamous cell carcinoma, and 0% of other cell types. Comparing the cell type percentage of all 169 cases to all of Taiwan, we found a significant difference ($P < 0.05$). As comparing the four districts' data separately with all of Taiwan, the ZY district presented significant difference ($P < 0.05$), while the other three districts presented no significant difference ($P > 0.05$; **Table 2**).

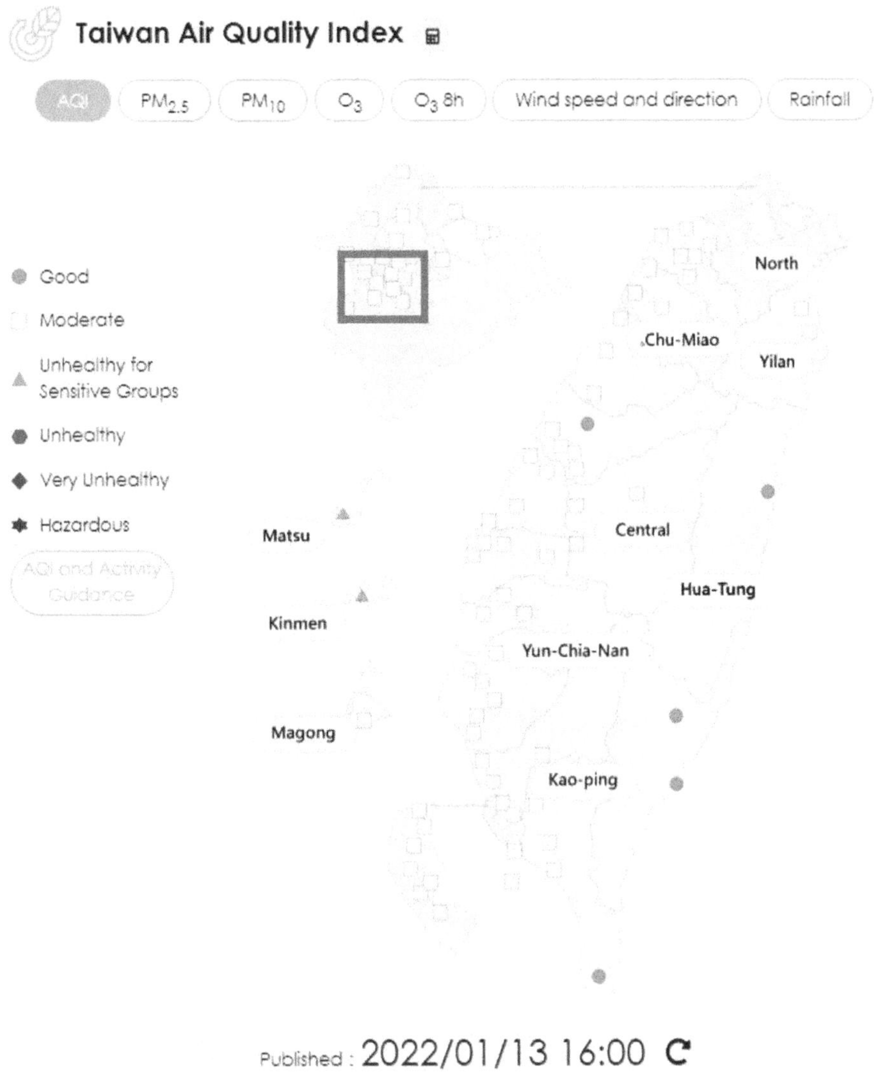

FIGURE 1 | Air quality index distribution in Taiwan, using the data on January 13, 2022 for example. The red block shows the areas involved in this study (29).

As for staging of lung cancer, the Taiwan data in 2018 presented 4.8% of stage 0 disease, 31.4% of stage I disease, 4.2% of stage II disease, 11.6% of stage III disease, and 46.7% of stage IV disease. The included 169 cases presented a total of 2.4% of stage 0 disease, 20.7% of stage I disease, 4.7% of stage II disease, 14.8% of stage III disease, and 57.3% of stage IV disease. The ZY district presented 3.2% of stage 0 disease, 15.8% of stage I disease, 4.7% of stage II disease, 14.8% of stage III disease, and 57.3% of stage IV disease. The BQ district presented 5.3% of stage 0 disease, 26.3% of stage I disease, 5.3% of stage II disease, 5.3% of stage III disease, and 57.9% of stage IV disease. The TC district presented 0% of stage 0 disease, 44.4% of stage I disease, 0% of stage II disease, 27.8% of stage III disease, and 27.8% of stage IV disease. The XZ district presented 0% of stage 0 disease, 25% of stage I disease, 0% of stage II disease, 0% of stage III disease, and 75% of stage IV disease. Comparing the staging percentage of all 169 cases to all of Taiwan, there was a significant difference ($P < 0.05$). As comparing the four-district data separately with all of Taiwan, the ZY district presented significant difference ($P < 0.05$), the other three districts presented no significant difference ($P > 0.05$; **Table 3**).

As for air quality, the average AQI (air quality index) of all air monitoring stations in Taiwan in 2020 was 57. The ZY district was 40, 48 in the BQ district, 56 in the TC district, and 54 in the XZ district (**Table 4**). The ambient air pollutants' concentrations include PM10, PM2.5, SO_2, NO_2, CO, and O_3 of all monitoring stations in Taiwan in 2020 as well as the individual data of monitoring stations at ZY, BQ, TC, and XZ districts are demonstrated in **Table 5**. The overall data of ambient air pollutants' concentrations of the four districts were compared to the overall data of Taiwan using the Z-test. The concentration of all pollutants presented no significant difference between the

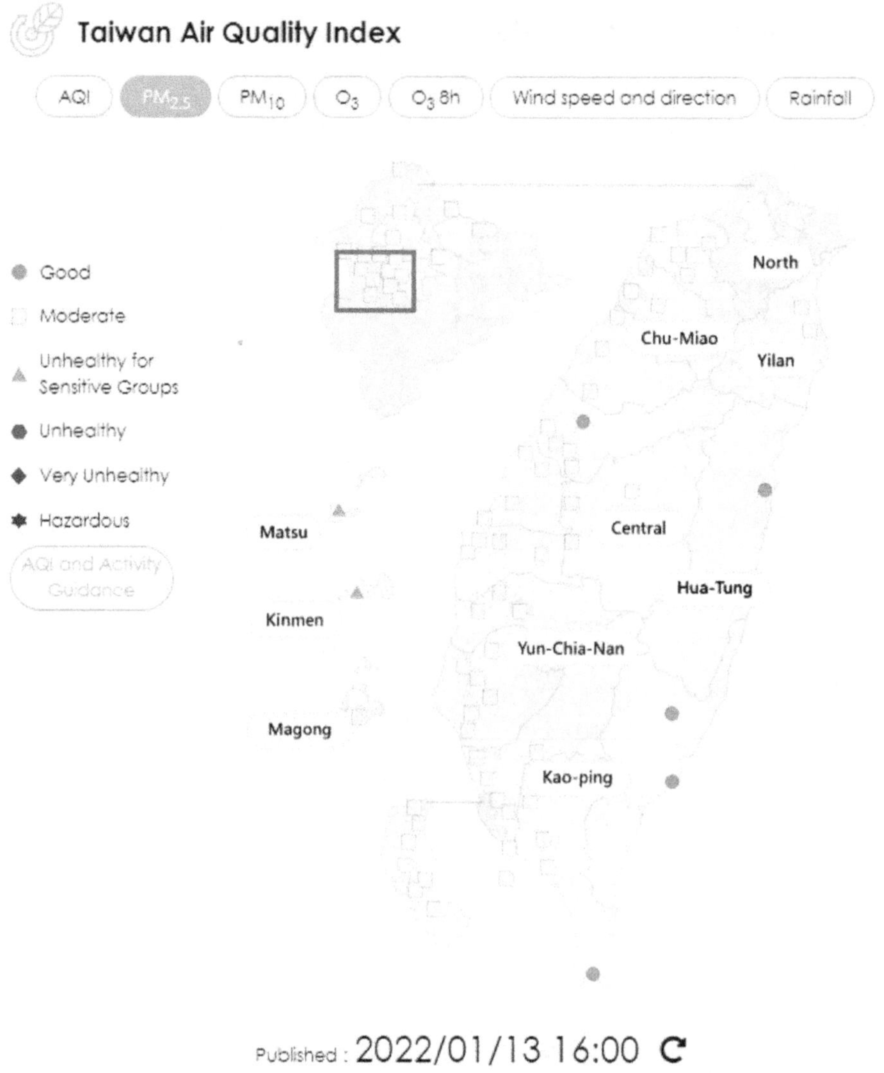

FIGURE 2 | Air quality index of PM2.5 distribution in Taiwan, using the data on January 13, 2022 for example. The red block shows the areas involved in this study (29).

two results. However, the PM10 and NO_2 presented low *P*-value (0.052 and 0.060, respectively) close to statistical significance. The PM10 presented generally lower levels in the four districts as compared to Taiwan in 2020. The NO_2 presented generally higher levels in the four districts as compared to Taiwan in 2020 (**Table 5**).

DISCUSSION

The data used in this study is from January 2020 to June 2020. There was a worldwide outbreak of COVID-19 infection in 2020, therefore, by shutting the borders early and requiring 2-week quarantines of nearly everyone who arrived from overseas, there was not a pandemic outbreak in Taiwan until May 2021, and most residents did not wear masks until May 2021. Therefore, the influences of COVID-19 infection on the study results are considered minor.

This study demonstrated significant difference between the subtypes of lung cancer in the ZY district and the total four districts when compared to the data of Taiwan in 2020. We detected that the ratio of adenocarcinoma was higher in these areas. At the same time, the PM10 concentration was significantly lower in the ZY district and in all four districts. On the other hand, we noted that the NO_2 concentration had much higher values. There were previous studies that suggested a certain correlation between air pollution and squamous cell carcinoma (31). However, the majority of studies found that ambient air pollution increased the incidence of adenocarcinoma with little to no effect on squamous cell carcinoma (25, 26, 32–34). As for the specific effect of each air pollutant, many studies reported previously that PM2.5 and PM10 are mostly associated with the increasing risk of adenocarcinoma, whereas the effects of NOx on lung cancer subtype were not sufficiently discussed (25–28, 33). This was somehow a paradoxical result when considering

TABLE 2 | The number and percentage of lung cancer subtype.

	Adenocarcinoma	Squamous	Other	Total	*P*-value	X^2
ZY	79 (82.3)	14 (14.6)	3 (3.1)	96	0.002	12.279
BQ	16 (84.2)	1 (5.3)	2 (10.5)	19	0.463	1.54
TC	15 (71.4)	4 (19.0)	2 (9.5)	21	0.485	1.449
XZ	3 (75)	1 (25)	0 (0)	4	0.544	1.217
Other	23 (79.3)	3 (10.3)	3 (10.3)	29	0.623	0.948
Total	136 (80.4)	23 (13.6)	10 (5.9)	169	0.001	13.367
Taiwan 2018	10,988 (71.6)	1,849 (12.0)	2,508 (16.3)	15,345		

TABLE 3 | The number and percentage of lung cancer stage.

	Stage 0	Stage 1	Stage 2	Stage 3	Stage 4	Total	*P*-value	X^2
ZY	3 (3.2)	15 (15.8)	6 (6.3)	14 (14.7)	57 (60)	95	0.011	13.0488
BQ	1 (5.3)	5 (26.3)	1 (5.3)	1 (5.3)	11 (57.9)	19	0.852	1.358
TC	0 (0)	8 (44.4)	0 (0)	5 (27.8)	5 (27.8)	18	0.0937	7.941
XZ	0 (0)	1 (25)	0 (0)	0 (0)	3 (75)	4	0.817	1.552
Other	0 (0)	6 (18.2)	1 (3.0)	5 (15.2)	21 (63.6)	33	0.208	5.878
Total	4 (2.4)	35 (20.7)	8 (4.7)	25 (14.8)	97 (57.3)	169	0.008	13.735
Taiwan 2018	656 (4.8)	4,230 (31.4)	577 (4.2)	1,563 (11.6)	6,281 (46.7)	13,444		

TABLE 4 | Air quality index.

AQI data					0–50		51–100		101–150	
Location	Average	SD	Lowest	Highest	Days	%	Days	%	Days	%
ZY	40	47	7	92	282	77.05	84	22.95	0	0
BQ	48	24	11	182	261	71.31	94	25.68	8	2.19
TC	56	30	12	200	224	61.2	117	31.97	17	4.64
XZ	54	26	13	190	223	60.93	123	33.61	15	4.1
Total Taiwan 2020	57				11,405	54.67	7,397	35.46	1,850	8.87

TABLE 5 | The concentration of ambient air pollutants in 2020.

Location	PM10 ($\mu g/m^3$)	PM2.5 ($\mu g/m^3$)	SO_2 (ppb)	NO_2 (ppb)	CO (ppm)	O_3 avg (ppb)
ZY	23	12.2	1.84	15.7	0.63	28.21
BQ	24.4	12.5	2.4	17.35	0.45	26.92
TC	24.1	12.9	1.93	14.03	0.39	30.7
XZ	26.5	13.8	2.6	15.11	0.43	30.49
Taiwan 2020	30.2	15.1	2.13	11.16	0.35	30.9
Taiwan 2020 SD	8.1	3.7	0.55	5.01	0.15	3.95
Regional SD	2.14	0.48	0.13	1.92	0.011	3.35
P-value	0.052	0.25	0.93	0.06	0.75	0.41

prior studies of biological effect of these substances. Nitrates and toxic agents formed from NOx were thought to be associated with adenocarcinoma formation, whereas the polycyclic aromatic hydrocarbons, one of the primary organic compound clusters in particulate matter, was thought to be associated with squamous cell carcinoma formation (35, 36). In this study, the increasing trend in adenocarcinoma ratio was accompanied with a trend of increase in NO_2 concentration, and with a decrease in PM10 concentration, a result that was more compatible with the biological effect of these substances, but inconsistent with some prior statistical studies (25, 27). More studies are needed to investigate the definite effect of each pollutant to lung cancer subtype.

The staging of lung cancer in the ZY district and in the total four districts presented significant differences compared to Taiwan in 2020. The ratio of late-stage disease was higher in the ZY district and in the total four districts. Prior study had presented that air pollution exposure shortens lung cancer survival (32). This effect was especially prominent with the early-stage patients and adenocarcinoma. The exposure of PM2.5, PM10, and NO_2 all presented increased risk of death (32, 34, 37, 38). In our study, the NO_2 concentration in the ZY district and in all the four districts were higher than in all of Taiwan in 2020 with a significant *P*-value. The PM2.5 presented no significant difference, while the PM10 presented a near significant decrease in the ZY district and in all four districts than Taiwan in 2020. The obtained results point at the possibility that NO_2 plays a key role in the increasing severity of lung cancer. Assessment of the evidence of NO_2 had been conducted by the US Environmental Protection Agency Integrated Science Assessment and Health Canada, and came out with the conclusion that the evidence was suggestive of, but not sufficient to infer, a causal relationship between long-term exposure to NO_2 and mortality among the adults (39). However, the existing reviews are limited by 2014. A more recent meta-analysis including new evidence focused on the effect of NO_2 presented a positive association between the NO_2 and the risk of mortality in several types of disease, including lung cancer (37). As a contribution to the existing case studies, the presented result supported the assumption that NO_2 might be causative to the increase of the mortality in cases of lung cancer by applying and investigating the additional data.

This study had several limitations. First, this was a single center study, not a population study. The ratio of lung cancer subtype and staging in a single center might not be totally compatible with the population ratio. Second, the air quality in the districts analyzed in this study was generally well, as well as in all of Taiwan. The highest AQI was only 56, and Taiwan was only 57, the results of this study might only be applicable in low air pollution areas. This was a study that demonstrated that even in concentrations lower than current EU limit values and below WHO Air Quality Guidelines (27, 40), particulate matter still increased the risk of lung cancer, and there was no threshold. However, the effect other than increasing risk and the effect of other air pollutants in low concentration was not clear. Being a limitation at the same time, this study might give additional information to the effect of air pollutants under low concentration, which was still a poor explored field. Third, the group size of this study was relatively small. Only 169 cases were included for analyzation. The small sample size might cause bias.

CONCLUSION

The detail impact of air pollution on lung cancer is still under investigation. This study adds more data to the field and shows that air pollution is related to an increase in the adenocarcinoma ratio and severity of lung cancer at initial presentation. The NO_2 was probably the leading pollutant causing this trend. However, more research is still needed to justify this correlation due to the inconsistency of results of currently published studies.

AUTHOR CONTRIBUTIONS

H-CL, Y-HL, and H-CC devised the project, the main conceptual ideas. H-CL performed the analytic calculations. All authors contributed to the final version of the manuscript. All authors provided critical feedback and helped shape the research, analysis and manuscript.

REFERENCES

1. Sung H, Ferlay J, Siegal RL, Laversanne M, Soerjomataram I, Jemal A, et al., Global cancer statistics 2020: GLOBOCAN estimates of incidence and mortality worldwide for 36 cancers in 185 countries. *CA Cancer J Clin.* (2021) 71:209–49. doi: 10.3322/caac.21492
2. de Groot P, Munden RF. Lung cancer epidemiology, risk factors, and prevention. *Radiol Clin North Am.* (2012) 50:863–76. doi: 10.1016/j.rcl.2012.06.006
3. Malhotra J, Malvezzi M, Negri E, La Vecchia C, Boffetta P. Risk factors for lung cancer worldwide. *Eur Respir J.* (2016) 48:889–902. doi: 10.1183/13993003.00359-2016
4. Mao Y, Yang D, He J, Krasna MJ. Epidemiology of lung cancer. *Surg Oncol Clin N Am.* (2016) 25:439–45. doi: 10.1016/j.soc.2016.02.001
5. Stapelfeld C, Dammann C, Maser E. Sex-specificity in lung cancer risk. *Int J Cancer.* (2020) 146:2376–82. doi: 10.1002/ijc.32716
6. Sigel K, Makinson A, Thaler J. Lung cancer in persons with HIV. *Curr Opin HIV AIDS.* (2017) 12:31–8. doi: 10.1097/COH.0000000000000326
7. Bade BC, Dela Cruz CS. Lung cancer 2020: epidemiology, etiology, and prevention. *Clin Chest Med.* (2020) 41:1–24. doi: 10.1016/j.ccm.2019.10.001
8. Rivera GA, Wakelee H. Lung cancer in never smokers. *Adv Exp Med Biol.* (2016) 893:43–57. doi: 10.1007/978-3-319-24223-1_3
9. Pallis AG, Syrigos KN. Lung cancer in never smokers: disease characteristics and risk factors. *Crit Rev Oncol Hematol.* (2013) 88:494–503. doi: 10.1016/j.critrevonc.2013.06.011
10. Lorenzo-Gonzalez M, Torres-Durán M, Barbosa-Lorenzo R, Provencio-Pulla M, Barros-Dios JM, Ruano-Ravina A. Radon exposure: a major cause of lung cancer. *Expert Rev Respir Med.* (2019) 13:839–50. doi: 10.1080/17476348.2019.1645599
11. Zamarron E, Prats E, Tejero E, Pardo P, Galera R, Casitas R, et al. Static lung hyperinflation is an independent risk factor for lung cancer in patients with chronic obstructive pulmonary disease. *Lung Cancer.* (2019) 128:40–6. doi: 10.1016/j.lungcan.2018.12.012
12. Tammemagi MC, Berg CD, Riley TL, Cunningham CR, Taylor KL. Impact of lung cancer screening results on smoking cessation. *J Natl Cancer Inst.* (2014) 106:dju084. doi: 10.1093/jnci/dju084
13. Proctor RN. The history of the discovery of the cigarette-lung cancer link: evidentiary traditions, corporate denial, global toll. *Tob Control.* (2012) 21:87–91. doi: 10.1136/tobaccocontrol-2011-050338
14. Loomis D, Grosse Y, Lauby-Secretan B, El Ghissassi F, Bouvard V, Benbrahim-Tallaa L, et al. The carcinogenicity of outdoor air pollution. *Lancet Oncol.* (2013) 14:1262–3. doi: 10.1016/S1470-2045(13)70487-X
15. Zare Sakhvidi MJ, Lequy E, Goldberg M, Jacquemin B. Air pollution exposure and bladder, kidney and urinary tract cancer risk: a systematic review. *Environ Pollut.* (2020) 267:115328. doi: 10.1016/j.envpol.2020.115328
16. White AJ, Gregoire AM, Niehoff NM, Bertrand KA, Palmer JR, Coogan PF, et al. Air pollution and breast cancer risk in the Black Women's Health Study. *Environ Res.* (2021) 194:110651. doi: 10.1016/j.envres.2020.110651
17. Vineis P, Husgafvel-Pursiainen K. Air pollution and cancer: biomarker studies in human populations. *Carcinogenesis.* (2005) 26:1846–55. doi: 10.1093/carcin/bgi216
18. Clofent D, Amigo MC, Loor K, Cruz M-J. Environmental pollution and lung cancer: the carcinogenic power of the air we breathe. *Arch Bronconeumol.* (2021) 57:317–8. doi: 10.1016/j.arbr.2021.03.002
19. Santibanez-Andrade M, Chirino YI, González-Ramírez I, Sánchez-Pérez Y, García-Cuellar CM. Deciphering the code between air pollution and disease: the effect of particulate matter on cancer hallmarks. *Int J Mol Sci.* (2019) 21:136. doi: 10.3390/ijms21010136

20. Fajersztajn L, Veras M, Barrozo LV, Saldiva P. Air pollution: a potentially modifiable risk factor for lung cancer. *Nat Rev Cancer.* (2013) 13:674–8. doi: 10.1038/nrc3572
21. Demetriou CA, Raaschou-Nielsen O, Loft S, Møller P, Vermeulen R, Palli D, et al. Biomarkers of ambient air pollution and lung cancer: a systematic review. *Occup Environ Med.* (2012) 69:619–27. doi: 10.1136/oemed-2011-100566
22. Turner MC, Krewski D, Diver WR, Pope CA III, Burnett RT, Jerrett M, et al. Ambient air pollution and cancer mortality in the cancer prevention study II. *Environ Health Perspect.* (2017) 125:087013. doi: 10.1289/EHP1249
23. Ou JY, Kirchhoff AC, Hanson HA. Air pollution across the cancer continuum: extending our understanding of the relationship between environmental exposures and cancer. *Cancer Epidemiol Biomarkers Prev.* (2020) 29:1876–9. doi: 10.1158/1055-9965.EPI-19-1588
24. Ou JY, Hanson HA, Ramsay JM, Kaddas HK, Pope CA III, Leiser CL, et al. Fine particulate matter air pollution and mortality among pediatric, adolescent, and young adult cancer patients. *Cancer Epidemiol Biomarkers Prev.* (2020) 29:1929–39. doi: 10.1158/1055-9965.EPI-19-1363
25. Raaschou-Nielsen O, Andersen ZJ, Beelen R, Samoli E, Stafoggia M, Weinmayr G, et al. Air pollution and lung cancer incidence in 17 European cohorts: prospective analyses from the European Study of Cohorts for Air Pollution Effects (ESCAPE). *Lancet Oncol.* (2013) 14:813–22. doi: 10.1016/S1470-2045(13)70279-1
26. Puett RC, Hart JE, Yanosky JD, Spiegelman D, Wang M, Fisher JA, et al. Particulate matter air pollution exposure, distance to road, and incident lung cancer in the nurses' health study cohort. *Environ Health Perspect.* (2014) 122:926–32. doi: 10.1289/ehp.1307490
27. Hvidtfeldt UA, Severi G, Andersen ZJ, Atkinson R, Bauwelinck M, Bellander T, et al. Long-term low-level ambient air pollution exposure and risk of lung cancer - A pooled analysis of 7 European cohorts. *Environ Int.* (2021) 146:106249. doi: 10.1016/j.envint.2020.106249
28. Bai L, Shin S, Burnett RT, Kwong JC, Hystad P, van Donkelaar A, et al., Exposure to ambient air pollution and the incidence of lung cancer and breast cancer in the Ontario Population Health and Environment Cohort. *Int J Cancer.* (2020) 146:2450–9. doi: 10.1002/ijc.32575
29. Taiwan Air Quality Monitoring Network. Available online at: https://airtw.epa.gov.tw/ (accessed September 19, 2021).
30. Taiwan Cancer Registry. Available online at: https://www.hpa.gov.tw/EngPages/List.aspx?nodeid=1061 (accessed September 19, 2021).
31. Lamichhane DK, Kim HC, Choi CM, Shin MH, Shim YM, Leem JH, et al., Lung cancer risk and residential exposure to air pollution: a Korean population-based case-control study. *Yonsei Med J.* (2017) 58:1111–8. doi: 10.3349/ymj.2017.58.6.1111
32. Eckel SP, Cockburn M, Shu YH, Deng H, Lurmann FW, Liu L, et al., Air pollution affects lung cancer survival. *Thorax.* (2016) 71:891–8. doi: 10.1136/thoraxjnl-2015-207927
33. Moon DH, Kwon SO, Kim S-Y, Kim WJ, Air pollution and incidence of lung cancer by histological type in Korean adults: a Korean National Health Insurance Service Health Examinee Cohort study. *Int J Environ Res Public Health.* (2020) 17:915. doi: 10.3390/ijerph17030915
34. Tseng CH, Tsuang BJ, Chiang CJ, Ku KC, Tseng JS, Yang TY, et al. The relationship between air pollution and lung cancer in nonsmokers in Taiwan. *J Thorac Oncol.* (2019) 14:784–92. doi: 10.1016/j.jtho.2018.12.033
35. Chen F, Cole P, Bina WF. Time trend and geographic patterns of lung adenocarcinoma in the United States, 1973-2002. *Cancer Epidemiol Biomarkers Prev.* (2007) 16:2724–9. doi: 10.1158/1055-9965.EPI-07-0455
36. Gabrielson E. Worldwide trends in lung cancer pathology. *Respirology.* (2006) 11:533–8. doi: 10.1111/j.1440-1843.2006.00909.x
37. Atkinson RW, Butland BK, Anderson HR, Maynard RL. Long-term concentrations of nitrogen dioxide and mortality: a meta-analysis of cohort studies. *Epidemiology.* (2018) 29:460–72. doi: 10.1097/EDE.0000000000000847
38. Bowe B, Xie Y, Yan Y, Al-Aly Z. Burden of cause-specific mortality associated with PM2.5 air pollution in the United States. *JAMA Netw Open.* (2019) 2:e1915834. doi: 10.1001/jamanetworkopen.2019.15834
39. U.S. EPA. *Integrated Science Assessment (ISA) for Oxides of Nitrogen - Health Criteria (Final Report, Jan 2016).* U.S. Environmental Protection Agency, Washington, DC, EPA/600/R-15/068 (2016).
40. Air Quality Guidelines. Available online at: https://www.eea.europa.eu/themes/air/air-quality-concentrations/air-quality-standards (accessed September 19, 2021).

13

Carcinoembryonic Antigen: A Potential Biomarker to Evaluate the Severity and Prognosis of COVID-19

Qianqian Chen[1†], Hui Kong[1†], Xu Qi[1], Wenqiu Ding[1], Ningfei Ji[1], Chaojie Wu[1], Chaolin Huang[2], Wenjuan Wu[2], Mao Huang[1], Weiping Xie[1*], Yun Liu[3*] and Jinhai Tang[4*]*

[1] Department of Respiratory and Critical Care Medicine, The First Affiliated Hospital of Nanjing Medical University, Nanjing, China, [2] Division of Intensive Care Unit, Wuhan Jin Yin-tan Hospital, Wuhan, China, [3] Department of Medical Informatics, School of Biomedical Engineering and Informatics, Nanjing Medical University, Nanjing, China, [4] Department of General Surgery, The First Affiliated Hospital of Nanjing Medical University, Nanjing, China

***Correspondence:**
Mao Huang
hm6114@126.com
Weiping Xie
wpxie@njmu.edu.cn
Yun Liu
liuyun@njmu.edu.cn
Jinhai Tang
jhtang@njmu.edu.cn

†These authors have contributed equally to this work

Background and Objectives: Corona Virus Disease 2019 (COVID-19) has become a serious pandemic disease worldwide. Identification of biomarkers to predict severity and prognosis is urgently needed for early medical intervention due to high mortality of critical cases with COVID-19. This retrospective study aimed to indicate the values of carcinoembryonic antigen (CEA) in evaluating the severity and prognosis of COVID-19.

Methods: We included 46 death cases from intensive care unit and 68 discharged cases from ordinary units with confirmed COVID-19 of Wuhan Jin Yin-tan Hospital from January 1 to March 22, 2020. Laboratory and radiologic data were analyzed retrospectively. All patients were followed up until April 10, 2020.

Results: COVID-19 patients in the death group had significantly higher CEA levels (ng/ml) than discharged group (14.80 ± 14.20 vs. 3.80 ± 2.43, $P < 0.001$). The risk of COVID-19 death increased 1.317 times for each additional 1 ng/ml CEA level (OR = 1.317, 95% CI: 1.099–1.579). The standardized and weighted receiver operating characteristic curve (ROC) analysis adjusted to age, sex, and ferritin levels suggested that the area under the curve (AUC) of the serum CEA levels was 0.808 in discrimination between death cases and discharged cases with COVID-19 ($P < 0.001$). We found mortality of COVID-19 is associated with elevated CEA levels increased (HR = 1.023, 95% CI: 1.005–1.042), as well as age (HR = 1.050, 95% CI: 1.016–1.086) and ferritin levels (HR = 1.001, 95% CI: 1.001–1.002) by survival analysis of Cox regression model. Among discharged patients, CEA levels were significant lower in moderate cases compared to the severe and critical cases ($P = 0.005$; OR = 0.488, 95% CI: 0.294–0.808) from binary logistic regression analysis. The AUC of CEA levels was 0.79 in distinguishing moderate cases from discharged COVID-19 patients by standardized and weighted ROC analysis ($P < 0.001$). A positive correlation between CEA levels and CT scores existed in discharged patients (Correlation Coefficient: 0.687; $P < 0.001$).

Conclusions: Elevated CEA levels increased the risk of death from COVID-19 and CEA levels were related to CT scores of the discharged patients positively.

Keywords: corona virus disease 2019, severe acute respiratory coronavirus 2, carcinoembryonic antigen, biomarker, prognosis

INTRODUCTION

Corona Virus Disease 2019 (COVID-19) is a disease caused by severe acute respiratory coronavirus 2 (SARS-CoV-2) (1). It has developed into a serious pandemic disease worldwide and become a burden borne by health care systems in many countries since its first outbreak in Wuhan, China in December, 2019 (2, 3). According to the latest COVID-2019 situation reports released by World Health Organization (WHO) (4), there were over 23 million patients with confirmed COVID-19 globally, along with over 806,000 death cases by August 24, 2020. It was reported that the case-fatality rates of critical cases were about 24-fold higher than those of confirmed cases with COVID-19 (49.0 vs. 2.3%) (5). In view of high mortality of critical cases, identifying specific biomarkers for estimate severity and prognosis of COVID-19 is in urgent need, especially when local health systems are overwhelmed. A few inflammatory factors, coagulation parameters or cytokines were considered as potential biomarkers of COVID-19 progression or severity (6–9). However, it is a long way to identify a simple biomarker with higher sensitivity or sensitivity for better comprehensive evaluation.

Carcinoembryonic antigen (CEA), also known as CEA-related cell adhesion molecule 5 (CEACAM5) or CD66e, is a kind of glycophosphatidylinositol-linked membrane glycoprotein anchored in a specific cell membrane microdomains (10). As a cell adhesion molecule, CEA functioned as a bridge linked to pathogens or stromal cells with other members of epithelial CEACAMs, triggers CEACAM-mediated signal communication and activated integrin signaling pathways in human endothelial cells (10–12). CEA is not only related to respiratory or digestive cancers but also some infectious diseases like gonorrhea or chronic inflammatory diseases like interstitial lung diseases (ILD) (13, 14). Immunohistochemical analysis of lung specimens from patients with pulmonary fibrosis indicated that strong expression of CEA in metaplastic bronchiolar and type II alveolar epithelia (15, 16). Formation of abnormal epithelial proliferation and renewal was seen as a possible source to elevated CEA levels in patients with pulmonary fibrosis (15). Similar to pathological changes of ILD, significant hyperplasia of type II alveolar epithelial cells and interstitial fibrosis were referred to from several reports of COVID-19 autopsies and biopsies (17, 18). To our knowledge, only one study about the serum cancer biomarkers including CEA levels of COVID-19 patients have been published (19). Whether elevated CEA levels are associated with poor prognosis or severity of COVID-19 remains unclear nevertheless.

Therefore, we conducted this study to present the serum CEA levels of COVID-19 patients and indicate the relation between serum CEA levels and prognosis or severity of COVID-19, which may be of great value for effective treatment.

MATERIALS AND METHODS

Data Sources and Extraction

A total of 46 death cases with confirmed COVID-19 were included in our study, which were admitted to an intensive care unit (ICU) for COVID-19 of Wuhan Jin Yin-tan Hospital from January 1 to March 22, 2020. Respectively, 68 discharged patients (13 from ICU, 55 from ordinary units) were included during the same period. All medical records of the patients we included were reviewed and related raw data were collected by the two authors independently. A senior investigator reviewed the raw data if there were any discrepancies. The following data of each patient we included were extracted: age, sex, smoking history, length of stay, comorbidities, white blood cell count, white blood cell count, lymphocyte count, neutrophil count, monocyte count, C-reactive protein (CRP), ferritin, interleukin 6 (IL-6), alpha fetoprotein (AFP), and CEA; radiology data including chest computed tomography (CT) or chest X-rays (for patients in ICU). Comorbidities of all patients were collected on admission. We only included the baseline data on admission if patients have the same kind of laboratory tests or radiology examination more than once. The survival time were defined as the time (days) from admission date to observation endpoint (death or April 10, 2020). Our study was approved by the Ethics Committee of Wuhan Jin Yin-tan Hospital (No. KY-2020-59.01).

Inclusion and Exclusion Criteria

All patients included met the following inclusion criteria: Confirmed COVID-19 cases was diagnosed by real-time fluorescent reverse transcription-polymerase chain reaction (RT-PCR) based on "Diagnosis and Treatment Protocol for Novel Coronavirus Pneumonia (Trial Version 7)" published by the National Health Commission of the People's Republic of China (20). Exclusion criteria were followed below: (1) Patients with a history of any cancer or any chronic disease related to elevated CEA levels like chronic kidney disease. (2) Patients infected with other viruses or bacteria.

Clinical Classification of COVID-19

The clinical classification of COVID-19 in our study was based on "Diagnosis and Treatment Protocol for Novel Coronavirus Pneumonia (Trial Version 7)" published by the National Health Commission of the People's Republic of China (20). Patients with COVID-19 are divided into four types: mild cases, moderate cases, severe cases, and critical cases (detailed descriptions on **Supplementary Material**).

Radiological Assessment by CT Scores

The CT scans of all discharged COVID-19 patients were assessed by two radiologists with more than 10 years of experience in a semi-quantitative way established by Xie et al. (21). Details of the criteria for the CT scores can be found on **Supplementary Material**. The definitions of lung lesions were specified in another study (22).

Statistical Analysis

Continuous variables were analyzed by Student's *t*-test while categorical variables were analyzed by Chi-square test. Binary logistic regression was applied for analysis of survival parameters. The variables with *P*-values < 0.05 in the univariate analysis were included in the binary logistic regression. The detailed descriptions of the model development and evaluation were mentioned in the previous study (23). We applied Nagelkerke

TABLE 1 | Demographic and clinical characteristics of the COVID-19 patients included.

	Total (n = 114)	Death group (n = 46)	Discharged group (n = 68)	P-values
Age (years)	61.74 ± 13.57	65.93 ± 8.49	58.60 ± 15.47	0.002
Sex				0.015
Female %	53 (46.50)	15 (32.61)	38 (55.88)	
Male %	61 (53.50)	31 (67.39)	30 (44.12)	
Smoker %	45 (39.47)	23 (50.00)	22 (32.35)	0.059
Comorbidities %	65 (57.02)	30 (65.22)	35 (51.47)	0.146
Diabetes mellitus	27 (23.68)	14 (30.43)	13 (19.12)	0.163
Cardiovascular disease	12 (10.53)	3 (6.52)	9 (13.24)	0.252
COPD	5 (4.39)	3(6.52)	2(2.94)	0.360
Hypertension	50(43.86)	23(50.00)	27(39.71)	0.277
Length of stay (days)	19.56 ± 15.91	11.48 ± 8.79	25.28 ± 17.34	<0.001
White blood cell count ($\times 10^9$/L)	7.90 ± 5.80	14.21 ± 8.18	5.87 ± 2.70	<0.001
Lymphocyte count ($\times 10^9$/L)	1.15 ± 0.57	0.77 ± 0.35	1.25 ± 0.59	<0.001
Neutrophil count ($\times 10^9$/L)	6.22 ± 5.98	13.04 ± 8.51	4.09 ± 2.66	0.001
Monocyte count ($\times 10^9$/L)	0.42 ± 0.20	0.44 ± 0.23	0.41 ± 0.19	0.766
C-reactive protein (mg/L)	44.58 ± 54.27	122.96 ± 62.13	28.44 ± 38.48	<0.001
Ferritin (ng/ml)	792.78 ± 684.73	1315.06 ± 653.17	423.81 ± 423.79	<0.001
Alpha fetoprotein (ng/ml)	2.48 ± 1.64	1.75 ± 0.85	2.98 ± 1.84	<0.001
Carcinoembryonic antigen (ng/ml)	8.23 ± 10.64	14.80 ± 14.20	3.80 ± 2.43	<0.001
Interleukin 6 (pg/ml)	22.30 ± 39.59	41.95 ± 40.11	20.10 ± 39.66	0.381

COPD, chronic obstructive pulmonary disease. Continuous variables are showed as mean ± SD.

TABLE 2 | Binary logistic regression analysis of factors related to covid-19 prognosis.

Variable		Model			
		1	2	3	4
Demographic factors	Age	1.072 (1.000–1.149)	1.062 (1.007–1.121)	1.104 (1.025–1.188)	1.057 (1.002–1.115)
	Sex	0.178 (0.029–1.113)	0.255 (0.048–1.347)	0.128 (0.018–0.918)	0.249 (0.048–1.284)
	Smoker	0.777 (0.146–4.125)	0.358 (0.070–1.838)	0.522 (0.088–3.100)	0.335 (0.066–1.706)
Inflammatory factors	CRP	1.023 (1.012–1.034)	1.024 (1.013–1.034)	-	-
	Ferritin	-	-	1.002 (1.001–1.003)	1.003 (1.002–1.004)
Tumor markers	CEA	1.311 (1.096–1.568)	-	1.317 (1.099–1.579)	-
	AFP	-	0.489 (0.272–0.879)	-	0.503 (0.281–0.899)
Model evaluation	Nagelkerke R^2	0.724	0.620	0.729	0.655
	AUC	0.936	0.914	0.940	0.924

Variables in the model are showed as OR (95% CI).

R^2 to measure overall model performance and the area under the receiver operating characteristic curve (AUC) to evaluate discriminative ability of each model (24). Hosmer–Lemeshow Test was used for Goodness of Fit Test. Only one inflammatory factor and one tumor marker were included in the same logistic model to avoid multicollinearity of interactive variables. We used standard and weighted receiver operating characteristic (ROC) curve analysis to assess the sensitivity and specificity of different parameters as biomarkers of COVID-19 prognosis or severity. The weighted ROC curve analysis was defined and performed as descriptions in a published article by the way of inverse probability weighting (25). The survival analysis was conducted by Cox regression model (proportional hazard model) and Kaplan–Meier analysis with Mantel–Cox Test. The relation between CEA levels and other factors in discharged cases was evaluated by Spearman's correlation coefficient. P-values < 0.05 in our study were statistically significant. We performed statistical analysis with IBM SPSS Statistics (Version 24.0).

RESULTS

Demographic and Clinical Characteristics of the Patients

According to the inclusion and exclusion criteria, we totally included 114 patients with COVID-19 (46 death cases and 68 discharged cases) in our study, with two patients with cancers, one with chronic kidney disease, and one without CEA

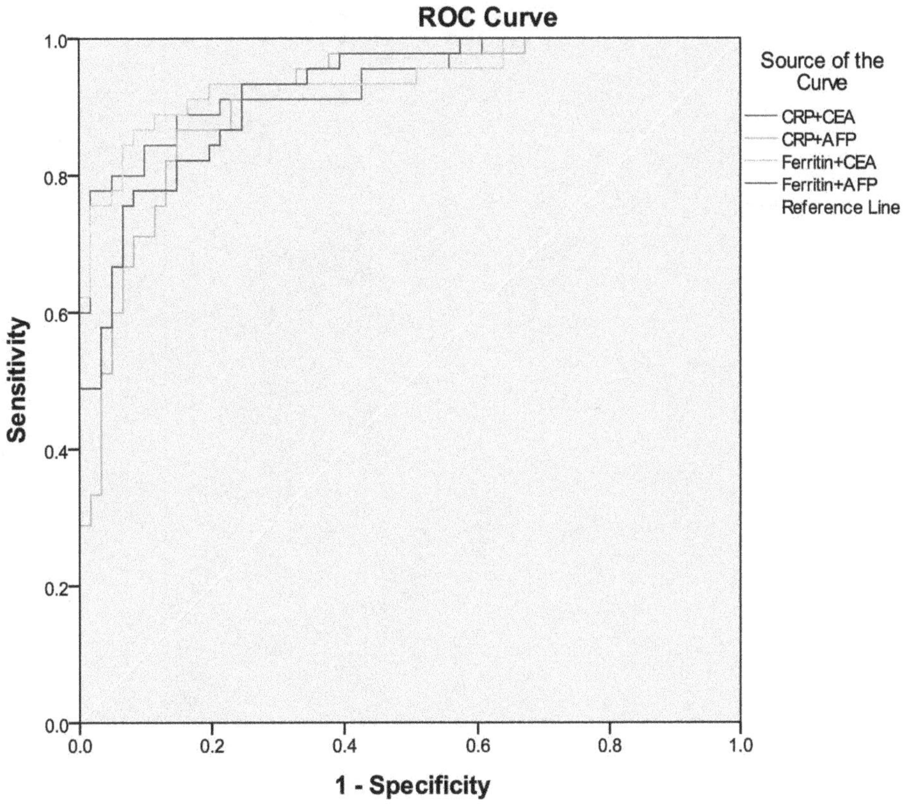

FIGURE 1 | The ROC curve analysis of different binary logistic regression models for the prediction of COVID-19 prognosis.

levels excluded. All demographic and clinical characteristics of the patients we included were demonstrated in **Table 1**. The mean age of all patients included was 61.74 ± 13.57. The patients in death group were older than those in discharged group (65.93 ± 8.49 vs. 58.60 ± 15.47, $P = 0.002$). There were 15 females in death group, which were less than those in discharged group (32.61 vs. 55.88%, $P = 0.015$). Death cases spent shorter time in hospital than discharged cases (11.48 ± 8.79 vs. 25.28 ± 17.34, $P < 0.001$). In complete blood count, white blood cell count (14.21 ± 8.18 vs. 5.87 ± 2.70, $P < 0.001$) and neutrophil count (13.04 ± 8.51 vs. 4.09 ± 2.66, $P = 0.001$) was increased significantly in death cases with COVID-19, while lymphocyte count decreased significantly (0.77 ± 0.35 vs. 1.25 ± 0.59, $P < 0.001$). We found CRP ($P < 0.001$) and ferritin levels ($P < 0.001$) were significantly higher in the death group than discharged group among inflammation indicators included in our study. No differences were found in IL-6 levels between the two groups ($P = 0.381$). Compared with the discharged group, the serum CEA levels were higher in the death group (14.80 ± 14.20 vs. 3.80 ± 2.43, $P < 0.001$).

Association Between CEA Levels and COVID-19 Prognosis

For multivariate analysis, we used binary logistic regression to build four models (**Table 2**). Variables with *P*-values < 0.05 in univariate analysis were included in our logistic regression models including demographic factors (sex, age, and smoking history), inflammatory factors (CRP or ferritin), and tumor markers (CEA or AFP). We found Model 3 including age, sex, smoking history, ferritin levels, and CEA levels showed the most discriminative ability among the four models we built in **Figure 1** (Nagelkerke $R^2 = 0.729$; AUC = 0.940). The Goodness of Fit Test of Model 3 was 0.408 by Hosmer–Lemeshow Test. From the binary logistic regression analysis of Model 3, age ($P = 0.009$), sex ($P = 0.041$), ferritin levels ($P < 0.001$) and CEA levels ($P = 0.003$) were significantly related to the prognosis of COVID-19. After adjustment to age, sex, and smoking history, the binary logistic regression equation (Model 3) demonstrated that the risk of COVID-19 death increased 1.002 times for each additional 1 mg/L ferritin level (OR = 1.002, 95% CI: 1.001–1.003) and 1.317 times for each additional 1 ng/ml CEA level (OR = 1.317, 95% CI: 1.099–1.579). The ROC curve analysis suggested that AUC of the serum CEA levels was 0.808 by standardized and weighted ROC curve analysis adjusted to other cofounding factors (age, sex, and ferritin levels). From survival analysis of proportional hazard model, we also found elevated CEA levels increased mortality of COVID-19 (HR = 1.023, 95% CI: 1.005–1.042), as well as age (HR = 1.050, 95% CI: 1.016–1.086) and ferritin levels. (HR = 1.001, 95% CI: 1.001–1.002). The COVID-19 patients were divided into two groups (high CEA levels group

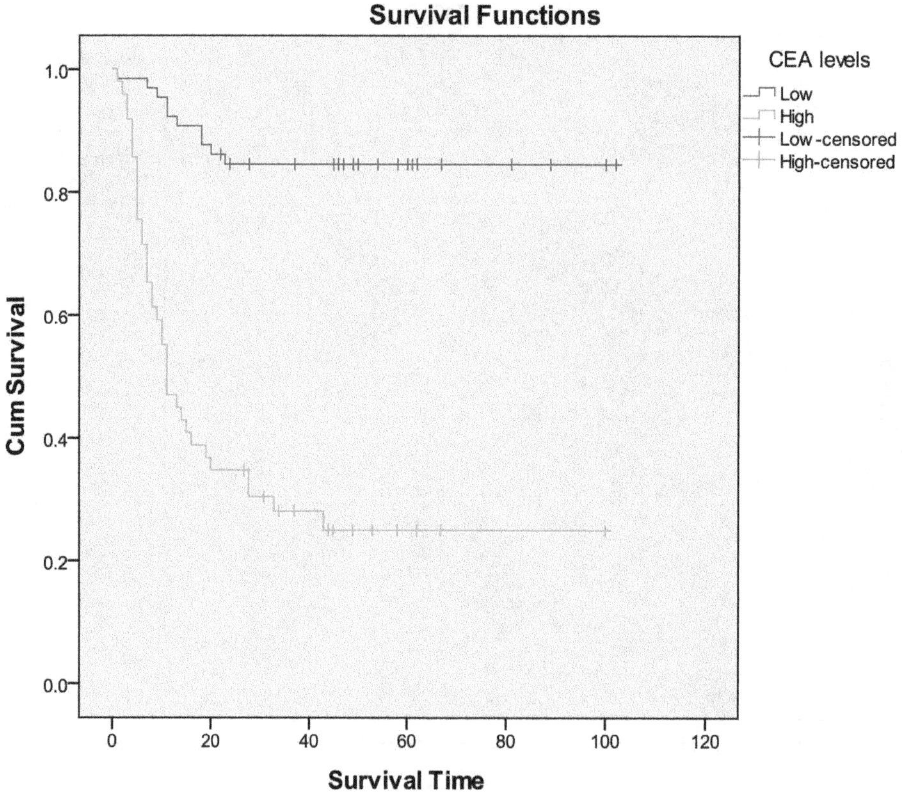

FIGURE 2 | Kaplan–Meier survival analysis of COVID-19 patients with different CEA levels.

and low CEA levels group) based on the cutoff value of CEA levels (5.2 ng/ml) calculated by time-dependent ROC curve. The COVID-19 patients with high CEA levels had higher risk of death than those with low CEA levels by Kaplan–Meier survival analysis (**Figure 2**). The Mantel–Cox Test of Kaplan–Meier survival analysis was $P < 0.001$.

Relation Between CEA Levels and COVID-19 Severity in Discharged Patients

A significant difference in CEA levels ($P < 0.001$) was found between the discharged patients with different clinical classifications, while age ($P = 0.001$) and other laboratory test including white blood cell count ($P = 0.008$), neutrophil count ($P = 0.012$), monocyte count ($P = 0.031$) and ferritin levels ($P = 0.039$) in **Table 3**. The results of binary logistic regression analysis (**Table 4**) revealed that CEA levels were lower ($P = 0.005$; OR = 0.488, 95% CI: 0.294–0.808) in moderate cases compared with the severe and critical cases after adjusted to age and the laboratory tests, which were statistic significantly in the univariate analysis. At the same time, moderate COVID-19 patients were younger than severe and critical cases from binary logistic regression analysis ($P = 0.039$; OR = 0.858, 95% CI: 0.742–0.993). **Figure 3** shows the ROC curves of CEA levels with the AUC of 0.790 ($P < 0.001$) in distinguishing moderate cases from discharged COVID-19 patients after considering age as a cofounding factor by weighted ROC analysis. The results of Spearman's correlation analyses (**Figure 4**) indicated that there was a positive correlation of CEA levels with CT scores in discharged patients (Correlation Coefficient: 0.687; $P < 0.001$). The **Figure 5** showed chest CT scans and CEA levels of three female patients in similar old age (69, 70, 71).

DISCUSSION

In our study, we found the serum CEA levels increased in non-survivors with COVID-19 compared to discharged patients statistically. Moreover, increasing levels of serum CEA were associated with more CT involvement scores in discharged COVID-19 patients. Till now, only one study reported the elevated serum CEA levels in COVID-19 patients (19). In that retrospective study, the authors found significant increases of CEA levels compared with health controls and a potential association between CEA and CRP levels. However, the role of CEA levels in clinical outcomes or CT involvements of COVID-19 patients was still unknown. This study validated the previous result that CEA levels were related to severity of COVID-19 reported by different research groups (Union Hospital of Tongji Medical College, Wuhan) (19). Furthermore,

TABLE 3 | Characteristics of 68 discharged patients with different disease severities.

	Moderate (*n* = 46)	Severe/critical (*n* = 22)	*P*-values
Age (years)	54.85 ± 15.78	66.95 ± 11.00	0.001
Sex			0.115
Female %	22 (47.83)	15 (68.18)	
Male %	24 (52.17)	7 (31.82)	
Smoker %	15 (32.61)	7 (31.82)	0.948
Comorbidities %	25 (54.35)	10 (45.45)	0.669
Diabetes mellitus	10 (21.74)	3 (13.64)	0.642
Cardiovascular disease	4 (8.70)	5 (22.73)	0.224
COPD	0 (0.00)	2 (9.10)	0.191
Hypertension	18 (39.13)	9 (40.91)	0.889
White blood cell count (×10^9/L)	5.31 ± 2.45	7.19 ± 2.94	0.008
Lymphocyte count (×10^9/L)	1.28 ± 0.58	1.17 ± 0.60	0.466
Neutrophil count (×10^9/L)	3.54 ± 2.27	5.80 ± 3.12	0.012
Monocyte count (×10^9/L)	0.39 ± 0.17	0.53 ± 0.27	0.031
CRP (mg/L)	27.53 ± 39.57	35.96 ± 37.14	0.424
Ferritin (ng/ml)	353.55 ± 295.24	578.94 ± 583.51	0.039
AFP (ng/ml)	2.96 ± 1.45	3.03 ± 2.51	0.895
CEA (ng/ml)	3.04 ± 1.97	5.35 ± 2.58	<0.001
IL-6 (pg/ml)	23.83 ± 44.05	10.72 ± 5.93	0.333
CT scores	12.57 ± 5.51	17.38 ± 5.53	0.002

COPD, chronic obstructive pulmonary disease. Continuous variables are showed as mean ± SD.

TABLE 4 | Binary logistic regression analysis of factors related to COVID-19 severities.

Valuable	*P*-value	OR	95% CI
Age	0.039	0.858	0.742–0.993
White blood cell count	0.833	1.246	0.161–9.662
Neutrophil count	0.729	0.708	0.100–5.005
Monocyte count	0.465	0.032	0.000–31.614
Ferritin	0.116	0.997	0.994–1.001
CEA	0.005	0.488	0.294–0.808
Constant	0.007	-	-

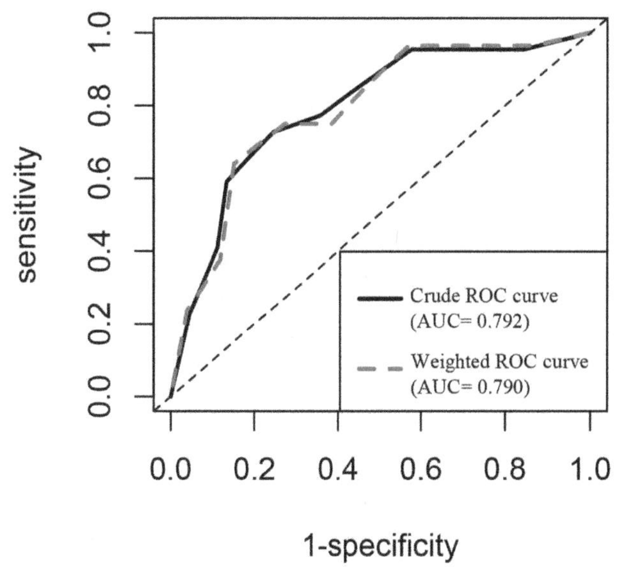

FIGURE 3 | ROC curve analysis of CEA levels in distinguishing moderate cases from discharged COVID-19 patients.

our study concentrated on different CEA levels in COVID-19 patients with different clinical outcomes (survivors or non-survivors) and potential correlations with CT involvement scores. We firstly found CEA levels are associated with prognosis and severity of COVID-19. We also calculated the value of CEA levels in evaluating the severity and prognosis of COVID-19.

Some hypotheses were formulated to explain the correlation between elevated CEA levels and poor prognosis or severity of COVID-19. Generally, CEA is considered to be a significant biomarker for adenocarcinoma in respiratory system or digestive system. Additionally, it should be noted that serum CEA levels were also significantly increased in some non-neoplastic lung diseases, especially in ILD or allergic bronchopulmonary aspergillosis (ABPA). In respiratory system, increased CEA expression of bronchiolar cells and type II pneumocytes (15) was responded to inflammation induced by mucus plug in ABPA (26) or atypical epithelial proliferation in idiopathic pulmonary fibrosis (IPF) (16). As human angiotensin-converting enzyme 2 (ACE2) is an entry receptor of SARS-CoV-2 (27, 28), bronchiolar epithelial cells and type II alveolar epithelial cells are the prime targets of SARS-CoV-2 in lung because of abundant expression on lung alveolar epithelial cells where SARS-CoV-2 particles were observed by electron microscopy (29, 30). Several autopsy studies have confirmed that bronchi were covered by mucus or mucus plug, as well as significant proliferating interstitial fibroblasts and type II pneumocyte hyperplasia (31) in COVID-19 patients. Since type II pneumocytes are considered as the stem cells or progenitors in alveoli (32), SARS-CoV-2 infection-induced massive alveolar epithelial cell death may lead to abnormal regeneration of type II pneumocytes for repair along with the production of CEA, which was similar to the uncontrolled proliferation of lung adenocarcinoma. Moreover, atypical epithelial proliferation and proliferating fibroblasts may also exacerbate obstruction of bronchioles and lung consolidation leading to refractory hypoxemia as well as worsen CT involvement scores. Therefore, it is reasonable that serum CEA levels correlate with the severity and prognosis of COVID-19.

Based on the relationship between CEA and type II pneumocyte hyperplasia and lung fibrosis, early medication focuses on atypical epithelial and fibrotic proliferation, such as Nintedanib, may be a potential therapeutic method to decrease

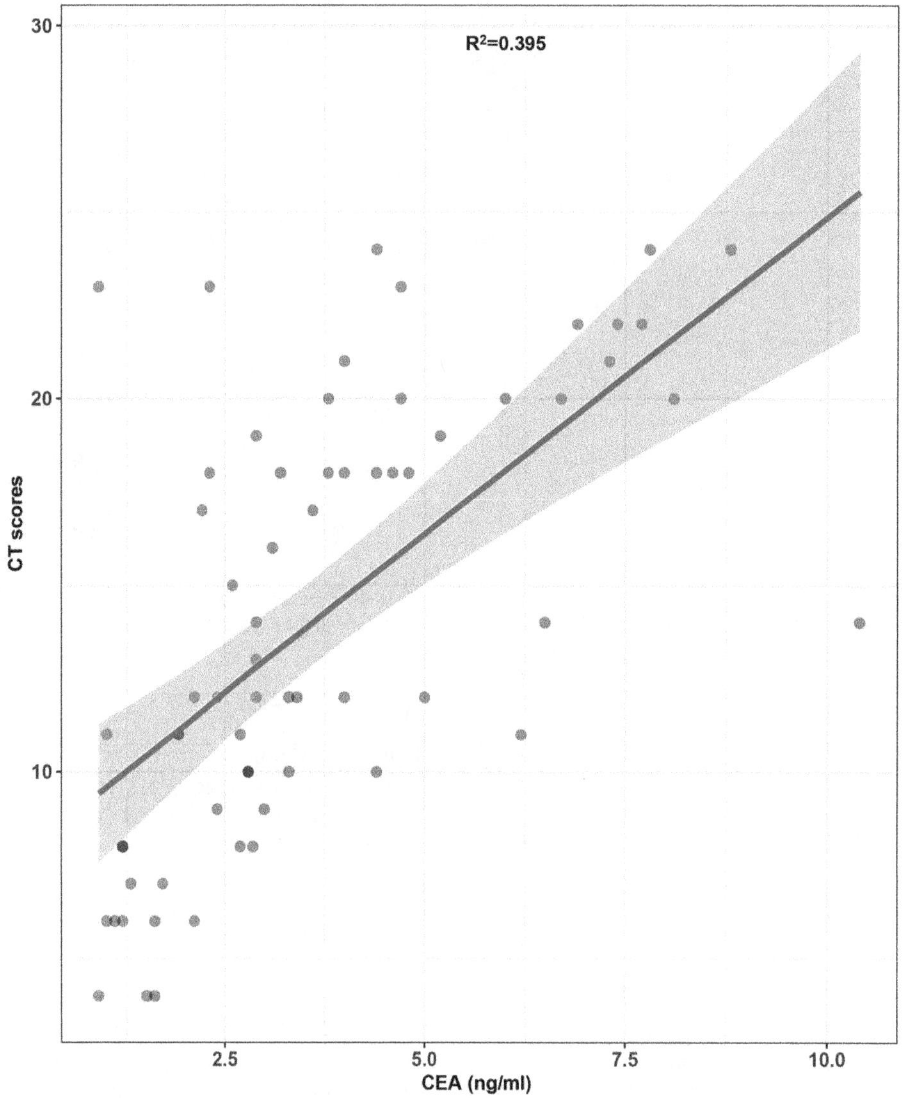

FIGURE 4 | Correlation of CEA levels with CT scores in discharged COVID-19 patients (the gray area on the figure means 95% confidence intervals).

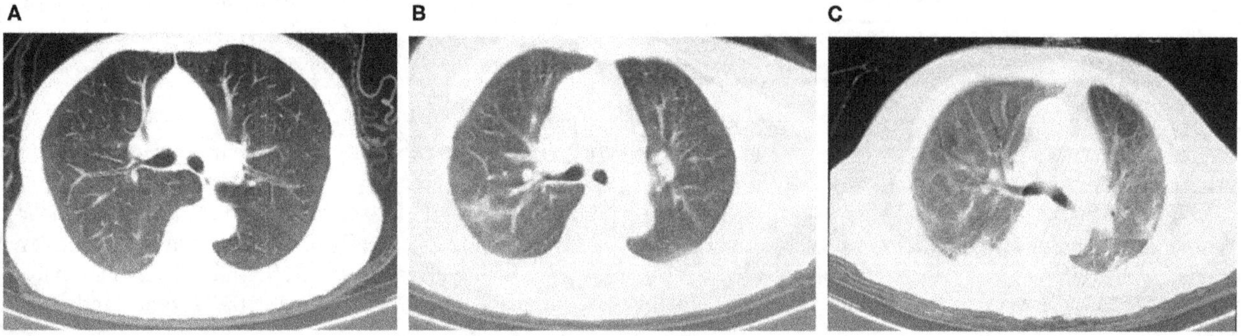

FIGURE 5 | Chest CT scans and CEA levels of three female patients. **(A)** Four points CT scores and 0.9 ng/ml CEA levels. (70 years old). **(B)** Sixteen points CT scores and 3.1 ng/ml CEA levels (70 years old). **(C)** Twenty two points CT scores and 7.7 ng/ml CEA levels (69 years old).

the mortality of COVID-19. Nintedanib is an inhibitor of multiple tyrosine kinases including vascular endothelial growth factor (VEGF), platelet-derived growth factor (PDGF) and fibroblast growth factor (FGF) (33), which is approved for the treatment of progressive fibrosing interstitial lung diseases (PF-ILD) (34) in March, 2020. It was reported that infection of SARS-CoV-2 resulted in significant elevation of many cytokines such as IL-2, VEGF, PDGF and FGF (35, 36). Hence, some hypotheses based on the potential effects of antifibrotic drugs like Nintedanib on COVID-19 was proposed in a Personal View published in May, 2020 (37). As an antifibrotic drug, Nintedanib also proved to have antiproliferative activity in non-small-cell lung cancer (NSCLC) (38) and its efficiency combined with other anti-tumor drugs on NSCLC was confirmed in clinical trials (39). Moreover, Nintedanib was reported to inhibit transforming growth factor-β (TGF-β) signaling pathway by suppressing phosphorylation of Smad2/3 and type II TGF-β receptor in human lung fibroblasts (33) and A549 cells (alveolar epithelial-type II cells models) (40), which were considered as novel antifibrotic mechanisms of Nintedanib. Meanwhile, another study found the relation between expression of CEA (CEACAM5) gene and TGF-β pathway genes (TGFBR1, TGFBR2, and SMAD3) in colorectal adenocarcinoma cells (41). Though there were few publications about the association in alveolar epithelial cells, it is possible that similar mechanisms existed in human alveolar epithelial cells, especially when CEA on the cell membrane functioned as microbial receptors for bacteria or viruses. In fact, TGF-β pathway plays a role in the pathogenesis of SARS-CoV-2 (42). However, the detailed mechanisms of CEA or effects of Nintedanib remains unknown in SARS-CoV-2 infected alveolar epithelial cells. More in-depth studies of related molecular mechanisms need to be conducted in the future. Overall, considering significant elevated CEA levels originating from atypical epithelial proliferation in non-survivors with COVID-19 of our study, we think Nintedanib may be one of therapeutic options for antifibrotic therapy in addition to other basic treatment (oxygen therapy, antiviral therapy etc.) for COVID-19 patients especially those critical cases with elevation of CEA levels. It is possible that additional antifibrotic therapy might be an effective supplement for the present COVID-19 treatment strategy. More pilot studies can be performed to validate the effects of antifibrotic therapy on COVID-19 in the future.

A few limitations existed in our study. Firstly, the number of the participants was not very large relatively. The patients with COVID-19 were from the same hospital and selection bias of the patients may exist in our study. The association should be validated in another cohort with larger sample size. Secondly, the CT scores of death cases in ICU were missing because these patients were impossible to have CT examinations in view of their critical condition. Thus, we cannot analyze the CT scores in the death group with COVID-19. Finally, the complications of other organs besides lung cannot be analyzed in discharged patients with COVID-19 due to a lack of data.

In conclusion, our study suggested that the elevation of serum CEA levels increased the risk of death from COVID-19 and serum CEA levels were related to CT scores of the discharged patients positively. Serum CEA levels might be a potential biomarker to evaluate the severity and prognosis of COVID-19. More prospective and multicenter studies with validation cohorts are needed to be conducted in the future.

AUTHOR CONTRIBUTIONS

JT, YL, MH, and WX contributed to funding acquisition, project administration, and supervision. QC and HK contributed to and writing original draft. XQ and WD contributed to software application and formal analysis. CH and WW contributed to data curation and investigation. NJ and CW contributed to methodology. MH and WX contributed to reviewing and editing original draft. All authors reviewed and approved the final manuscript.

FUNDING

This work was funded by grants from National Key Research & Development Plan of the Ministry of Science and Technology of the People's Republic of China (Grant Nos. 2018YFC1314900 and 2018YFC1314901), Project of Science and Technology Department of Jiangsu Province (Grant No. BE2016002-4), 2019 Provincial Special Guide Fund Project for the Development of Modern Service Industry (Grant No. 2019 [783]), 2016 Projects of Nanjing Science Bureau (Grant No. 201608003), National Health and Family Planning Commission Statistical Information Center Project, National Natural Science Foundation of China (NSFC) (Grant Nos. 81870054 and 81800011), and Key Project of National Science & Technology for Infectious Diseases of China (Grant No. 2018ZX10722301-002).

ACKNOWLEDGMENTS

The authors thank all colleagues from Division of Intensive Care Unit in Wuhan Jin Yin-tan Hospital for their support during the preparation of this manuscript.

REFERENCES

1. Coronaviridae Study Group of the International Committee on Taxonomy of Viruses. The species severe acute respiratory syndrome-related coronavirus: classifying 2019-nCoV and naming it SARS-CoV-2. *Nature Microbiol.* (2020) 5:536–44. doi: 10.1038/s41564-020-0695-z
2. Zhou F, Yu T, Du R, Fan G, Liu Y, Liu Z, et al. Clinical course and risk factors for mortality of adult inpatients with COVID-19 in Wuhan, China: a retrospective cohort study. *Lancet.* (2020) 395:1054–62. doi: 10.1016/S0140-6736(20)30566-3
3. Sohrabi C, Alsafi Z, O'Neill N, Khan M, Kerwan A, Al-Jabir A, et al. World Health Organization declares global emergency: a review of the 2019 novel coronavirus (COVID-19). *Int J Surg.* (2020) 76:71–6. doi: 10.1016/j.ijsu.2020.02.034
4. WHO. *Coronavirus Disease (COVID-19) Situation Reports* 2020. Available online at: https://www.who.int/emergencies/diseases/novel-coronavirus-2019/situation-reports (accessed August 24, 2020).
5. Wu Z, McGoogan JM. Characteristics of and important lessons from the coronavirus disease 2019 (COVID-19) outbreak in China: summary of a report of 72314 cases from the Chinese Center for Disease Control and Prevention. *JAMA.* (2020) 323:1239–42. doi: 10.1001/jama.2020.2648

6. Tan C, Huang Y, Shi F, Tan K, Ma Q, Chen Y, et al. C-reactive protein correlates with computed tomographic findings and predicts severe COVID-19 early. *J Med Virol.* (2020)92:856–62. doi: 10.1002/jmv.25871
7. Li H, Xiang X, Ren H, Xu L, Zhao L, Chen X, et al. Serum amyloid A is a biomarker of severe coronavirus disease and poor prognosis. *J Infect.* (2020) 80:646–55. doi: 10.1016/j.jinf.2020.03.035
8. Arachchillage DR, Laffan M. Abnormal coagulation parameters are associated with poor prognosis in patients with novel coronavirus pneumonia. *J Thromb Haemost.* (2020) 18:844–7. doi: 10.1111/jth.14768
9. Ulhaq ZS, Soraya GV. Interleukin-6 as a potential biomarker of COVID-19 progression. *Med Mal Infect.* (2020) 50:382–3. doi: 10.1016/j.medmal.2020.04.002
10. Tchoupa AK, Schuhmacher T, Hauck CR. Signaling by epithelial members of the CEACAM family—mucosal docking sites for pathogenic bacteria. *Cell Commun Signal.* (2014) 12:27. doi: 10.1186/1478-811X-12-27
11. Beauchemin N, Arabzadeh A. Carcinoembryonic antigen-related cell adhesion molecules (CEACAMs) in cancer progression and metastasis. *Cancer Metastasis Rev.* (2013) 32:643–71. doi: 10.1007/s10555-013-9444-6
12. Camacho-Leal P, Zhai AB, Stanners CP. A co-clustering model involving alpha5beta1 integrin for the biological effects of GPI-anchored human carcinoembryonic antigen (CEA). *J Cellular Physiol.* (2007) 211:791–802. doi: 10.1002/jcp.20989
13. Hao C, Zhang G, Zhang L. Serum CEA levels in 49 different types of cancer and noncancer diseases. *Prog Mol Biol Transl Sci.* (2019) 162:213–27. doi: 10.1016/bs.pmbts.2018.12.011
14. Islam EA, Anipindi VC, Francis I, Shaik-Dasthagirisaheb Y, Xu S, Leung N, et al. Specific binding to differentially expressed human carcinoembryonic antigen-related cell adhesion molecules determines the outcome of neisseria gonorrhoeae infections along the female reproductive tract. *Infect Immun.* (2018) 86:e00092. doi: 10.1128/IAI.00092-18
15. Abbona GC, Papotti M, Gugliotta P, Pecchio F, Rapellino M. Immunohistochemical detection of carcinoembryonic antigen (CEA) in non-neoplastic lung disease. *Int J Biol Markers.* (1993) 8:240–3. doi: 10.1177/172460089300800407
16. Fahim A, Crooks MG, Wilmot R, Campbell AP, Morice AH, Hart SP. Serum carcinoembryonic antigen correlates with severity of idiopathic pulmonary fibrosis. *Respirology.* (2012) 17:1247–52. doi: 10.1111/j.1440-1843.2012.02231.x
17. Liu Q, Wang RS, Qu GQ, Wang YY, Liu P, Zhu YZ, et al. Gross examination report of a COVID-19 death autopsy. *Fa yi xue za zhi.* (2020) 36:21–3. doi: 10.12116/j.issn.1004-5619.2020.01.005
18. Tian S, Xiong Y, Liu H, Niu L, Guo J, Liao M, et al. Pathological study of the 2019 novel coronavirus disease (COVID-19) through postmortem core biopsies. *Mod Pathol.* (2020) 33:1007–14. doi: 10.1038/s41379-020-0536-x
19. Wei X, Su J, Yang K, Wei J, Wan H, Cao X, et al. Elevations of serum cancer biomarkers correlate with severity of COVID-19. *J Medical Virol.* (2020) 92:2036–41. doi: 10.1002/jmv.25957
20. Zhao JY, Yan JY, Qu JM. Interpretations of "diagnosis and treatment protocol for novel coronavirus pneumonia (trial version 7)". *Chin Med J.* (2020) 133:1347–49. doi: 10.1097/CM9.0000000000000866
21. Xie X, Zhong Z, Zhao W, Zheng C, Wang F, Liu J. Chest CT for typical 2019-nCoV pneumonia: relationship to negative RT-PCR testing. *Radiology.* (2020) 296:E41–5. doi: 10.1148/radiol.2020200343
22. Ajlan AM, Ahyad RA, Jamjoom LG, Alharthy A, Madani TA. Middle East respiratory syndrome coronavirus (MERS-CoV) infection: chest CT findings. *AJR American J Roentgenol.* (2014) 203:782–7. doi: 10.2214/AJR.14.13021
23. Sharif-Askari FS, Syed Sulaiman SA, Saheb Sharif-Askari N, Al Sayed Hussain A. Development of an adverse drug reaction risk assessment score among hospitalized patients with chronic kidney disease. *PLoS ONE.* (2014) 9:e95991. doi: 10.1371/journal.pone.0095991
24. Steyerberg EW, Vickers AJ, Cook NR, Gerds T, Gonen M, Obuchowski N, et al. Assessing the performance of prediction models: a framework for traditional and novel measures. *Epidemiology.* (2010) 21:128–38. doi: 10.1097/EDE.0b013e3181c30fb2
25. Le Borgne F, Combescure C, Gillaizeau F, Giral M, Chapal M, Giraudeau B, et al. Standardized and weighted time-dependent receiver operating characteristic curves to evaluate the intrinsic prognostic capacities of a marker by taking into account confounding factors. *Stat Methods Med Res.* (2018) 27:3397–410. doi: 10.1177/0962280217702416
26. Noguchi T, Yamamoto K, Moriyama G, Saito Y, Kyoyama H, Mikami S, et al. Evaluation of serum levels of carcinoembryonic antigen in allergic bronchopulmonary aspergillosis. *J Nippon Med Sch = Nippon Ika Daigaku zasshi.* (2013) 80:404–09. doi: 10.1272/jnms.80.404
27. Zhou P, Yang XL, Wang XG, Hu B, Zhang L, Zhang W, et al. A pneumonia outbreak associated with a new coronavirus of probable bat origin. *Nature.* (2020) 579:270–3. doi: 10.1038/s41586-020-2012-7
28. Wang Q, Zhang Y, Wu L, Niu S, Song C, Zhang Z, et al. Structural and functional basis of SARS-CoV-2 entry by using human ACE2. *Cell.* (2020) 181:894–904. doi: 10.1016/j.cell.2020.03.045
29. Yao XH, Li TY, He ZC, Ping YF, Liu HW, Yu SC, et al. [A pathological report of three COVID-19 cases by minimal invasive autopsies]. *Zhonghua bing li xue za zhi = Chin J Pathol.* (2020) 49:411–7. doi: 10.3760/cma.j.cn112151-20200312-00193
30. Fox SE, Akmatbekov A, Harbert JL, Li G, Quincy Brown J, et al. Pulmonary and cardiac pathology in African American patients with COVID-19: an autopsy series from New Orleans. *Lancet Respir Med.* (2020) 8:681–6. doi: 10.1016/S2213-2600(20)30243-5
31. Tian S, Hu W, Niu L, Liu H, Xu H, Xiao SY. Pulmonary pathology of early-phase 2019 novel coronavirus (COVID-19) pneumonia in two patients with lung cancer. *J Thorac Oncol.* (2020) 15:700–4. doi: 10.1016/j.jtho.2020.02.010
32. Barkauskas CE, Cronce MJ, Rackley CR, Bowie EJ, Keene DR, Stripp BR, et al. Type 2 alveolar cells are stem cells in adult lung. *J Clin Invest.* (2013) 123:3025–36. doi: 10.1172/JCI68782
33. Rangarajan S, Kurundkar A, Kurundkar D, Bernard K, Sanders YY, Ding Q, et al. Novel mechanisms for the antifibrotic action of nintedanib. *Am J Respir Cell Mol Biol.* (2016) 54:51–9. doi: 10.1165/rcmb.2014-0445OC
34. Flaherty KR, Wells AU, Cottin V, Devaraj A, Walsh SLF, Inoue Y, et al. Nintedanib in progressive fibrosing interstitial lung diseases. *N Engl J Med.* (2019) 381:1718–27. doi: 10.1056/NEJMoa1908681
35. Nile SH, Nile A, Qiu J, Li L, Jia X, Kai G. COVID-19: pathogenesis, cytokine storm and therapeutic potential of interferons. *Cytokine Growth Factor Rev.* (2020) 53:66–70. doi: 10.1016/j.cytogfr.2020.05.002
36. Huang C, Wang Y, Li X, Ren L, Zhao J, Hu Y, et al. Clinical features of patients infected with 2019 novel coronavirus in Wuhan, China. *Lancet.* (2020) 395:497–506. doi: 10.1016/S0140-6736(20)30183-5
37. George PM, Wells AU, Jenkins RG. Pulmonary fibrosis and COVID-19: the potential role for antifibrotic therapy. *Lancet Respir Med.* (2020) 8:807–15. doi: 10.1016/S2213-2600(20)30225-3
38. Hilberg F, Tontsch-Grunt U, Baum A, Le AT, Doebele RC, Lieb S, et al. Triple angiokinase inhibitor nintedanib directly inhibits tumor cell growth and induces tumor shrinkage via blocking oncogenic receptor tyrosine kinases. *J Pharmacol Exp Ther.* (2018) 364:494–503. doi: 10.1124/jpet.117.244129
39. Capelletto E, Migliorino MR, Morabito A, Chiari R, Grossi F, Tiseo M, et al. Final results of the SENECA (SEcond line NintEdanib in non-small cell lung CAncer) trial. *Lung Cancer.* (2019) 134:210–7. doi: 10.1016/j.lungcan.2019.06.028
40. Ihara H, Mitsuishi Y, Kato M, Takahashi F, Tajima K, Hayashi T, et al. Nintedanib inhibits epithelial-mesenchymal transition in A549 alveolar epithelial cells through regulation of the TGF-β/Smad pathway. *Respir Investig.* (2020) 58:275–84. doi: 10.1016/j.resinv.2020.01.003
41. Gu S, Zaidi S, Hassan MI, Mohammad T, Malta TM, Noushmehr H, et al. Mutated CEACAMs disrupt transforming growth factor beta signaling and alter the intestinal microbiome to promote colorectal carcinogenesis. *Gastroenterology.* (2020) 158:238–52. doi: 10.1053/j.gastro.2019.09.023
42. Delpino MV, Quarleri J. SARS-CoV-2 Pathogenesis: imbalance in the renin-angiotensin system favors lung fibrosis. *Front Cell Infect Microbiol.* (2020) 10:340. doi: 10.3389/fcimb.2020.00340

14

Lung Cancer Death Attributable to Long-Term Ambient Particulate Matter ($PM_{2.5}$) Exposure in East Asian Countries During 1990–2019

Xiaoxue Liu [1], *Sumaira Mubarik* [1], *Fang Wang* [1], *Yong Yu* [2], *Yafeng Wang* [1], *Fang Shi* [1], *Haoyu Wen* [1] *and Chuanhua Yu* [1,3*]

[1] *Department of Epidemiology and Biostatistics, School of Public Health, Wuhan University, Wuhan, China,* [2] *School of Public Health and Management, University of Medicine, Shiyan, China,* [3] *Global Health Institute, Wuhan University, Wuhan, China*

***Correspondence:**
Chuanhua Yu
yuchua@163.com

Background: Ambient particulate matter is a public health concern in East Asia as it contributes to a growing number of all-cause and cancer deaths. This study aimed to estimate lung cancer death attributable to ambient particulate matter (PM) $< 2.5\,\mu m$ ($PM_{2.5}$) in East Asia countries.

Methods: The attributable death rates of lung cancer were estimated based on the calculation of population attributable fraction. We performed joinpoint regression analysis and age-period-cohort (APC) model to estimate temporal trends of the attributable death to $PM_{2.5}$.

Results: In 2019, $PM_{2.5}$ was estimated to have caused 42.2% (nearly 0.13 million) of lung cancer deaths in East Asia men. During 1990–2019, the increase in age-standardized death rates of lung cancer attributable to $PM_{2.5}$ was highest in China, which increased by 3.50% in males and 3.71% in females. The death rate caused by $PM_{2.5}$ also significantly increased in the Democratic People's Republic of Korea (2.16% in males; 3.06% in females). Joinpoint analysis showed that the rates generally increased in younger and older people in both the Democratic People's Republic of Korea and Mongolia, while it only increased in elderly people in other countries'. Age effect from APC analysis demonstrated the risk of lung cancer death attributable to $PM_{2.5}$ generally increased from young to old age. Period effect indicated that from 1994–1998 to 2019–2023 period risk continuously increased by 1.77, 1.68, and 1.72 times in China, the Democratic People's Republic of Korea, and Japan, respectively. The period risk decreased from 1999 to 2009 and subsequently increased from 2009 to 2019 in both the Republic of Korea and Mongolia.

Conclusions: The death rate of lung cancer attributable to $PM_{2.5}$ is increasing in the Democratic People's Republic of Korea, Mongolia, and China. In East Asia, China is facing the highest attributable death rate in recent decades. The period effect suggested a remarkably increased risk of lung cancer death caused by $PM_{2.5}$ in China, the Democratic People's Republic of Korea, and Japan during the long-term period. It is recommended that the governments of these countries should continuously concentrate on particulate matter pollution governance and improvement.

Keywords: death, lung cancer, YLL, $PM_{2.5}$, elder, population attributable fraction (PAF)

INTRODUCTION

Ambient particulate matter of <2.5 µm ($PM_{2.5}$) pollution is recognized as a major health concern worldwide. $PM_{2.5}$ was associated with an increased risk of disease mortality and morbidities (1–4), and a 10-µg/m^3 increment in $PM_{2.5}$ was associated with a 4.3% increment in total mortality (5). However, ambient particulate matter pollution continues to be one of the largest increases in risk exposures from 1990 to 2019 worldwide (6).

In 2019, according to the Global Burden of Disease (GBD) 2019 study, among the 87 risk factors identified, long-term exposure to $PM_{2.5}$ caused 118.2 million disability-adjusted life-years (DALYs), representing 4.7% of global DALYs in 204 countries and territories (7). Approximately 4,140,971 all-causes deaths and 307,680 lung cancer deaths in 2019 were attributed to ambient $PM_{2.5}$ globally. However, the ambient $PM_{2.5}$ risk-oriented health problems have mainly occurred in low- and middle-income countries (LMICs) according to previous studies (1, 8). In 2017, ambient particulate matter pollution ranked as the eighth leading risk for death, with a total of 2.94 million deaths globally and 1.05 million deaths in Southeast Asia, East Asia, and Oceania (2). Based on a newly published global comparative risk assessment in 2019, nearly all locations in south Asia, many parts of Southeast Asia, and most provinces in China had 10–15% of DALYs attributable to air pollution (6).

Lung cancer has been the leading cause of cancer deaths for many years worldwide, with the incidence and mortality markedly varying between countries (9, 10). Asia has extremely diverse lung cancer incidences, and it is the leading cause of cancer death in China (10, 11). The major risk factor for the burden of lung cancer was tobacco smoking, followed by air pollution-related age-standardized rates (12). This study aims to focus on lung cancer death caused by particulate matter pollution. Previous studies have evaluated the association of ambient air pollution with lung cancer (13–15). Few studies have been conducted regarding ambient air pollutant-related lung cancer death (16), while no national study has comprehensively evaluated the long-term trend in lung cancer death due to long-term exposure to ambient particulate matter in East Asia countries. Although a recent study reported that the age-standardized death rate attributable to air pollution decreased by 60.6% for China overall between 1990 and 2017 (17), the temporal trend in lung cancer death attributable to air pollution was not clearly analyzed. Therefore, this study aimed to estimate the trend and risk for long-term exposure to $PM_{2.5}$ caused by lung cancer death from 1990 to 2019 among East Asia countries, including China, Mongolia, the Democratic People's Republic of Korea, the Republic of Korea, and Japan.

MATERIALS AND METHODS

Data Sources and Methods for Quantifying the Health Burden

The attributable burden of lung cancer data (1990–2019) for China, the Democratic People's Republic of Korea, the Republic of Korea, Japan, and Mongolia was collected from the most recent GBD project. The datasets analyzed during the current study are published and available in the Global Burden of Disease Database repository. Due to the publicly available nature of data, ethical approval and patient consent to participate were not required in this study.

The GBD 2019 provides a systematic scientific assessment of published, publicly available, and contributed data on incidence, prevalence, mortality, and risk factors for a mutually exclusive and collectively exhaustive list of diseases and injuries. It contains data on 87 behavioral, environmental, occupational, and metabolic risks or clusters of risks, 369 diseases and injuries, and the healthy life expectancy (HALE) for 204 countries and territories (http://ghdx.healthdata.org/).

The original data on lung cancer death were obtained from the local Center for Disease Control and Prevention (CDC), Disease Surveillance Points (DSPs), and the Maternal and Child Surveillance System. Ambient air quality was estimated by extracting the annual average mass concentration data of ambient $PM_{2.5}$ from the multiple-source data, including satellite observation, ground measurement, and chemical migration model simulation, etc., and the grid-level exposure to ambient $PM_{2.5}$ was estimated by data integration model for air quality (DIMAQ) (6, 18). The relative risks (RR) of ambient particulate matter pollution at different exposure levels for different health outcomes were estimated as the Integrated Exposure Response function of exposure based on 81 published systematic reviews, the specific methods are outlined in a previous study (6).

Population attributable fraction (PAF) was defined as if the exposure of a certain risk factor was reduced to the theoretical minimum exposure level in a certain population, the proportion of related diseases or deaths in the population would reduce (2, 19). In this study, the exposure level associated with minimum risk, known as the theoretical minimum risk exposure level, for ambient particulate matter pollution was between 2.4 and 5.9 µg/m^3. Lung cancer deaths caused by $PM_{2.5}$ were estimated based on defining PAF through combining the distribution of exposure to air pollution with exposure-risk estimates at each level of exposure.

$$PAF = \frac{\sum_i^n p_i(RR_i - 1)}{\sum_i^n p_i(RR_i - 1) + 1} \quad (1)$$

where P_i is the percentage of the population exposed to level i of ambient air exposure, RR_i is the relative risk at exposure level i, and n is the total number of exposure levels.

Attributable death numbers were computed by multiplying PAFs by the relevant outcome quantity for each age-sex-location-year (6, 20). For example, the attributable deaths (AD) were calculated by multiplying the number of the deaths for lung cancer (N) and the PAF:

$$AD = PAF \times N \quad (2)$$

The age-standardized rate of attributable deaths caused by $PM_{2.5}$ was calculated by the world standard population (21).

Statistical Analysis

Joinpoint Regression Analysis

Temporal trends for lung cancer death rates attributable to $PM_{2.5}$ were assessed using the joinpoint regression analysis (Joinpoint regression software, Version 4.5.0.1, available through the Surveillance Research Program of the United States National Cancer Institute). Joinpoint analysis was based on regression with age-standardized mortality rates as the dependent variables and with year as the independent variable. Gender and age group were the by-variables. In the model, logarithmic transformation of the rates was carried out and the standard errors were calculated based on binomial approximation (22). An average annual percentage of change (AAPC), along with the corresponding 95% confidence interval (95%CI), was calculated for each trend. The statistically significant AAPC values indicated a temporal change in mortality trend over the time period. We used the Monte Carlo Permutation method for tests of significance. In this analysis, age groups under 25 years old were excluded due to very low probabilities.

Age-Period-Cohort Analysis

APC analysis could decompose the accumulation of health risks for incidence and death of disease (23). This analysis is developed to reflect the relative risks of disease by estimates on age, period, and cohort effects. Age effect indicates that the risk of death from disease increases with the process of aging. The period effect represents influential factors that simultaneously affect all age groups with advanced periods. The cohort effect represents variations across groups of individuals born in the same year or years. These effects influence morbidity and mortality risk of diseases in specific ways. An intrinsic estimator (IE) method used in this APC analysis could decompose the three effects simultaneously. In this model, the death rates of lung cancer attributed $PM_{2.5}$ were recoded into successive 5-year age groups (25–29, 30–34, ..., 90–94), consecutive 5-year periods (1994–1998, 1999–2003, 2004–2008, 2009–2013, 2014–2018, 2019–2023) and correspondingly consecutive 5-year birth cohort groups (1904–1908, 1909–1913, ..., 1994–1998).

The estimated coefficients of age, period, and cohort effects are plotted in **Figure 2**, and their exponential values [exp(coef.) = $e^{coef.}$] denote the relative risk (RR) of the age, period, or birth cohort effect. Age, period, and cohort effects were analyzed by Stata 12.0 software (StataCorp, College Station, TX, USA). Deviance, Akaike Information Criterion (AIC), and Bayesian Information Criterion (BIC), and represent the loss of information caused by using models to represent the process of generating the actual data.

RESULTS

Lung Cancer Attributable Death to $PM_{2.5}$ in East Asia Countries for Males and Females

In 2019, there were 2,042,639 deaths and 2,259,998 new cases of lung cancer worldwide, with a 25.18/100,000 ASDR and 27.66/100,000 ASIR. Importantly, a significant number of these 1,508,993 deaths were attributed to ambient particulate matter pollution that occurred in these East Asia countries, accounting for 36.4% of the global deaths attributed to ambient particulate matter pollution, and 12.3% of the attributed deaths were due to lung cancer. The death rate of lung cancer attributable to $PM_{2.5}$ among men was 2.34 times higher than that in women.

The global number of lung cancer deaths due to ambient particulate matter pollution were 307,680, 60.1% (185,041 deaths) of which were concentrated in East Asia countries, especially in male patients (42.2%). **Table 1** shows lung cancer attributable death to $PM_{2.5}$ in East Asia countries for both male and female patients.

Figure 1 shows the secular trends of the age-standardized rate of lung cancer death attributable to $PM_{2.5}$ in East Asia during 1990–2019. We observed a significant increase in the death rate among patients in China, the Democratic People's Republic of Korea, and Mongolia. We found a continuously decreasing trend in Japan for both male and female patients. In contrast, the death rate from the Republic of Korea peaked in 1999 while a slight rise in female patients has been observed since 2005.

Results of Joinpoint Regression Analysis

We conducted Joinpoint regression analysis to estimate the average annual percent changes in age-standardized and age-specific death rates of lung cancer attributable to $PM_{2.5}$ in East Asia (**Table 2**). Between 1990 and 2019, the increase in the death rate to $PM_{2.5}$ was highest in China [AAPC: 3.50 [95% CI, 3.05–3.94] in male and 3.71 [95% CI, 3.26–4.17] in female patients], and a small decrease was observed in Japan (AAPC: −0.76 [95% CI, −0.92 to −0.60] in male and −0.43 [−0.67 to −0.18] in female patients). As a high SDI country, the Republic of Korea showed no obvious change in the death rate. Similar to China, there was also a substantial increase in the Democratic People's Republic of Korea over the past 30 years (AAPC: 2.16 [95% CI, 2.01–2.32] in male and 3.06 [2.83–3.30] in female patients). We observed a slight increase in Mongolia, and the average percent changes increased by 1.63 (1.19–2.07) annually.

We also estimated changes in the age-specific rates of lung cancer death attributed to $PM_{2.5}$ across age groups (from 25–29 to 90–94 age group) (**Table 2**). We noted that the death rates in all age groups rose significantly in both the Democratic People's Republic of Korea and Mongolia. Other East Asia counties showed declines in the death rate for younger age groups but increases in older age groups. In China, the death rate to $PM_{2.5}$ rose significantly among people aged 65 years and over for male patients, and among people aged 75 years and over for female patients. In Japan, for both sexes, the rate generally declined for most age groups except for 85–89 and 90–94 age groups. In the Republic of Korea, an increase in the rate was also observed in elderly age groups (≥75 years in males and ≥80 years in females). Therefore, lung cancer death due to $PM_{2.5}$ generally increased in the Democratic People's Republic of Korea and Mongolia but decreased for all age groups in Japan. We almost observed a significant increase among elderly people aged 75 years and above in China and the Republic of Korea.

Results of Age-Period-Cohort Analysis

The coefficients of age effect on lung cancer death attributed to $PM_{2.5}$ increased from the 25–29 to 90–94 age group in

TABLE 1 | Lung cancer death and YLL attributable to $PM_{2.5}$ in East Asia in 1990 and 2019.

East Asia	1990				2019			
	Death		YLL*		Death		YLL*	
	Number	Age-standardized Per 100,000	Number	Age-standardized Per 100,000	Number	Age-standardized Per 100,000	Number	Age-standardized Per 100,000
Male								
China	20,576.26	5.42	548,863.25	123.69	120,186.42	13.36	2,704,360.07	271.65
Democratic People's Republic of Korea	243.67	4.09	7,097.63	99.15	899.90	7.04	23,694.74	164.94
Republic of Korea	862.99	7.06	24,070.02	167.94	3,085.32	8.31	60,056.13	147.69
Japan	2,709.53	3.89	57,200.87	76.31	5,513.54	3.21	88,070.16	58.29
Mongolia	28.30	6.55	695.62	144.09	95.61	11.43	2,518.83	240.23
Female								
China	7,060.43	1.69	183,062.82	40.27	51,113.34	4.99	1,107,912.93	105.28
Democratic People's Republic of Korea	85.01	0.89	2,288.95	22.18	367.73	1.94	8,661.43	47.23
Republic of Korea	300.29	1.82	7,878.83	42.89	1,240.90	2.43	21,475.66	44.36
Japan	1,054.48	1.09	21,248.93	22.47	2,516.99	1.02	34,851.02	19.27
Mongolia	6.40	1.17	149.19	26.21	24.35	2.28	577.58	45.55

YLL, Years of Life Lost.

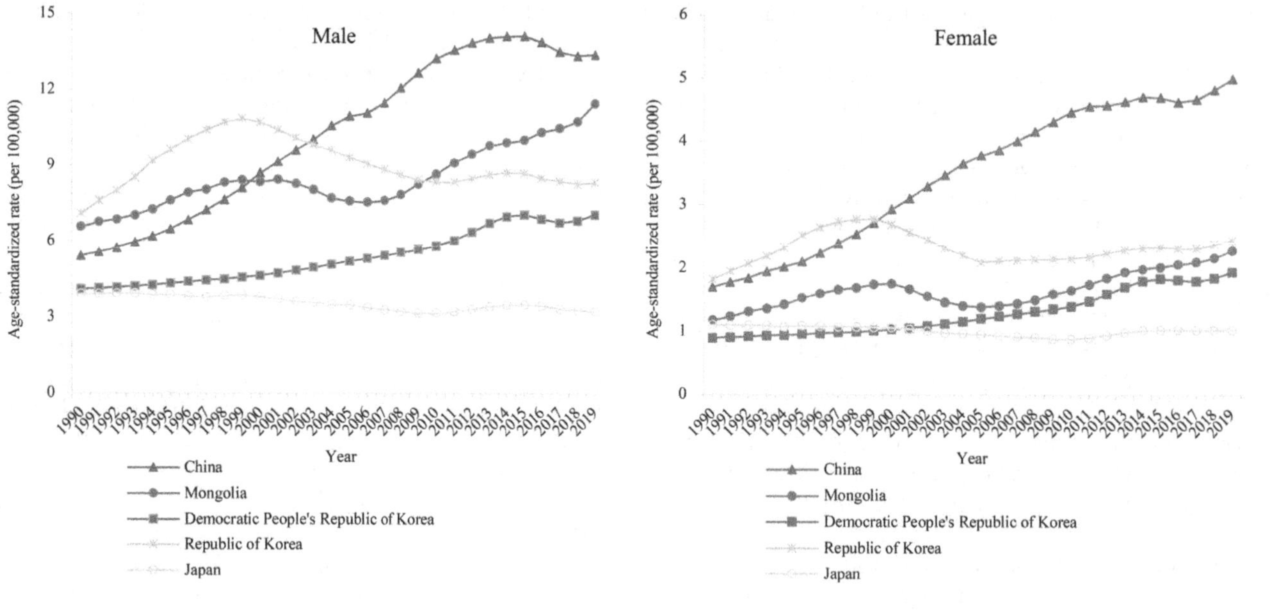

FIGURE 1 | The age-standardized rates of lung cancer attributable death to $PM_{2.5}$ in East Asia for both sexes at all ages, during 1990–2019.

East Asia countries, except for in the Democratic People's Republic of Korea, where the age risk peaked in the 70–74 age group (**Figure 2A**). The age effect showed that in the from 25–29 to 90–94 age group, the risk for lung cancer death attributed to $PM_{2.5}$ increased by 58.99, 36.51, 113.04, 190.68, and 101.86 times in China, the Democratic People's Republic of Korea, Republic of Korea, Japan, and Mongolia, respectively.

The period effect showed different trends in the death rates among East Asia countries (**Figure 2B**). In the from 1994–1998 to 2019–2023 period, the risk increased by 1.77, 1.68, and 1.72 times in China, the Democratic People's Republic of Korea, and Japan, respectively. The period effect in the Republic of Korea and Mongolia showed an N-shape trend, which decreased from 1999 to 2009 and increased from 2009 to 2019.

The cohort effect showed an ongoing decreasing trend from 1904–1908 to 1994–1998 birth cohort in all these countries (**Figure 2C**). From the earliest birth cohort to the most recent cohorts, the risk decreased by around 90% for all East Asia counties.

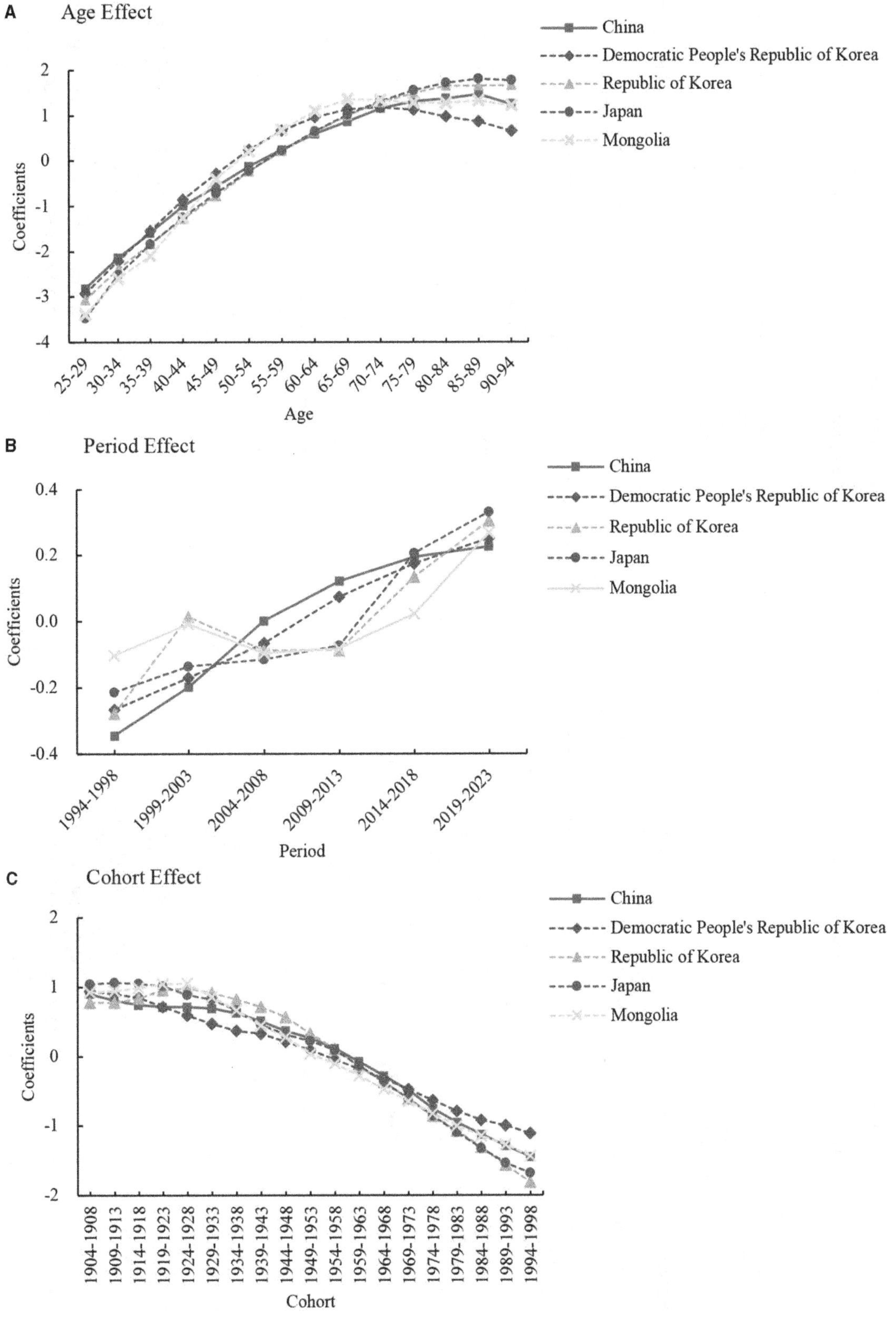

FIGURE 2 | Lung cancer death attributable to $PM_{2.5}$ estimated coefficients for the age **(A)**, period **(B)**, and cohort effects **(C)**.

TABLE 2 | The average annual percent changes (AAPC) in lung cancer deaths attributable to $PM_{2.5}$ in East Asia during 1990–2019 for male and female patients.

ASR* and Age-group (year)	Average annual percent changes (AAPC), male					Average annual percent changes (AAPC), female				
	China (95% CI)	Democratic people's republic of korea (95% CI)	Republic of korea (95% CI)	Japan (95% CI)	Mongolia (95% CI)	China (95% CI)	Democratic people's republic of korea (95% CI)	Republic of korea (95% CI)	Japan (95% CI)	Mongolia (95% CI)
ASR	3.50 (3.05, 3.94)	2.16 (2.01, 2.32)	−0.35 (−0.81, 0.12)	−0.76 (−0.92, −0.60)	1.52 (1.23, 1.81)	3.71 (3.26, 4.17)	3.06 (2.83, 3.30)	−0.07 (−0.52, 0.39)	−0.43 (−0.67, −0.18)	1.63 (1.19, 2.07)
25–29	−1.28 (−1.52, −1.04)	1.63 (1.35, 1.92)	−4.46 (−4.99, −3.94)	−2.07 (−2.26, −1.87)	1.09 (0.56, 1.62)	−2.83 (−3.77, −1.87)	2.84 (2.57, 3.11)	−3.55 (−4.02, −3.08)	−1.64 (−1.87, −1.40)	2.92 (2.68, 3.16)
30–34	−1.25 (−1.49, −1.01)	1.24 (0.95, 1.53)	−3.65 (−4.07, −3.23)	−2.81 (−3.05, −2.57)	2.93 (2.62, 3.23)	−2.73 (−3.43, −2.02)	2.66 (2.42, 2.90)	−2.86 (−3.18, −2.53)	−2.09 (−2.37, −1.80)	0.79 (0.31, 1.28)
35–39	−1.88 (−2.18, −1.58)	0.87 (0.68, 1.06)	−3.47 (−3.83, −3.11)	−2.78 (−2.98, −2.58)	1.97 (1.63, 2.30)	−2.01 (−2.33, −1.70)	2.55 (2.34, 2.76)	−1.84 (−2.04, −1.63)	−2.22 (−2.43, −2.00)	1.11 (0.57, 1.65)
40–44	−1.81 (−2.08, −1.54)	1.01 (0.85, 1.18)	−3.50 (−3.69, −3.30)	−2.66 (−2.93, −2.38)	1.54 (1.21, 1.87)	−1.87 (−2.13, −1.61)	2.52 (2.29, 2.76)	−1.89 (−2.12, −1.66)	−2.27 (−2.59, −1.95)	0.62 (1.12, 2.56)
45–49	−1.07 (−1.33, −0.81)	1.39 (1.22, 1.57)	−3.66 (−3.89, −3.44)	−2.29 (−2.58, −1.99)	1.78 (1.45, 2.11)	−2.01 (−2.47, −1.54)	2.71 (2.49, 2.94)	−1.25 (−1.35, −1.15)	−2.06 (−2.37, −1.74)	1.32 (0.80, 1.85)
50–54	−1.15 (−1.42, −0.88)	1.61 (1.44, 1.77)	−3.56 (−3.75, −3.38)	−1.31 (−1.60, −1.01)	2.00 (1.85, 2.16)	−1.44 (−1.72, −1.15)	2.86 (2.62, 3.10)	−1.32 (−1.60, −1.04)	−1.53 (−1.82, −1.23)	−0.12 (−0.74, 0.51)
55–59	−0.61 (−0.78, −0.43)	1.96 (1.82, 2.10)	−3.11 (−3.39, −2.82)	−0.92 (−1.07, −0.77)	1.63 (1.33, 1.94)	−0.78 (−1.12, −0.44)	2.99 (2.74, 3.24)	−1.44 (−1.65, −1.24)	−0.93 (−1.07, −0.79)	−0.31 (−0.96, 0.35)
60 - 64	0.05 (−0.14, 0.24)	2.03 (1.89, 2.18)	−2.42 (−2.71, −2.12)	−0.84 (−1.13, −0.56)	1.61 (1.16, 2.05)	−0.45 (−0.57, −0.34)	2.96 (2.70, 3.22)	−1.36 (−1.51, −1.20)	−0.37 (−0.55, −0.19)	0.10 (−0.49, 0.69)
65–69	0.26 (0.07, 0.45)	2.29 (2.13, 2.44)	−1.59 (−1.97, −1.21)	−1.05 (−1.39, −0.70)	0.45 (−0.09, 0.99)	−0.25 (−0.44, −0.08)	2.99 (2.73, 3.25)	−1.35 (−1.69, −1.00)	−0.28 (−0.58, 0.02)	0.63 (0.06, 1.21)
70–74	0.57 (0.32, 0.83)	2.44 (2.25, 2.62)	−0.53 (−1.08, 0.02)	−1.29 (−1.61, −0.97)	0.69 (0.19, 1.19)	0.30 (−0.04, 0.65)	3.07 (2.83, 3.31)	−0.82 (−1.36, −0.28)	−0.64 (−0.98, −0.29)	2.03 (1.56, 2.51)
75–79	1.13 (0.81, 1.46)	2.51 (2.35, 2.67)	0.46 (−0.29, 1.22)	−1.32 (−1.47, −1.17)	0.79 (0.35, 1.23)	0.99 (0.64, 1.33)	3.22 (2.98, 3.46)	−0.18 (−0.89, 0.54)	−0.97 (−1.30, −0.65)	1.64 (1.25, 2.04)
80–84	1.77 (1.39, 2.15)	2.46 (2.29, 2.62)	1.62 (0.74, 2.52)	−0.44 (−0.58, −0.29)	2.20 (1.83, 2.58)	1.78 (1.43, 2.13)	3.37 (3.16, 3.57)	0.80 (−0.17, 1.78)	−0.38 (−0.68, −0.07)	2.86 (2.55, 3.17)
85–89	2.57 (2.15, 2.98)	2.37 (2.22, 2.53)	2.88 (2.19, 3.57)	0.46 (0.28, 0.64)	3.87 (3.67, 4.07)	1.65 (1.36, 1.95)	3.59 (3.42, 3.77)	2.50 (1.93, 3.09)	0.31 (0.08, 0.54)	4.28 (4.01, 4.56)
90–94	2.08 (1.66, 2.50)	2.17 (2.06, 2.29)	1.97 (1.36, 2.59)	1.15 (1.04, 1.25)	4.19 (3.89, 4.49)	1.37 (1.17, 1.56)	3.75 (3.56, 3.94)	2.72 (2.18, 3.26)	1.53 (1.38, 1.68)	5.52 (5.08, 5.96)

**ASR, age-standardized rate, which was age-standardized by the GBD 2019 global age-standard population; CI, Confidence interval.*

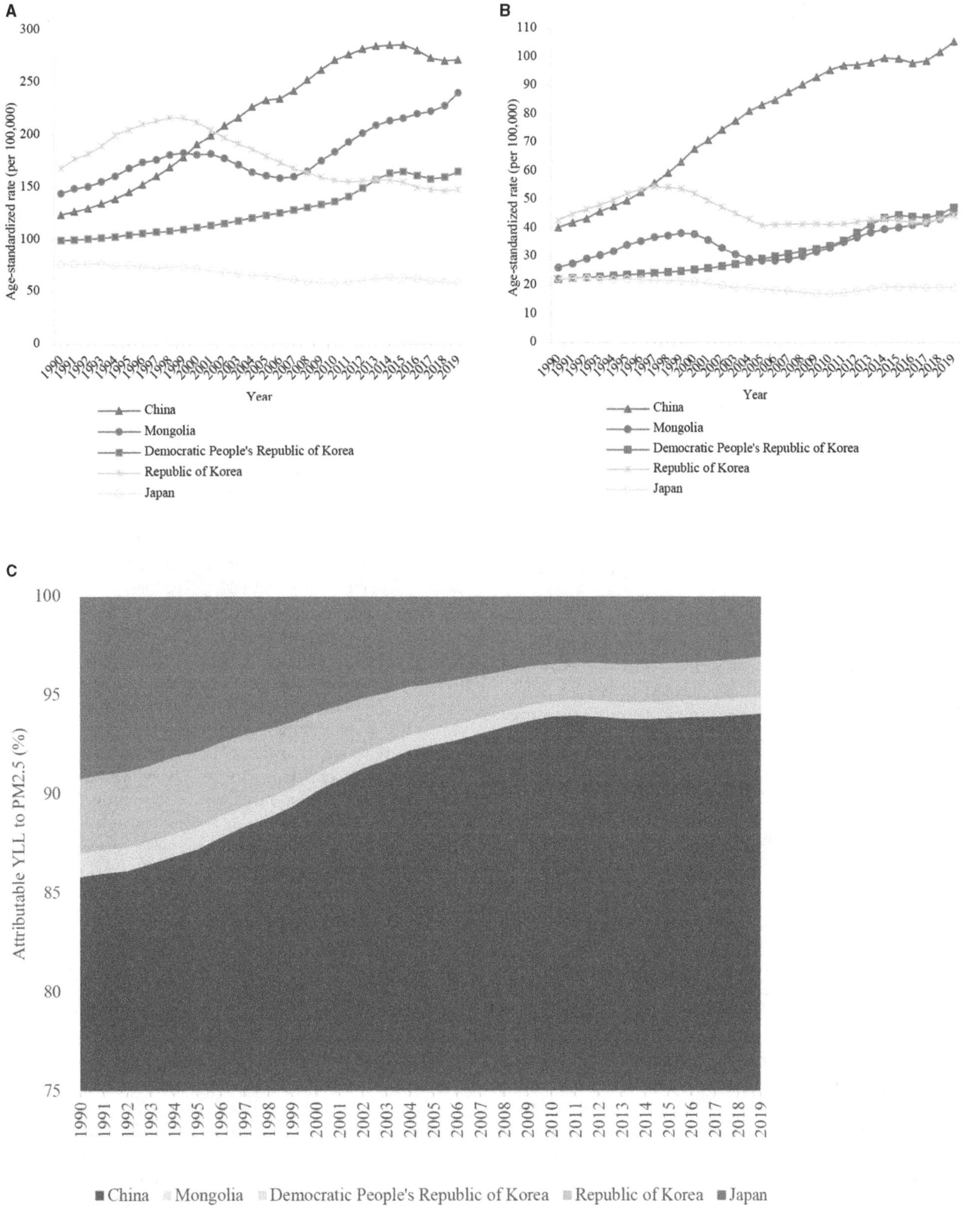

FIGURE 3 | The age-standardized rates of lung cancer attributable YLL to $PM_{2.5}$ in East Asia for both sexes at all ages, during 1990–2019. **(A)** male patients; **(B)** female patients; **(C)** The proportion of lung cancer YLL attributed to ambient $PM_{2.5}$ in East Asia countries from 1990 to 2019.

Lung Cancer Attributable YLL to $PM_{2.5}$ in East Asia Countries

The YLL rate of lung cancer attributable to $PM_{2.5}$ also showed a significant increase for male and female patients in the three regions (**Figure 3**).

In 2019, in male patients, the age-standardized YLL rate of lung cancer attributed to $PM_{2.5}$ was highest in China (271.65/100,000), closely followed by Mongolia (240.23/100,000) (**Table 1**). The YLL rate to $PM_{2.5}$ was relatively lower in the Democratic People's Republic of Korea (164.94/100,000) and the Republic of Korea (147.69/100,000). The YLL rate to $PM_{2.5}$ was lowest in Japan (58.29/100,000). In females, the highest YLL rate was observed in China (105.28/100,000) and the lowest rate in Japan (19.27/100,000). Overall, the YLL rates of lung cancer due to $PM_{2.5}$ were much lower in females than males among all East Asia countries. Compared with 1990, the age-standardized YLL rate of lung cancer attributed to $PM_{2.5}$ increased by 1.20 and 1.61 times in male and female patients in China, respectively (**Table 1**). However, the age-standardized YLL rate of lung cancer attributed to $PM_{2.5}$ decreased in male (24.0%) and female (14.0%) patients in Japan. In the Republic of Korea, the rate decreased by 12.0% in male and increased by 3.0% in female patients.

We also plotted the distribution proportion of lung cancer YLL attributed to ambient $PM_{2.5}$ in East Asia from 1990 to 2019 (**Figure 3C**). The YLLs from East Asia were mainly driven by China. Indeed, 94.08, 0.08, 0.80, 2.01, and 3.03% of YLLs attributable to $PM_{2.5}$ in 2019 were due to lung cancer in China, Mongolia, the Democratic People's Republic of Korea, the Republic of Korea, and Japan, respectively. Overall, apart from death, China also has a substantially increased lung cancer YLL attributed to $PM_{2.5}$ and mainly contributed to the YLLs from East Asia.

Lung Cancer Attributable Death and YLL to $PM_{2.5}$ in East Asia Compared With the Global Level in 2019

Compared with the global level, we plotted the ASDR, ASIR, and death and YLL attributable to the $PM_{2.5}$ of lung cancer in East Asia countries (**Figure 4** and **Supplemental Table 1**). The ASDR and ASIR of lung cancer in these East Asia countries were about 1.0–1.5 times higher than those of the global average in both sexes, while the low ASDR of Japan was 0.84 times that of the global average. In addition, the ASDR and ASIR of lung cancer were higher in male than female patients. In 2019, the death and YLL rates of lung cancer attributable to $PM_{2.5}$ in China were more than 2.0 times higher than those of the world average. In Mongolia, the rates were around 1.5 times that of global levels. It was 1.0–1.3 times more than global levels in the Democratic People's Republic of Korea and the Republic of Korea than the global level, while the level differed in the two countries. There were about 0.4 and 0.5 times higher levels in Japan for lung cancer death and YLL attributable to $PM_{2.5}$. In terms of genders, the death and YLL rates of lung cancer attributed to $PM_{2.5}$ in male patients were higher than that in female patients for most East Asia countries when compared with global levels. The gender difference was exactly different for China (Attributable to death: 231.15% in male patients, and 239.46% in female patients; Attributable to YLL: 217.31% in male patients, 229.92% in female patients). Generally, compared with the global level, China had the highest attributable death and YLL of lung cancer due to $PM_{2.5}$ in East Asia.

DISCUSSION

This study comprehensively estimates on temporal trends in lung cancer death caused by long-term exposure to ambient $PM_{2.5}$ in East Asia. We found that the lung cancer attributable death caused by $PM_{2.5}$ generally increased in younger and older people in both the Democratic People's Republic of Korea and Mongolia by Joinpoint analysis. APC analysis demonstrated that the risk of lung cancer death attributed to $PM_{2.5}$ generally increased from young to old age, and the risk increased continuously in China, the Democratic People's Republic of Korea, and Japan from 1994–1998 to 2019–2023 period. The Republic of Korea and Mongolia showed a different period risk trend. The cohort effect declined to the most recent birth cohorts, which demonstrated a decreasing risk from the old generation to the new generation.

This section discusses the attributable death of lung cancer due to ambient particulate matter. Among East Asia countries, we found that China and Mongolia had high mortality and YLL rates attributable to ambient $PM_{2.5}$. The high population density in China exhibited a huge lung cancer burden attributed to ambient $PM_{2.5}$ and was a major contributor to the death and YLL burden caused by $PM_{2.5}$ in East Asia. This finding was related to the fact that more than a quarter of global deaths caused by ambient particulate matter pollution occurred in China, which is the third risk factor affecting the health of Chinese people (16). A huge proportion of attributable YLL to $PM_{2.5}$ was related to China, which is consistent with studies by the World Bank and the WHO. The Chinese Academy for Environmental Planning on the effect of air pollution on health concluded that between 350,000 and 500,000 people die prematurely each year as a result of outdoor air pollution in China (18, 24). This finding could be contributed to the fact that $PM_{2.5}$ pollution in the winter is worse in China (4), in addition to the increasing high mortality of lung cancer in China (7). Mongolia has a relatively high level of age-standardized attributable death and YLL rates. This is because, during the cold wintertime in Mongolia, a lot of coal is burnt for domestic heating. As reported, ambient particulate levels frequently exceed 100 times the WHO-recommended safety level for sustained periods and account for the majority of personal particulate matter exposure (25). Reducing home heating emissions in traditional housing areas has been the primary focus of air pollution control efforts for Mongolian cities (26). Moreover, we observed that Mongolia still has a much higher level of lung cancer mortality in 2019, which is only second to China, although it has been decreasing over the past decades. Differing from China and Mongolia, Japan's age-standardized attributable death and YLL rates were the lowest from 1990 to 2019. This may be related to the fact that Japan has a declining relatively low level of air pollution, and its mortality rate from lung cancer is relatively low compared with other Asian

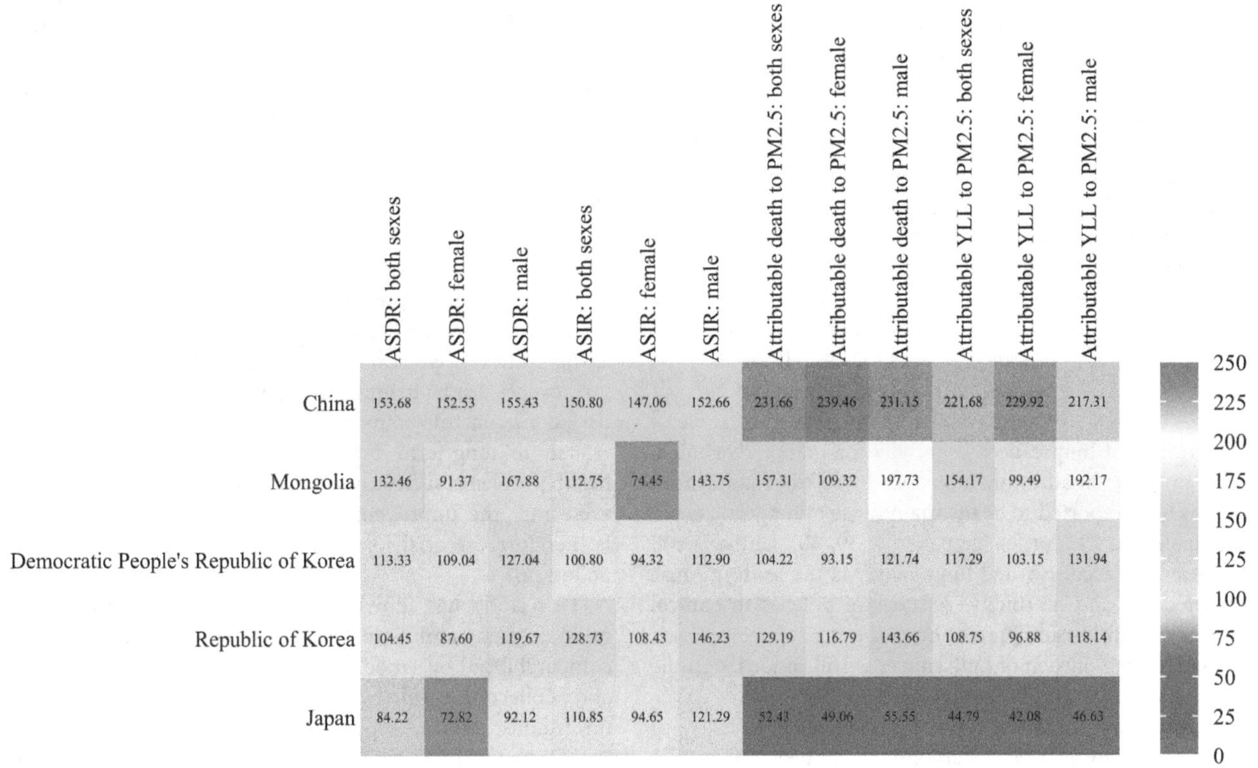

FIGURE 4 | Age-standardized rates of lung cancer attributable death and YLL to $PM_{2.5}$ in East Asia compared with those globally in 2019.

countries (14, 27). A relatively low level of attributable burden was observed in both the Democratic People's Republic of Korea and the Republic of Korea, while the difference was that the death and YLL rate of lung cancer due to $PM_{2.5}$ increased in the former but declined in the latter. Ambient air pollution is recognized as a major environmental health hazard in the Republic of Korea and the average $PM_{2.5}$ exposure concentration for the whole period was estimated to be 30.2 $\mu g/m^3$ during 1990–2013 (28). However, the mortality rate from lung cancer was much lower than in other countries. Therefore, although the Republic of Korea's air pollution is relatively high, the lung cancer attributable burden related to $PM_{2.5}$ is not at a high level. During 1990–2019, lung cancer death and YLL rates to $PM_{2.5}$ have increased in China, the Democratic People's Republic of Korea, and Mongolia, and decreased in Japan and the Republic of Korea. In East Asia countries, these trends were consistent with mean $PM_{2.5}$ concentrations, which showed substantial increases in China, with decreases observed in Japan during 1990–2013 (29).

We observed gender and area-specific distributions of lung cancer attributable burdens due to $PM_{2.5}$. Lung cancer deaths caused by ambient particulate matter were 2.34 times higher in East Asia men than women in 2019. Furthermore, the age-standardized death and YLL rates of lung cancer attributed to $PM_{2.5}$ were much higher in men than women in all countries, which was consistent with the gender difference in trends of lung cancer mortality. A previous study also reported that long-term $PM_{2.5}$ exposure has led to a much higher number of lung cancer premature death in male patients than in female patients (28).

In East Asia, the YLL burden of lung cancer caused by $PM_{2.5}$ was also mainly driven by China, especially in men. This finding was consistent with another previous study, which indicated that the elderly and men had higher health risks than younger people and women. When the $PM_{2.5}$ concentrations meet the WHO air quality guidelines of 10 $\mu g/m^3$, 84% of the premature deaths would be avoided (30). Compared to 1990, the age-standardized death rate of lung cancer attributed to $PM_{2.5}$ increased in 2019, while the increase rate was smaller in males than females in the Democratic People's Republic of Korea, Republic of Korea, and Mongolia. Outdoor air pollution occurs predominantly in developing countries, particularly in Asia (1, 31). In China, industrial and residential sources were the two leading sources of mortality due to exposure to ambient $PM_{2.5}$ (32), and annual concentrations of ambient $PM_{2.5}$ are more than 5 times higher than the WHO guideline values in many populous cities. In Mongolia, sources concentrated on increased coal consumption in the cold season (33). Whether females were exposed to a higher risk of death in these countries, need to be further explored in relation to the different sources of mortality caused by ambient $PM_{2.5}$. In Japan, we observed that lung cancer death attributable to $PM_{2.5}$ decreased in both sexes.

Increasing automobile traffic has caused considerable increases in concentrations of particulate matter, and concentrations have gradually decreased since control measures based on the automobile PM law were enforced in 2001 (34).

It is well-known that the major risk factor for lung cancer is tobacco smoking (12). Reactive oxygen or nitrogen species (ROS, RNS) and oxidative stress in the respiratory system could initiate or promote mechanisms of carcinogenesis, and the lungs are likely exposed to oxidants generated exogenously (air pollutants, cigarette smoke, etc.) daily (35). As reported, inhalable quartz, metal powders, mineral asbestos fibers, ozone, soot from gasoline and diesel engines, tobacco smoke, and ambient PM are involved in various oxidative stress mechanisms (35–38). It seems to be highly possible that $PM_{2.5}$ not only adds to lung cancer risk but also smoking habits over the years might be related to some of the differences of lung cancer, especially for men and women. Because smoking significantly increases the risk of lung cancer, which has been reported to be the main cause of lung cancers in 90% of male and 79% of female patients (39, 40). China is still facing heavy tobacco use, and lung cancer is the leading cause of cancer death and morbidity. A series of policies to control tobacco consumption and prevent lung cancer have been carried out. However, the burden of lung cancer is still serious, and the smoking rate in men is still very high (41).

In terms of age difference, the attributable death to $PM_{2.5}$ of lung cancer generally increased among elderly people (age $\geq$75 years) in both China and the Republic of Korea. This finding was also observed in other studies, which showed that long-term exposure to $PM_{2.5}$ was associated with an increased risk of disease death among people aged 65 years and older (42, 43). However, it is noteworthy that lung cancer death attributable to $PM_{2.5}$ increased for all age groups in the Democratic People's Republic of Korea and Mongolia. We also found that the percentage change of ASR of lung cancer death caused by $PM_{2.5}$ for China was significantly higher than that in any age groups in **Table 2**. This result was related to the age-standardized rate, which eliminates the influence of different age components of the population, and ensures the comparability of the lung cancer death rate.

Days of heavy pollution regularly occur in Asian megacities (23). China and the Democratic People's Republic of Korea had increasing attributable deaths rates of lung cancer caused by $PM_{2.5}$, and the period risk has also increased over the past few decades. According to the most up-to-date risk factor assessment, global exposure to harmful environmental risks has been declining, with the notable exception of ambient particulate matter pollution (6). In China, a large proportional increase in $PM_{2.5}$ was observed between 1990 and 2013 (29). While the early air pollution policies were ineffective at reducing emissions since the 1980s, and air pollution problems dominated by $PM_{2.5}$ have emerged and worsened since 2005 (44). As $PM_{2.5}$ was not been included in the National Air Reporting System until 2013, we collected data on the national annual mean $PM_{2.5}$ concentrations in China and found that it declined with a range of 72–36 $\mu g/m^3$ from 2013 to 2019 (**Supplemental Figure 1**). Another previous study also reported that the average annual population-weighted $PM_{2.5}$ exposure in China was 52.7 $\mu g/m^3$ in 2017, which is 9% lower than in 1990 (17). This decline is because of effective air pollution control policies after the winter-long $PM_{2.5}$ episode in China (44). However, the annual average $PM_{2.5}$ concentration in China was 36 $\mu g/m^3$ in 2019 and the planned reductions in annual average $PM_{2.5}$ concentration from the current level to 10 $\mu g/m^3$ still have not been achieved. As early as 2013, 87% of the global population lived in areas exceeding the WHO air quality guideline of 10 $\mu g/m^3$ $PM_{2.5}$ (annual average) (29). Thus, the changes derived from the policy evolution have implications for future studies, as well as further reforming the management of health risk and air quality control. More interventions are required to achieve the guideline levels of $PM_{2.5}$ as the Chinese population is still facing a high exposure level. The lung cancer death attributable to $PM_{2.5}$ declined in Japan but the period risk in this country still be increasing. This is possibly related to long-term exposure to particulate matter causing health problems, such as normal lung function not being restored even after the improvement of air pollution in Japan (45). It is therefore essential for countries in East Asia to prevent air pollution.

This study has limitations. Although GBD 2019 collected missing data and improved the quality of data and its comparability by modifying and adjusting data sources and collection and evaluation methods, there might be uncertainty about exposure estimates, as there was no measurement in some areas or the data was not available in the GBD 2019 study. Therefore, the results should be carefully interpreted for these countries. Second, the majority of air quality monitoring stations were located in urban areas where air pollution mean concentrations are expected to be high. Third, the APC analysis only takes the effects of age, period, and cohort into account and does not further analyze other risk factors underlying lung cancer death.

CONCLUSIONS

Our study showed that ambient air pollution could impose a substantial burden in terms of lung cancer death in East Asia, where China is facing the highest attributable death rate for lung cancer caused by $PM_{2.5}$. An increasing trend of lung cancer death attributed to $PM_{2.5}$ was observed in East Asia from 1990 to 2019, except for Japan and the Republic of Korea. However, the period effect nevertheless suggests a remarkably increasing risk in China, the Democratic People's Republic of Korea, and Japan in the long-term, and overall reduction of air pollution would have significant benefits for the health of the populations in these countries.

AUTHOR CONTRIBUTIONS

CY conceived of the study and participated in its design and coordination. XL led data collection and analysis, wrote the original draft, and oversaw editing of the final manuscript. All authors contributed to the drafting and revision of the article, read, and approved the final manuscript.

ACKNOWLEDGMENTS

We appreciate the work undertaken by collaborators on the 2019 Global Burden of Disease study.

SUPPLEMENTARY MATERIAL

Supplemental Figure 1 | National exposure in China to $PM_{2.5}$ for 12 months during 2013-2019.

Supplemental Table 1 | The age standardized rates of death and incidence lung cancer and its attributable burden to $PM_{2.5}$ in East Asia countries compared with the global's in 2019 (%).

REFERENCES

1. Lelieveld J, Evans JS, Fnais M, Giannadaki D, Pozzer A. The contribution of outdoor air pollution sources to premature mortality on a global scale. *Nature.* (2015) 525:367–71. doi: 10.1038/nature15371
2. GBD 2017 Risk Factor Collaborators. Global, regional, and national comparative risk assessment of 84 behavioural, environmental and occupational, and metabolic risks or clusters of risks for 195 countries and territories, 1990–2017: a systematic analysis for the Global Burden of Disease Study 2017. *Lancet.* (2018) 392:1923–94. doi: 10.1016/S0140-6736(18)32225-6
3. Burnett R, Chen H, Szyszkowicz M, Fann N, Hubbell B, Pope CA III, et al. Global estimates of mortality associated with long-term exposure to outdoor fine particulate matter. *Proc Natl Acad Sci USA.* (2018) 115:9592–7. doi: 10.1073/pnas.1803222115
4. Song C, Wu L, Xie Y, He J, Chen X, Wang T, et al. Air pollution in China: status and spatiotemporal variations. *Environ Pollut.* (2017) 227:334–47. doi: 10.1016/j.envpol.2017.04.075
5. Xue T, Zhu T, Zheng YX, Liu J, Li X, Zhang Q. Change in the number of PM2.5-attributed deaths in China from 2000 to 2010: comparison between estimations from census-based epidemiology and pre-established exposure-response functions. *Environ Int.* (2019) 129:430–7. doi: 10.1016/j.envint.2019.05.067
6. Collaborators GBDRF. Global burden of 87 risk factors in 204 countries and territories, 1990–2019: a systematic analysis for the Global Burden of Disease Study 2019. *Lancet.* (2020) 396:1223–49. doi: 10.1016/S0140-6736(20)30752-2
7. GBD 2019 Diseases and Injuries Collaborators. Global burden of 369 diseases and injuries in 204 countries and territories, 1990–2019: a systematic analysis for the Global Burden of Disease Study 2019. *Lancet.* (2020) 396:1204–22. doi: 10.1016/S0140-6736(20)30925-9
8. Brook RD, Newby DE, Rajagopalan S. The global threat of outdoor ambient air pollution to cardiovascular health: time for intervention. *JAMA Cardiol.* (2017) 2:353–4. doi: 10.1001/jamacardio.2017.0032
9. Miranda-Filho A, Pineros M, Bray F. The descriptive epidemiology of lung cancer and tobacco control: a global overview 2018. *Salud Publica Mex.* (2019) 61:219–29. doi: 10.21149/10140
10. Barta JA, Powell CA, Wisnivesky JP. Global epidemiology of lung cancer. *Ann Glob Health.* (2019) 85:8. doi: 10.5334/aogh.2419
11. Cao M, Chen W. Epidemiology of lung cancer in China. *Thorac Cancer.* (2019) 10:3–7. doi: 10.1111/1759-7714.12916
12. Deng YJ, Zhao P, Zhou LH, Xiang D, Hu JJ, Liu Y, et al. Epidemiological trends of tracheal, bronchus, and lung cancer at the global, regional, and national levels: a population-based study. *J Hematol Oncol.* (2020) 13:98. doi: 10.1186/s13045-020-00915-0
13. Raaschou-Nielsen O, Andersen ZJ, Beelen R, Samoli E, Stafoggia M, Weinmayr G, et al. Air pollution and lung cancer incidence in 17 European cohorts: prospective analyses from the European Study of Cohorts for Air Pollution Effects (ESCAPE). *Lancet Oncol.* (2013) 14:813–22. doi: 10.1016/S1470-2045(13)70279-1
14. Katanoda K, Sobue T, Satoh H, Tajima K, Suzuki T, Nakatsuka H, et al. An association between long-term exposure to ambient air pollution and mortality from lung cancer and respiratory diseases in Japan. *J Epidemiol.* (2011) 21:132–43. doi: 10.2188/jea.JE20100098
15. Schraufnagel DE, Balmes JR, Cowl CT, De Matteis S, Jung SH, Mortimer K, et al. Air pollution and noncommunicable diseases: a review by the Forum of International Respiratory Societies' Environmental Committee, Part 1: the damaging effects of air pollution. *Chest.* (2019) 155:409–16. doi: 10.1016/j.chest.2018.10.041
16. Yang J, Yin P, Zeng XY, You JL, Zhao YF, Wang ZQ, et al. [Deaths attributed to ambient air pollution in China between 2006 and 2016]. *Zhonghua Liu Xing Bing Xue Za Zhi.* (2018) 39:1449–53. doi: 10.3760/cma.j.issn.0254-6450.2018.11.006
17. Yin P, Brauer M, Cohen AJ, Wang H, Li J, Burnett RT, et al. The effect of air pollution on deaths, disease burden, and life expectancy across China and its provinces, 1990–2017: an analysis for the Global Burden of Disease Study 2017. *Lancet Planet Health.* (2020) 4:e386–98. doi: 10.1016/S2542-5196(20)30161-3
18. Chen Z, Wang JN, Ma GX, Zhang YS. China tackles the health effects of air pollution. *Lancet.* (2013) 382:1959–60. doi: 10.1016/S0140-6736(13)62064-4
19. Burnett RT, Pope CA, 3rd, Ezzati M, Olives C, Lim SS, Mehta S, et al. An integrated risk function for estimating the global burden of disease attributable to ambient fine particulate matter exposure. *Environ Health Perspect.* (2014) 122:397–403. doi: 10.1289/ehp.1307049
20. GBD 2017 Causes of Death Collaborators. Global, regional, and national age-sex-specific mortality for 282 causes of death in 195 countries and territories, 1980–2017: a systematic analysis for the Global Burden of Disease Study 2017. *Lancet.* (2018) 392:1736–88. doi: 10.1016/S0140-6736(18)32203-7
21. Rudd KE, Johnson SC, Agesa KM, Shackelford KA, Tsoi D, Kievlan DR, et al. Global, regional, and national sepsis incidence and mortality, 1990–2017: analysis for the Global Burden of Disease Study. *Lancet.* (2020) 395:200–11. doi: 10.1016/S0140-6736(19)32989-7
22. Kim HJ, Fay MP, Feuer EJ, Midthune DN. Permutation tests for joinpoint regression with applications to cancer rates. *Stat Med.* (2000) 19:335–51. doi: 10.1002/(sici)1097-0258(20000215)19:3<335::aid-sim336>3.0.co;2-z
23. Cheng Z, Luo L, Wang S, Wang Y, Sharma S, Shimadera H, et al. Status and characteristics of ambient PM2.5 pollution in global megacities. *Environ Int.* (2016) 89–90:212–21. doi: 10.1016/j.envint.2016.02.003
24. Yang G, Wang Y, Zeng Y, Gao GF, Liang X, Zhou M, et al. Rapid health transition in China, 1990–2010: findings from the Global Burden of Disease Study 2010. *Lancet.* (2013) 381:1987–2015. doi: 10.1016/S0140-6736(13)61097-1
25. Warburton D, Warburton N, Wigfall C, Chimedsuren O, Lodoisamba D, Lodoysamba S, et al. Impact of seasonal winter air pollution on health across the lifespan in mongolia and some putative solutions. *Ann Am Thorac Soc.* (2018) 15(Suppl. 2):S86–90. doi: 10.1513/AnnalsATS.201710-758MG
26. Allen RW, Gombojav E, Barkhasragchaa B, Byambaa T, Lkhasuren O, Amram O, et al. An assessment of air pollution and its attributable mortality in Ulaanbaatar, Mongolia. *Air Qual Atmos Health.* (2013) 6:137–50. doi: 10.1007/s11869-011-0154-3
27. Global Burden of Disease Cancer Collaboration, Fitzmaurice C, Akinyemiju TF, Al Lami FH, Alam T, Alizadeh-Navaei R, et al. Global, regional, and national cancer incidence, mortality, years of life lost, years lived with disability, and disability-adjusted life-years for 29 cancer groups, 1990 to 2016: a systematic analysis for the global burden of disease study. *JAMA Oncol.* (2018) 4:1553–68. doi: 10.1001/jamaoncol.2018.2706
28. Kim JH, Oh IH, Park JH, Cheong HK. Premature deaths attributable to long-term exposure to ambient fine particulate matter in the Republic of Korea. *J Korean Med Sci.* (2018) 33:e251. doi: 10.3346/jkms.2018.33.e251
29. Brauer M, Freedman G, Frostad J, van Donkelaar A, Martin RV, Dentener F, et al. Ambient air pollution exposure estimation for the global burden of disease 2013. *Environ Sci Technol.* (2016) 50:79–88. doi: 10.1021/acs.est.5b03709
30. Nie D, Chen M, Wu Y, Ge X, Hu J, Zhang K, et al. Characterization of fine particulate matter and associated health burden in Nanjing. *Int J Environ Res Public Health.* (2018) 15:602. doi: 10.3390/ijerph15040602

31. Cohen AJ, Anderson HR, Ostro B, Pandey KD, Krzyzanowski M, Kunzli N, et al. The global burden of disease due to outdoor air pollution. *J Toxicol Env Heal A.* (2005) 68:1301–7. doi: 10.1080/15287390590936166
32. Hu J, Huang L, Chen M, Liao H, Zhang H, Wang S, et al. Premature mortality attributable to particulate matter in china: source contributions and responses to reductions. *Environ Sci Technol.* (2017) 51:9950–9. doi: 10.1021/acs.est.7b03193
33. Nakao M, Yamauchi K, Ishihara Y, Omori H, Ichinnorov D, Solongo B. Effects of air pollution and seasons on health-related quality of life of Mongolian adults living in Ulaanbaatar: cross-sectional studies. *BMC Public Health.* (2017) 17:594. doi: 10.1186/s12889-017-4507-1
34. Shima M. Health effects of air pollution: a historical review and present status. *Nihon Eiseigaku Zasshi.* (2017) 72:159–65. doi: 10.1265/jjh.72.159
35. Valavanidis A, Vlachogianni T, Fiotakis K, Loridas S. Pulmonary oxidative stress, inflammation and cancer: respirable particulate matter, fibrous dusts and ozone as major causes of lung carcinogenesis through reactive oxygen species mechanisms. *Int J Environ Res Public Health.* (2013) 10:3886–907. doi: 10.3390/ijerph100 93886
36. Nagai H, Toyokuni S. Biopersistent fiber-induced inflammation and carcinogenesis: lessons learned from asbestos toward safety of fibrous nanomaterials. *Arch Biochem Biophys.* (2010) 502:1–7. doi: 10.1016/j.abb.2010.06.015
37. Strak M, Janssen NA, Godri KJ, Gosens I, Mudway IS, Cassee FR, et al. Respiratory health effects of airborne particulate matter: the role of particle size, composition, and oxidative potential-the RAPTES project. *Environ Health Perspect.* (2012) 120:1183–9. doi: 10.1289/ehp.1104389
38. Valavanidis A, Vlachogianni T, Fiotakis K. Tobacco smoke: involvement of reactive oxygen species and stable free radicals in mechanisms of oxidative damage, carcinogenesis and synergistic effects with other respirable particles. *Int J Environ Res Public Health.* (2009) 6:445–62. doi: 10.3390/ijerph6020445
39. Hansen MS, Licaj I, Braaten T, Lund E, Gram IT. The fraction of lung cancer attributable to smoking in the Norwegian Women and Cancer (NOWAC) Study. *Br J Cancer.* (2021) 124:658–62. doi: 10.1038/s41416-020-01131-w
40. Ozlu T, Bulbul Y. Smoking and lung cancer. *Tuberk Toraks.* (2005) 53:200–9.
41. Zou X, Jia M, Wang X, Zhi X. [Changing epidemic of lung cancer & tobacco and situation of tobacco control in China]. *Zhongguo Fei Ai Za Zhi.* (2017) 20:505–10. doi: 10.3779/j.issn.1009-3419.2017.08.01
42. Li T, Zhang Y, Wang J, Xu D, Yin Z, Chen H, et al. All-cause mortality risk associated with long-term exposure to ambient PM2.5 in China: a cohort study. *Lancet Public Health.* (2018) 3:e470–7. doi: 10.1016/S2468-2667(18)30144-0
43. Pun VC, Kazemiparkouhi F, Manjourides J, Suh HH. Long-term PM2.5 exposure and respiratory, cancer, and cardiovascular mortality in older US adults. *Am J Epidemiol.* (2017) 186:961–9. doi: 10.1093/aje/kwx166
44. Jin Y, Andersson H, Zhang S. Air pollution control policies in China: a retrospective and prospects. *Int J Environ Res Public Health.* (2016) 13:1219. doi: 10.3390/ijerph13121219
45. Yanagita Y, Senjyu H, Asai M, Tanaka T, Yano Y, Miyamoto N, et al. Air pollution irreversibly impairs lung function: a twenty-year follow-up of officially acknowledged victims in Japan. *Tohoku J Exp Med.* (2013) 230:177–84. doi: 10.1620/tjem.230.177

15

Circulating D-Dimers Increase the Risk of Mortality and Venous Thromboembolism in Patients with Lung Cancer: A Systematic Analysis Combined with External Validation

Jing Li[1†], Shanle Yan[2†], Xiaohui Zhang[3†], Mengqi Xiang[4], Chuanhua Zhang[5], Ling Gu[3], Xiaoying Wei[1], Chuanyun You[3], Shenhua Chen[3], Daxiong Zeng[1] and Junhong Jiang[1*]*

[1] Department of Medicine, Respiratory, Emergency and Intensive Care Medicine, The Affiliated Dushu Lake Hospital of Soochow University, Suzhou, China, [2] Department of Rheumatology and Immunology, The Affiliated Dushu Lake Hospital of Soochow University, Suzhou, China, [3] Department of Medicine, Respiratory, Emergency and Intensive Care Medicine, The First Affiliated Hospital of Soochow University, Suzhou, China, [4] Department of Medical Oncology, Sichuan Cancer Hospital, Medical School, University of Electronic Science and Technology of China, Chengdu, China, [5] Department of Thoracic Surgery, Sichuan Cancer Hospital, Medical School, University of Electronic Science and Technology of China, Chengdu, China

***Correspondence:**
Daxiong Zeng
darxzeng@126.com
Junhong Jiang
jiangjunhong1969@suda.edu.cn

[†] These authors have contributed equally to this work

Background: D-dimer is a fibrin-degrading substance that is soluble and whose degradation is produced by plasma protein-mediated degradation of cross-linked fibrin. Previous investigations have shown a link between D-dimer and the mortality in lung cancer patients. However, different investigations varied whether D-dimer could predict prognosis in these patients.

Methods: A meta-analysis and systematic review of all available cohort studies were performed on the link between circulating D-dimer levels and survival of lung cancer patients. Relevant studies were searched in Embase, Cochrane Library, and PubMed databases. Data from 540 lung cancer patients from the First Hospital of Soochow University and Sichuan Cancer Hospital were used for external validation.

Results: We finally obtained 19 eligible cohort studies with pooled HR showing that high D-dimer levels contribute to death in tumor group (HR 1.62, 95% CI: 1.39–1.88, $I^2 = 75.0\%$). Further stratified analysis showed that higher circulating D-dimer in the advanced lung cancer group was linked to a 1.91-fold risk (HR = 2.91, 95% CI: 2.24–3.78, $I^2 = 6.0\%$). Incorporation of other variables, including days of follow-up, country, design, public year, population, disease status, and quality score, into the meta-regression model, indicated that disease status was an additional source of heterogeneity (p <0.001). External validation of 540 patients also showed that high levels of D-dimer showed a higher risk of overall mortality (HR 1.39, 95% CI: 1.13–1.72, $p = 0.002$) and VTE events (HR 3.98, 95% CI: 1.99–8.70, $p = 0.002$) in lung cancer patients.

Conclusions: High circulating plasma D-dimer levels independently predict long-term prognosis and the risk of venous thromboembolism in lung cancer.

Keywords: D-dimer, lung cancer, mortality, meta-analysis, VTE

INTRODUCTION

Malignant tumors of the respiratory system are the most frequently occurring malignancies and the primary cause of mortality in patients over 65 years old (1). Statistically, 1.8 million people are diagnosed with NSCLC or SCLC, while nearly 1.6 million dies of this disease in the world per year (2). The 5-year overall survival of NSCLC is only 17.7%, which is much lower than other cancers (3). Complications of lung cancer, especially coagulation disorders, are needed to be focused on. Previous studies confirmed that coagulation disorders occurred in those patients Incidence of hypercoagulability in malignant tumors often increased, such as venous thrombosis (VTE), disseminated intravascular coagulation (DIC), compared with the patients without cancer (4). Cancer-associated thrombosis predicted poor clinical prognosis and was regarded as the 2nd cause of mortality among patients with tumors (5). Besides, the risk of arterial and venous thromboembolism is significantly increased in patients with tumors. Pulmonary embolism (PE) is one of the most severe complications in those patients, and it is also a significant risk factor of cancer-related mortality worldwide (6, 7).

D-dimer is a fibrin-degrading substance that is soluble and whose degradation is produced by plasma protein-mediated degradation of cross-linked fibrin. It is regarded as a marker of fibrinolysis and coagulation (8). As a sign of hypercoagulability, D-dimer has been clinically used to evaluate the risk of VTE, DVT, and PE (9–11). D-dimer levels raised in patients with hypercoagulability and elevated while inflammation, malignancy, sepsis, recent surgery, trauma, severe burns, chronic kidney failure, and pregnancy (10). Previous research showed that elevated D-dimer levels predict poor prognosis in most types of tumors, such as lung, colorectal, pancreatic, or gastric cancer (4, 5, 12, 13).

However, the link between D-dimer and OS of these patients is still controversial. Several studies have shown that lung cancer cases with elevated levels of D-dimer had a poor prognosis (4, 14, 15). Some other research suggested no clear relationship between D-dimer levels and the prognosis statistically (16). Some studies show that patients with elevated D-dimer have a better prognosis (17, 18). Our ultimate purpose is to figure out the predictive value of D-dimer in these patients and provide better guidance for clinical intervention. We launched a meta-analysis to assess the value of D-dimer levels in patients with lung carcinomas. Data from multi-centers were used for external validation.

METHODS

Patients

We accordingly conducted a cohort study to collect data including 540 NSCLC patients at our medical center and Sichuan Cancer Hospital between February 1, 2014, and March 1, 2016. The deadline for follow-up was December 1, 2021. The diagnosis of lung cancer was regarding pathological diagnostic criteria. Death data were obtained from the hospital registry, and the time of death was confirmed by telephone follow-up or by reviewing electronic medical records. The median follow-up period was 22.3 months. Informed consent was got from the patients themselves or their immediate family members. All research projects conformed to the guidelines of the ethics committees of Soochow University and Sichuan Cancer Hospital and followed the Declaration of Helsinki.

Search Method

Databases from the Cochrane Library Embase and PubMed were categorized and searched from inception to December 31, 2021. The methods used followed the Meta-Analysis of Observational Studies in Epidemiology (MOOSE) and PRISMA guidelines for systematic analysis reporting statements (19). **Supplementary Material** shows data extraction, selection criteria, PRISMA checklist, search terms, and quality evaluation.

Selection Strategy

The inclusion criteria for this meta-analysis and systematic review were as follows. (1) the subjects were human; (2) the data contained plasma or serum D-dimer levels; (3) death was shown as the primary endpoint and VTE events as a secondary endpoint; and (4) confidence intervals (CI) and hazard ratios (HRs) were obtained between D-dimer levels and patient death. We excluded case reports, animal studies, studies that provided insufficient data, or narrative reviews. Three independent reviewers performed literature reviews and database searches. A senior researcher consulted to resolve the above issues in case of disputes.

Data Collection

For each potential inclusion, the first author's last country of origin, name, year of publication, gender, sample size, study design, age, serum or plasma D-dimer, adjustment variables, follow-up period, disease outcome, and their corresponding 95% CI and disease status were extracted. The primary endpoint analyzed in the meta-analysis was patient death. Three reviewers also performed data extraction, and senior investigator input was sought when disputes were encountered.

Quality Assessment

We tested the risk of bias of the selected projects according to the Newcastle-Ottawa scale (20), including identifying exposure or outcome and group comparability. The GRADE scoring system analyzed the quality of evidence from the included studies in Grade Pro 4.05, and the relevant results are shown in **Supplementary Table 1**. Three reviewers independently assessed this process.

Statistical Analysis

We analyzed the correlation of different levels of plasma D-dimer with patient death endpoints by confidence intervals and HR. We referred to various literature's original definitions as the quartiles of baseline plasma D-dimer. Cochran's Q test, I^2 statistic, and P-value were used to assess the overall heterogeneity

Abbreviations: NSCLC, non-small-cell lung cancer; NALC, non-advanced lung cancer; ALC, advanced lung cancer; PCS, prospective cohort study; LC, lung cancer; IA, immunoturbidimetric assay; ELISA, enzyme-linked immunosorbent assay; SCLC, small cell lung cancer; RS, retrospective study; RCT, randomized controlled trial, HR, hazard ratio.

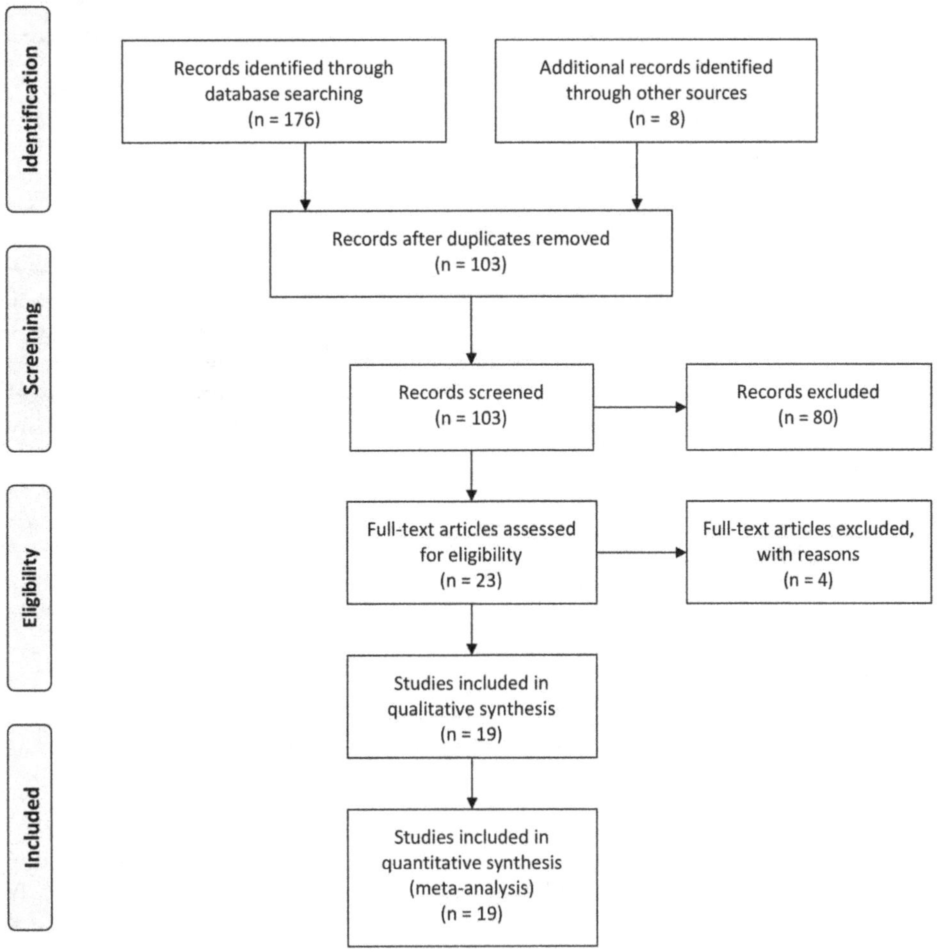

FIGURE 1 | Flow chart of projects' selection designed by PRISMA.

of the included studies. The merging process used a random-effects model for groups with several studies less than or equal to 5 in the subgroup analysis. In contrast, both random-effects models and fixed effects were used to calculate pooled HR or OR when heterogeneity was zero. A fixed-effects model was used. We further investigate the issue of the source of heterogeneity through stratified analysis. Our study also analyzed meta-regression models consistent with standard variables (including grade score, design, country, sample, days of follow-up, public years, clinical adherence, population, and adjusted covariates) to analyze heterogeneity similarly. We examined the effect of individual studies on overall heterogeneity by sensitivity analysis. We similarly analyzed funnel plot asymmetries to analyze publication and selective reporting bias. We also performed linear regression analysis by Egger and Begg to determine the statistical significance of the included studies when combined (21). Fill and trim methods were used to identify the number of additional items needed to provide adjusted effects and overcome potential biases. The mean $\pm$ standard deviation was presented as customarily distributed data, and the median and the IQR were presented as skewed data. Unpaired t-tests and Mann-Whitney U tests were used for comparison. Categorical variables were tested using the κ^2-test and shown as percentages. Survival analysis was presented by Kaplan-Meier curves and analyzed using the log-rank test. Cox regression models examined multivariate and univariate survival analyses of overall survival (OS). Forest plots demonstrated the significance of the multifactorial analysis variables on prognosis. All statistical analyses were performed with RStudio (R version 4.0.2). Bilateral $P < 0.05$ were regarded as statistically significant.

RESULT

Literature Selection

We retrieved 176 records from Cochrane Library, Embase, and PubMed databases. Seventy-three of these records were duplicates, and for the remaining 103 records, we made further checks of the abstracts and titles. Of these records, 13 were not clinical studies, and 67 were unrelated to the subject. After the full-text screening of the final 23 records and removing the four

TABLE 1 | Characteristics of included studies.

Authors	Year	Country	Population	Stage	Follow-up months	Subjects	male(%)	Age	Assay	sample	Design	Quality score
Fan, S.	2019	China	SCLC	NALC	60	82	81.7	60 (28–82)	IA	Plssma	RS	3
Minglei, Y.	2019	China	NSCLC	NALC	24	376	60.6	58 (27–81)	IA	Plssma	RCT	8
Hou, C.	2019	China	NSCLC	NALC	13.2	395	60.0	61 (35–81)	IA	Plssma	PCS	6
Huagang, L.	2019	China	NSCLC	NALC	42	456	69.7	65 (56–69)	IA	Plssma	RS	4
Edyta I. W.	2018	Poland	LC	ALC	30	95	75.0	67 (40–81)	IA	Plssma	PCS	6
Cuicui, Z.	2018	China	SCLC	NALC	60	160	80.6	59 (23–83)	IA	Plssma	RS	3
Wenwen, S.	2017	China	NSCLC	ALC	56	785	60.0	≥65 (41.6%)	IA	Plssma	PCS	5
Kaoru, S.	2017	Japan	NSCLC	ALC	60	237	59.1	69 ± 9.7	IA	Plssma	PCS	7
Zhu, L.-R.	2016	China	SCLC	NALC	60	74	77.0	57 (42–80)	IA	Plssma	PCS	6
Magdalena, Z.	2016	Poland	NSCLC	NALC	11.5	52	38.5	63 (58–70)	IA	Plssma	PCS	7
Koichi, F.	2015	Japan	NSCLC	ALC	60	247	61.5	69 (31–85)	IA	Plssma	PCS	6
Yuezhen, W.	2015	China	NSCLC	NALC	60	1931	70.0	≥65 (39.9%)	ELISA	Plssma	RS	5
Tuba, I.	2015	Turkey	LC	ALC	60	72	77.8	≥60 (37.5%)	IA	Plasma	PCS	6
Ge, L.-P.	2014	China	NSCLC	NALC	36	82	67.0	64 (44–72)	IA	Plasma	PCS	6
Heguo, J.	2014	China	NSCLC	ALC	36	184	45.2	≥60 (34.1%)	IA	Plasma	PCS	5
Zhang, P.-P.	2013	China	NSCLC	NALC	60	232	64.2	61 (30–86)	IA	Plasma	PCS	6
Cihan, A.	2012	Austria	LC	NALC	24	182	56.5	62 (52–68)	IA	Plasma	PCS	7
Katsuhiro, M.	2011	Japan	NSCLC	NALC	60	99	71.8	72 (35–88)	ELISA	Plasma	PCS	6
Altiay, G.	2007	Turkey	LC	ALC	78	78	93.6	61 (37–82)	ELISA	Plasma	PCS	7

SCLC, small cell lung cancer; NSCLC, non-small-cell lung cancer; LC, lung cancer; NALC, non-advanced lung cancer; ALC, advanced lung cancer; IA, immunoturbidimetric assay; ELISA, enzyme-linked immunosorbent assay; RS, retrospecitive study; PCS, prospective cohort study; RCT, randomized controlled trial.

studies that could not extract data (Three lacked data from D-dimer-related HRs, and one other primary source was children), we obtained 19 studies for final analysis. We show a flow chart of the projects' selection process in **Figure 1**.

Study Baseline Data

The baseline information of the 19 projects published from 2007 to 2019 is displayed in **Table 1**. Eleven were launched in China (9, 14–18, 22–26), while others were performed in Poland (27, 28), Japan (4, 29, 30), Austria (31) and Turkey (13, 32), respectively. The follow-up time for these programs ranged from 11.5 to 60 months. Adjusted covariates of different studies are shown in **Supplementary Table 2**. Overall, the sample sizes of the project cohorts ranged from 52 to 1931, with a final sample size of 5,819 included in the meta-analysis. The study endpoint for all these projects was patient death. All included projects were ranked according to study quality, with projects scoring between 5 and 8 on the Newcastle-Ottawa Scale (NOS).

D-Dimer and Mortality

The 19 projects we included, with an overall sample size of 5,819, were all studies that addressed the association between circulating blood D-dimer and the risk of death in patients with lung cancer (4, 9, 13–15, 22–32). Meta-analysis results from these 19 studies demonstrated that elevated circulating blood D-dimer levels were linked to an increased risk of death in patients with lung cancer (random-effects model. HR 1.62, 95% CI: 1.39–1.88; fixed-effects model. HR 1.31, 95% CI: 1.24–1.37). However, substantial heterogeneity remained between the different items included ($I^2 = 75.0\%$, $p < 0.01$; **Figure 2**). To analyze the sources of heterogeneity, we performed subgroup analyses to assess the effect of sample, country, design, population, public year, days of follow-up, disease status, and quality score on heterogeneity. The results showed that subgrouping by this classification resulted in the highest level of I^2 decline in non-advanced lung cancer (HR = 1.29, 95% CI: 1.15–1.44, $I^2 = 58.0\%$) and advanced lung cancer (HR = 2.91, 95% CI: 2.24–3.78, $I^2 = 6.0\%$), indicating that this is likely the main source of heterogeneity (**Figure 2**). Studies of patients with either SCLC or NSCLC showed that high D-dimer levels increased the risk of death in patients with lung cancer (SCLC: HR = 1.86, 95% CI: 1.33–2.61, $I^2 = 85.0\%$; NSCLC: HR = 1.60, 95% CI: 1.33–1.92, $I^2 = 65.0\%$; **Table 2**). The number of studies in most subgroups was less than 5, so we used fixed-effects models to calculate pooled HRs (RS: HR = 1.21, 95% CI: 0.96–1.53; PCS: OR = 1.93, 95% CI: 1.57–2.37). In addition, the pooled HR (HR = 2.22, 95% CI: 1.58–3.13) was not statistically significant in the group from other countries than China, while the study from China showed a 44% risk of death in patients with increased D-dimer (HR = 1.44, 95% CI: 1.19–1.75). Analysis of other subgroups showed that the risk of death varied with the duration of follow-up (follow-up <60 months. HR = 1.52, 95% CI: 1.26–1.83, $I^2 = 64.0\%$; follow-up ≥60 months. HR = 1.89, 95% CI: 1.42–2.51, $I^2 = 82.0\%$). In addition, the association between plasma D-dimer and death persisted after inclusion in the new study, as can be shown by data from meta-regression ($P = 0.794$). The

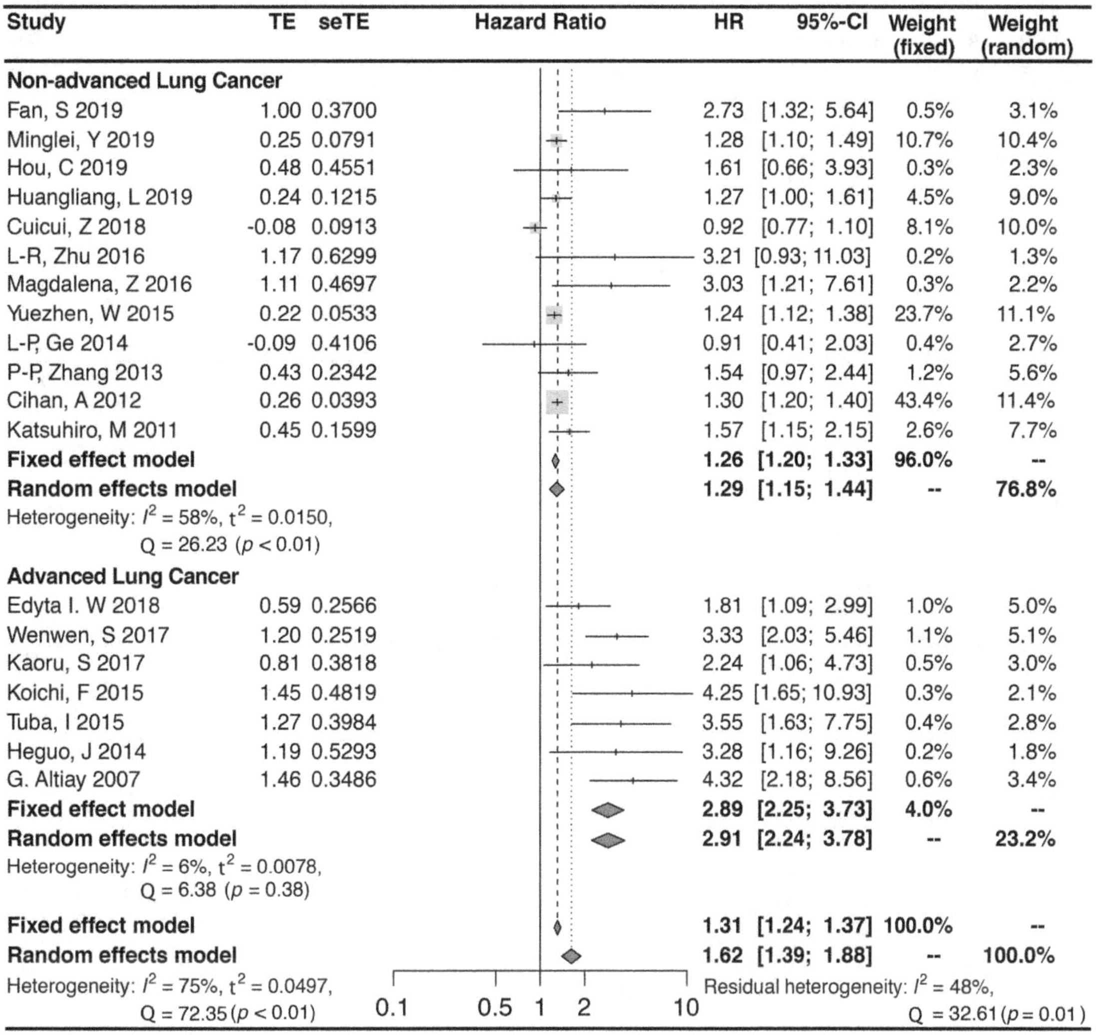

FIGURE 2 | Forest plot (Fixed and random-effects model) for the link between plasma D-dimer levels (highest *vs.* lowest category) and lung cancer-associated mortality. Subgroup analysis is grouped by disease states (non-advanced lung cancer and advanced lung cancer).

inclusion of other variables, including the year of disclosure, country, days of follow-up, population, quality score, disease status, and design in the meta-regression model, showed that disease status was likely the main source of heterogeneity (P <0.001; **Table 2**). Data from sensitivity analyses showed that individual studies had little effect on overall heterogeneity (**Supplementary Figure 1**).

The data from the funnel plot showed an asymmetry, indicating that publication bias still exists (**Figure 3A**). Application of the fill and trim model suggested that the inclusion of three new items may eliminate publication bias (**Figure 3B**). The results of the regression analysis using Begg's (p = 0.036) and Egger's (p = 0.002) regressions showed the presence of publication bias (**Supplementary Figure 2**). In addition to this, NOS and standard "risk of bias" tools were used to assess bias (**Table 1**, **Supplementary Figures 3A,B** and **Supplementary Table 3**).

External Validation

Five hundred forty patients with lung cancer were included in this project. The median age was 64 (58, 70). Of these, 165 (31.0%) were female and 375 (69.0%) were male. The mean BMI level was 22.64 ± 3.16. 169 (31.0%) cases were squamous carcinomas, and 346 (64.0%) were adenocarcinomas. Smokers accounted for 52.0% of the included population, with 279 cases (**Table 3**). Kaplan-Meier curves showed that patients with increased levels of VTE events (**Figure 4A**) or D-dimers (**Figure 4B**) had a poor prognosis in patients with NSCLC. We chose the median D-dimer of 6.53 as the cut-off value. To explore the effect of D-dimer on long-term prognosis and VTE events in NSCLC patients, we performed a univariate analysis of potential factors. The data showed that stage, D-dimer, hyperlipidemia, type of pathology, KPS score, smoking, gender, VTE events, and age were risk factors for death, whereas ACS, D-dimer, and stage were risk factors for VTE events (**Table 4**). Based on the statistical

TABLE 2 | Stratified analysis of pooled hazard ratio risks of D-dimer in LC patients.

Stratified analysis	Pooled HR (95% CI)	Heterogenety	Meta regression (*P*-value)
Public year			0.794
After 2015	1.70 [1.38–2.10]	Q = 54.51, $P < 0.01$, $I^2 = 78.0\%$	
Before 2015	1.67 (1.22–2.29)	Q = 16.95, $P < 0.01$, $I^2 = 71.0\%$	
Country			0.121
China	1.44 [1.19–1.75]	Q = 38.22, $P < 0.01$, $I^2 = 74.0\%$	
Non-China	2.22 [1.58–3.13]	Q = 30.27, $P < 0.01$, $I^2 = 77.0\%$	
Population			0.683
SCLC	1.86 [1.33–2.61]	Q = 40.12, $P < 0.01$, $I^2 = 85.0\%$	
NSCLC	1.60 [1.33–1.92]	Q = 31.52, $P < 0.01$, $I^2 = 65.0\%$	
Follow-up months			0.519
≥60 months	1.89 [1.42–2.51]	Q = 49.03, $P < 0.01$, $I^2 = 82.0\%$	
<60 months	1.52 [1.26–1.83]	Q = 22.44, $P < 0.01$, $I^2 = 64.0\%$	
Design			0.074
RS	1.21 [0.96–1.53]	Q = 13.8, $P < 0.01$, $I^2 = 78.0\%$	
PCS	1.93 [1.57–2.37]	Q = 49.21, $P < 0.01$, $I^2 = 72.0\%$	
Quality Score			0.537
<6	1.55 [1.15–2.09]	Q = 33.88, $P < 0.01$, $I^2 = 85.0\%$	
≥6	1.74 [1.43–2.12]	Q = 34.18, $P < 0.01$, $I^2 = 65.0\%$	
Stage			<0.001
NALC	1.29 [1.15–1.44]	Q = 26.23, $P < 0.01$, $I^2 = 58.0\%$	
ALC	2.91 [2.24–3.78]	Q = 6.38, $P = 0.38$, $I^2 = 6.0\%$	

SCLC, small cell lung cancer; NSCLC, non-small-cell lung cancer; LC, lung cancer; NALC, non-advanced lung cancer; ALC, advanced lung cancer; RS, retrospecitive study; PCS, prospective cohort study; HR, hazard ratio.

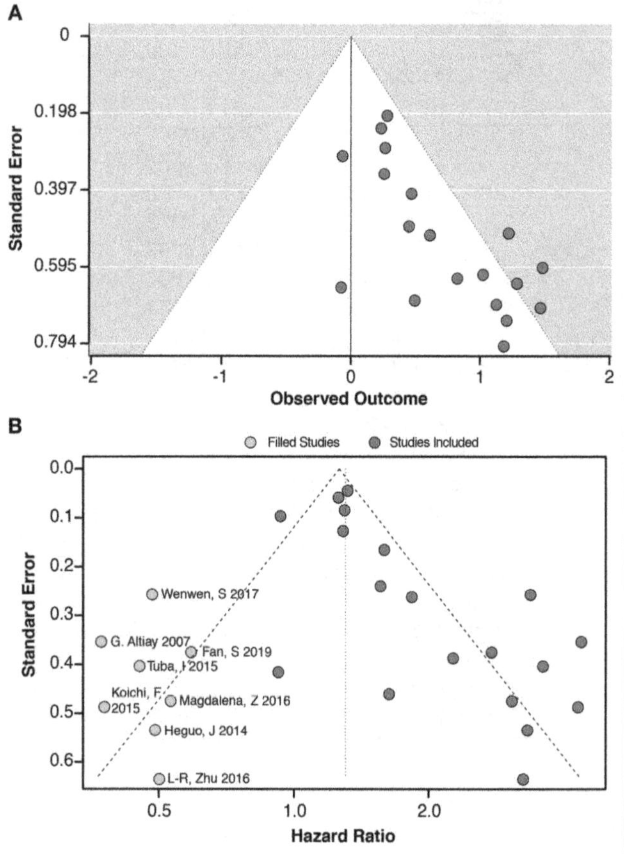

FIGURE 3 | (A) Funnel plot for the link between plasma D-dimer levels (highest *vs.* lowest category) and lung cancer-associated mortality. **(B)** Filled funnel plot and meta trim-and-fill model. The blue dots indicate that these included studies require a corresponding study for correction, thus reducing bias.

results and clinical experience, we included factors with potential predictive value in the multifactorial analysis. The results showed that mortality (HR 1.39, 95% CI: 1.13–1.72, $p = 0.002$; **Figure 5A**) and VTE events (HR 3.98, 95% CI: 1.99–8.70, $p = 0.002$) in patients with high D-dimer levels (**Figure 5B**).

DISCUSSION

In this project, by pooling 19 cohort studies on D-dimer and lung cancer involving a total of 5819 patients, we found that high circulating plasma D-dimer levels were associated with the risk of death in lung cancer patients. And external validation not only demonstrated the above correlation and found that its elevated levels were equally related to the occurrence of long-term VTE events. During the analysis, we detected significant heterogeneity, and further subgroup analysis revealed that disease status might be the primary source of heterogeneity ($p < 0.001$). Characteristics such as days of follow-up, country, public year, design, quality score, and population were not strongly correlated for the association of plasma D-dimer with the endpoint event of death in lung cancer patients. The above data suggest that lung cancer patients with higher plasma D-dimer have a poor long-term prognosis.

D-dimer is regarded as a biomarker of intravascular fibrin degradation and formation (33). It is also a biomarker of the activation of coagulation (34). Previous studies showed that the production of D-dimer might be stimulated by hypercoagulability, such as cancer, chronic inflammation, aging, as well as atrial fibrillation (35).

D-dimers are produced during the generation of fibrin monomers in fibrinogen, which consists of two peripheral D-structural domains and E-structural domain linkage centers. The fibrin network is formed. After conversion, the D-domain is cross-linked by factor XIII, strengthening the fibrin network. Thrombin bound to fibrin is degraded from the

TABLE 3 | Study Participant Characteristics at Enrollment.

Variables	Total (n = 540)	Cohort, median (IQR)		p-value
		D-dimer ≤ 6.53 (n = 270)	D-dimer > 6.53 (n = 270)	
Baseline data				
Age, Median (Q1,Q3)	64 (58, 70)	63 (58, 69)	64 (59, 70)	0.144
Gender, n (%)				0.575
female	165 (31)	79 (29)	86 (32)	
male	375 (69)	191 (71)	184 (68)	
BMI, Mean ± SD	22.64 ± 3.16	22.62 ± 3.23	22.66 ± 3.1	0.881
Pathological type, n (%)				0.089
Adenocarcinoma	346 (64)	161 (60)	185 (69)	
Mixed lung cancer	25 (5)	13 (5)	12 (4)	
Squamous carcinoma	169 (31)	96 (36)	73 (27)	
Stage				0.269
I	88 (16)	52 (19)	36 (13)	
II	59 (11)	30 (11)	29 (11)	
III	103 (19)	47 (17)	56 (21)	
IV	290 (54)	141 (52)	149 (55)	
Smoking, n (%)				0.605
No	261 (48)	127 (47)	134 (50)	
Yes	279 (52)	143 (53)	136 (50)	
KPS, Median (Q1,Q3)	90 (80, 90)	90 (80, 90)	90 (80, 90)	0.133
D-dimer, Median (Q1,Q3) (U/L)	6.53 (3.94, 8.48)	3.93 (2.85, 5.42)	8.49 (7.4, 10.34)	<0.001
Complications				
Hypertension, n (%)				0.037
No	366 (62)	49 (53)	47 (76)	
Yes	224 (38)	44 (47)	15 (24)	
Diabetes, n (%)				0.323
No	533 (90)	82 (88)	57 (92)	
Yes	57 (10)	11 (12)	5 (8)	
Hyperlipidemia, n (%)				0.024
No	538 (91)	88 (95)	57 (92)	
Yes	52 (9)	5 (5)	5 (8)	
Heart.failure, n (%)				0.111
No	579 (98)	89 (96)	61 (98)	
Yes	11 (2)	4 (4)	1 (2)	
ACS, n (%)				0.813
No	575 (97)	90 (97)	60 (97)	
Yes	15 (3)	3 (3)	2 (3)	
Outcomes				
Status, n (%)				<0.001
alive	174 (29)	43 (46)	23 (37)	
dead	416 (71)	50 (54)	39 (63)	
Overall survival time, Median (Q1,Q3)	24.17 (9.9, 50.99)	38.9 (12.87, 59.8)	18.05 (7.53, 50.99)	0.012
VTE events				<0.001
	494 (91)	260 (96)	234 (87)	
	46 (9)	10 (4)	36 (13)	

IQR, interquartile range; BMI, Body Mass Index; KPS, Karnofsky Performance Status; AQI, air quality index; ACS, Acute Coronary Syndromes; VTE, venous thromboembolism.

fibrin network to soluble fragments. Thereby D dimers are produced. Thus, D-dimer in peripheral blood reflects the degree of fibrinolysis and coagulation and is elevated during thrombosis (34).

The process of coagulation is the conversion of blood from a liquid to a gel, which then forms a blood clot. Recent investigations suggested that patients with lung cancer showed disorders in activating both fibrinolysis and coagulation. Over

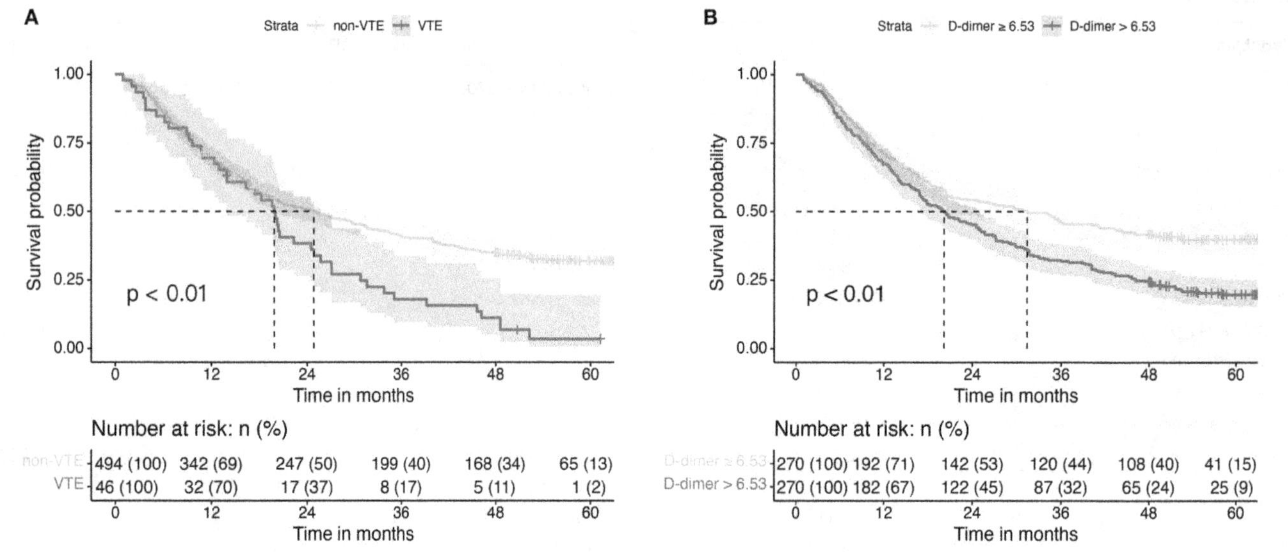

FIGURE 4 | Kaplan-Meier curves for NSCLC patients with different factors. **(A)** Kaplan-Meier curves for OS in patients in the VTE and non-VTE groups. **(B)** Kaplan-Meier curves for OS in different D-dimer levels.

TABLE 4 | Univariate regression analysis on NSCLC patients for different endpoints.

Variants	OS		VTE events	
	HR	*p*-value	OR	*p*-value
VTE events, yes vs. no	1.72 [1.25, 2.36]	0.001	-	-
Age (year), >65 vs. ≤65	1.39 [1.13, 1.70]	0.002	0.79 [0.42, 1.47]	0.466
Gender, male vs. female	1.45 [1.15, 1.82]	0.001	1.27 [0.66, 2.62]	0.492
Pathological type, adenocarcinoma vs. others	0.80 [0.65, 0.99]	0.036	1.06 [0.57, 2.03]	0.866
Stage III or IV, yes vs. no	1.32 [1.04, 1.68]	0.024	2.66 [1.19, 7.12]	0.029
Smoking, yes vs. no	1.23 [1.00, 1.51]	0.045	1.24 [0.68, 2.30]	0.491
KPS score, <90, vs. >90	2.34 [1.91, 2.88]	<0.001	1.45 [0.79, 2.67]	0.228
D-dimer, >6.53 vs. ≤6.53	1.51 [1.23, 1.85]	<0.001	4.00 [2.01, 8.68]	<0.001
Hypertension, yes vs. no	1.04 [0.84, 1.27]	0.743	1.17 [0.62, 2.14]	0.626
Diabetes, yes vs. no	1.10 [0.78, 1.54]	0.591	-	-
Hyperlipidemia, yes vs. no	0.66 [0.45, 0.98]	0.037	1.08 [0.31, 2.85]	0.887
Heart failure, yes vs. no	1.25 [0.59, 2.63]	0.563	1.20 [0.06, 6.59]	0.866
ACS, yes vs. no	1.45 [0.77, 2.72]	0.245	3.06 [0.67, 10.26]	0.095
BMI, >24 vs. ≤24	0.94 [0.75, 1.17]	0.554	0.81 [0.39, 1.57]	0.545

IQR, interquartile range; BMI, Body Mass Index; KPS, Karnofsky Performance Status; AQI, air quality index; ACS, Acute Coronary Syndromes.

the past few years, many studies explored the mechanism of hypercoagulability and thrombogenesis in tumor status. Cancer cells cause coagulation relying on their apparent procoagulant activity to activate the coagulation system and deposit fibrin (36). Meanwhile, cancer cells could induce hypercoagulable status by secreting procoagulant factors, circulating microparticles, enhancing endothelial function, and altering platelet activity (37).

Moreover, some chemotherapeutics, especially platinum compounds, have been reported to increase the risk of thrombosis (7). Recent investigations have found that regulating hemostatic protein expression depends on oncogenes. The tumor-derived tissue factor-positive microparticles play a critical role in thrombosis (38). There is evidence that membrane vesicles of tumor cells can activate the coagulation system. In contrast, microvesicles (MV) released from the membranes of apoptotic cells can stimulate coagulation via negatively charged membrane phospholipids or tissue factors (TF). Several types of cancer cells can release MV-derived TF *in vitro*, but the function of cancer cells *in vivo* still needs to be further explored (39, 40).

The incidence of thrombosis in patients is increased. In addition, the initiation of the hemostatic system affects every stage of the tumor (14). Tumors can activate coagulation factors and induce a procoagulant state, promoting tumor invasion, angiogenesis, growth, and metastasis (41, 42). Deposition of fibrin in lung cancer tissues may promote the generation of new blood vessels and the proliferation of cancer cells. These deposits could protect the tumor cells against chemotherapy drugs and immune elimination (43, 44). Besides, tumor cells

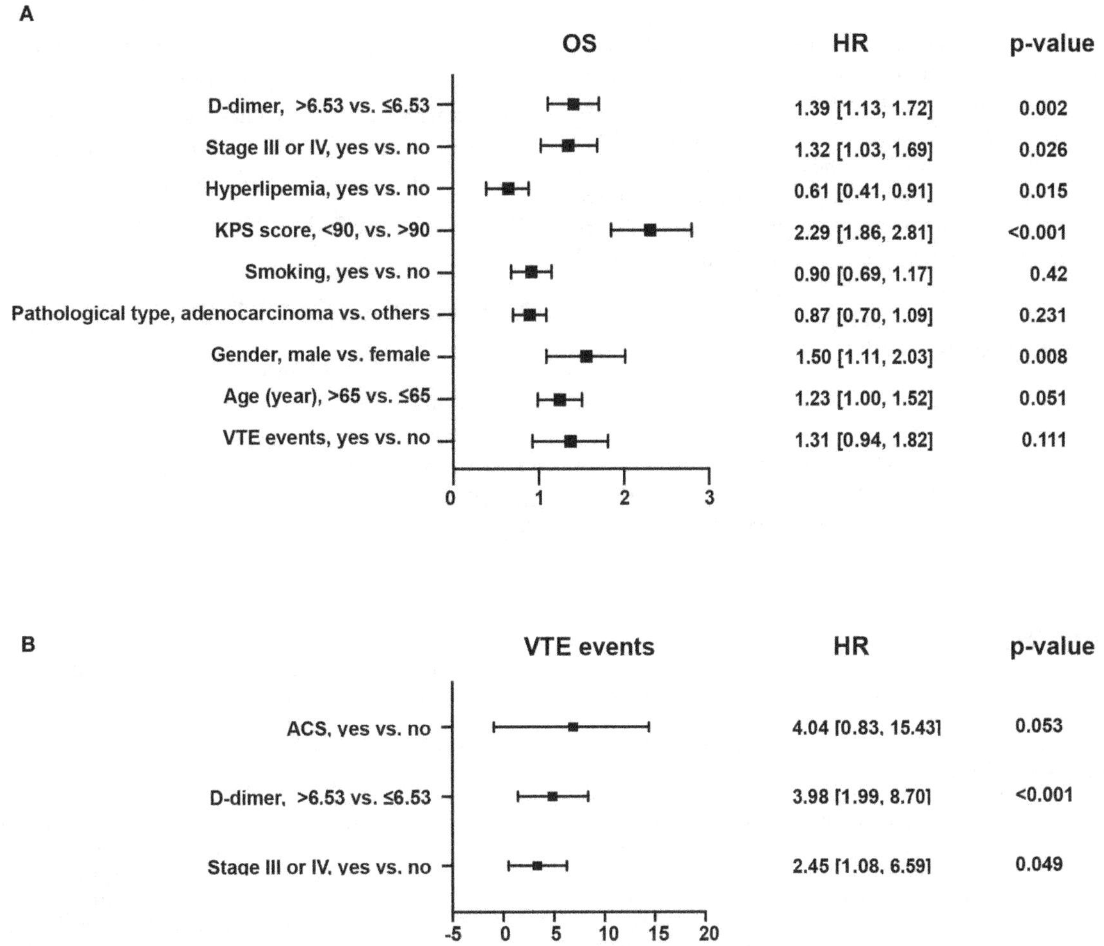

FIGURE 5 | Forest plot for multifactorial analysis of different endpoints in patients with NSCLC. **(A)** Forest plot for multifactor analysis of the risk of overall mortality. **(B)** Forest plot for multifactor analysis of the risk of VTE events.

may cause intravascular clotting when entering the blood and promoting metastasis (45). Osamu T et al. reported that circulating biomarkers of the fibrinolysis system play a significant role in response to chemotherapy, tumor burden, and clinical progression in lung cancer (46). Previous studies have shown that a history of hyperlipidemia and serum D-dimer can together predict the probability of stroke events in oncology patients, and this may also be promising for lung cancer patients (47).

VTE is a recognized complication of cancer, and the incidence of VTE in cancer patients is more than four times that of normal controls. d-dimer has been used as a predictor of VTE in lung cancer patients, so we hypothesized that it could also be used as a biomarker for lung cancer (48). Cancer patients have a high risk of developing VTE, which leads to severe consequences that cover the need for long-term anticoagulant therapy (49). The risk of VTE is further increased by chemotherapeutic or immunomodulatory drugs (50). Besides venous thrombosis, arterial thrombosis is also a common complication of lung cancer and predicts a poor prognosis in common cancers (7, 51). Also, DIC further complicates the spectrum of hemostatic complications in malignancy, which is fatal (41).

However, among the papers we analyzed in this meta-analysis, two studies showed an increased D-dimer predicts a good prognosis (17, 18). Moreover, these two studies were also a source of heterogeneity. The study conducted by Zhang et al. (17) collected the plasma before chemotherapy for D-dimer detection. It may be responsible for the negative result of the link between D-dimer and the prognosis. In another investigation by Ge et al. (18), they only compared the patients in the B0 stage, so their result also displayed a negative link between D-dimer and mortality of patients with lung cancer.

LIMITATIONS AND STRENGTH

We found the prognostic, predictive value of D-dimer in different pathological types of lung cancer by meta-analysis. Few previous studies have meta-analyses showing the correlation between D-dimer and lung cancer mortality endpoints. Our study included only prospective cohorts and followed MOOSE and PRISMA guidelines. Sources of heterogeneity were analyzed using different pathways, including subgroup analysis, meta-regression, and padding and trimming methods were used to explore the publication bias.

However, our study has limitations. First, not all study items were included because data could not be extracted for some studies, which may raise the risk of bias. Most of the studies we included were of NSCLC patients and the number of SCLC patients was small, so there will be some bias. Future prospective studies are needed for relevant validation. In addition, there was considerable bias in the underlying clinical characteristics of each program, including race, sex, and age in the individual studies. Therefore, whether increased D-dimer is associated with the occurrence of lung cancer mortality endpoints requires a large sample size of clinical trials to verify.

CONCLUSION

Elevated circulating D-dimer levels correlate with the endpoint of death and VTE development in lung cancer patients. However, large sample size clinical trials are still needed in the future to validate this argument.

AUTHOR CONTRIBUTIONS

JL and SY designed and performed research studies, analyzed the data, and wrote the manuscript. XZ, MX, CZ, LG, CY, and XW performed research studies and analyzed data. SC, DZ, and JJ contributed to the research design, data analysis, manuscript writing, and study supervision. All authors contributed to the article and approved the submitted version.

ACKNOWLEDGMENTS

Thanks to Dr. Linya Qiu of Gusu District Center for Disease Control and Prevention, Soochow for her critical reading and comments. She was not compensated for this assistance. The Department of Medicine supported Respiratory, Emergency, and Intensive Care Medicine, The Affiliated Dushu Lake Hospital of Soochow University.

REFERENCES

1. Siegel RL, Miller KD, Jemal A. Cancer statistics, 2019. *CA Cancer J Clin.* (2019) 69:7–34. doi: 10.3322/caac.21551
2. Hirsch FR, Scagliotti GV, Mulshine JL, Kwon R, Curran WJ, Jr., et al. Lung cancer: current therapies and new targeted treatments. *Lancet.* (2017) 389:299–311. doi: 10.1016/S0140-6736(16)30958-8
3. Vachani A, Sequist LV, Spira A. AJRCCM: 100-year anniversary. The shifting landscape for lung cancer: past, present, and future. *Am J Respir Crit Care Med.* (2017) 195:1150–60. doi: 10.1164/rccm.201702-0433CI
4. Fukumoto K, Taniguchi T, Usami N, Kawaguchi K, Fukui T, Ishiguro F, et al. Preoperative plasma D-dimer level is an independent prognostic factor in patients with completely resected non-small cell lung cancer. *Surg Today.* (2015) 45:63–7. doi: 10.1007/s00595-014-0894-4
5. Demers M, Krause DS, Schatzberg D, Martinod K, Voorhees JR, Fuchs TA, et al. Cancers predispose neutrophils to release extracellular DNA traps that contribute to cancer-associated thrombosis. *Proc Natl Acad Sci U S A.* (2012) 109:13076–81. doi: 10.1073/pnas.1200419109
6. Xiong W, Zhao Y, Xu M, Guo J, Pudasaini B, Wu X, et al. The relationship between tumor markers and pulmonary embolism in lung cancer. *Oncotarget.* (2017) 8:41412–21. doi: 10.18632/oncotarget.17916
7. Navi BB, Reiner AS, Kamel H, Iadecola C, Okin PM, Elkind MSV, et al. Risk of arterial thromboembolism in patients with cancer. *J Am Coll Cardiol.* (2017) 70:926–38. doi: 10.1016/j.jacc.2017.06.047
8. Favresse J, Lippi G, Roy PM, Chatelain B, Jacqmin H, Ten Cate H, et al. D-dimer: Preanalytical, analytical, postanalytical variables, and clinical applications. *Crit Rev Clin Lab Sci.* (2018) 55:548–77. doi: 10.1080/10408363.2018.1529734
9. Liang HG, Gao K, Jia R, Li J, Wang C. Prognostic significance of the combination of preoperative fibrinogen and the neutrophil-lymphocyte ratio in patients with non-small cell lung cancer following surgical resection. *Oncol Lett.* (2019) 17:1435–44. doi: 10.3892/ol.2018.9760
10. Kruger PC, Eikelboom JW, Douketis JD, Hankey GJ. Deep vein thrombosis: update on diagnosis and management. *Med J Aust.* (2019) 210:516–24. doi: 10.5694/mja2.50201
11. Pabinger I, Thaler J, Ay C. Biomarkers for prediction of venous thromboembolism in cancer. *Blood.* (2013) 122:2011–8. doi: 10.1182/blood-2013-04-460147
12. Liu L, Zhang X, Yan B, Gu Q, Zhang X, Jiao J, et al. Elevated plasma D-dimer levels correlate with long term survival of gastric cancer patients. *PLoS ONE.* (2014) 9:e90547. doi: 10.1371/journal.pone.0090547
13. Altiay G, Ciftci A, Demir M, Kocak Z, Sut N, Tabakoglu E, et al. High plasma D-dimer level is associated with decreased survival in patients with lung cancer. *Clin Oncol (R Coll Radiol).* (2007) 19:494–498. doi: 10.1016/j.clon.2007.04.002
14. Fan S, Zhao G, An G. High pretreatment plasma D-dimer levels are associated with shorter overall survival in patients with small cell lung cancer. *J Int Med Res.* (2019) 47:215–24. doi: 10.1177/0300060518799869
15. Sun WW, Hu JA, Niu WQ, Gao BL, Xu ZH. Significance of NLDA, the commixed index of inflammation, immune responses, hemostasis, and nutrition, for predicting metastatic non-small cell lung cancer prognosis and metastases. *Oncotarget.* (2017) 8:81978–93. doi: 10.18632/oncotarget.18184
16. Hou C, Jiang F, Ma H, Zhu Q, Wang Z, Zhao B, et al. Prognostic role of preoperative platelet, fibrinogen, and D-dimer levels in patients with non-small cell lung cancer: a multicenter prospective study. *Thorac Cancer.* (2019) 10:304–11. doi: 10.1111/1759-7714.12956
17. Zhang C, Jia Y, Jia Y, Zhang X, Li K. Prognostic and predictive value of plasma D-dimer levels in patients with small-cell lung cancer. *Int J Clin Oncol.* (2018) 23:1070–5. doi: 10.1007/s10147-018-1320-5
18. Ge LP, Li J, Bao QL, Chen P, Jiang Q, Zhu LR. Prognostic and predictive value of plasma D-dimer in advanced non-small cell lung cancer patients undergoing first-line chemotherapy. *Clin Transl Oncol.* (2015) 17:57–64. doi: 10.1007/s12094-014-1198-2
19. Stroup DF, Berlin JA, Morton SC, Olkin I, Williamson GD, Rennie D, et al. Meta-analysis of observational studies in epidemiology: a proposal for reporting. Meta-analysis of observational studies in epidemiology (MOOSE) group. *JAMA.* (2000) 283:2008–12. doi: 10.1001/jama.283.15.2008
20. Stang A. Critical evaluation of the Newcastle-Ottawa scale for the assessment of the quality of nonrandomized studies in meta-analyses. *Eur J Epidemiol.* (2010) 25:603–5. doi: 10.1007/s10654-010-9491-z
21. Chaimani A, Mavridis D, Salanti G. A hands-on practical tutorial on performing meta-analysis with Stata. *Evid Based Ment Health.* (2014) 17:111–6. doi: 10.1136/eb-2014-101967
22. Jiang HG, Li J, Shi SB, Chen P, Ge LP, Jiang Q, et al. Value of fibrinogen and D-dimer in predicting recurrence and metastasis after radical surgery for non-small cell lung cancer. *Med Oncol.* (2014) 31:22. doi: 10.1007/s12032-014-0022-8
23. Wang Y, Wang Z. Predictive value of plasma D-dimer levels in patients with advanced non-small-cell lung cancer. *Onco Targets Ther.* (2015) 8:805–8. doi: 10.2147/OTT.S78154
24. Yang M, Xu W, Liu T, Yang X, Wang P, Wu S, et al. Development and validation of a novel survival prediction model in patients with spinal

metastasis from non-small cell lung cancer. *Spine (Phila Pa 1976).* (2019) 44:246–57. doi: 10.1097/BRS.0000000000002816
25. Zhang PP, Sun JW, Wang XY, Liu XM, Li K. Preoperative plasma D-dimer levels predict survival in patients with operable non-small cell lung cancer independently of venous thromboembolism. *Eur J Surg Oncol.* (2013) 39:951–6. doi: 10.1016/j.ejso.2013.06.008
26. Zhu LR, Li J, Chen P, Jiang Q, Tang XP. Clinical significance of plasma fibrinogen and D-dimer in predicting the chemotherapy efficacy and prognosis for small cell lung cancer patients. *Clin Transl Oncol.* (2016) 18:178–88. doi: 10.1007/s12094-015-1350-7
27. Zaborowska-Szmit M, Kowalski DM, Piorek A, Krzakowski M, Szmit S. A decrease in D-dimer concentration and an occurrence of skin rash as iatrogenic events and complementary predictors of survival in lung cancer patients treated with EGFR tyrosine kinase inhibitors. *Pharmacol Rep.* (2016) 68:1140–8. doi: 10.1016/j.pharep.2016.07.003
28. Wolny-Rokicka EI, Wydmanski J, Tukiendorf A, Mroz P, Zembron-Lacny A. Appraisal of basic-hemostatic markers in lung cancer patients during follow-up care after radiotherapy treatment. *Med Sci Monit.* (2018) 24:8577–82. doi: 10.12659/MSM.910280
29. Masago K, Fujita S, Mio T, Togashi Y, Kim YH, Hatachi Y, et al. Clinical significance of the ratio between the alpha 2 plasmin inhibitor-plasmin complex and the thrombin-antithrombin complex in advanced non-small cell lung cancer. *Med Oncol.* (2011) 28:351–6. doi: 10.1007/s12032-010-9454-y
30. Kaseda K, Asakura K, Kazama A, Ozawa Y. Prognostic significance of preoperative plasma D-dimer level in patients with surgically resected clinical stage I non-small cell lung cancer: a retrospective cohort study. *J Cardiothorac Surg.* (2017) 12:102. doi: 10.1186/s13019-017-0676-3
31. Ay C, Dunkler D, Pirker R, Thaler J, Quehenberger P, Wagner O, et al. High D-dimer levels are associated with poor prognosis in cancer patients. *Haematologica.* (2012) 97:1158–64. doi: 10.3324/haematol.2011.054718
32. Inal T, Anar C, Polat G, Unsal I, Halilcolar H. The prognostic value of D-dimer in lung cancer. *Clin Respir J.* (2015) 9:305–13. doi: 10.1111/crj.12144
33. Chen F, Wang MJ, Li J, Yan CE, Han XH, Wu ZY, et al. Plasma D-dimer value as a predictor of malignant lymph node involvement in operable non-small cell lung cancer. *Tumour Biol.* (2015) 36:9201–7. doi: 10.1007/s13277-015-3526-8
34. Kyrle PA, Eichinger S. D-Dimer for long-term risk prediction in patients after acute coronary syndrome. *Circulation.* (2018) 138:724–6. doi: 10.1161/CIRCULATIONAHA.118.033670
35. Weitz JI, Fredenburgh JC, Eikelboom JW. A test in context: D-dimer. *J Am Coll Cardiol.* (2017) 70:2411–20. doi: 10.1016/j.jacc.2017.09.024
36. Rong G, Fan W, Shen J. High pretreatment plasma D-dimer levels predict poor prognosis in gastrointestinal cancers: a meta-analysis. *Medicine (Baltimore).* (2019) 98:e16520. doi: 10.1097/MD.0000000000016520
37. Gomes M, Khorana AA. Risk assessment for thrombosis in cancer. *Semin Thromb Hemost.* (2014) 40:319–24. doi: 10.1055/s-0034-1370770
38. Falanga A, Russo L, Milesi V. The coagulopathy of cancer. *Curr Opin Hematol.* (2014) 21:423–9. doi: 10.1097/MOH.0000000000000072
39. Davila M, Robles-Carrillo L, Unruh D, Huo Q, Gardiner C, Sargent IL, et al. Microparticle association and heterogeneity of tumor-derived tissue factor in plasma: is it important for coagulation activation? *J Thromb Haemost.* (2014) 12:186–96. doi: 10.1111/jth.12475
40. Yu JL, Rak JW. Shedding of tissue factor (TF)-containing microparticles rather than alternatively spliced TF is the main source of TF activity released from human cancer cells. *J Thromb Haemost.* (2004) 2:2065–7. doi: 10.1111/j.1538-7836.2004.00972.x
41. Falanga A, Marchetti M, Vignoli A. Coagulation and cancer: biological and clinical aspects. *J Thromb Haemost.* (2013) 11:223–33. doi: 10.1111/jth.12075
42. Kvolik S, Jukic M, Matijevic M, Marjanovic K, Glavas-Obrovac L. An overview of coagulation disorders in cancer patients. *Surg Oncol.* (2010) 19:e33–46. doi: 10.1016/j.suronc.2009.03.008
43. Nakaki T, Nakayama M, Kato R. Inhibition by nitric oxide and nitric oxide-producing vasodilators of DNA synthesis in vascular smooth muscle cells. *Eur J Pharmacol.* (1990) 189:347–53. doi: 10.1016/0922-4106(90)90031-R
44. Gasic GJ, Tuszynski GP, Gorelik E. Interaction of the hemostatic and immune systems in the metastatic spread of tumor cells. *Int Rev Exp Pathol.* (1986) 29:173–212.
45. Dvorak HF. Thrombosis and cancer. *Hum Pathol.* (1987) 18:275–84. doi: 10.1016/S0046-8177(87)80010-2
46. Taguchi O, Gabazza EC, Yasui H, Kobayashi T, Yoshida M, Kobayashi H. Prognostic significance of plasma D-dimer levels in patients with lung cancer. *Thorax.* (1997) 52:563–5. doi: 10.1136/thx.52.6.563
47. Jiang J, Shang X, Zhao J, Cao M, Wang J, Li R, et al. Score for predicting active cancer in patients with ischemic stroke: a retrospective study. *Biomed Res Int.* (2021) 2021:5585206. doi: 10.1155/2021/5585206
48. Ay C, Unal UK. Epidemiology and risk factors for venous thromboembolism in lung cancer. *Curr Opin Oncol.* (2016) 28:145–9. doi: 10.1097/CCO.0000000000000262
49. Ay C, Vormittag R, Dunkler D, Simanek R, Chiriac AL, Drach J, et al. D-dimer and prothrombin fragment 1 + 2 predict venous thromboembolism in patients with cancer: results from the vienna cancer and thrombosis study. *J Clin Oncol.* (2009) 27:4124–9. doi: 10.1200/JCO.2008.21.7752
50. Zwicker JI, Bauer KA. How long is long enough? Extended anticoagulation for the treatment of cancer-associated deep vein thrombosis. *J Clin Oncol.* (2014) 32:3596–9. doi: 10.1200/JCO.2014.56.5184
51. Sundboll J, Veres K, Horvath-Puho E, Adelborg K, Sorensen HT. Risk and prognosis of cancer after lower limb arterial thrombosis. *Circulation.* (2018) 138:669–77. doi: 10.1161/CIRCULATIONAHA.117.032617

16

Blood and Salivary Amphiregulin Levels as Biomarkers for Asthma

Mahmood Yaseen Hachim[1,2], *Noha Mousaad Elemam*[2], *Rakhee K. Ramakrishnan*[2], *Laila Salameh*[3], *Ronald Olivenstein*[4], *Ibrahim Yaseen Hachim*[2,5], *Thenmozhi Venkatachalam*[2], *Bassam Mahboub*[3,5], *Saba Al Heialy*[1,4], *Rabih Halwani*[2,5], *Qutayba Hamid*[2,4,5] *and Rifat Hamoudi*[2,5,6*]

[1] *College of Medicine, Mohammed Bin Rashid University of Medicine and Health Sciences, Dubai, United Arab Emirates,* [2] *Sharjah Institute for Medical Research, College of Medicine, University of Sharjah, Sharjah, United Arab Emirates,* [3] *Rashid Hospital, Dubai Health Authority, Dubai, United Arab Emirates,* [4] *Meakins-Christie Laboratories, McGill University, Montreal, QC, Canada,* [5] *Department of Clinical Sciences, College of Medicine, University of Sharjah, Sharjah, United Arab Emirates,* [6] *Division of Surgery and Interventional Science, UCL, London, United Kingdom*

Correspondence:
Rifat Hamoudi
rhamoudi@sharjah.ac.ae

Background: Amphiregulin (AREG) expression in asthmatic airways and sputum was shown to increase and correlate with asthma. However, no studies were carried out to evaluate the AREG level in blood and saliva of asthmatic patients.

Objective: To measure circulating AREG mRNA and protein concentrations in blood, saliva, and bronchial biopsies samples from asthmatic patients.

Methods: Plasma and Saliva AREG protein concentrations were measured using ELISA while PBMCs, and Saliva mRNA expression was measured by RT qPCR in non-severe, and severe asthmatic patients compared to healthy controls. Primary asthmatic bronchial epithelial cells and fibroblasts were assessed for AREG mRNA expression and released soluble AREG in their conditioned media. Tissue expression of AREG was evaluated using immunohistochemistry of bronchial biopsies from asthmatic patients and healthy controls. Publicly available transcriptomic databases were explored for the global transcriptomic profile of bronchial epithelium, and PBMCs were explored for AREG expression in asthmatic vs. healthy controls.

Results: Asthmatic patients had higher AREG protein levels in blood and saliva compared to control subjects. Higher mRNA expression in saliva and primary bronchial epithelial cells plus higher AREG immunoreactivity in bronchial biopsies were also observed. Both blood and saliva AREG levels showed positive correlations with allergic rhinitis status, atopy status, eczema status, plasma periostin, neutrophilia, Montelukast sodium use, ACT score, FEV1, and FEV1/FVC. *In silico* analysis showed that severe asthmatic bronchial epithelium with high AREG gene expression is associated with higher neutrophils infiltration.

Conclusion: AREG levels measured in a minimally invasive blood sample and a non-invasive saliva sample are higher in non-allergic severe asthma.

Clinical Implications

This is the first report to show the higher level of AREG levels in blood and saliva of non-allergic severe asthma.

Keywords: asthma, biomarkers, saliva, amphiregulin (AREG), non-invasive

INTRODUCTION

Asthma is characterized by chronic airway inflammation, mucus hyper-production, airway hyper-responsiveness, and variable airway obstruction (1). The prevalence of asthma has increased in the last few years, reaching alarming levels (2). Understanding the complexity of asthma will help in establishing management strategies aiming for better asthma patients stratification for personalized therapeutic options (3). Current biomarkers include eosinophil counts, a fraction of exhaled nitric oxide (Feno) values, periostin, IgE levels, and T-helper2 related cytokines (4). The identification of novel, cost-effective, reliable, and measurable non-invasive markers (5) is the goal for many research projects (6–8).

The epidermal growth factor receptor (EGFR) signaling is vital to epithelial cell physiology, and its dysregulation is involved in different pathologies (9), including pathogenesis of early stage of asthma (10). Many asthma triggers like allergens, viruses, and pollutants activate EGFR signaling, which seems to be a common pathway shared by different asthma phenotypes (11). EGFR signaling mediates airway hyper-responsiveness (AHR), tissue remodeling (12) and is implicated in lung fibrosis (10). Amphiregulin (Areg), an EGFR ligand, and a widely expressed transmembrane tyrosine kinase (13, 14), was shown to be upregulated upon inflammation, hormones, growth factors, and xenobiotics stimuli (13). Previously, high AREG expression was related to lung inflammation (15), specifically in damaged lung tissues in patients with chronic obstructive pulmonary disease (COPD) and asthma (16). AREG expression in structural cells (15) and sputum was associated with asthma severity (17), and it was shown to be increased in airways during an acute asthma attack (18).

Interestingly, hematopoietic cells that infiltrate inflamed lung tissue were shown to locally upregulate AREG expression and influence its local concentrations (15). While human monocytes were found to express AREG upon activation (19), eosinophils still represent the primary producers of AREG when compared to other types of blood cells (19) and can be reprogrammed to an inflammatory state by AREG- EGFR-mediated signaling (20). For all the above reasons, AREG was suggested to be linked to severe eosinophilic asthma with less response to asthma therapy (21). Such sensitized individual develops eosinophilic airway inflammation after the exposure to allergens through IgE antibody-mediated mast cell degranulation is labeled as allergic asthmatic. On the other hand, a non-allergic asthmatic is a non-sensitized individual who can develop eosinophilic inflammation without exposure to an allergen through the activation of ILC2 cells that do not need allergen-specific IgE (22). ILC2s and lung activated alveolar macrophages can control lung inflammation by producing AREG to promote repair of the airway epithelium, that is why depletion of these cells can result in diminished lung function after the loss of airway epithelial integrity which can be restored by adding AREG (23–26).

Non-allergic patients may have innate immunity or neutrophilic airway inflammation independent of Th2 cells (27). Triggers of asthma in non-allergic patients can vary from external triggers like viral infections, cigarette smoke, diesel particles, and ozone to patient's intrinsic factors like stress, exercise, and obesity (1). Following epithelial damage, the epidermal growth factor (EGF) can enhance the neutrophil accumulation to stimulate neutrophil defenses during acute injury (28).

Of note, T cells in peripheral blood mononuclear cells (PBMC) can also produce AREG in response to signals of tissue damage and repair (29). The association of a protective AREG with disease progression, and whether there is cell to cell variation in production and response to AREG remain unknown.

Some circulating plasma proteins originating from tissue leakage (30) and thus being detected in saliva and can reflect their upregulation in serum/plasma (31). Because saliva is easy to collect, innocuous, acceptable by patients, thus it represents a potential tool for measuring disease biomarkers (32). Therefore, measuring the expression of AREG in plasma and saliva from asthmatic patients can provide a minimally invasive approach for the assessment of AREG, which may provide a more reliable tool complementary to existing measures.

METHODS

Patient Population (Cohort 1)

From January 2017 to May 2019, individuals were recruited consecutively from the Asthma Clinic in Rashid Hospital, Pulmonary Medicine Department. Thirty-two asthmatic patients were included, 19 were non-severe asthmatic patients (mild to moderate), and 13 were severe asthmatic subjects (fulfilling the criteria for asthma as per American Thoracic Society) (**Table 1**). According to GINA and ERS/ATS Task Force on severe asthma, guidelines define asthma severity as "those who require continuous high-dose treatment, as their asthma is refractory or difficult-to-treat plus a second controller (and/or systemic corticosteroids) to prevent it from becoming uncontrolled or which remains uncontrolled despite this therapy" (33). Those patients were compared to 12 non-asthmatic volunteer subjects who had no recent infection of the respiratory tract and no histories of allergy or asthma. Participants completed the Asthma Control Test self-assessment. The Ethics Committee of Dubai Health Authority and the University of Sharjah approved the study with REC (Research Ethics Committee) approval number DSREC-11/2017_04, and each subject gave written informed consent after a thorough explanation by the treating physician and the researchers. This study was conducted in accordance with the Declaration of Helsinki. The demographic characteristics of the asthmatic patients and control subjects are shown in **Table 4**.

Abbreviations: ACT, asthma control test; ADAM, a disintegrin and metalloproteases; AHR, airway hyperresponsiveness; AREG, amphiregulin; COPD, chronic obstructive pulmonary disease; DMEM, Dulbecco's Modified Eagle's medium; EDTA, ethylenediaminetetraacetic acid; EGF, epidermal growth factor; EGFR, the epidermal growth factor receptor; ELISA, enzyme-linked immunoassay; ErbB, erythroblastic leukemia viral oncogene; FBS, fetal bovine serum; Feno, fraction of exhaled nitric oxide; GEO, Gene Expression Omnibus; HDM, house dust mite; IgE, immunoglobulin E; IL17A, Interleukin 17 A; mRNA, Messenger RNA; PBMC, peripheral blood mononuclear cells; qRT-PCR, Real-Time qRT-PCR; ROC, Receiver Operating Characteristic curve; TH2, T helper cell type 2; TNFα, TNF-alpha.

TABLE 1 | Characteristics of the cohort 1 subjects with asthma and healthy controls.

	Control	Non-severe asthma	Severe asthma	*P*-value
Number of subjects	12	19	13.00	
Age (Years)	37.00 ± 11.73	40.19 ± 15.65	48.42 ± 17.95	NS
Age of onset (adult to childhood ratio)				
Childhood asthma		11	5	
Adult asthma		5	8	
Female to male ratio	8:4	13:3	7:6	NS
BMI	24.60 ± 3.19	27.63 ± 6.40	27.03 ± 6.56	NS
ACT score	–	20.75 ± 4.31	17.55 ± 6.15	NS
Oral steroid use per day/week	–	0.6563 ± 1.06	2.083 ± 1.459	0.01
Exacerbations/year	–	1.688 ± 2.575	2.133 ± 1.482	NS
History of atopy				
Yes	0	0	4	<0.01
No	10	16	9	
History of allergic rhinitis				
Yes	1	10	9	<0.01
No	9	6	4	
Peak flow (l/min)	453.80 ± 101.00	299.30 ± 78.20	302.50 ± 139.90	<0.01
FEV1 (% predicted)	–	55.46 ± 42.42	54.06 ± 45.53	NS
FEV1/FVC	–	56.87 ± 40.30	49.13 ± 35.35	NS
Total serum IgE (IU/mL)	–	280.30 ± 358.40	1167.00 ± 1428.00	<0.01
Blood eosinophil (%)	–	4.54 ± 3.24	6.88 ± 9.57	NS
Blood neutrophil (%)	–	58.29 ± 12.34	60.04 ± 13.86	NS
Blood basophil (%)	–	0.53 ± 0.36	0.52 ± 0.24	NS
Blood lymphocytes (%)	–	28.89 ± 11.05	26.67 ± 12.15	NS
Absolute eosinophil counts (cells/μL)	–	181.6 ± 129.6	275.2 ± 382.8	NS

Patient Population (Cohort 2)

A matched cohort of severe asthmatics ($n = 17$) vs. non-severe asthmatics ($n = 21$) was recruited for fresh saliva collections and RNA extractions was performed to explore the feasibility of detecting AREG mRNA in the saliva.

Blood Collection Protocol and Plasma Isolation

Twelve milliliters of whole blood were collected from each sample in EDTA-containing blood collection tubes (3 mL each) and transferred immediately within 2 h to Sharjah Institute for Medical Research (SIMR), Sharjah for further processing to isolate PBMCs as previously described (34). Twelve milliliters of Histopaque-1077 (Sigma, #10771, Germany) were added to a 50 mL centrifuge tube and brought to room temperature (RT), then 12 mL of whole blood were carefully layered on top of the Histopaque and centrifuged at 400 × g for precisely 30 min at room temperature. After centrifugation, the plasma layer and the buffy layer interface were carefully collected with separate Pasteur pipettes and transferred to clean 15 mL conical centrifuge tubes separately, to be frozen at −80°C till future use.

Unstimulated Whole Saliva Collection Protocol

Participants were asked to fast for at least 1 h and not to brush their teeth or smoke for 30 min, accompanied by gargling and rinsing of the mouth with water 5 min before proceeding with saliva collection. One milliliter of unstimulated whole saliva via passive drool was collected in a pre-prepared 50 mL tube containing 1 mL of RNAlater (Invitrogen). Collected saliva samples were transported on ice and stored at - 80°C until analysis. Sample measurements were undertaken within 3 months of storage.

Primary Cell Lines and Bronchial Biopsies (Cohort 3)

Primary cells from healthy and asthmatic patients were isolated from bronchial biopsies in Meakins-Christie Laboratories, The Centre for Respiratory Research at McGill University and the Research Institute of McGill University Health Centre as previously described (35). In total, 17 primary cells were exploited: 7 healthy primary cells: epithelial ($n = 3$) and fibroblasts ($n = 4$), and 10 primary asthmatic cells: epithelial cells ($n = 3$), non-severe asthmatic fibroblasts ($n = 4$), and severe asthmatic fibroblasts ($n = 3$). Twelve bronchial biopsies were taken from control ($n = 3$) and asthmatic ($n = 9$, 3 in each clinical stage: mild, moderate, and severe) were used for immunohistochemical assessment. Epithelial cells were revived and maintained using epithelial growth medium PneumaCult™-Ex Medium (Stem Cell Technology, Canada), supplemented with 100 units/mL penicillin/streptomycin (Gibco, USA). Primary fibroblasts were maintained in complete Dulbecco's

Modified Eagle's medium (DMEM) (Sigma-Aldrich, Germany) with 10% fetal bovine serum (FBS) (Sigma-Aldrich, Germany) supplemented with 100 units/mL penicillin/streptomycin (Gibco, USA).

mRNA Gene Expression Using qRT-PCR

RNA was extracted using RNAeasy mini kit (Qiagen, Germany) as per the manufacturer instructions. The purified RNA was reverse transcribed into cDNA using High Capacity cDNA Reverse Transcription (Applied Biosystems, USA) as per the manufacturer instructions. 5X Hot FIREPol EvaGreen qPCR Supermix (Solis BioDyne, Estonia) was used to quantify mRNA of the selected genes using QuantStudio3 (Applied Biosystems, USA). Details of used primers are in **Table 2**.

Enzyme-Linked Immunoassay (ELISA) Quantification

Human amphiregulin was measured in plasma and saliva of healthy controls and asthmatic patients as well as the conditioned media of primary bronchial cells using the Human Amphiregulin Quantikine and Duoset ELISA Kits (R&D Systems, USA) according to the manufacturer's instructions. Periostin (POSTN) and IL-17A were assessed in plasma using human Periostin/OSF-2 and human IL-17A DuoSet ELISA Kits (R&D Systems, USA),respectively, according to the manufacturer's instructions.

Soluble Receptors Array

To assess any difference in the shedding of AREG in the conditioned media of the asthmatics vs. healthy primary fibroblasts, Non-Hematopoietic Array and the Common Analytes Array (R&D Systems, Catalog # ARY011) was used as per the manufacturer instructions. The conditioned media of healthy bronchial fibroblasts and non-severe asthmatic fibroblasts were collected, centrifuged and 1.5 mL of each were added to the array wells separately and incubated overnight on a rocking shaker. On the next day, the membranes were washed to remove any unbound material and incubated with the specific cocktail of biotinylated detection antibodies. Streptavidin-horseradish peroxidase and chemiluminescent detection reagents were added, and a chemiluminescent signal was produced in proportion to the amount of receptor-bound. Dot blots were registered with ChemiDoc Imaging System (BioRad, USA). The average pixel density of duplicate spots on the membrane was determined using ImageJ software (36). After background subtraction, the relative amounts of individual proteins were calculated as previously reported (37).

Immunohistochemical Assessment of Bronchial Biopsies

Immunohistochemical evaluation of bronchial biopsies from healthy and asthmatic patients was done on a 3 μm section of the tissue block mounted on positively charged slides. After routine deparaffination and rehydration, antigen retrieval using Tris EDTA buffer (pH 9.0) in a microwave oven at 95°C for 15 min was done. Horse radish peroxidase (HRP) kit (760-700, Optiview DAB IHC Detection kit, Ventana) was used as per the manufacturer instructions, along with neutralizing antibody for AREG (15 μg/mL) (R&D Systems, USA) for AREG detection.

In silico Validation in Lung and Blood Transcriptomic Datasets

Twenty-five publicly available transcriptomics datasets ($n = 2,666$) of Bronchial Epithelium, Bronchial Fibroblasts, Whole Lung, Bronchial Biopsy, Induced Sputum, Nasal, Bronchioalveolar lavage, Blood, Whole Blood, PBMCs, and CD4 cells from asthmatic patients vs. healthy subjects in different settings were downloaded from Gene Expression Omnibus (https://www.ncbi.nlm.nih.gov/geo). The raw data was extracted according to Hachim et al. (38) and the normalized gene expression of the AREG was compared between patients with different asthma severities as shown in **Table 3**.

In silico Prediction of the Percentage and Status of Immune Cells

We used the transcriptomic data to predict the percentage and status of immune cells in the bronchial epithelium or blood of severe asthmatics patients compared to the healthy controls using CIBERSORT computational method (https://cibersort.stanford.edu/) to quantify cell fractions from samples gene expression profiles as previously described (39).

Statistical Methods

GraphPad Prism version 8.00 for Windows (GraphPad Software, La Jolla, CA, USA) was used for statistical analysis. First, the D'Agostino-Pearson normality test was used to determine whether to perform parametric or non-parametric tests. One-way ANOVA test was performed to determine whether there are any statistically significant differences between the mean values of the controls and different asthma groups for the gene expression and protein levels. The same software was used to examine the correlations between the different parameters using Pearson correlation test in GraphPad Prism. Student t-test was used to look for the difference between two groups under a given experiment or treatment. A $p < 0.05$ is considered to be statistically significant.

RESULTS

Severe Asthmatic Patients PBMCs Express Less AREG mRNA but Higher Protein Compared to Non-severe Asthmatics

PBMCs AREG mRNA was lower in severe asthmatics compared to non-severe asthmatics ($p = 0.05$), (**Figure 1A**). PBMCs AREG mRNA correlated positively with IL17A plasma level (0.43, $p < 0.05$). Also, the expression correlated negatively with age (−0.38, $p < 0.05$), the use of oral corticosteroids (−0.58, $p < 0.05$), the number of exacerbations per year (−0.39, $p < 0.05$), and atopic status (−0.40, $p < 0.05$).

TABLE 2 | List of forward and reverse primers for each of the genes assessed by qRT-PCR.

Gene	NCBI reference sequence	Primer	Sequence (5′-3′)	Amplicon size (bp)
Areg	NM_001657.4	Forward primer	GAGCACCTGGAAGCAGTAAC	151
		Reverse primer	GGATCACAGCAGACATAAAGGC	
18S rRNA	NR_145820.1	Forward primer	TGACTCAACACGGGAAACC	114
		Reverse primer	TGCCTCCACCAACTAAGAAC	

TABLE 3 | List of datasets extracted from GEO omnibus for the in silico analysis.

Dataset ID	Tissue/sample	Study title	Samples
GSE4302	Bronchial epithelium	Genome-Wide Profiling of Airway Epithelial Cells in Asthmatics, Smokers and Healthy Controls	70
GSE18965	Bronchial epithelium	Decreased Fibronectin Production Significantly Contributes to Dysregulated Repair of Asthmatic Epithelium	16
GSE43696	Bronchial epithelium	Asthma	108
GSE51392	Bronchial epithelium	Expression Data From Airway Epithelial Cells Stimulated With Poly(I:C) From Patients With Asthma, Rhinitis, and Healthy Controls	12
GSE67472	Bronchial epithelium	Airway Epithelial Gene Expression in Asthma Versus Healthy Controls	105
GSE64913	Bronchial epithelium	Altered Epithelial Gene Expression in Peripheral Airways of Severe Asthma	36
GSE76227	Bronchial epithelium	Expression Data of Bronchial Biopsies and Epithelial Brushing From Unbiased Biomarkers in Prediction of Respiratory Disease Outcomes (U-BIOPRED) Project	190
GSE13785	Bronchial epithelium	Novel Mediators of Eicosanoid and Epithelial Nitric Oxide Production in Asthma	22
GSE30063	Bronchial epithelium	Epithelial Expression of Toll-like Receptor 5 is Modulated in Healthy Smokers and Smokers With Chronic Obstructive Lung Disease	63
GSE27335	Bronchial fibroblasts	Genomic Differences Distinguish the Myofibroblast Phenotype of the Distal Lung From Airway Fibroblasts	24
GSE21369	Whole lung	Gene Expression Profiles of Interstitial Lung Disease (ILD) Patients	6
GSE41649	Bronchial biopsy	Comparison of Two Sets of Microarray Experiments to Define Allergic Asthma Expression Pattern	8
GSE56396	Induced sputum	Non-invasive Analysis of the Airway Transcriptome Discriminates Clinical Phenotypes of Asthma	112
GSE41863	Induced sputum	Sputum Gene Expression Profiling in Asthmatics	56
GSE41861	Nasal	Upper Airway Gene Expression Is an Effective Surrogate Biomarker for Th2-Driven Inflammation in the Lower Airway	84
GSE41862	Nasal	Nasal Scrape Gene Expression Profiling in Asthmatics	116
GSE67940	Bronchioalveolar lavage	Asthma III	104
GSE115823	Blood	A Network of Transcriptome Modules Demonstrates Mechanistic Pathways of Both Virus-Induced and Non-viral Asthma Exacerbations in Children [Blood]	208
GSE69683	Blood	Expression Profiling in Blood From Subjects With Severe Asthma, Moderate Asthma, and Non-asthmatics Collected in the U-BIOPRED Study	498
GSE35571	Blood	Gene Expression Data From 131 Human Subjects in Detroit, Michigan	131
GSE137394	Whole blood	Genome-Wide Profiling of Allergic Asthma Peripheral Blood	309
GSE123750	Whole blood	U-BIOPRED Blood Transcriptomics From children With Asthma or Wheeze	216
GSE31773	PBMC	Comparison of mRNA Expression in Circulating T-Cells From Patients With Severe Asthma	40
GSE16032	PBMC	Gene Expression Data From Severe Asthmatic Children: PBMC Profiles During Acute Exacerbation Versus Convalescence	10
GSE73482	CD4	Gene Expression Patterns in Allergen-Driven CD4 T Cell Responses From Human Atopics With or Without Asthma	144
Total	2,666		

AREG Was Higher in Well-Controlled Asthma

Asthma Control Test (ACT) is a patient self-administered tool for identifying those with poorly controlled asthma. The scores range from 5 (poor control of asthma) to 25 (complete control of asthma), with higher scores reflecting greater asthma control. An ACT score > 20 indicates well-controlled asthma. When we divided our patients accordingly, AREG mRNA expression in PBMC correlated positively with higher ACT scores, as shown in **Figure 1B**.

AREG mRNA Was Higher in the Saliva of Severe Asthmatics Compared to Non-severe Asthmatics

A matched cohort of severe asthmatics ($n = 17$) vs. non-severe asthmatics ($n = 21$) was recruited for fresh saliva collections and RNA was extracted to detect AREG mRNA in the saliva. AREG showed significant upregulation in severe asthmatics compared to non-severe asthmatics, as shown in **Figure 1C**.

Asthmatic Patients' Plasma and Saliva AREG Protein Level Is Higher Than Healthy Controls

Plasma AREG level, as measured by ELISA, was higher in non-severe and severe asthmatic patients (333.24 ± 133.14 pg/mL, $p < 0.01$) compared to healthy controls (265.05 ± 29.49 pg/mL) as shown in **Figure 2A**. Interestingly, the saliva AREG level was also higher in severe asthmatic patients (247.35 ± 271.4 pg/mL, $p = 0.02$), as shown in **Figure 2B**. Indeed, plasma AREG correlated positively to saliva AREG level ($r = 0.3671$, $p = 0.02$), indicating the feasibility of using saliva to reflect the plasma level of AREG. AREG plasma level correlated negatively with PBMC AREG mRNA expression ($r = -0.37$, $p < 0.05$).

Blood and Saliva AREG Protein Levels Correlate With Patient's Atopy Status and Allergic Rhinitis

Plasma AREG levels had a positive correlation with ACT ($r = 0.32$, $p < 0.05$), allergic rhinitis status ($r = 0.35$, $p =$

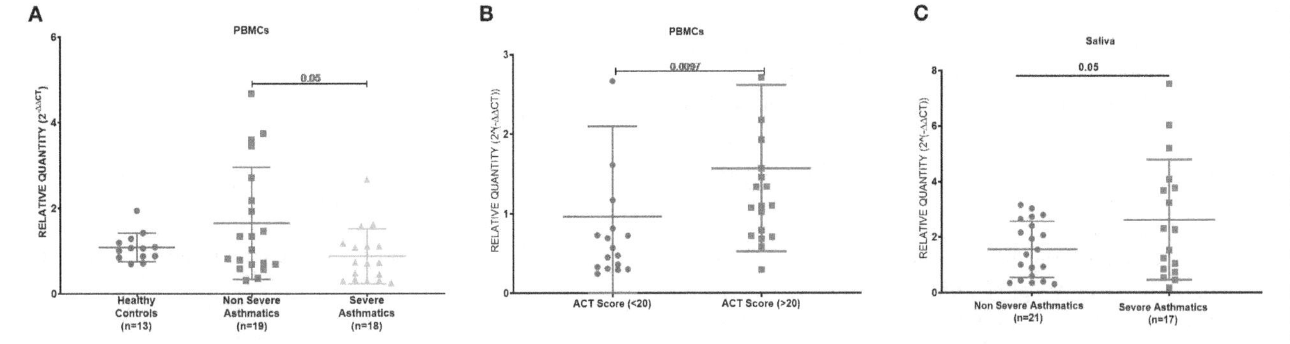

FIGURE 1 | AREG mRNA expression as measured by RT qPCR in PBMCs and saliva of cohort of asthmatic vs. healthy control. **(A)** AREG mRNA level in PBMCs of the locally recruited cohort (cohort 1), healthy controls ($n = 13$), non-severe asthmatics ($n = 20$), and severe asthmatic ($n = 18$). **(B)** AREG mRNA gene expression in PBMC of a locally recruited cohort divided according to the ACT score into two groups: a well-controlled group (ACT > 20) and those with poor control (ACT < 20). **(C)** AREG mRNA gene expression in the saliva of independent validation locally recruited cohort (cohort 2), which includes non-severe asthmatics ($n = 21$) and severe asthmatic who are not on biological treatment ($n = 17$).

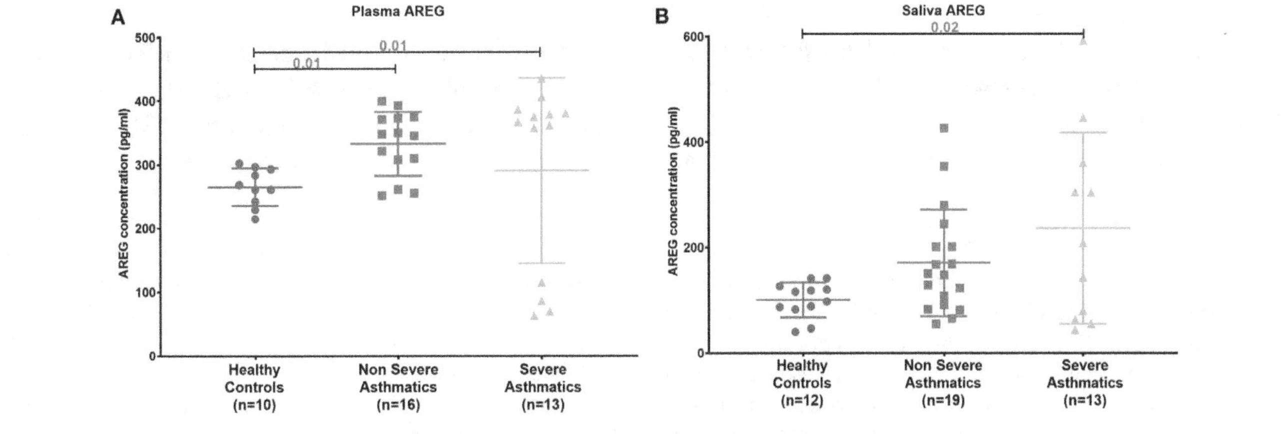

FIGURE 2 | AREG protein level in **(A)** plasma and **(B)** saliva of the locally recruited cohort (cohort 1), including healthy controls, non-severe and severe asthmatic patients.

0.03, **Figure 3A**), atopy status ($r = 0.35$, $p = 0.03$), neutrophil percentage in patients' blood ($r = 0.45$, $p = 0.01$), and the use of Montelukast sodium (Singulair) ($r = 0.39$, $p = 0.04$, **Figure 3B**). Interestingly, plasma AREG levels correlated positively with plasma POSTN levels ($r = 0.34$, $p = 0.03$). Correlation between Plasma AREG concentrations, and the cohort demographics and laboratory tests are listed in **Table 4**.

On the other hand, saliva AREG levels correlated significantly with key clinical indicators for asthma assessment compared to plasma AREG, as listed in **Table 5**. Beside allergic rhinitis ($r = 0.42$, $p = 0.02$) and atopy status ($r = 0.37$, $p = 0.02$), saliva AREG level correlated positively with ACT score ($r = 0.38$, $p = 0.04$), FEV1 (% predicted) ($r = 0.47$, $p = 0.001$), FEV1/FVC ($r = 0.48$, $p = 0.02$) and eczema status ($r = 0.35$, $p = 0.03$). Interestingly, saliva AREG level correlated positively with the age of onset as adult asthmatics showed higher levels ($r = 0.31$, $p < 0.05$).

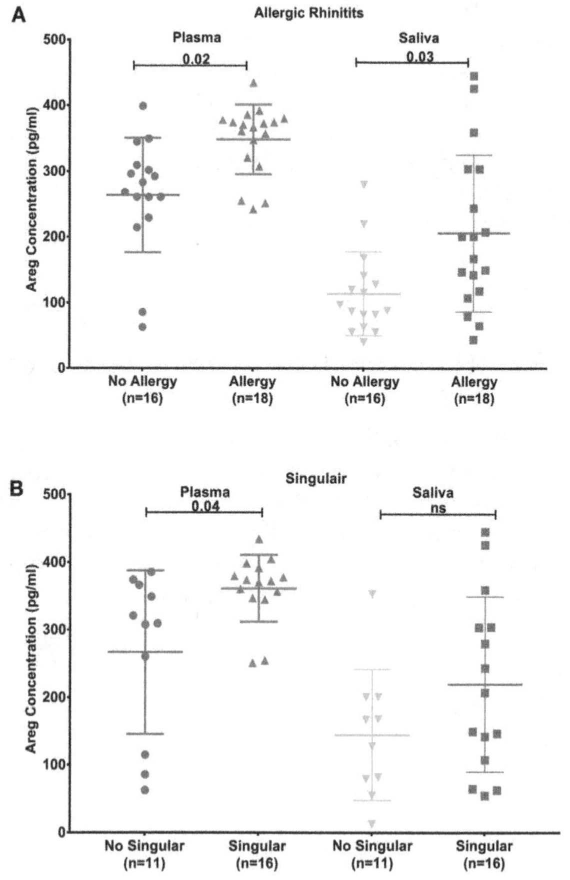

FIGURE 3 | AREG protein levels in plasma and saliva. **(A)** in asthmatic with allergic rhinitits compared to those who are not and **(B)** in asthmatics currently on Montelukast sodium (Singulair) compared to those who are not on Singulair.

AREG Protein Expression Was Higher in Bronchial Epithelial Cells of Mild Asthmatics Compared to Those of Moderate and Severe Patients as Well as Healthy Controls

AREG expression in lung tissue and its cellular localization were investigated using bronchial biopsies from asthmatic patients ($n = 13$) and healthy controls ($n = 4$), as shown in **Figure 4**. The asthmatic samples were from mild ($n = 5$), moderate ($n = 4$), and severe ($n = 4$) patients. Immunohistochemical expression of AREG was high in bronchial epithelial pseudostratified cells, while lower expression was observed in fibroblasts and other cells, including infiltrating immune cells. Interestingly, AREG expression in a healthy epithelium was nuclear while it was cytoplasmic in asthmatic samples. As expected, AREG expression was positive (6 out of 13, 46.15%) in asthmatic patient's samples compared to only 1 out of 4 samples in the control group (25%). Interestingly, AREG expression was positive in 4 out of the five mild asthmatic samples (80%) compared to only 1 case out of the four moderate (25%) and severe asthmatic samples (25%), $p = 0.0495$.

AREG mRNA Level Was Higher in Non-severe Asthmatic Bronchial Epithelial Cells Compared to Healthy Controls and Severe Asthmatic

AREG mRNA and protein levels were measured in primary bronchial epithelial cells and fibroblasts from asthmatic patients and healthy controls. AREG mRNA expression was upregulated in non-severe asthmatic bronchial epithelial cells compared to healthy controls ($p = 0.05$), and severe asthmatics ($p = 0.04$), **Figure 5A**. Using ELISA, secreted AREG levels detected in the conditioned media of bronchial epithelium using ELISA showed no significant difference between asthmatics and healthy controls, as shown in **Figure 5B**. Nevertheless, asthmatic bronchial epithelial cells secrete higher amounts (more than five times) of soluble AREG in their conditioned media compared to their asthma severity matching fibroblasts, indicating that epithelial cells are the primary source of pulmonary AREG in asthma. Moreover, bronchial fibroblasts of severe asthmatics ($n = 3$) showed lower expression of AREG mRNA compared to healthy fibroblasts ($n = 4$) ($p = 0.04$), which goes in line with the ELISA results ($p = 0.01$), **Figures 5C,D**.

Asthmatic Fibroblasts Secrete More AREG Ectoderm Shedders ADAM8, ADAM9, ADAM10 Compared to Healthy Fibroblasts

As the secreted levels of AREG matched its mRNA expression in severe asthmatic fibroblasts, we investigated the reason behind the low secreted levels of AREG in non-severe asthmatic fibroblasts despite of its high mRNA expression levels (**Figure 6**). We profiled the shredded proteins in their conditioned media and found that asthmatic fibroblasts secrete higher AREG ectoderm shedders ADAM8 ($p = 0.01$), ADAM9 ($p = 0.001$), ADAM10 ($p < 0.0001$) and ADAM17 ($p < 0.0001$) compared to healthy fibroblasts (**Figure 6A**). Another interesting finding is that non-severe asthmatic fibroblasts shed less ErbB1 ($p = 0.003$) and ErbB3 ($p = 0.003$) receptors compared to healthy fibroblasts (**Figure 6B**).

TABLE 4 | Correlation between plasma AREG concentrations, and the cohort demographics and laboratory tests.

AREG plasma (pg/mL)	vs. AREG saliva (pg/mL)	vs. Atopy status	vs. Allergic rhinitis status	vs. Blood neutrophil (%)	vs. POSTN plasma (pg/mL)
Pearson correlation test *r*	0.3671	0.3547	0.351	0.4494	0.3436
95% confidence interval	0.04391–0.6207	0.02475–0.615	0.02544–0.6092	0.07192–0.7143	0.01704–0.6039
P (two-tailed)	0.0234	0.0312	0.0307	0.0187	0.0347
Number of XY pairs	38	37	38	27	38

TABLE 5 | Correlation between saliva AREG concentrations, and the cohort demographics and laboratory tests.

AREG saliva (pg/mL)	vs. ACT score	vs. Atopy status	vs. Allergic rhinitis status	vs. Eczema status	vs. FEV1 (% predicted)	vs. FEV1/FVC
Pearson correlation test *r*	0.3895	0.3744	0.4216	0.3554	0.6458	0.487
95% confidence interval	−0.009556–0.6815	0.04223–0.632	0.1032–0.6616	0.02557–0.6155	0.2959–0.8429	0.06913–0.7595
P (two-tailed)	0.0492	0.0245	0.0094	0.0309	0.0012	0.0215
Number of XY pairs	26	36	37	37	22	22

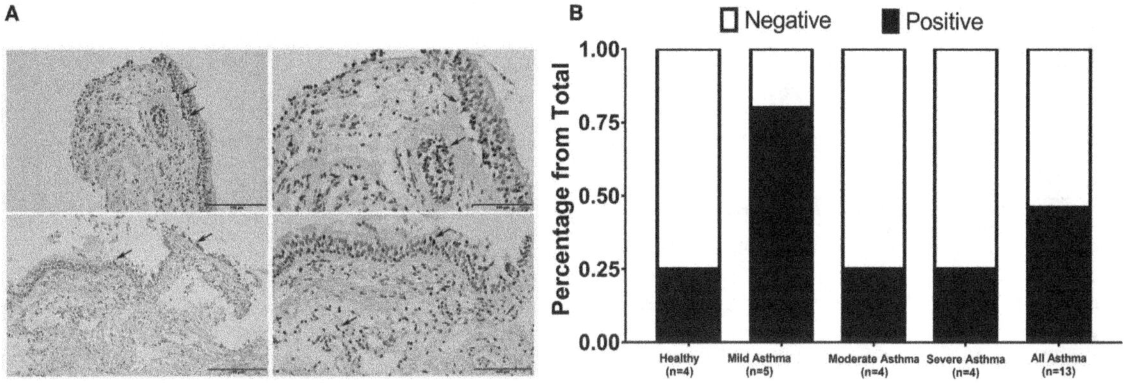

FIGURE 4 | Immunohistochemical staining of AREG in bronchial biopsies of healthy, non-severe (mild and moderate) and severe asthmatic patients. **(A)** Arrows showing positively stained epithelial cells, **(B)** percentage of positive AREG IHC staining sample among all samples examined in each group.

IN SILICO VALIDATION

AREG mRNA Expression Was Significantly Different in Asthmatic Bronchial Epithelium, Fibroblasts Using Biopsy or Brush

AREG showed consistent differential expression in asthmatic lung epithelium and fibroblasts using biopsy or brush in publicly available bronchial epithelium datasets and confirmed *in vitro* (**Table 6**).

AREG mRNA Expression Was Significantly Different in Severe Asthmatic Compared to Severe Wheezing Children Only

In order to explore the correlation of AREG mRNA in wheezing in asthmatic vs. non-asthmatic children, (GSE123750) gene set was explored. AREG mRNA expression in whole blood of children with non-severe and severe wheezes was compared to non-severe and severe asthmatics. As shown in **Figure 7A**, AREG mRNA expression was only significantly higher in severe asthmatic compared to severe wheezing children ($p = 0.03$). However, there was no significant difference in the gene expression of AREG between non-severe and severe asthmatic, indicating it is asthma specific markers.

AREG mRNA Expression in Whole Blood of Eosinophilic Asthma Was Significantly Lower Compared to Non-eosinophilic

In order to explore the correlation of AREG mRNA to the eosinophilic phenotype of asthma, (GSE137394) gene set was, as shown in **Figure 7B**. AREG was significantly lower in eosinophilic asthmatics ($p = 0.004$). This indicates that AREG can identify a non-eosinophilic subtype of a severe asthma phenotype.

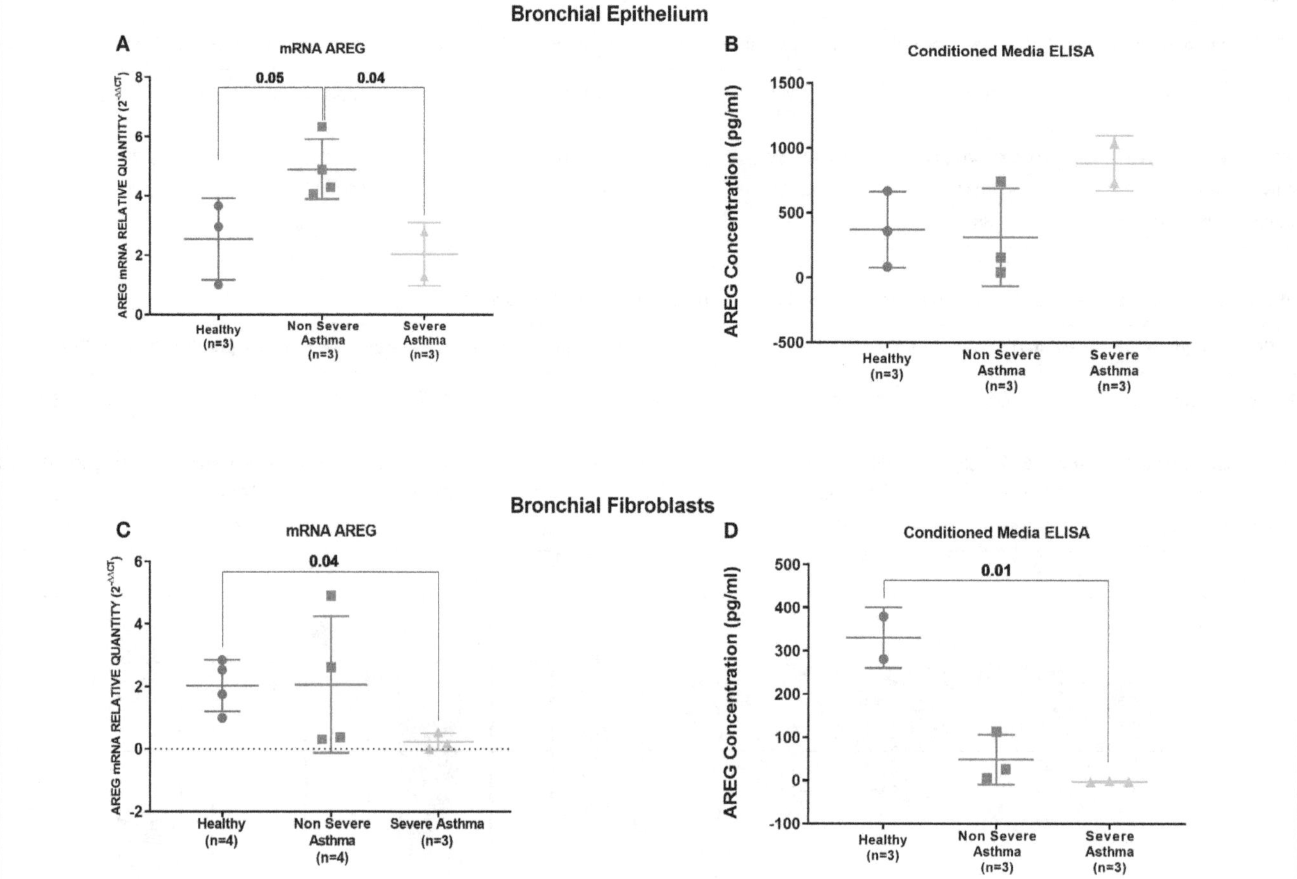

FIGURE 5 | AREG mRNA and secreted protein in bronchial epithelium cells and fibroblasts of healthy, non-severe, and severe asthmatic individuals. Assessment of AREG in asthmatic bronchial epithelium compared to the healthy epithelium on the **(A)** mRNA level measured by qRT-PCR, **(B)** secreted AREG protein levels by ELISA. Similarly, AREG was assessed in asthmatic fibroblasts compared to the healthy fibroblasts for the **(C)** AREG mRNA levels by qRT-PCR and **(D)** secreted AREG protein levels by ELISA.

PBMCs of Asthmatic Patients During Exacerbation Phase Express Higher AREG Compared to Convalescent Phase

GSE16032 dataset was chosen to identify the differential expression of the selected genes in PBMCs taken from asthmatic patients during the acute/exacerbation phase and the convalescent phase, as shown in **Figure 7C**. Interestingly, AREG was upregulated in the acute/exacerbation phase of asthma and returned back to the basal level when the attack subsides. This highlights the possible use of AREG as a marker for this specific disease phase.

SUMMARY IN BLOOD

Since, PBMCs mRNA expression was associated with asthma control score and AREG saliva mRNA was upregulated in severe asthma compared to non-severe asthmatics, we decided to explore its dynamics to understand its role in initiating and progression of the disease. AREG mRNA in the blood of drug naïve asthmatics compared to healthy, can differentiate severe asthmatic wheezes from others, can differentiate eosinophilic from non-eosinophilic, can differentiate acute attacks from convalescent-phase, and its expression was not affected by viruses (**Table 7**).

AREG Has Never been Linked to SNPs in Asthma

Genome-wide association studies (GWASs) of asthma have identified many risk alleles and loci that can be a potential source for diagnostic biomarkers. NHGRI-EBI GWAS Catalog was explored to identify 1,174 SNPs with the strongest Asthma-related SNP-risk allele. Interestingly, none of these SNPs were reported in AREG.

Severe Asthmatics Epithelium and Blood That Showed Higher AREG Expression Showed Different Immune Cells Populations Than Healthy Controls

We investigated if immune cell populations are different between asthmatic and healthy controls using the transcriptomic expression of the bronchial epithelium to predict the cell type and their state of activation. CIBERSORT tool, a digital cytometry

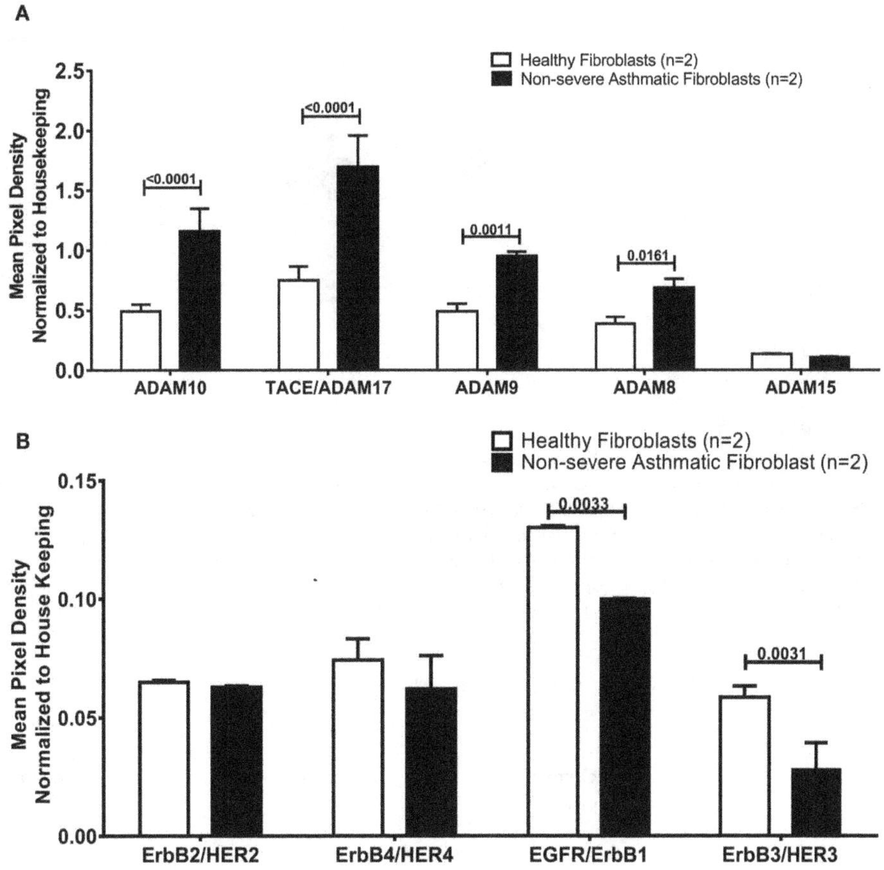

FIGURE 6 | Levels of soluble receptors shed in the conditioned media of healthy and non-severe asthmatic fibroblasts using non-hematopoietic and the common analytes array. **(A)** Protein expression of AREG shredders: ADAM 8, 9, 10, 15, and 17 in non-severe asthmatic fibroblasts compared to healthy fibroblasts. **(B)** Protein expression of shed ErbBI-4/HER1-4 in non-severe asthmatic fibroblasts compared to healthy fibroblasts.

TABLE 6 | Summary of *in silico* and *in vitro* analysis of AREG mRNA expression in different settings of asthma.

Genes	Bronchial epithelium		Bronchial fibroblasts		Biopsy vs. brush		OS = Oral Steroids	Th2 high	Th2 low
	In silico	*In vitro*	*In silico*	*In vitro*	Healthy	Asthma			
AREG	UP	UP	UP (the dataset available was with no details on severity)	Down in severe asthma	Both	-	-	-	-

that can determine cell type abundance and expression from bulk tissues (40), was used for that purpose. We used CIBERSORT tool on Bronchial epithelium transcriptomic data of (GSE64913 and GSE67472) datasets and blood transcriptomic dataset (GSE69683) of a well-characterized and a large cohort of patients with different asthma severity compared to healthy controls to estimate the percentage of the immune cells (**Figure 8**).

Bronchial Epithelium of Severe Asthmatic With Higher AREG mRNA Expression Showed a Lower Percentage of Gamma Delta (γδ) T and T Regulatory Cells but Higher Percentage of Neutrophils

In severe asthmatic bronchial epithelium with higher AREG mRNA expression, the percentage of infiltrating Gamma Delta (γδ) T and Regulatory T cells was lower than healthy controls, while there was an increase in the percentage of neutrophils (**Figure 8**).

Peripheral Blood of Severe Asthmatics Showed a Higher Percentage of Eosinophils, Neutrophils and Activated NK Cells Compared to Healthy Controls

Estimating the immune cells population in the blood of a large cohort of asthmatic patients with different severities compared to healthy controls using the transcriptomics data from (GSE69683) dataset revealed a similar trend of cells abundance of that in bronchial epithelium in terms of neutrophils and macrophages. As shown in **Figure 9**, eosinophilia was more evident in severe asthmatic blood than in local bronchial epithelium. Severe

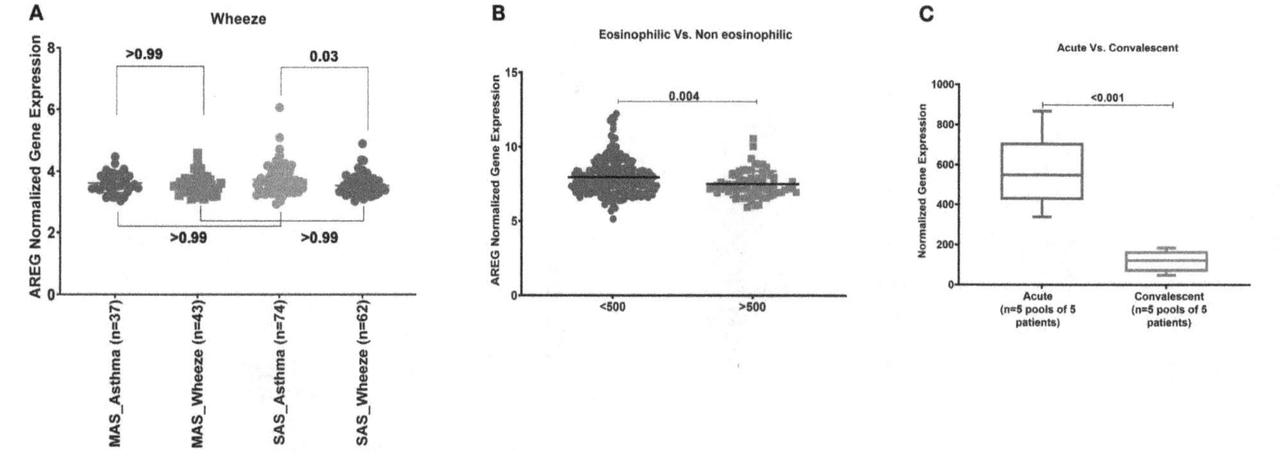

FIGURE 7 | (A) AREG normalized gene expression in whole blood of children with non-severe and severe wheezes were compared to non-severe and severe asthmatics extracted from the expression profile of publically available datasets (GSE123750), where non-severe asthmatic (MAS_Asthma) and severe asthmatic (SAS_Asthma) patients were compared to patients presented with non-severe wheezes (MAS_Wheeze) and severe wheezes (SAS_Wheeze). **(B)** Normalized gene expression of genes identified in whole blood of eosinophilic asthma (>500 cells) compared to non-eosinophilic (eosinophils count less than 500) extracted from the expression profile of publicly available datasets (GSE137394). **(C)** Normalized Gene Expression of Gènes Identified in PBMC5 taken from asthmatic patients during the acute/exacerbation phase and the convalescent phase extracted from the expression profile of publicly available datasets(6SE16032).

TABLE 7 | Summary of *in silico* analysis of the AREG genes in blood of asthmatic patients in different settings compared to healthy controls.

Genes	Whole blood				
	Asthma	Asthma wheezes	Eosinophilic	Acute	Viral
AREG	–	UP	Down	UP	–

AREG expression in whole blood of asthmatics in different phenotypes, in asthmatic with wheezes vs. non-asthmatics wheezers, in eosinophilic asthmatic vs. non-eosinophilic, in acute vs. convalescent (acute) and during viral infection.

asthmatic patients showed a higher percentage of eosinophils in their blood than healthy controls ($p = 0.02$). However, the percentages of monocytes and macrophages percentages were not statistically different between the groups. Surprisingly, memory B cells showed a significant difference in severe asthmatics compared to non-severe asthmatics ($p = 0.04$) and healthy controls ($p < 0.01$).

Interestingly, peripheral neutrophilia and activated NK was consistent with airway findings. Blood neutrophils and activated NK percentages were higher in severe asthmatics compared to non-severe asthmatics and healthy controls ($p < 0.05$).

DISCUSSION

To our knowledge, no studies used saliva, while very few studies used blood levels to discover markers related to asthma pathogenesis. This is the first study to investigate AREG blood and saliva expression levels and associate them to asthma. Other studies focused on AREG expression in sputum (17), damaged bronchial epithelium (41), fibroblasts (42), smooth muscle cells (43, 44) from bronchial biopsies and hematopoietic cells such as eosinophils (19), and basophils (45) in asthma and allergic conditions.

As illustrated in **Figures 1**, **2**, our results showed that AREG plasma and saliva levels were higher in asthmatic patients compared to healthy controls. AREG plasma level was significantly different between healthy and non-severe asthmatic ($p < 0.0001$).

Currently, in asthma research, there is a growing interest in replacing the available invasive bronchoscopy sampling and sputum induction with less invasive options like blood, urine, and exhaled gas biomarkers (4). These biomarkers can aid in a personalized and targeted approach to manage asthmatic patients, especially those with severe refractory asthma (46).

Our results confirmed that AREG level in plasma and saliva are simple, minimally invasive tools that can be used as biomarkers to assess asthma pathogenesis. Salivary marker measurements of various diseases is a new concept and currently is carried out mostly in head and neck cancers (47) and oral diseases (48). However, these assays are mostly DNA based. More recently, a predictive genetic assay measuring salivary mRNA was used to predict the onset of esophageal cancer (patent no: WO2017137427A1). As saliva sampling is non-invasive and is easy to collect, it represents an attractive tool for measuring asthma biomarkers (25).

This promising discriminating power of our results can be an additional bedside marker to help the managing physician in

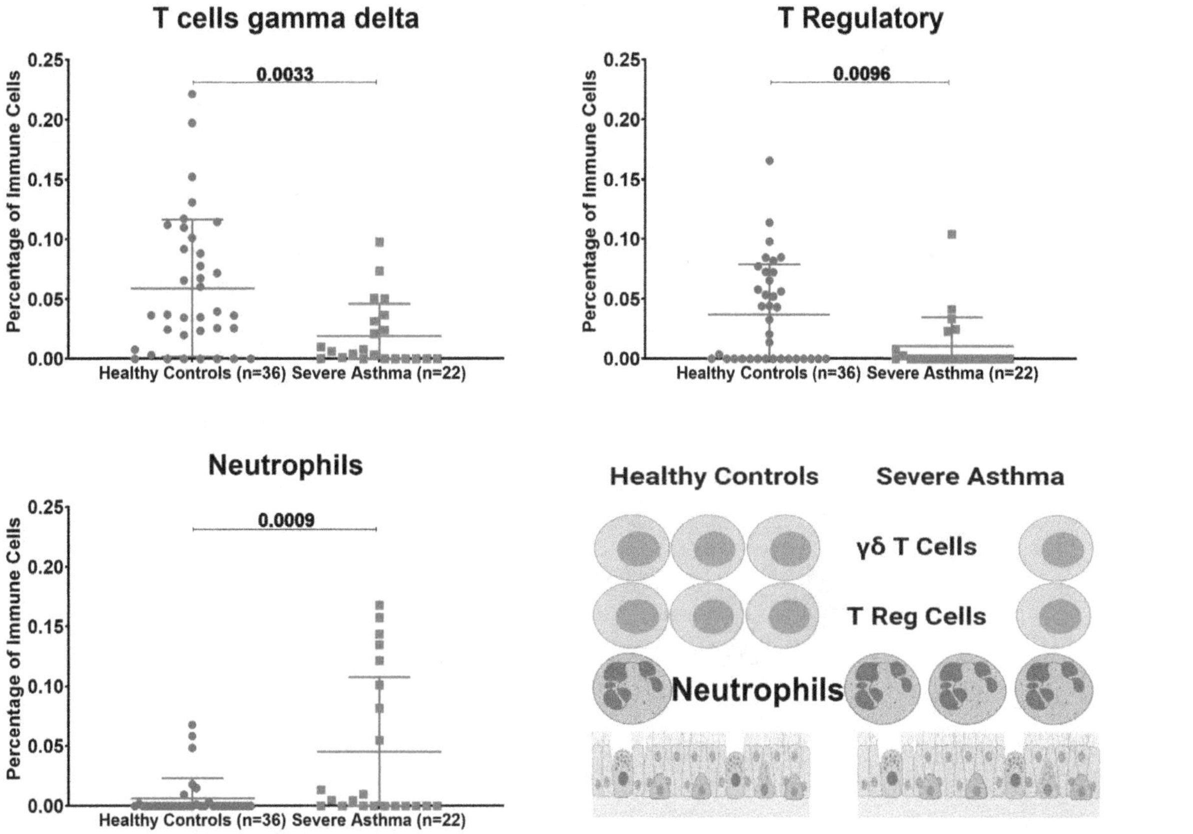

FIGURE 8 | Estimating immune cells populations in the bronchial epithelium of (c3SE64913) dataset in healthy controls ($n = 36$) compared to severe asthmatics ($n = 22$). Bronchial epithelium genes expression was loaded to CIBERSORT *in silico* flow cytometry.

diagnosing early stages of asthma with borderline clinical criteria. As for plasma, AREG saliva level was not able to differentiate between different asthma severity indicating its association with asthma as a disease; this might be explained by the limitation of the sample size and the effect of aggressive asthma medication on AREG levels in severe asthmatics.

Determining the presence of eosinophilic inflammation, or high Th2 cytokines phenotype is essential for patient stratification for targeted asthma therapy (49). Currently, peripheral blood eosinophil count is considered as a surrogate marker for eosinophilic inflammation of the airways (50); hence, finding a new reliable biomarker to predict eosinophilic asthma is needed (4). Therefore, correlating AREG expression with other pathological parameters, specifically those related to eosinophilic inflammation or high Th2 cytokines phenotype is essential.

Our results showed that AREG protein level in asthmatic patients' plasma and saliva correlate with clinical allergic phenotypes such as allergic rhinitis and atopy. Patients with a history of allergic rhinitis showed specifically a higher plasma AREG level compared to those with no history of allergic rhinitis. Allergic rhinitis is a common comorbidity of asthma and contributes to asthma severity (51) and poor asthma control (52). Asthma and allergic rhinitis share similar local and systemic eosinophil inflammation (53). AREG was shown to be secreted by eosinophils to participate in some physiological and pathological conditions *in vivo* (19). Asthma specific memory Th2 cells were shown to induce AREG to reprogram eosinophils to produce osteopontin leading to enhanced airway fibrosis (20).

On the other hand, AREG protein level in plasma correlates with the level of periostin, a known marker for Th2 high asthma phenotype (54), which can predict airway eosinophilia in patients with severe asthma (55). Periostin was found to be involved in atopic conditions such as dermatitis, rhinitis/rhinosinusitis, allergic skin inflammations; and its upregulation was shown to induce extracellular matrix (ECM) tissue remodeling (56). Beside eosinophils and mast cells, increased levels of periostin have also been detected in relation to neutrophils (56). On the other hand, periostin, was shown to play a vital role in chemokines induction to recruit neutrophils and macrophages that participate in pulmonary fibrosis in mouse model (57). Positive correlation between AREG and periostin might augment the role of neutrophils in non-eosinophilic severe asthma.

Of note, plasma AREG levels correlated positively with neutrophil levels in patients' blood. It is known that neutrophilia correlates with asthma that is refractory to the mainstay of asthma treatment (corticosteroids) (58). It was shown that during epithelial damage and repair, neutrophils enhance AREG production by epithelial cells to promote tissue repair (59). It can be suggested that patients with high circulating AREG might

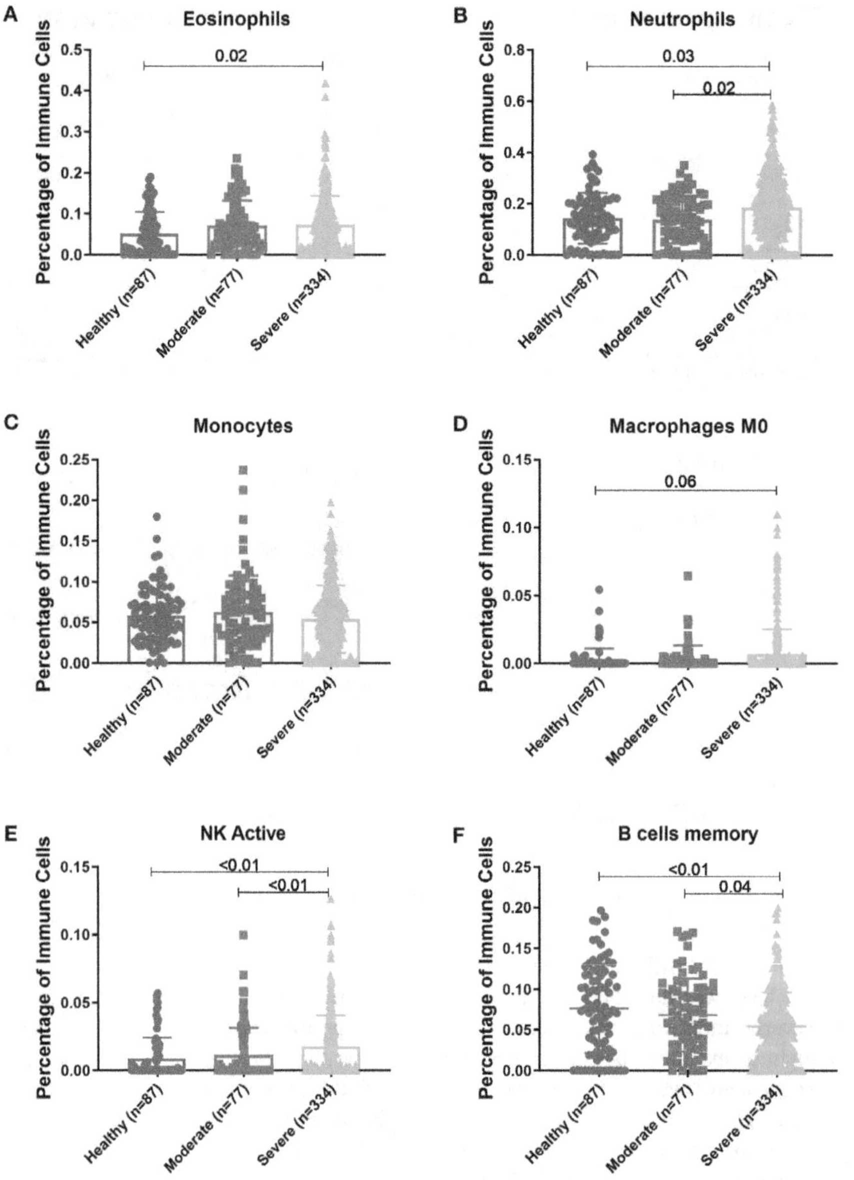

FIGURE 9 | Estimating immune cells populations in blood of (GSE69683) dataset to compare healthy controls ($n = 87$), non-severe asthma ($n = 77$), and severe asthmatics ($n = 334$). Blood genes expression was loaded to CIBERSORT *in silico* flow cytometry and immune cells which showed significant differences between the groups are shown. **(A)** Eosinophils, **(B)** Neutrophils, **(C)** Monocytes, **(D)** Macrophages M0, **(E)** NK active, and **(F)** B cells memory.

be in need of that level to be used for the massive tissue repair process ongoing during asthma.

A non-allergic asthmatic is a non-sensitized individual who can develop eosinophilic inflammation without exposure to an allergen through the activation of ILC2 cells that do not need allergen-specific IgE (22). Non-allergic patients may have innate immunity or neutrophilic airway inflammation independent of Th2 cells (27). Triggers of asthma in non-allergic patients can vary from external triggers like viral infections, cigarette smoke, diesel particles, and ozone to patient's intrinsic factors like stress, exercise, and obesity (1).

The type and quantity of inflammatory cells in the airway of asthma is an attractive research area now as it can guide the selection of biological treatment (60). Differentiating neutrophilic asthma (usually characterized by acute severe asthma exacerbations and steroid-resistant) from the eosinophilic phenotype is very important as the later phenotype can respond to corticosteroids and targeted therapies (61).

During acute lung injury, AREG was shown to suppress ICAM-1 expression and neutrophil accumulation (62). However, if neutrophils infiltration occurs, their elastase can promote myofibroblast differentiation that ends up with lung fibrosis; thus, AREG can limit fibrosis by limiting neutrophil arrival earlier in inflammation (63). This model is opposite to the skin model of psoriasis, where AREG enhanced the transmigration of human neutrophils through epithelial cell monolayers (64).

Our results showed that in severe asthmatic bronchial epithelium, the percentage of infiltrating Gamma Delta (γδ) T and Regulatory T cells was lower than in those of healthy controls. The high content of neutrophils in severe asthmatic bronchial epithelium compared to healthy controls matches the decrease in γδ T and Tregs as it might indicate more inflammatory consequences of lack of the primary tolerogenic and regulators of an immune response.

Estimating the immune cells population in the blood of a large cohort of asthmatic patients with different severities compared to healthy controls revealed a similar trend of cells abundance of that in bronchial epithelium in terms of neutrophils and macrophages. Eosinophilia was more evident in severe asthmatic blood than in local bronchial epithelium.

Interestingly, peripheral neutrophilia was consistent with airway neutrophilia. Increased local airway neutrophils count in asthma in neutrophilic asthma is associated with steroid resistance, suggesting that the neutrophil plays a role in asthma pathophysiology (65). Increased airway neutrophils in severe asthma and Th2 low phenotype might indicate specific endotype of asthma that share neutrophilia and eosinophilia but not Th2-high phenotype. In response to allergens, activation of LPS receptor TLR4 on lung epithelial cells can stimulate CXCL8 chemokine secretion to recruit neutrophil to the lung in association with increased eosinophilic inflammation, IgE, Th2 cytokines and mucus secretion (66). TLR signaling activation during the sensitization phase recruit neutrophils and inflammatory monocytes, to attenuate allergic symptoms by promoting the Th1-associated cytokines (67).

High levels of IL17 are linked to both eosinophils and neutrophils infiltrates in the airways of severe asthmatics (68). In neutrophilic asthma, Th17 cells released interleukins can recruit macrophages, and lymphocytes alongside neutrophils (69). Despite being glucocorticoid sensitive in some autoimmune diseases, Th17 cells are glucocorticoid resistant in asthma (70).

During allergen exposure, the first immune cells arriving the airways are the neutrophils that usually have a short life before it undergoes apoptosis, except in severe asthmatics who showed defective neutrophil apoptosis and/or clearance (71).

Another interesting finding was the correlation between plasma AREG level and the use of Montelukast sodium (Singulair); a selective and orally active leukotriene receptor antagonist that inhibits the cysteinyl leukotriene CysLT1 receptor (72). Our results showed that asthmatic patients who are on regular Singulair treatment have a higher level of AREG in their plasma compared to those who are not using Singulair. CysLTs as a potent contractile agonist of airways smooth muscles can stimulate their amphiregulin release and enhance their proliferation (73). Moreover, cysteinyl leukotriene was recently found to activate human ILC2s to secrete amphiregulin (72). This can have an important translational impact on patients' stratifications and appropriate drug selection.

Immunohistochemistry staining of bronchial biopsies showed that AREG staining intensity was higher in non-severe mild asthmatic epithelium when compared to healthy controls (**Figure 4**). These findings confirm the role of AREG in the sequence of events in asthma pathogenesis involving both bronchial epithelial cells and fibroblasts. Our results agree with previous studies where AREG level in sputum was associated with asthma severity (17) and was found to be increased in airways during an acute asthma attack (18).

Our results confirmed that AREG is locally upregulated in the asthmatic lung. AREG is constitutively expressed during development and physiologic processes but rapidly upregulated in damaged epithelium to restore tissue integrity (15). Asthmatic bronchial epithelial cells had higher AREG mRNA expression and protein levels than healthy ones but no significant difference in the secreted levels. However, AREG secretion in conditioned media was higher in bronchial epithelial cells compared to their asthma severity matching bronchial fibroblasts confirming that epithelial cells are the primary source of local lung cells in asthma (**Figure 5**). The insignificant difference between AREG secreted levels of healthy and asthmatic epithelial cells despite the overexpression of its mRNA levels can be explained by the complex regulatory network controlling AREG synthesis and secretion.

AREG was reported to show the ability to restore tissue integrity (15), through the mechanism of shedding to bind to autocrine or paracrine EGF receptor family. AREG ectodomain shedding is mediated by ADAM17 (74) and under some conditions ADAM8 and ADAM15 that are called sheddases (75). Most of these enzymes are secreted proteins (76). This processing adds another layer of regulation of AREG (77). Our results showed that asthmatic fibroblasts showed higher shedding of AREG ectoderm shedders (ADAM8, 9, 10, and 17). This goes with previous reports that in asthmatics airways, ADAMs, and ADAMTSs and their inhibitors are involved in asthma development (76).

As illustrated in **Figure 6A**, asthmatic fibroblasts showed higher shedding of AREG ectoderm shedders (ADAM8, 9, 10, and 17). The loss of the shedders can decrease the amount of the shed protein in the conditioned media. These shedders can still act on the adjacent cells to shed more AREG and increase its soluble forms. ADAM8 plays a proinflammatory role in asthma airway inflammation, and ADAM8-deficient mice failed to develop an experimental model of asthma (78). Nevertheless, there is a controversy about its function in asthma, ADAM8 can induce or inhibit the transmigration of leukocytes in airway inflammation of asthma (79). Also, ADAM8 was shown to mediate the infiltration of eosinophils and Th2 lymphocytes to airways of asthmatic patients (80). On the other hand, some reports showed that ADAM8 facilitates neutrophil migration to the airways in severe asthma and COPD (81).

Moreover, as illustrated in **Figure 6B**, our results revealed that non-severe asthmatic fibroblasts shed less ErbB1 and ErbB3 EGFR receptors compared to healthy ones. The indispensability of ErbB1/EGFR for AREG-mediated responses was previously reported in lung structural cells, and it was suggested that ErbB1-ErbB3 and/or ErbB2-ErbB3 heterodimers are involved in the AREG-mediated responses (82). AREG soluble form can act in an autocrine fashion to increase the stability and accumulation of its active EGFR (83). Alternatively, it was recently documented that in stressed cells (like the case of asthma), mRNA concentrations can transiently escalate in pulse-like pattern and return to basal level, while protein concentrations establish a new steady-state (84). It was reported that upon stimulation, cells would release soluble ADAM17 in exosomes to reach more distant substrates or cells (85).

AREG can activate intracellular signaling network that controls cell survival, proliferation, and motility (13). AREG binding to EGFR induced EGFR homodimerization or heterodimerization with ErbB2, ErbB3, and ErbB4 to trigger intracellular signals (13). The membrane proteoglycan, CD44, is a cofactor for the interaction of AREG with EGFR (86).

In contrast to most of EGFR ligands, AREG did not generate nuclear translocation of EGFR but showed markedly different patterns of EGFR internalization and trafficking (87). The ubiquitination of pro-AREG accelerated its half-life on the cell surface with the subsequent trafficking to intracellular organelles (88). The remaining cytoplasmic carboxy-terminal domain of AREG plays a vital role in regulating autocrine growth through the EGFR (77). The released AREG can circulate in a recently discovered type of extracellular nanoparticle called exomeres can modulate EGFR trafficking and prolong EGFR downstream signaling in recipient cells (89). Cells lacking AREG showed growth arrest that is restored by proAREG and AREG-CTD (90). AREG has "geographically" specific and unique intracellular signaling pathways that can determine whether cells grow or differentiate (77).

Helminth-induced type 2 inflammation enhance EGFR expression and AREG production under the effect of IL33 cytokine; later, AREG-EGFR activation will stimulate IL13 secretion needed for host resistance (15, 91). The upregulated AREG can reprogram infiltrating eosinophils to an inflammatory phenotype that produces an excess of profibrotic immunomodulatory protein osteopontin (20). IL5 stimulated eosinophils can contribute to the progression of airway remodeling, through the production of AREG (19).

There is translational evidence indicating upregulated expression of EGFR appears in the airways of asthmatics and activity of this signaling pathway is enhanced in relation to asthma severity (92). Specifically mucus hypersecretion is induced by EGFR activation to promote goblet-cell metaplasia in severe asthma (12). EGFR signaling of the asthmatic epithelium has been reported to be increased in relation to disease severity through the capacity of driving neutrophil fate and function through elaboration of neutrophil-specific factors in relation to disease severity (28). Others have reported a strong correlation between EGFR expression and neutrophilic-specific chemokines in the epithelium of patients with severe asthma (93, 94).

The high AREG expression in blood and saliva of asthmatic patients can be linked to the local increase in AREG expression secreted by structural cells into the extracellular spaces. AREG will then enter the systemic circulation due to the increased microvascular permeability during tissue inflammation (95, 96). The increased AREG blood levels will most likely diffuse into saliva and hence used as a reflective marker for upregulated plasma levels (31).

One limitation of our study is the small size of the participants, although we tried to include all patients who fulfill the criteria, many of the patients refused to participate in the study. Since asthma is a heterogeneous disease, having larger cohort can be more informative about the applicability of the new biomarkers. The number of females in each group was higher than males, previous reports showed that mice males differentially produce and utilize AREG in their lungs in response to viral infections, with greater EGFR internalization and was linked to the combinational effect of testosterone and AREG, that can improve the repair and recovery of damaged tissue in males compared with females (97). On the other hand circulating AREG was undetectable with no significant variation during the menstrual cycle (98). On the other hand, AREG mRNA expression was peaked in the pregnant females and correlated positively with number of good-quality embryos under the induction by diverse luteinizing hormones (99).

In conclusion, our findings suggest circulating AREG expression level can be a reliable, non-invasive, and cost-effective biomarker that can provide additional discriminating power to the available clinical and laboratory tests of asthma.

AUTHOR CONTRIBUTIONS

MH, RHam, and QH: conception and design of the study, data and sample collection, analysis and interpretation of data, and writing the manuscript. BM and RHam: conception and design of the study, clinical samples selections, and collections. MH and IH: *in silico* validation and analysis. SA, IH, and RHal: reviewing the manuscript. RO: primary lung cell lines and bronchial biopsies provision. NE, MH, and RHam: data collection and interpretation of ELISA and reviewing the manuscript. RR and MH: sample collections and cell lines maintenance. TV and LS: samples and data collections. All authors contributed to the article and approved the submitted version.

REFERENCES

1. Kim HY, DeKruyff RH, Umetsu DT. The many paths to asthma: phenotype shaped by innate and adaptive immunity. *Nat Immunol.* (2010) 11:577–84. doi: 10.1038/ni.1892
2. Thomsen SF. Genetics of asthma: an introduction for the clinician. *Eur Clin Respir J.* (2015) 2. doi: 10.3402/ecrj.v2.24643
3. Thomas M. Why aren't we doing better in asthma: time for personalised medicine? *NPJ Prim Care Respir Med.* (2015) 25:15004. doi: 10.1038/npjpcrm.2015.4
4. Wan XC, Woodruff PG. Biomarkers in severe asthma. *Immunol Allergy Clin North Am.* (2016) 36:547–57. doi: 10.1016/j.iac.2016.03.004
5. Byrnes SA, Weigl BH. Selecting analytical biomarkers for diagnostic applications: a first principles approach. *Expert Rev Mol Diagn.* (2018) 18:19–26. doi: 10.1080/14737159.2018.1412258
6. Chiappori A, De Ferrari L, Folli C, Mauri P, Riccio AM, Canonica GW. Biomarkers and severe asthma: a critical appraisal. *Clin Mol Allergy.* (2015) 13:20. doi: 10.1186/s12948-015-0027-7
7. Dawson SJ, Tsui DW, Murtaza M, Biggs H, Rueda OM, Chin SF, et al. Analysis

of circulating tumor DNA to monitor metastatic breast cancer. *N Engl J Med.* (2013) 368:1199–209. doi: 10.1056/NEJMoa1213261
8. Yoshizawa JM, Schafer CA, Schafer JJ, Farrell JJ, Paster BJ, Wong DTW. Salivary biomarkers: toward future clinical and diagnostic utilities. *Clin Microbiol Rev.* (2013) 26:781–91. doi: 10.1128/CMR.00021-13
9. Wee P, Wang Z. Epidermal growth factor receptor cell proliferation signaling pathways. *Cancers.* (2017) 9:52. doi: 10.3390/cancers9050052
10. Vallath S, Hynds RE, Succony L, Janes SM, Giangreco A. Targeting EGFR signalling in chronic lung disease: therapeutic challenges and opportunities. *Eur Respir J.* (2014) 44:513–22. doi: 10.1183/09031936.00146413
11. Acciani TH, Suzuki T, Trapnell BC, Le Cras TD. Epidermal growth factor receptor signalling regulates granulocyte-macrophage colony-stimulating factor production by airway epithelial cells and established allergic airway disease. *Clin Exp Allergy.* (2016) 46:317–28. doi: 10.1111/cea.12612
12. Le Cras TD, Acciani TH, Mushaben EM, Kramer EL, Pastura PA, Hardie WD, et al. Epithelial EGF receptor signaling mediates airway hyperreactivity and remodeling in a mouse model of chronic asthma. *Am J Physiol Lung Cell Mol Physiol.* (2011) 300:L414–21. doi: 10.1152/ajplung.00346.2010
13. Berasain C, Avila MA. Amphiregulin. *Semin Cell Dev Biol.* (2014) 28:31–41. doi: 10.1016/j.semcdb.2014.01.005
14. Amin K, Yaqoob U, Schultz B, Vaughn BP, Khoruts A, Howard JR, et al. Amphiregulin in intestinal acute graft-versus-host disease: a possible diagnostic and prognostic aid. *Mod Pathol.* (2019) 32:560–7. doi: 10.1038/s41379-018-0170-z
15. Zaiss DMW, Gause WC, Osborne LC, Artis D. Emerging functions of amphiregulin in orchestrating immunity, inflammation, and tissue repair. *Immunity.* (2015) 42:216–26. doi: 10.1016/j.immuni.2015.01.020
16. Manzo ND, Foster WM, Stripp BR. Amphiregulin-dependent mucous cell metaplasia in a model of nonallergic lung injury. *Am J Respir Cell Mol Biol.* (2012) 47:349–57. doi: 10.1165/rcmb.2011-0257OC
17. Kim KW, Jee HM, Park YH, Choi BS, Sohn MH, Kim KE. Relationship between amphiregulin and airway inflammation in children with asthma and eosinophilic bronchitis. *Chest.* (2009) 136:805–10. doi: 10.1378/chest.08-2972
18. Takamasu T, Enomoto Y, Orihara K, Matsuda A, Gon Y, Saito H, et al. An acute asthma attack induces tissue remodeling by hypersecretion of epidermal growth factor (egf) and amphiregulin (areg) in the airway. *J Allergy Clin Immunol.* (2011) 127:AB59. doi: 10.1016/j.jaci.2010.12.245
19. Matsumoto K, Fukuda S, Nakamura Y, Saito H. Amphiregulin production by human eosinophils. *Int Arch Allergy Immunol.* (2009) 149(Suppl. 1):39–44. doi: 10.1159/000210652
20. Morimoto Y, Hirahara K, Kiuchi M, Wada T, Ichikawa T, Kanno T, et al. Amphiregulin-producing pathogenic memory T helper 2 cells instruct eosinophils to secrete osteopontin and facilitate airway fibrosis. *Immunity.* (2018) 49:134–50.e6. doi: 10.1016/j.immuni.2018.04.023
21. Buhl R, Humbert M, Bjermer L, Chanez P, Heaney Liam G, Pavord I, et al. Severe eosinophilic asthma: a roadmap to consensus. *Eur Respir J.* (2017) 49:1700634. doi: 10.1183/13993003.00634-2017
22. Yamauchi K, Ogasawara M. The role of histamine in the pathophysiology of asthma and the clinical efficacy of antihistamines in asthma therapy. *Int J Mol Sci.* (2019) 20:1733. doi: 10.3390/ijms20071733
23. Kim HY, Umetsu DT, Dekruyff RH. Innate lymphoid cells in asthma: will they take your breath away? *Eur J Immunol.* (2016) 46:795–806. doi: 10.1002/eji.201444557
24. Monticelli LA, Sonnenberg GF, Abt MC, Alenghat T, Ziegler CG, Doering TA, et al. Innate lymphoid cells promote lung-tissue homeostasis after infection with influenza virus. *Nat Immunol.* (2011) 12:1045–54. doi: 10.1038/ni.2131
25. Minutti CM, Modak RV, Macdonald F, Li F, Smyth DJ, Dorward DA, et al. A macrophage-pericyte axis directs tissue restoration via amphiregulin-induced transforming growth factor beta activation. *Immunity.* (2019) 50:645–54e6. doi: 10.1016/j.immuni.2019.01.008
26. Xu Y, Meng C, Liu G, Yang D, Fu L, Zhang M, et al. Classically activated macrophages protect against lipopolysaccharide-induced acute lung injury by expressing amphiregulin in mice. *Anesthesiology.* (2016) 124:1086–99. doi: 10.1097/ALN.0000000000001026
27. Pasha MA, Patel G, Hopp R, Yang Q. Role of innate lymphoid cells in allergic diseases. *Allergy Asthma Proc.* (2019) 40:138–45. doi: 10.2500/aap.2019.40.4217
28. Uddin M, Lau LC, Seumois G, Vijayanand P, Staples KJ, Bagmane D, et al. EGF-induced bronchial epithelial cells drive neutrophil chemotactic and anti-apoptotic activity in asthma. *PLoS ONE.* (2013) 8:e72502. doi: 10.1371/journal.pone.0072502
29. Lourenço O, Fonseca AM, Taborda-Barata L. Human CD8$^+$ T cells in asthma: possible pathways and roles for NK-like subtypes. *Front Immunol.* (2016) 7:638. doi: 10.3389/fimmu.2016.00638
30. Geyer PE, Holdt LM, Teupser D, Mann M. Revisiting biomarker discovery by plasma proteomics. *Mol Syst Biol.* (2017) 13:942. doi: 10.15252/msb.20156297
31. Castagnola M, Scarano E, Passali GC, Messana I, Cabras T, Iavarone F, et al. Salivary biomarkers and proteomics: future diagnostic and clinical utilities. *Acta Otorhinolaryngol It.* (2017) 37:94–101. doi: 10.14639/0392-100X-1598
32. Koh GC-H, Pei-Chi Shek L, Kee J, Wee A, Ng V, Koh D. Saliva and serum eosinophil cationic protein in asthmatic children and adolescents with and without allergic sensitization. *J Asthma.* (2010) 47:61–5. doi: 10.3109/02770900903350499
33. Chung KF, Wenzel SE, Brozek JL, Bush A, Castro M, Sterk PJ, et al. International ERS/ATS guidelines on definition, evaluation and treatment of severe asthma. *Eur Respir J.* (2014) 43:343–73. doi: 10.1183/09031936.00202013
34. Dagur PK, McCoy JP Jr. Collection, storage, and preparation of human blood cells. *Curr Protoc Cytom.* (2015) 73:5.1.1–16. doi: 10.1002/0471142956.cy0501s73
35. Wang SW, Oh CK, Cho SH, Hu G, Martin R, Demissie-Sanders S, et al. Amphiregulin expression in human mast cells and its effect on the primary human lung fibroblasts. *J Allergy Clin Immunol.* (2005) 115:287–94. doi: 10.1016/j.jaci.2004.11.037
36. Schneider CA, Rasband WS, Eliceiri KW. NIH Image to ImageJ: 25 years of image analysis. *Nat Methods.* (2012) 9:671. doi: 10.1038/nmeth.2089
37. Szatmári T, Mundt F, Heidari-Hamedani G, Zong F, Ferolla E, Alexeyenko A, et al. Novel genes and pathways modulated by syndecan-1: implications for the proliferation and cell-cycle regulation of malignant mesothelioma cells. *PLoS ONE.* (2012) 7:e48091. doi: 10.1371/journal.pone.0048091
38. Hachim MY, Mahboub B, Hamid Q, Hamoudi R, editors. Identifying Asthma genetic signature patterns by mining Gene Expression BIG Datasets using Image Filtering Algorithms. In: *2019 IEEE International Conference on Imaging Systems and Techniques (IST).* Abu Dhabi (2019).
39. Chen B, Khodadoust MS, Liu CL, Newman AM, Alizadeh AA. Profiling tumor infiltrating immune cells with CIBERSORT. *Methods Mol Biol.* (2018) 1711:243–59. doi: 10.1007/978-1-4939-7493-1_12
40. Newman AM, Steen CB, Liu CL, Gentles AJ, Chaudhuri AA, Scherer F, et al. Determining cell type abundance and expression from bulk tissues with digital cytometry. *Nat Biotechnol.* (2019) 37:773–82. doi: 10.1038/s41587-019-0114-2
41. Lambrecht BN, Hammad H. The airway epithelium in asthma. *Nat Med.* (2012) 18:684. doi: 10.1038/nm.2737
42. Vermeer PD, Panko L, Karp P, Lee JH, Zabner J. Differentiation of human airway epithelia is dependent on erbB2. *Am J Physiol Lung Cell Mol Physiol.* (2006) 291:L175–80. doi: 10.1152/ajplung.00547.2005
43. Deacon K, Knox AJ. Human airway smooth muscle cells secrete amphiregulin via bradykinin/COX-2/PGE2, inducing COX-2, CXCL8, and VEGF expression in airway epithelial cells. *Am J Physiol Lung Cell Mol Physiol.* (2015) 309:L237–49. doi: 10.1152/ajplung.00390.2014
44. Hirota N, Risse P-A, Novali M, McGovern T, Al-Alwan L, McCuaig S, et al. Histamine may induce airway remodeling through release of epidermal growth factor receptor ligands from bronchial epithelial cells. *FASEB J.* (2012) 26:1704–16. doi: 10.1096/fj.11-197061
45. Qi Y, Operario DJ, Oberholzer CM, Kobie JJ, Looney RJ, Georas SN, et al. Human basophils express amphiregulin in response to T cell-derived IL-3. *J Allergy Clin Immunol.* (2010) 126:1260-6.e4. doi: 10.1016/j.jaci.2010.08.040
46. Kim H, Ellis AK, Fischer D, Noseworthy M, Olivenstein R, Chapman KR, et al. Asthma biomarkers in the age of biologics. *Allergy Asthma Clin Immunol.* (2017) 13:48. doi: 10.1186/s13223-017-0219-4

47. Nonaka T, Wong DTW. Liquid biopsy in head and neck cancer: promises and challenges. *J Dent Res.* (2018) 97:701–8. doi: 10.1177/0022034518762071
48. Roi A, Rusu LC, Roi CI, Luca RE, Boia S, Munteanu RI. A new approach for the diagnosis of systemic and oral diseases based on salivary biomolecules. *Dis Markers.* (2019) 2019:8761860. doi: 10.1155/2019/8761860
49. Bhakta NR, Woodruff PG. Human asthma phenotypes: from the clinic, to cytokines, and back again. *Immunol Rev.* (2011) 242:220–32. doi: 10.1111/j.1600-065X.2011.01032.x
50. Kostikas K, Brindicci C, Patalano F. Blood eosinophils as biomarkers to drive treatment choices in asthma and COPD. *Curr Drug Targets.* (2018) 19:1882–96. doi: 10.2174/1389450119666180212120012
51. Egan M, Bunyavanich S. Allergic rhinitis: the "Ghost Diagnosis" in patients with asthma. *Asthma Res Pract.* (2015) 1:8. doi: 10.1186/s40733-015-0008-0
52. de Groot EP, Nijkamp A, Duiverman EJ, Brand PLP. Allergic rhinitis is associated with poor asthma control in children with asthma. *Thorax.* (2012) 67:582–7. doi: 10.1136/thoraxjnl-2011-201168
53. Kämpe M, Stolt I, Lampinen M, Janson C, Stålenheim G, Carlson M. Patients with allergic rhinitis and allergic asthma share the same pattern of eosinophil and neutrophil degranulation after allergen challenge. *Clin Mol Allergy.* (2011) 9:3. doi: 10.1186/1476-7961-9-3
54. Jia G, Erickson RW, Choy DF, Mosesova S, Wu LC, Solberg OD, et al. Periostin is a systemic biomarker of eosinophilic airway inflammation in asthmatic patients. *J Allergy Clin Immunol.* (2012) 130:647–54e10. doi: 10.1016/j.jaci.2012.06.025
55. Noguchi T, Nakagome K, Kobayashi T, Uchida Y, Soma T, Nakamoto H, et al. Periostin upregulates the effector functions of eosinophils. *J Allergy Clin Immunol.* (2016) 138:1449–52e5. doi: 10.1016/j.jaci.2016.05.020
56. Li W, Gao P, Zhi Y, Xu W, Wu Y, Yin J, et al. Periostin: its role in asthma and its potential as a diagnostic or therapeutic target. *Respir Res.* (2015) 16:57. doi: 10.1186/s12931-015-0218-2
57. Uchida M, Shiraishi H, Ohta S, Arima K, Taniguchi K, Suzuki S, et al. Periostin, a matricellular protein, plays a role in the induction of chemokines in pulmonary fibrosis. *Am J Respir Cell Mol Biol.* (2012) 46:677–86. doi: 10.1165/rcmb.2011-0115OC
58. Ray A, Kolls JK. Neutrophilic inflammation in asthma and association with disease severity. *Trends Immunol.* (2017) 38:942–54. doi: 10.1016/j.it.2017.07.003
59. Chen F, Yang W, Huang X, Cao AT, Bilotta AJ, Xiao Y, et al. Neutrophils promote amphiregulin production in intestinal epithelial cells through TGF-beta and contribute to intestinal homeostasis. *J Immunol.* (2018) 201:2492–501. doi: 10.4049/jimmunol.1800003
60. Nishio T, Wakahara K, Suzuki Y, Nishio N, Majima S, Nakamura S, et al. Mixed cell type in airway inflammation is the dominant phenotype in asthma patients with severe chronic rhinosinusitis. *Allergol Int.* (2019) 68:515–20. doi: 10.1016/j.alit.2019.05.004
61. Pillai RA, Calhoun WJ. Introduction to asthma and phenotyping. In: Brasier AR, editor. *Heterogeneity in Asthma.* Boston, MA: Springer US (2014). p. 5–15.
62. Ogata-Suetsugu S, Yanagihara T, Hamada N, Ikeda-Harada C, Yokoyama T, Suzuki K, et al. Amphiregulin suppresses epithelial cell apoptosis in lipopolysaccharide-induced lung injury in mice. *Biochem Biophys Res Commun.* (2017) 484:422–8. doi: 10.1016/j.bbrc.2017.01.142
63. Gregory AD, Kliment CR, Metz HE, Kim KH, Kargl J, Agostini BA, et al. Neutrophil elastase promotes myofibroblast differentiation in lung fibrosis. *J Leukoc Biol.* (2015) 98:143–52. doi: 10.1189/jlb.3HI1014-493R
64. Chung E, Cook PW, Parkos CA, Park YK, Pittelkow MR, Coffey RJ. Amphiregulin causes functional downregulation of adherens junctions in psoriasis. *J Invest Dermatol.* (2005) 124:1134–40. doi: 10.1111/j.0022-202X.2005.23762.x
65. Jasper AE, McIver WJ, Sapey E, Walton GM. Understanding the role of neutrophils in chronic inflammatory airway disease. *F1000Res.* (2019) 8:F1000 Faculty Rev-557. doi: 10.12688/f1000research.18411.1
66. Radermecker C, Louis R, Bureau F, Marichal T. Role of neutrophils in allergic asthma. *Curr Opin Immunol.* (2018) 54:28–34. doi: 10.1016/j.coi.2018.05.006
67. Huang C, Wang J, Zheng X, Chen Y, Wei H, Sun R, et al. Activation of TLR signaling in sensitization-recruited inflammatory monocytes attenuates OVA-induced allergic asthma. *Front Immunol.* (2018) 9:2591. doi: 10.3389/fimmu.2018.02591
68. Morishima Y, Ano S, Ishii Y, Ohtsuka S, Matsuyama M, Kawaguchi M, et al. Th17-associated cytokines as a therapeutic target for steroid-insensitive asthma. *Clin Dev Immunol.* (2013) 2013:609395. doi: 10.1155/2013/609395
69. Wu X, Tian J, Wang S. Insight into non-pathogenic Th17 cells in autoimmune diseases. *Front Immunol.* (2018) 9:1112. doi: 10.3389/fimmu.2018.01112
70. Banuelos J, Cao Y, Shin SC, Lu NZ. Immunopathology alters Th17 cell glucocorticoid sensitivity. *Allergy.* (2017) 72:331–41. doi: 10.1111/all.13051
71. Uddin M, Nong G, Ward J, Seumois G, Prince LR, Wilson SJ, et al. Prosurvival activity for airway neutrophils in severe asthma. *Thorax.* (2010) 65:684–9. doi: 10.1136/thx.2009.120741
72. Salimi M, Stöger L, Liu W, Go S, Pavord I, Klenerman P, et al. Cysteinyl leukotriene E4 activates human group 2 innate lymphoid cells and enhances the effect of prostaglandin D2 and epithelial cytokines. *J Allergy Clin Immunol.* (2017) 140:1090–100.e11. doi: 10.1016/j.jaci.2016.12.958
73. Holgate ST, Peters-Golden M, Panettieri RA, Henderson WR Jr. Roles of cysteinyl leukotrienes in airway inflammation, smooth muscle function, and remodeling. *J Allergy Clin Immunol.* (2003) 111(1 Suppl.):S18–34; discussion S-6. doi: 10.1067/mai.2003.25
74. Kasina S, Scherle PA, Hall CL, Macoska JA. ADAM-mediated amphiregulin shedding and EGFR transactivation. *Cell Prolif.* (2009) 42:799–812. doi: 10.1111/j.1365-2184.2009.00645.x
75. Hosur V, Farley ML, Burzenski LM, Shultz LD, Wiles MV. ADAM17 is essential for ectodomain shedding of the EGF-receptor ligand amphiregulin. *FEBS Open Bio.* (2018) 8:702–10. doi: 10.1002/2211-5463.12407
76. Paulissen G, Rocks N, Quesada-Calvo F, Gosset P, Foidart JM, Noel A, et al. Expression of ADAMs and their inhibitors in sputum from patients with asthma. *Mol Med.* (2006) 12:171–9. doi: 10.2119/2006-00028.Paulissen
77. Seykora JT. Grabbing amphiregulin by the tail to better understand keratinocyte growth. *J Invest Dermatol.* (2010) 130:1966–8. doi: 10.1038/jid.2010.199
78. Naus S, Blanchet MR, Gossens K, Zaph C, Bartsch JW, McNagny KM, et al. The metalloprotease-disintegrin ADAM8 is essential for the development of experimental asthma. *Am J Respir Crit Care Med.* (2010) 181:1318–28. doi: 10.1164/rccm.200909-1396OC
79. Chen J, Jiang X, Duan Y, Long J, Bartsch JW, Deng L. ADAM8 in asthma. Friend or foe to airway inflammation? *Am J Respir Cell Mol Biol.* (2013) 49:875–84. doi: 10.1165/rcmb.2013-0168TR
80. Chen J, Deng L, Dreymuller D, Jiang X, Long J, Duan Y, et al. A novel peptide ADAM8 inhibitor attenuates bronchial hyperresponsiveness and Th2 cytokine mediated inflammation of murine asthmatic models. *Sci Rep.* (2016) 6:30451. doi: 10.1038/srep30451
81. Oreo KM, Gibson PG, Simpson JL, Wood LG, McDonald VM, Baines KJ. Sputum ADAM8 expression is increased in severe asthma and COPD. *Clin Exp Allergy.* (2014) 44:342–52. doi: 10.1111/cea.12223
82. Enomoto Y, Orihara K, Takamasu T, Matsuda A, Gon Y, Saito H, et al. Tissue remodeling induced by hypersecreted epidermal growth factor and amphiregulin in the airway after an acute asthma attack. *J Allergy Clin Immunol.* (2009) 124:913–20.e7. doi: 10.1016/j.jaci.2009.08.044
83. Kappler CS, Guest ST, Irish JC, Garrett-Mayer E, Kratche Z, Wilson RC, et al. Oncogenic signaling in amphiregulin and EGFR-expressing PTEN-null human breast cancer. *Mol Oncol.* (2015) 9:527–43. doi: 10.1016/j.molonc.2014.10.006
84. Cheng Z, Teo G, Krueger S, Rock TM, Koh HW, Choi H, et al. Differential dynamics of the mammalian mRNA and protein expression response to misfolding stress. *Mol Syst Biol.* (2016) 12:855. doi: 10.15252/msb.20156423
85. Groth E, Pruessmeyer J, Babendreyer A, Schumacher J, Pasqualon T, Dreymueller D, et al. Stimulated release and functional activity of surface expressed metalloproteinase ADAM17 in exosomes. *Biochim Biophy Acta.* (2016) 1863:2795–808. doi: 10.1016/j.bbamcr.2016.09.002
86. Nylander N, Smith LT, Underwood RA, Piepkorn M. Topography of amphiregulin expression in cultured human keratinocytes: colocalization with the epidermal growth factor receptor and CD44. *In Vitro Cell Dev Biol Anim.* (1998) 34:182–8. doi: 10.1007/s11626-998-0103-0
87. Faria J, de Andrade C, Goes AM, Rodrigues MA, Gomes DA. Effects of different ligands on epidermal growth factor receptor

(EGFR) nuclear translocation. *Biochem Biophys Res Commun.* (2016) 478:39–45. doi: 10.1016/j.bbrc.2016.07.097

88. Fukuda S, Nishida-Fukuda H, Nakayama H, Inoue H, Higashiyama S. Monoubiquitination of pro-amphiregulin regulates its endocytosis and ectodomain shedding. *Biochem Biophys Res Commun.* (2012) 420:315–20. doi: 10.1016/j.bbrc.2012.02.156
89. Zhang Q, Higginbotham JN, Jeppesen DK, Yang YP, Li W, McKinley ET, et al. Transfer of functional cargo in exomeres. *Cell Rep.* (2019) 27:940–54e6. doi: 10.1016/j.celrep.2019.01.009
90. Stoll SW, Stuart PE, Lambert S, Gandarillas A, Rittié L, Johnston A, et al. Membrane-tethered intracellular domain of amphiregulin promotes keratinocyte proliferation. *J Invest Dermatol.* (2016) 136:444–52. doi: 10.1016/j.jid.2015.10.061
91. Minutti CM, Drube S, Blair N, Schwartz C, McCrae JC, McKenzie AN, et al. Epidermal growth factor receptor expression licenses type-2 helper T cells to function in a T cell receptor-independent Fashion. *Immunity.* (2017) 47:710-22e6. doi: 10.1016/j.immuni.2017.09.013
92. El-Hashim AZ, Khajah MA, Renno WM, Babyson RS, Uddin M, Benter IF, et al. Src-dependent EGFR transactivation regulates lung inflammation via downstream signaling involving ERK1/2, PI3Kδ/Akt and NFκB induction in a murine asthma model. *Sci Rep.* (2017) 7:9919. doi: 10.1038/s41598-017-09349-0
93. Burgel PR, Nadel JA. Epidermal growth factor receptor-mediated innate immune responses and their roles in airway diseases. *Eur Respir J.* (2008) 32:1068–81. doi: 10.1183/09031936.00172007
94. Hamilton LM, Torres-Lozano C, Puddicombe SM, Richter A, Kimber I, Dearman RJ, et al. The role of the epidermal growth factor receptor in sustaining neutrophil inflammation in severe asthma. *Clin Exp Allergy.* (2003) 33:233–40. doi: 10.1046/j.1365-2222.2003.01593.x
95. Chung K, Rogers D, Barnes P, Evans T. The role of increased airway microvascular permeability and plasma exudation in asthma. *Eur Respir J.* (1990) 3:329–37.
96. Zanini A, Chetta A, Imperatori AS, Spanevello A, Olivieri D. The role of the bronchial microvasculature in the airway remodelling in asthma and COPD. *Respir Res.* (2010) 11:132. doi: 10.1186/1465-9921-11-132
97. Vermillion MS, Ursin RL, Kuok DIT, Vom Steeg LG, Wohlgemuth N, Hall OJ, et al. Production of amphiregulin and recovery from influenza is greater in males than females. *Biol Sex Differ.* (2018) 9:24. doi: 10.1186/s13293-018-0184-8
98. Peterson EA, Shabbeer S, Kenny PA. Normal range of serum Amphiregulin in healthy adult human females. *Clin Biochem.* (2012) 45:460–3. doi: 10.1016/j.clinbiochem.2011.12.029
99. Huang Y, Zhao Y, Yu Y, Li R, Lin S, Zhang C, et al. Altered amphiregulin expression induced by diverse luteinizing hormone receptor reactivity in granulosa cells affects IVF outcomes. *Reprod Biomed Online.* (2015) 30:593–601. doi: 10.1016/j.rbmo.2015.03.001

17

Monitoring Long Term Noninvasive Ventilation: Benefits, Caveats and Perspectives

Jean-Paul Janssens [1,2,3]****, Chloé Cantero*** [4]***, Patrick Pasquina*** [1]***, Marjolaine Georges*** [5] ***and Claudio Rabec*** [5]

[1] Division of Pulmonary Diseases, Department of Medicine, Geneva University Hospitals, Geneva, Switzerland, [2] Hôpital de La Tour, Centre Cardio-Respiratoire, Geneva, Switzerland, [3] Faculty of Medicine, University of Geneva, Geneva, Switzerland, [4] Service de Pneumologie, Hôpital Pitié-Salpêtrière AP-HP – Sorbonne Université, Paris, France, [5] Pulmonary Department and Respiratory Critical Care Unit, University Hospital Dijon, Dijon, France

****Correspondence:***
Jean-Paul Janssens
jp.janssens56@gmail.com

Long term noninvasive ventilation (LTNIV) is a recognized treatment for chronic hypercapnic respiratory failure (CHRF). COPD, obesity-hypoventilation syndrome, neuromuscular disorders, various restrictive disorders, and patients with sleep-disordered breathing are the major groups concerned. The purpose of this narrative review is to summarize current knowledge in the field of monitoring during home ventilation. LTNIV improves symptoms related to CHRF, diurnal and nocturnal blood gases, survival, and health-related quality of life. Initially, patients with LTNIV were most often followed through elective short in-hospital stays to ensure patient comfort, correction of daytime blood gases and nocturnal oxygenation, and control of nocturnal respiratory events. Because of the widespread use of LTNIV, elective in-hospital monitoring has become logistically problematic, time consuming, and costly. LTNIV devices presently have a built-in software which records compliance, leaks, tidal volume, minute ventilation, cycles triggered and cycled by the patient and provides detailed pressure and flow curves. Although the engineering behind this information is remarkable, the quality and reliability of certain signals may vary. Interpretation of the curves provided requires a certain level of training. Coupling ventilator software with nocturnal pulse oximetry or transcutaneous capnography performed at the patient's home can however provide important information and allow adjustments of ventilator settings thus potentially avoiding hospital admissions. Strategies have been described to combine different tools for optimal detection of an inefficient ventilation. Recent devices also allow adapting certain parameters at a distance (pressure support, expiratory positive airway pressure, back-up respiratory rate), thus allowing progressive changes in these settings for increased patient comfort and tolerance, and reducing the requirement for in-hospital titration. Because we live in a connected world, analyzing large groups of patients through treatment of "big data" will probably improve our knowledge of clinical pathways of our patients, and factors associated with treatment success or failure, adherence and efficacy. This approach provides a useful add-on to randomized controlled studies and allows generating hypotheses for better management of HMV.

Keywords: non-invasive ventilation, chronic hypercapnic respiratory failure, monitoring, home ventilation, long term mechanical ventilation

INTRODUCTION

Long term noninvasive ventilation (LTNIV) is widely accepted for treatment of chronic hypercapnic respiratory failure (CHRF) related to obstructive or restrictive disorders. Its development was triggered in the early 1980's by the report by Sullivan et al. of the use of CPAP for obstructive sleep apnea syndrome (1). Since then devices have undergone major evolutions, with a progressive shift from volume-cycled to pressure-cycled then multimodal devices, and appearance of auto-titrating modes which can adapt to changes in airway resistance, reactance, or compliance of the respiratory system and aim to ensure a target tidal volume and minute ventilation (2). One of the major contributions of medical engineering for these devices has been the development of built-in software, allowing to monitor in detail items such as compliance, leaks, tidal volume, residual respiratory events, or percentage of cycles triggered/cycled by the device (3–7). Moreover, for some devices, analysis of raw data for flow, pressure and even thoraco-abdominal movements on a breath-by-breath basis is possible. Strategies for monitoring LTNIV have also evolved: historically, elective evaluations of patients on LTNIV were initially most often hospital-based or even ICU-based; at present, they rely more and more on tools such as pulse oximetry, transcutaneous capnography ($PtcCO_2$) and built-in software that can be assessed at home (4). New developments in telemedicine and the growing contribution of health care providers make these data easily available, allowing to remotely assess quality of ventilation.

In this review, we will discuss the benefits, but also the possible pitfalls of monitoring patients under LTNIV, and perspectives as to future options. This review will focus on an adult population under LTNIV.

Why Monitor LTNIV?

The goals of long-term NIV (LTNIV) are to improve symptoms related to chronic hypercapnia and—when present—sleep-related breathing disorders (SRBD), to improve health-related quality of life (HRQL), decrease hospital admissions, correct hypoventilation and optimize SpO_2 in order to prevent the development of pulmonary hypertension and cor pulmonale, and improve survival (8). In several indications (chronic obstructive pulmonary diseases (COPD), amyotrophic lateral sclerosis (ALS), restrictive thoracic disorders), improvement of ABG and control of nocturnal hypoventilation are significantly associated with a better prognosis (9–13). In order to achieve these goals, it is mandatory to ensure that: 1/ LTNIV improves daytime and nocturnal arterial blood gases, 2/ compliance to LTNIV is sufficient to have a significant physiological effect, 3/ LTNIV does not generate *per se* undesired respiratory events or side effects and discomfort, and 4/ HRQL and symptom scores improve over time. Guidelines usually recommend at least one annual elective assessment for patients under LTNIV: the frequency of evaluations depends however on the underlying pathology, its severity and rate of progression, and may be required as often as every 3 months (8, 14, 15).

Monitoring LTNIV: A Step by Step Approach

Daytime and Nocturnal Blood Gases: Capillary, Transcutaneous or Arterial Samples

Normalizing daytime arterial blood gases (ABG) is a major physiological goal for patients under LTNIV (9, 10). Thus, performing daytime measurements of ABG—by puncture of the radial artery—is a standard procedure when monitoring LTNIV. Measurements are performed without NIV, at least 30 min after interrupting NIV (when possible), preferably in a sitting position. Capillary arterialized samples, taken at the earlobe after application of a vasodilating gel, are considered reliable surrogates of arterial ABG for pH and $PaCO_2$ (16–19). Results for PaO_2 are less reliable, with a possible underestimation by the capillary technique (20).

In stable chronic respiratory failure, pH is usually within a normal range (2, 21–24). The contribution of bicarbonates to the detection of residual nocturnal hypoventilation is debated because of the impact of a large panel of drugs and comorbidities on HCO_3 levels (25, 26). HCO_3 levels should not be used as an isolated criterion for detecting nocturnal hypoventilation, but can be indicative of nocturnal hypoventilation and should lead to nocturnal capnography if available.

Daytime ABG measurements under NIV are indicative of correction of $PaCO_2$ by NIV but have been shown to be a poor reflection of correction of nocturnal hypoventilation (27–29). Thus, assessing nocturnal pCO_2 is essential for identifying periods of hypoventilation related to leaks, undesired respiratory events including patient-ventilator asynchrony or inappropriate settings.

Nocturnal arterial punctures are a source of discomfort, awaken the patient, and are not recommended. Surrogates of nocturnal ABG assessment are end-tidal CO_2 ($ETCO_2$) and transcutaneous capnography ($TcPCO_2$). Reliability of $ETCO_2$ measurements is subject to V/Q mismatch, physiological dead space and ventilatory mode. Importantly, a normal $ETCO_2$ does not exclude hypercapnia, while an elevated $ETCO_2$ is strongly suggestive of hypercapnia but may underestimate actual $PaCO_2$ value (4, 30). Thus, the use of $ETCO_2$ as a surrogate measurement for nocturnal $PaCO_2$ is not recommended in most circumstances (4).

Transcutaneous capnography ($TcPCO_2$) is considered reliable for continuous (nocturnal) monitoring of $PaCO_2$ when patients are hemodynamically stable, and devices are used by an experienced team. A probe temperature of 42°C is tolerated for 8 h without any risk of skin burns in adults (31). Several studies have reviewed the performances of commercialized capnographs and show acceptable biases and limits of agreement (27, 29). A review of the recent literature on transcutaneous capnography suggested that bias values up to ± 1 kPa (7.5 mmHg), and limits of agreement up to ± 1.33 kPa (10 mmHg) were acceptable (27). $PtcCO_2$ however has a few drawbacks: 1/ its lag time which precludes the detection of very short events (32) and 2/ the occurrence of occasional errand values, largely dependent on the expertise of the users.

Consensual—although arbitrary—definitions for hypoventilation have been published by the American

Association for Sleep Medicine (33). However, minor changes in definitions of hypoventilation can have a major impact on clinical assessment (34–36).

Pulse oximetry has the advantage of simplicity and low cost: its major drawback is the lack of specificity of desaturations, which do not allow to distinguish hypoventilation from other causes of drops in SpO_2.

Contribution of Built-In Monitoring Devices

Compliance

Compliance is directly related to efficacy of NIV (on ABG and symptom control), and prognosis; it may also reflect patient discomfort, which impairs health related quality of life. Analysis of use of LTNIV (compliance) has 3 components: total time spent with the ventilator, pattern of use and evolution of these parameters (**Figure 1**). Total time spent under NIV has to be long enough for NIV to have a beneficial impact on daytime and nocturnal ABG, and, in some cases, on total energy expenditure (37, 38). It is usually considered that using NIV <3:30 h per 24 h is insufficient and does not allow resetting of respiratory centers and resting of respiratory muscles. Borel et al. described a "U-shaped curve" relationship between compliance and prognosis (39). Too low values provide insufficient benefit, while higher values indicate more severe respiratory impairment (39). In COPD, a meta-analysis by Struik et al. suggests that a daily use of NIV for at least 5 h is required to improve $PaCO_2$ (40). In neuromuscular disorders such as amyotrophic lateral sclerosis or myotonic dystrophy, there is a clear relation between adherence to treatment and survival (41–44). Thus, the best compromise between patient comfort and efficacy must be sought for. Pattern of use (fragmentation vs. continuous use) can be an indicator of discomfort and side-effects (leaks, pain or discomfort related to interface), co-morbidities (nycturia, use of diuretics) or symptomatic patient-ventilator asynchrony (**Figure 1**) (7, 45, 46). Evolution of total time spent under NIV and changes in pattern of use may be indicative of an exacerbation with a risk of hospital admission (47).

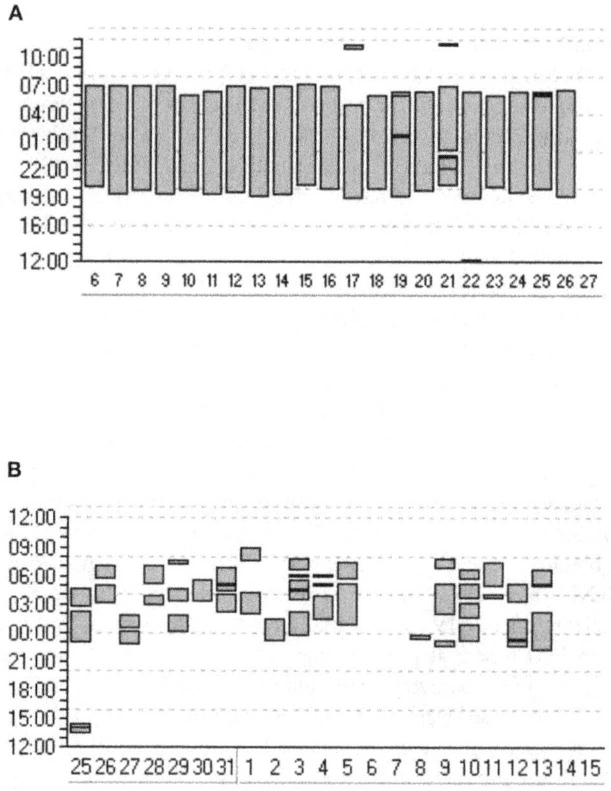

FIGURE 1 | Adherence to NIV. Graphic transcription of ventilator use provided by ventilator software. Y axis: time of the day/night; X axis: days. Each vertical bar represents time spent using the ventilator for a given day. **(A)** Very regular use suggesting that patient is adherent and comfortable with his/her treatment. **(B)** Frequent interruptions and irregular use of ventilator suggesting discomfort and/or comorbidity.

Leaks

Leaks in LTNIV are either intentional (i.e., related to exhalation valves to avoid rebreathing) or unintentional (i.e., caused for instance by a poorly adapted interface, too high insufflation pressures, or mouth leaks). Intentional leaks depend on the type of mask and insufflation pressures: interfaces have their predefined leak vs. pressure curves (48). In barometric modes, which are presently by far the most frequently used, ventilators adapt the airflow generated by the turbine to the intentional leak to ensure that the pressure attained in the airways reflects settings determined by the clinicians. Unintentional leaks are by definition unpredictable, most often variable, may differ between inspiratory and expiratory phases, and can be influenced by elements such as facial morphology, type of interface (facial *vs.* nasal mask), body position, sleep stages or ventilator settings. More importantly, they may interfere with the detection of patient's changes in inspiratory flow (which triggers pressurization or induces cycling). Leaks are thus the most frequent etiology of patient-ventilator asynchrony. They may induce significant and sometimes severe desaturations due to hypoventilation or to a "dilution effect" in patients with supplemental oxygen and can impact on quality of sleep (49). Also, leaks have a detrimental effect on reliability of data provided by ventilator software such as tidal volume, minute ventilation, or percentage of cycles triggered or cycled by the ventilator (3). This may be particularly problematic in automated modes with volume targeting or providing a continuous assessment of airway resistance.

Most built-in monitoring systems coupled to LTNIV ventilators provide data about leaks. However, leaks are estimated and reported differently according to manufacturers, which may misguide the clinician (i.e., average leaks, average leak only during expiratory phase, average leaks with or without intentional leaks) (3, 50, 51). Bench test studies have shown that reliability of reported leaks may vary considerably according to device used and to absolute value of leaks (3, 5, 52). Arbitrary threshold values for acceptable leaks are commonly reported by several manufacturers: the threshold of 24 L/min often referred to was first mentioned in a study by Teschler et al. (53): the relevance of this value is questionable today since the efficacy

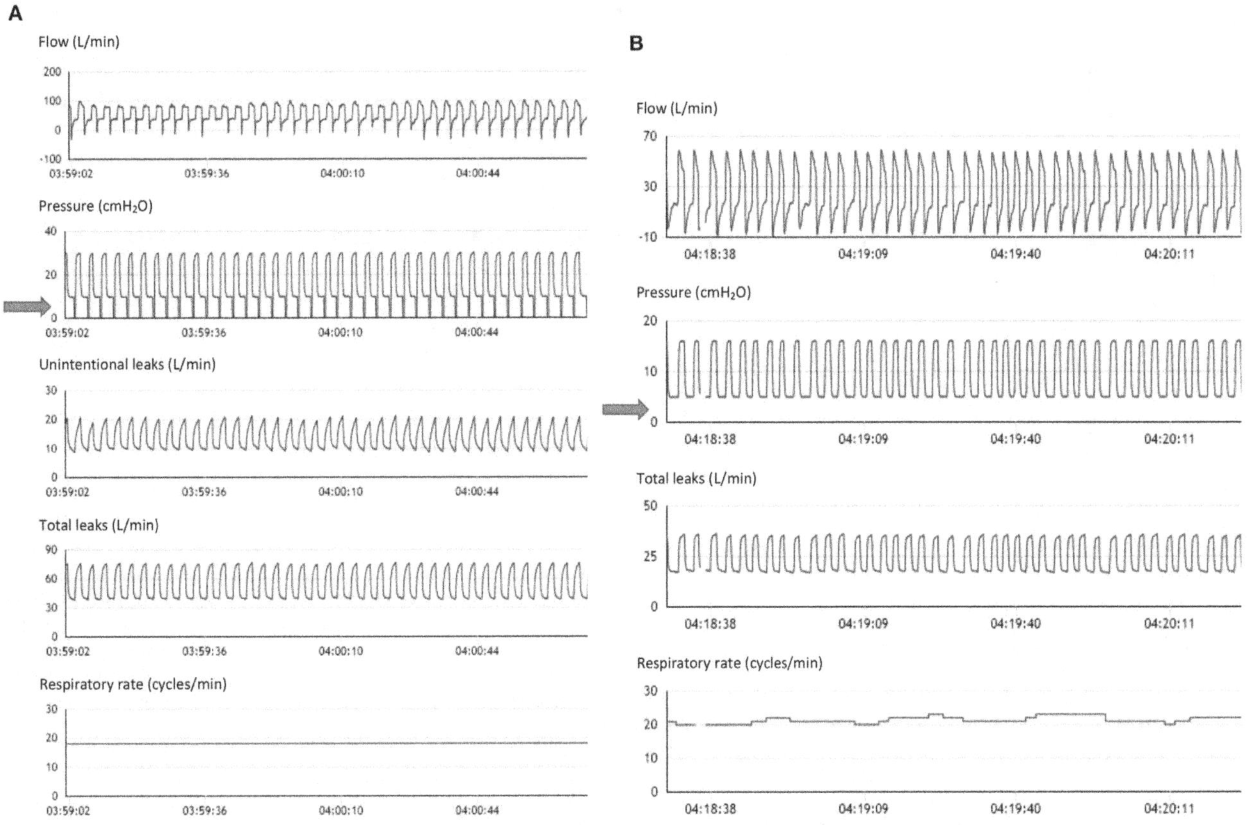

FIGURE 2 | Spontaneous vs. controlled cycles. **(A)** From top to bottom: flow (including leaks), pressure, unintentional leaks (i.e.: difference between total leak flow and estimated flow through the leak valve (small holes) of the mask), total leaks, and respiratory rate. Seventy six-year-old female subject with kyphoscoliosis, obstructive sleep apnea and obesity; ventilator settings: ST mode (spontaneous/timed); IPAP (Inspiratory positive airway pressure): 30 cmH_2O; EPAP: 10 cmH_2O (Expiratory positive airway pressure); Back-up respiratory rate (BURR): 18 cycles/min. Nasal mask (facial mask not tolerated). Flow tracing shows intermittent flattening of inspiratory curve suggesting persisting flow limitation (upper airway collapse to be compensated by increasing EPAP). Blue arrow: pressure tracing shows vertical marks associated with each cycle indicating controlled cycle (i.e., delivered by ventilator). On this segment, patient is continuously on back-up respiratory rate. Low level of intentional leaks. **(B)** From top to bottom: flow (including leaks), pressure, total leaks, and respiratory rate. Fifty four-year-old male subject with restrictive disorder. Ventilator settings: ST mode (spontaneous/timed); IPAP (Inspiratory positive airway pressure): 16 cmH_2O; EPAP: 5 cmH_2O (Expiratory positive airway pressure); Back-up respiratory rate (BURR): 16 cyc/min; nasal mask. Blue arrow: as opposed to **(A)**, all cycles are triggered by the patient (i.e., spontaneous). Normal aspect of flow and pressure tracings. DirectView software, Philips Respironics.

of ventilator turbines and their capacity to compensate for leaks has improved substantially. A statement by the French GAV-O_2 group suggested that leaks are considered troublesome essentially 1/ if they impact on patient comfort and compliance and 2/ if they cause recurrent nocturnal desaturations and episodes of hypercapnia (46).

For the patient, the variability of leaks and peak levels even of short duration may be a more important source of discomfort than the mean or median leak level.

Tidal Volume and Minute Ventilation

Tidal volume (V_T) and minute ventilation (MV) are important goals for the clinician when determining ventilator settings: a usual target for V_T is 8–10 ml/kg of ideal body weight. The accuracy of V_T, and thus MV, depends on the reliability of ventilator software, on pressure values and on leaks (54, 55). In a bench study of 7 home ventilators, bias between measured and reported V_T ranged from 66 to 236 ml (3). This may be problematic in automated volume-targeted modes. A high variability of tidal volume may *per se* be suggestive of leaks.

Cycles Triggered or Cycled by the Device

Quantifying the percentage of cycles triggered by the patient is theoretically an important information. It allows to determine to what extent the patient's respiratory rate (RR) is captured by the ventilator, i.e., to what extent ventilatory support approaches a controlled mode (**Figure 2**). This may be a goal for clinicians in neuromuscular disorders for instance, to rest inspiratory muscles, or to decrease residual apneas in obesity hypoventilation (56). However, in the presence of leaks, and/or upper airway obstruction, a low percentage of triggered cycles may reflect the fact that the ventilator does not detect the patient's inspiratory efforts. Conversely, a high percentage of cycles triggered by the patient, i.e., a spontaneous mode, may be an indicator of patient-ventilatory synchronization. This parameter must

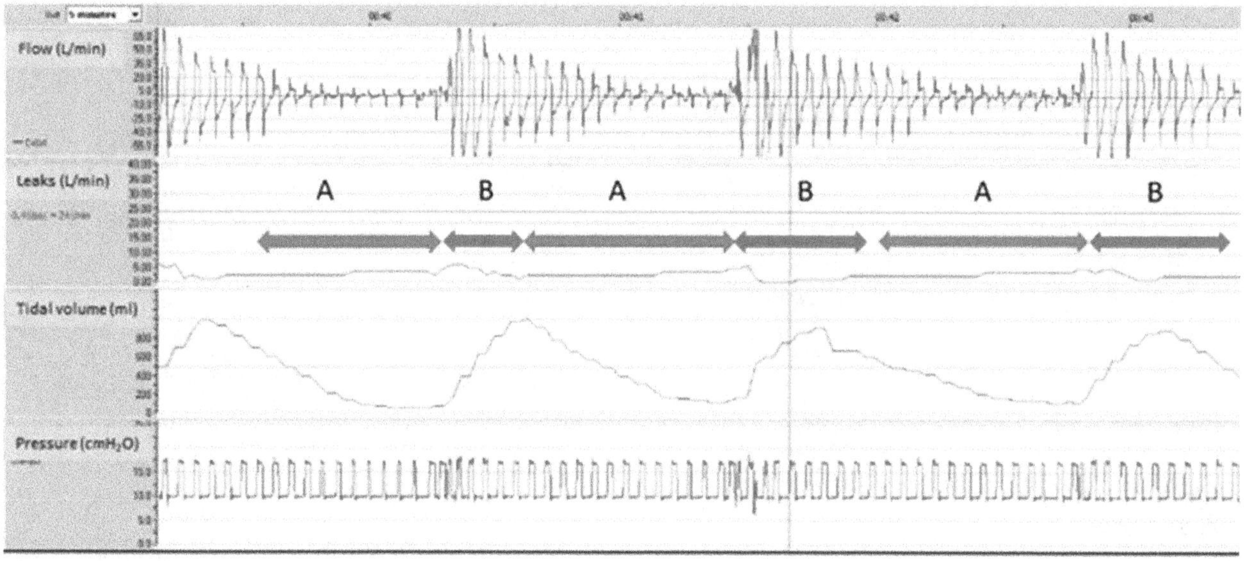

FIGURE 3 | Upper airway obstruction under NIV. 65-year-old male subject, obesity-hypoventilation with obstructive sleep apnea syndrome (OSAS). Bi-level pressure support ventilator, ResScan software, ResMed. Facial mask. Ventilator settings: ST Mode (spontaneous/timed), IPAP (Inspiratory positive airway pressure): 20 cmH_2O; EPAP (Expiratory positive airway pressure): 10 cmH_2O; BURR (Back-up respiratory rate): 16 cycles/min. From top to bottom: flow, unintentional leaks (i.e.: difference between total leak flow and estimated flow through the leak valve of the mask), tidal volume, pressure. 5 min window. Red line on leaks tracing (24L/min) is a threshold value suggested by manufacturer for upper limit of acceptable leaks (see text for comments). Event **A**: marked decrease in flow with tracing suggesting increase in upper airway resistance (leading to intermittent complete obstruction); simultaneous decrease in tidal volume without increase in leaks. Event **B**: sudden transient resumption of flow with a simultaneous increase in tidal volume. Increase in upper airway resistance could be related to an insufficient "pneumatic splint" effect in spite of rather high insufflation pressures, or to glottic closure (further characterization would require respiratory polygraphy). In a patient with a known OSAS, a pragmatic trial of increasing EPAP is an option. Value of IPAP should be increased accordingly to maintain same level of pressure support (if tolerated). Use of a facial mask may also contribute to these events, and may be replaced by nasal mask with chin strap if tolerated.

therefore be interpreted with caution, especially in the presence of leaks.

Ventilators also provide the percentage of respiratory cycles cycled by the patient i.e., for which the predefined percentage of peak inspiratory flow is reached. A high percentage of respiratory cycles cycled by the patient may be considered as evidence of appropriate patient ventilator synchronization. Conversely, a high percentage of cycling by the device may reflect either a "controlled mode" or leaks with or without patient ventilator asynchrony.

Residual Respiratory Events Under LTNIV

The presence of residual respiratory events is frequent and has a documented impact on quality of sleep and sleep structure (23, 57–60) (**Figures 3–5**). Severe patient-ventilator asynchrony may compromise the efficacy of NIV. Also, events such as recurrent upper airway obstruction may affect survival in ALS (9). It is thus important to evaluate, and correct these events.

Most devices report residual respiratory events occurring under NIV: they are labeled as apnea, hypopnea, and sometimes even classified as "central" or "obstructive" according to complex algorithms and estimation of upper airway resistance using the force oscillation technique, the shape of the flow curves or both. The relevance of these parameters in LTNIV is not well-established: these parameters are derived mainly from the use of CPAP in sleep-related disordered breathing (SRDB), and do not take into account the higher level of complexity of undesired residual (or *de novo*) respiratory events associated with LTNIV. Very few studies have assessed the reliability of these data. Georges et al. showed that the apnea-hypopnea index (AHI) reported by one specific device in patients with obesity-hypoventilation was well-correlated with a manually read polysomnographic assessment, and that a threshold value of 10/hour for AHI allowed to discriminate with a high sensitivity and specificity subjects who were correctly ventilated vs. those for whom adjustments were required (61). In a similar study, Alvarez et al. compared manually scored polygraphy with built-in software data in 26 patients with obesity-hypoventilation: automated analysis of residual events was well-correlated with polygraphy; however, manually scored tracings from ventilator software provided more consistent results than automated software (62). More recently Aarrestad et al. compared manually scored polygraphy and data from ventilator software in 67 subjects on LTNIV for restrictive disorders: a value of AHI above 7.2/hour reported by ventilator software had a sensitivity of 93% (95%CI: 68–100) and a specificity of 92% (95%CI: 81–98) for detecting patients with an AHI > 10/hour scored by polygraphy (34).

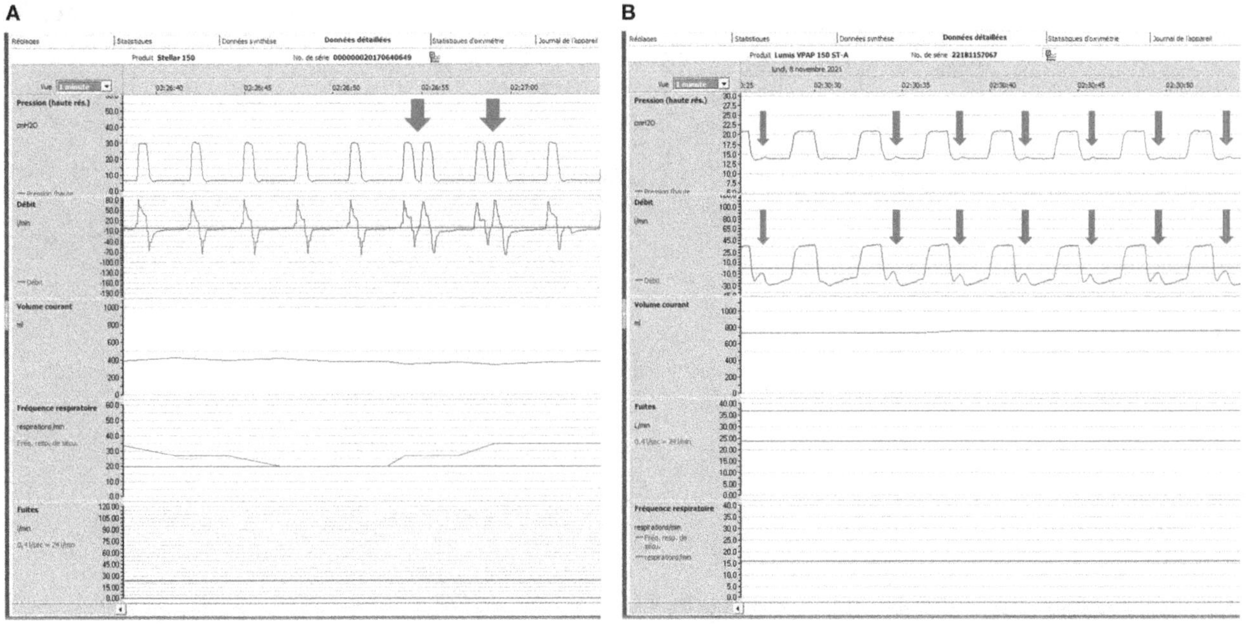

FIGURE 4 | Patient ventilator asynchrony (PVA): illustrative ventilator tracings. One-minute windows. From top to bottom: pressure, flow, tidal volume, respiratory rate and unintentional leaks (i.e., without intentional leak through exhalation valve of mask). Rescan software, ResMed. **(A)** 74-year-old male subject with severe COPD (FEV1: 20% of predicted). Bi-level pressure support ventilator, Rescan software, Resmed. Ventilator settings: ST (spontaneous/timed) mode; IPAP (Inspiratory positive airway pressure): 30 cmH_2O; EPAP (Expiratory positive airway pressure): 7 cmH_2O; BURR (back-up respiratory rate) 20 cycles/min. Red arrows show intermittent double-triggering. In this case, leaks are not in cause. Possible causes are dysfunction of ventilator, too high inspiratory trigger sensitivity, too short minimal inspiratory time (TI_{MIN}) with prolonged inspiratory efforts. Adjustments of settings (if required) to be considered are: to increase TI_{MIN}; to adapt cycling sensitivity (at a lower percentage of peak inspiratory flow, which delays cycling); to increase IPAP and reduce rise time; or to decrease sensitivity of inspiratory trigger. **(B)** 67-year-old male subject with obesity hypoventilation and severe OSAS. Bi-level pressure support ventilator, Rescan software, Resmed. Ventilator settings: ST (spontaneous/timed) mode; IPAP (Inspiratory positive airway pressure): 21 cmH_2O; EPAP (Expiratory positive airway pressure): 14 cmH_2O; BURR (back-up respiratory rate) 16 cycles/min. Red arrows show low amplitude repeated increases in flow and pressure which represent unrewarded efforts (i.e., inspiratory efforts by the patient which do not trigger the ventilator). Among possible causes are: inappropriate setting of inspiratory trigger sensitivity, increase in upper airway resistance, leaks, intrinsic PEEP (Positive end expiratory pressure), decrease in inspiratory muscle function. For all PVA, control of leaks is mandatory before adjusting other settings.

Detailed Analysis of Flow and Pressure Curves and Coupling With Pulse Oximetry and Leaks

Ventilator software provides the possibility of a detailed cycle-by-cycle analysis of pressure and flow curves, while simultaneously providing curves of estimated leaks and tidal volume. Oximetry can be added to most devices to complete this analysis. This allows the detection of residual obstructive events with or without persistence of respiratory drive (63), may show periodic breathing, and patient ventilator asynchronies (rate asynchrony such as multiple triggering, auto-triggering, ineffective efforts, or intracycle asynchronies such as underassistance, or overshoot) (49). Coupling the detailed analysis of ventilator curves with oximetry and leaks allows a better assessment of relevance and mechanisms involved, and provides a rationale to adapt ventilator settings. Illustrative cases of contribution of pressure and flow curves are shown in **Figures 2–5**.

Contribution of Respiratory Polygraphy or Polysomnography

Respiratory polygraphy (PG) or polysomnography (PSG), preferably coupled with $TcPCO_2$, are considered as gold-standard for documenting undesired respiratory events occurring under LTNIV. These events have been reported by several studies (34, 45, 57, 58, 64, 65) and defined in detail by the SomnoNIV group (63). However, PG or PSG under NIV requires expertise. PSG is not easily available in many countries, and thus use of PSG for titrating and/or monitoring LTNIV, although recommended by the AASM (American Association of Sleep Medicine), is not standard practice (66). Some specialized centers use PSG for titration and follow-up (67). Proposed algorithms recommend PSG or PG only after a thorough analysis of symptoms, $PtcCO_2$, ventilator software and correction of leaks (4, 68) (**Figure 6**).

Symptom Scores and Assessment of Health-Related Quality of Life (HRQL)

Specific HRQL questionnaires have been designed for patients under LTNIV, such as the SRI (Severe Respiratory Insufficiency Questionnaire) which is the most widely used in this setting, with 16 translations and an "App" version available (69, 70). This type of questionnaire is however mostly designed for clinical studies, and not for follow-up of individuals.

A disease-specific symptom score (S^3-NIV) has been recently developed (71) and is undergoing several translations: it is an

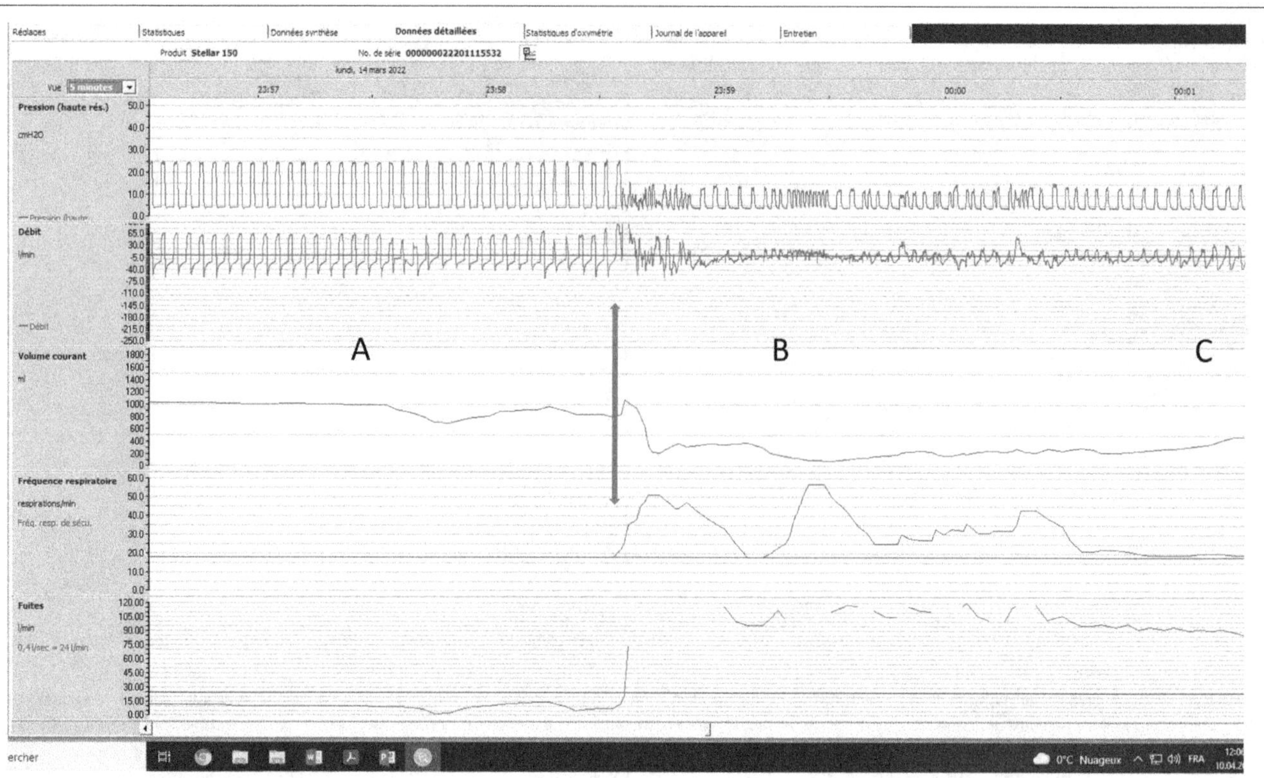

FIGURE 5 | Impact of major leaks. Seventy five-year old male subject with severe COPD (GOLD D; FEV1: 17% of predicted). Bi-level pressure support ventilator, S/T mode (spontaneous/timed); IPAP (Inspiratory positive airway pressure): 24 cmH_2O; EPAP (Expiratory positive airway pressure): 4 cmH_2O; Back-up respiratory rate (BURR): 18 cycles/min. Facial mask. Five-minute window, Rescan software, ResMed. **(A)** normal tracing albeit for a few cycles with decrease in flow; **(B)** Vertical arrow marks appearance of major leaks (could be related to transient displacement of interface). Pressure tracing shows episodes of auto-triggering, and double triggering. Marked drop in pressure, flow and V_T (explained by magnitude of leaks). **(C)** As leaks progressively decrease, breathing pattern becomes more regular; pressure and flow increase progressively.

11-item Lickert scale type questionnaire which can be auto-administered, and provides 2 sub-scores: "respiratory symptoms" and "sleep and NIV-related side effects." This score is perfectly suitable for clinical practice. It can be coupled with simple tools for assessing mood disturbances such as the Hospital Anxiety and Depression scale (72). These tools do not replace however the necessary face-to-face exchange with the patient and/or his/her caregivers to appreciate the relevance of findings downloaded from ventilator software and mentioned in symptom scores such as the S3-NIV.

Strategies to Detect Ineffective Control of Nocturnal Hypoventilation by NIV

NIV should be systematically monitored (4, 46). As mentioned previously, residual nocturnal hypoventilation, unintentional leaks, patient-ventilator asynchrony or abnormal respiratory events are frequent under NIV and have a negative impact on patient-related outcomes such as symptoms, HRQL and survival. It has been estimated that approximately one third of ventilated patients with normal daytime ABG and nocturnal SpO_2 had residual nocturnal hypoventilation under NIV (28, 35, 73). Withholding from performing regular testing of NIV efficacy could therefore be detrimental.

Optimal modalities for monitoring of long-term ventilated patients remain a matter of debate. As previously mentioned, complete polysomnography (PSG) under NIV is performed by some groups, but is not feasible in most centers on a routine basis (74).

Alternative tools (such as oximetry, $TcPCO_2$, or ventilator software) can be used alone or in combination. A step-by-step strategy starting by ABG and nocturnal SpO_2 has been proposed by the SomnoNIV group (4) (**Figure 6**).

Over the past years, the use of $TcPCO_2$ has been simplified (less frequent changes of probes, improved software and estimation of drift). Failure to retrieve data is rare (75) and instrumental drift of $TcPCO_2$ is a minor problem when used by an experienced team (27). Several studies have shown that continuous $TcPCO_2$ recording provides an accurate picture of the overnight time course of $PaCO_2$ in CHRF under NIV. Experts propose different thresholds to define significant nocturnal hypercapnia: maximal $TcPCO_2$ >49 mmHg, $TcPCO_2$ >49 mmHg for >10% of recording time, $TcPCO_2$ >55 mmHg for ≥10 min or an increase in $TcPCO_2$ ≥10 mmHg above awake supine value to a value exceeding 50 mmHg for ≥10 min (33). The choice of a clinically relevant threshold may be influenced by 1/the bias between arterial and transcutaneous

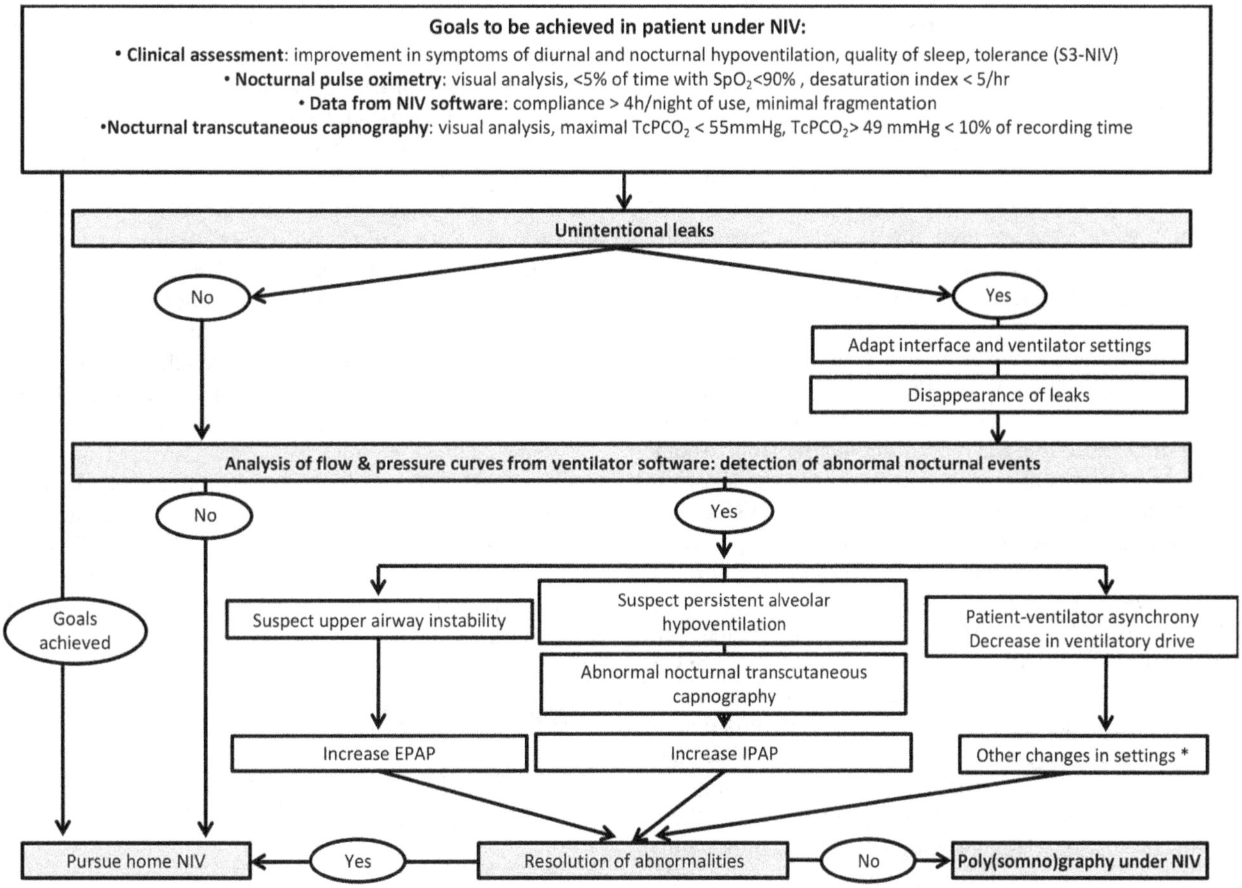

FIGURE 6 | Proposed algorithm for a systematic approach to monitoring of patients under LNIV and analysis of ventilator software. *: the reader is referred to references 4 and 8 for further details.

PCO_2 according to the device used, 2/the etiology of the underlying chronic respiratory failure and 3/$PaCO_2$ levels when NIV is started. Beyond this debate, capnography is currently a well-accepted surrogate procedure for diagnosing nocturnal residual hypoventilation in ventilated patients. Simultaneous recording of SpO_2 with the same ear probe improves the clinical contribution of nocturnal transcutaneous capnography. Indeed, sampling rate and averaging of SpO_2 and $TcPCO_2$ recordings are different. Therefore, SpO_2 traces can detect brief desaturations related to short ventilatory events while $TcPCO_2$ traces allow evaluating overnight trends because of a longer lag time (4).

Significant leaks and/or abnormal residual respiratory events (i.e., flow reduction or patient-ventilator asynchronism) are frequently detected in patients with normal nocturnal $TcPCO_2$ and SpO_2 (23, 59, 64).

In a study comparing different tools and their combination, Georges et al. demonstrated that combining the signals provided by $TcPCO_2$ and data from ventilator software provides the best noninvasive assessment of NIV efficacy (73). This approach allows monitoring of LTNIV at the hospital or at home without complex logistics. Interpretation of the results is simple and further analysis of detailed raw data provided by ventilator software can help clarify the underlying mechanism to optimize NIV settings, thus limiting the use of PSG to more complex cases.

A suggested strategy for nocturnal NIV monitoring and parameter optimization is summarized in **Figure 6**.

Patient-Ventilator Asynchrony and Its' Relevance

Several studies have reported the—sometimes frequent—occurrence of patient ventilator asynchrony (PVA) in patients under LTNIV (23, 57–59, 63, 64, 76) (**Figures 4, 5**). Their specific semiology and a suggested framework for their analysis has been proposed by the SomnoNIV group (49). Briefly, after correction of leaks and obstructions, which are the major contributors to PVA, a visual analysis of tracings is necessary to detect the presence of rate asynchrony and/or intracycle asynchrony. Rate asynchrony is further subdivided into multiple triggering, uncoupling and ineffective efforts, while intracycle asynchrony can reveal either flow asynchrony (under-assistance) or phase asynchrony (premature or delayed cycling). Clinical relevance of PVA is still a matter of debate, especially if not associated with discomfort and hypoventilation and/or nocturnal desaturation. Scoring of PVA is not yet standardized in the medical literature, and prevalence can vary considerably according to working definitions (23). Seeking for PVA seems however appropriate after correction of leaks in the presence of symptoms and/or unexplained desaturations.

Tele-Monitoring

Although the use of tele-monitoring has become in many countries standard practice for following patients treated by CPAP and Sleep-related breathing disorders (SRBD), and, in some countries, is even required for its reimbursement, this is not the case for LTNIV. Many devices used for LTNIV have the necessary technology built-in, but each manufacturer has its software, and way of reporting certain parameters, representing a challenge for clinicians. Reliability of data remains an issue for some data, as previously discussed (77). In spite of these limitations, home titration and follow-up of LTNIV are emerging strategies. Use of tele-monitoring as an adjunct to home initiation of LTNIV is also an option, and has been shown to be cost-effective in selected indications such as CHRF related to neuromuscular disorders or other restrictive lung diseases (78, 79). Several studies suggest a benefit on healthcare utilization (emergency visits, hospital admissions) and cost-effectiveness of tele-monitoring in ALS (80–82). Preliminary studies have explored the possibility of early detection of exacerbations of COPD under LTNIV (47). For instance, changes in number of hours of NIV use may be a sign of imminent exacerbation, of worsening of underlying disease, or of discomfort, and can be a useful signal for early home intervention (7, 47). On-going trials (reviewed by Borel et al.) (77) will help clarify the modalities of a cost-effective use of tele-monitoring in NIV, and importantly, its benefit (or absence of) on relevant outcomes (such as HRQL, survival, hospital admissions). Points of potential interest for telemonitoring are: follow-up after initiation of NIV following an acute episode of respiratory failure (effective daily use, leaks etc.), progressive titration of NIV after home initiation of LTNIV, and, once specific algorithms will have been validated, early detection of exacerbations or deterioration of disorder causing CRF. The present tools for tele-monitoring already provide a limited "traffic light system" (red, yellow and green icons) usually based on leaks, AHI and compliance. A more elaborate signaling system, using limits for tidal volume, minute ventilation, respiratory rate etc. has yet to be validated in clinical practice, the risk being an unwarranted increase of "red lights." The possibility of adapting certain parameters at a distance (pressure support, expiratory positive airway pressure, or back-up respiratory rate) allows progressive changes in these settings for increased patient comfort and tolerance, and reduces the requirement for in-hospital titration (83).

The Contribution of "Big Data"

The concept of "Big data" refers to access to a massive quantity of data, its speed of acquisition, and the diversity and heterogeneity of data sources, with potential uncertainties regarding data quality (84). The widespread use of telemonitoring for CPAP has opened the way to a new approach for exploring patient pathways, identifying potentially relevant phenotypes, and elements impacting on adherence and efficacy. For instance, Liu et al. provided very useful data for a better understanding of trajectories of patients with central sleep apnea (emergent, transient, persistent) after initiation of CPAP (85). Technical information such as the impact of changes of interface can be easily assessed through daily longitudinal follow-up data at a large scale. Detailed analysis of day by day use of devices reveals behavioral patterns which improve our understanding of how patients adhere and accept their treatment (86, 87). Recently, it has been possible through telemonitoring to evaluate the impact of the lockdown during the COVID pandemic on adherence to CPAP or NIV (88, 89). Undoubtedly, in a near future, this type of information will become increasingly available and provide a useful adjunct to clinical trials.

CONCLUSIONS

The relevance and necessity of a regular monitoring of patients under LTNIV is clearly established, and has an impact on prognosis and HRQL. The progressive shift from hospital-based to home-based assessment over the past years is important for patient comfort and cost-effectiveness of LTNIV. Strategies for monitoring LTNIV include clinical assessment, symptom scores, simple tools such as $TcPCO_2$ or oximetry, ventilator software, and in specific situations, respiratory polygraphy or polysomnography. Although telemonitoring of patients treated by CPAP for SRBD is widely accepted, its use in LTNIV still has to be explored and shown to be cost-effective. Access to big data may provide additional information to better clarify phenotypes of responders and non-responders to LTNIV.

AUTHOR CONTRIBUTIONS

J-PJ, CC, PP, MG, and CR have contributed to the writing, designing, and revision of the final version of this manuscript and are accountable for the content of this manuscript. All authors contributed to the article and approved the submitted version.

REFERENCES

1. Sullivan CE, Issa FG, Berthon-Jones M, Eves L. Reversal of obstructive sleep apnoea by continuous positive airway pressure applied through the nares. *Lancet.* (1981) 1:862–5. doi: 10.1016/S0140-6736(81)92140-1
2. Cantero C, Adler D, Pasquina P, Uldry C, Egger B, Prella M, et al. Long term noninvasive ventilation in the Geneva Lake area: indications, prevalence and modalities. *Chest.* (2020) 158:279–91. doi: 10.1016/j.chest.2020.02.064
3. Contal O, Vignaux L, Combescure C, Pepin JL, Jolliet P, Janssens JP. Monitoring of noninvasive ventilation by built-in software of home bilevel ventilators: a bench study. *Chest.* (2012) 141:469–76. doi: 10.1378/chest.11-0485
4. Janssens JP, Borel JC, Pepin JL, Somno NIVG. Nocturnal monitoring of home non-invasive ventilation: the contribution of simple tools such as pulse oximetry, capnography, built-in ventilator software and autonomic markers of sleep fragmentation. *Thorax.* (2011) 66:438–45. doi: 10.1136/thx.2010.139782

5. Rabec C, Georges M, Kabeya NK, Baudouin N, Massin F, Reybet-Degat O, et al. Evaluating noninvasive ventilation using a monitoring system coupled to a ventilator: a bench-to-bedside study. *Eur Respir J.* (2009) 34:902–13. doi: 10.1183/09031936.00170508
6. Mansell SK, Cutts S, Hackney I, Wood MJ, Hawksworth K, Creer DD, et al. Using domiciliary non-invasive ventilator data downloads to inform clinical decision-making to optimise ventilation delivery and patient compliance. *BMJ Open Respir Res.* (2018) 5:e000238. doi: 10.1136/bmjresp-2017-000238
7. Pasquina P, Adler D, Farr P, Bourqui P, Bridevaux PO, Janssens JP. What does built-in software of home ventilators tell us? An observational study of 150 patients on home ventilation. *Respiration.* (2012) 83:293–9. doi: 10.1159/000330598
8. Janssens JP, Michel F, Schwarz EI, Prella M, Bloch K, Adler D, et al. Long-term mechanical ventilation: recommendations of the swiss society of pulmonology. *Respiration.* (2020) 99:867–902. doi: 10.1159/000510086
9. Georges M, Attali V, Golmard JL, Morelot-Panzini C, Crevier-Buchman L, Collet JM, et al. Reduced survival in patients with ALS with upper airway obstructive events on non-invasive ventilation. *J Neurol Neurosurg Psychiatry.* (2016) 87:1045–50. doi: 10.1136/jnnp-2015-312606
10. Gonzalez-Bermejo J, Morelot-Panzini C, Arnol N, Meininger V, Kraoua S, Salachas F, et al. Prognostic value of efficiently correcting nocturnal desaturations after one month of non-invasive ventilation in amyotrophic lateral sclerosis: a retrospective monocentre observational cohort study. *Amyotroph Lateral Scler Frontotemporal Degener.* (2013) 14:373–9. doi: 10.3109/21678421.2013.776086
11. Murphy PB, Rehal S, Arbane G, Bourke S, Calverley PMA, Crook AM, et al. Effect of home noninvasive ventilation with oxygen therapy vs oxygen therapy alone on hospital readmission or death after an acute COPD exacerbation: a randomized clinical trial. *JAMA.* (2017) 317:2177–86. doi: 10.1001/jama.2017.4451
12. Kohnlein T, Windisch W, Kohler D, Drabik A, Geiseler J, Hartl S, et al. Non-invasive positive pressure ventilation for the treatment of severe stable chronic obstructive pulmonary disease: a prospective, multicentre, randomised, controlled clinical trial. *Lancet Respir Med.* (2014) 2:698–705. doi: 10.1016/S2213-2600(14)70153-5
13. Tsuboi T, Oga T, Sumi K, Machida K, Ohi M, Chin K. The importance of controlling PaCO(2) throughout long-term noninvasive ventilation. *Respir Care.* (2014) 59:1671–8. doi: 10.4187/respcare.02829
14. Windisch W, Geiseler J, Simon K, Walterspacher S, Dreher M, on behalf of the Guideline C. German national guideline for treating chronic respiratory failure with invasive and non-invasive ventilation: revised edition 2017 - part 1. *Respiration.* (2018) 96:66–97. doi: 10.1159/000488001
15. Windisch W, Geiseler J, Simon K, Walterspacher S, Dreher M, on behalf of the Guideline C. German national guideline for treating chronic respiratory failure with invasive and non-invasive ventilation - revised edition 2017: part 2. *Respiration.* (2018) 96:171–203. doi: 10.1159/000488667
16. Ekkernkamp E, Welte L, Schmoor C, Huttmann SE, Dreher M, Windisch W, et al. Spot check analysis of gas exchange: invasive versus noninvasive methods. *Respiration.* (2015) 89:294–303. doi: 10.1159/000371769
17. Zavorsky GS, Cao J, Mayo NE, Gabbay R, Murias JM. Arterial versus capillary blood gases: a meta-analysis. *Respir Physiol Neurobiol.* (2007) 155:268–79. doi: 10.1016/j.resp.2006.07.002
18. Mollard P, Bourdillon N, Letournel M, Herman H, Gibert S, Pichon A, et al. Validity of arterialized earlobe blood gases at rest and exercise in normoxia and hypoxia. *Respir Physiol Neurobiol.* (2010) 172:179–83. doi: 10.1016/j.resp.2010.05.017
19. Sauty A, Uldry C, Debetaz LF, Leuenberger P, Fitting JW. Differences in PO2 and PCO2 between arterial and arterialized earlobe samples. *Eur Respir J.* (1996) 9:186–9. doi: 10.1183/09031936.96.09020186
20. Magnet FS, Majorski DS, Callegari J, Schwarz SB, Schmoor C, Windisch W, et al. Capillary PO2 does not adequately reflect arterial PO2 in hypoxemic COPD patients. *Int J Chron Obstruct Pulmon Dis.* (2017) 12:2647–53. doi: 10.2147/COPD.S140843
21. Masa JF, Mokhlesi B, Benitez I, Gomez de Terreros FJ, Sanchez-Quiroga MA, Romero A, et al. Long-term clinical effectiveness of continuous positive airway pressure therapy versus non-invasive ventilation therapy in patients with obesity hypoventilation syndrome: a multicentre, open-label, randomised controlled trial. *Lancet.* (2019) 393:1721–32. doi: 10.1016/S0140-6736(18)32978-7
22. Masa JF, Corral J, Caballero C, Barrot E, Teran-Santos J, Alonso-Alvarez ML, et al. Non-invasive ventilation in obesity hypoventilation syndrome without severe obstructive sleep apnoea. *Thorax.* (2016) 71:899–906. doi: 10.1136/thoraxjnl-2016-208501
23. Aarrestad S, Qvarfort M, Kleiven AL, Tollefsen E, Skjonsberg OH, Janssens JP. Sleep related respiratory events during non-invasive ventilation of patients with chronic hypoventilation. *Respir Med.* (2017) 132:210–6. doi: 10.1016/j.rmed.2017.10.025
24. Janssens JP, Derivaz S, Breitenstein E, De Muralt B, Fitting JW, Chevrolet JC, et al. Changing patterns in long-term noninvasive ventilation: a 7-year prospective study in the Geneva Lake area. *Chest.* (2003) 123:67–79. doi: 10.1378/chest.123.1.67
25. Borel JC, Guerber F, Jullian-Desayes I, Joyeux-Faure M, Arnol N, Taleux N, et al. Prevalence of obesity hypoventilation syndrome in ambulatory obese patients attending pathology laboratories. *Respirology.* (2017) 22:1190–8. doi: 10.1111/resp.13051
26. Jullian-Desayes I, Borel JC, Guerber F, Borel AL, Tamisier R, Levy P, et al. Drugs influencing acid base balance and bicarbonate concentration readings. *Expert Rev Endocrinol Metab.* (2016) 11:209–16. doi: 10.1586/17446651.2016.1147951
27. Aarrestad S, Tollefsen E, Kleiven AL, Qvarfort M, Janssens JP, Skjonsberg OH. Validity of transcutaneous PCO2 in monitoring chronic hypoventilation treated with non-invasive ventilation. *Respir Med.* (2016) 112:112–8. doi: 10.1016/j.rmed.2016.01.017
28. Paiva R, Krivec U, Aubertin G, Cohen E, Clement A, Fauroux B. Carbon dioxide monitoring during long-term noninvasive respiratory support in children. *Intensive Care Med.* (2009) 35:1068–74. doi: 10.1007/s00134-009-1408-5
29. Georges M, Nguyen-Baranoff D, Griffon L, Foignot C, Bonniaud P, Camus P, et al. Usefulness of transcutaneous PCO2 to assess nocturnal hypoventilation in restrictive lung disorders. *Respirology.* (2016) 21:1300–6. doi: 10.1111/resp.12812
30. Nassar BS, Schmidt GA. Estimating arterial partial pressure of carbon dioxide in ventilated patients: how valid are surrogate measures? *Ann Am Thorac Soc.* (2017) 14:1005–14. doi: 10.1513/AnnalsATS.201701-034FR
31. Janssens JP, Perrin E, Bennani I, de Muralt B, Titelion V, Picaud C. Is continuous transcutaneous monitoring of PCO2 (TcPCO2) over 8 h reliable in adults? *Respir Med.* (2001) 95:331–5. doi: 10.1053/rmed.2001.1045
32. Janssens JP, Howarth-Frey C, Chevrolet JC, Abajo B, Rochat T. Transcutaneous PCO2 to monitor noninvasive mechanical ventilation in adults: assessment of a new transcutaneous PCO2 device. *Chest.* (1998) 113:768–73. doi: 10.1378/chest.113.3.768
33. Berry RB, Budhiraja R, Gottlieb DJ, Gozal D, Iber C, Kapur VK, et al. Rules for scoring respiratory events in sleep: update of the 2007 AASM manual for the scoring of sleep and associated events. Deliberations of the sleep apnea definitions Task Force of the American Academy of Sleep Medicine. *J Clin Sleep Med.* (2012) 8:597–619. doi: 10.5664/jcsm.2172
34. Aarrestad S, Qvarfort M, Kleiven AL, Tollefsen E, Skjonsberg OH, Janssens JP. Diagnostic accuracy of simple tools in monitoring patients with chronic hypoventilation treated with non-invasive ventilation; a prospective cross-sectional study. *Respir Med.* (2018) 144:30–5. doi: 10.1016/j.rmed.2018.09.015
35. Ogna A, Quera Salva MA, Prigent H, Mroue G, Vaugier I, Annane D, et al. Nocturnal hypoventilation in neuromuscular disease: prevalence according to different definitions issued from the literature. *Sleep Breath.* (2016) 20:575–81. doi: 10.1007/s11325-015-1247-2
36. Orlikowski D, Prigent H, Quera Salva MA, Heming N, Chaffaut C, Chevret S, et al. Prognostic value of nocturnal hypoventilation in neuromuscular patients. *Neuromusc Disord.* (2017) 27:326–30. doi: 10.1016/j.nmd.2016.12.006
37. Gonzalez-Bermejo J, Lofaso F, Falaize L, Lejaille M, Raphael JC, Similowski T, et al. Resting energy expenditure in Duchenne patients using home mechanical ventilation. *Eur Respir J.* (2005) 25:682–7. doi: 10.1183/09031936.05.00031304
38. Georges M, Morelot-Panzini C, Similowski T, Gonzalez-Bermejo J. Noninvasive ventilation reduces energy expenditure in amyotrophic lateral sclerosis. *BMC Pulm Med.* (2014) 14:17. doi: 10.1186/1471-2466-14-17

39. Borel JC, Pepin JL, Pison C, Vesin A, Gonzalez-Bermejo J, Court-Fortune I, et al. Long-term adherence with non-invasive ventilation improves prognosis in obese COPD patients. *Respirology.* (2014) 19:857–65. doi: 10.1111/resp.12327
40. Struik FM, Lacasse Y, Goldstein RS, Kerstjens HA, Wijkstra PJ. Nocturnal noninvasive positive pressure ventilation in stable COPD: a systematic review and individual patient data meta-analysis. *Respir Med.* (2014) 108:329–37. doi: 10.1016/j.rmed.2013.10.007
41. Pinto A, de Carvalho M, Evangelista T, Lopes A, Sales-Luis L. Nocturnal pulse oximetry: a new approach to establish the appropriate time for non-invasive ventilation in ALS patients. *Amyotroph Lateral Scler Other Motor Neuron Disord.* (2003) 4:31–5. doi: 10.1080/14660820310006706
42. Seijger C, Raaphorst J, Vonk J, van Engelen B, Heijerman H, Stigter N, et al. New insights in adherence and survival in myotonic dystrophy patients using home mechanical ventilation. *Respiration.* (2021) 100:154–63. doi: 10.1159/000511962
43. Walsh LJ, Deasy KF, Gomez F, O'Sullivan E, Eustace J, Ryan AM, et al. Use of non-invasive ventilation in motor neuron disease - a retrospective cohort analysis. *Chron Respir Dis.* (2021) 18:1–9. doi: 10.1177/14799731211063886
44. Aboussouan LS, Khan SU, Meeker DP, Stelmach K, Mitsumoto H. Effect of noninvasive positive-pressure ventilation on survival in amyotrophic lateral sclerosis. *Ann Intern Med.* (1997) 127:450–3. doi: 10.7326/0003-4819-127-6-199709150-00006
45. Fanfulla F, Delmastro M, Berardinelli A, Lupo ND, Nava S. Effects of different ventilator settings on sleep and inspiratory effort in patients with neuromuscular disease. *Am J Respir Crit Care Med.* (2005) 172:619–24. doi: 10.1164/rccm.200406-694OC
46. Rabec C, Cuvelier A, Cheval C, Jaffre S, Janssens JP, Mercy M, et al. [Noninvasive ventilation. The 2015 guidelines from the Groupe Assistance Ventilatoire (GAV) of the Societe de Pneumologie de Langue Francaise (SPLF)]. *Rev Mal Respir.* (2016) 33:905–10. doi: 10.1016/j.rmr.2016.07.003
47. Borel JC, Pelletier J, Taleux N, Briault A, Arnol N, Pison C, et al. Parameters recorded by software of non-invasive ventilators predict COPD exacerbation: a proof-of-concept study. *Thorax.* (2015) 70:284–5. doi: 10.1136/thoraxjnl-2014-206569
48. Borel JC, Sabil A, Janssens JP, Couteau M, Boulon L, Levy P, et al. Intentional leaks in industrial masks have a significant impact on efficacy of bilevel noninvasive ventilation: a bench test study. *Chest.* (2009) 135:669–77. doi: 10.1378/chest.08-1340
49. Gonzalez-Bermejo J, Janssens JP, Rabec C, Perrin C, Lofaso F, Langevin B, et al. Framework for patient-ventilator asynchrony during long-term non-invasive ventilation. *Thorax.* (2019) doi: 10.1136/thoraxjnl-2018-213022
50. Lujan M, Lalmolda C, Ergan B. Basic concepts for tidal volume and leakage estimation in non-invasive ventilation. *Turk Thorac J.* (2019) 20:140–6. doi: 10.5152/TurkThoracJ.2018.177
51. Lujan M, Sogo A, Grimau C, Pomares X, Blanch L, Monso E. Influence of dynamic leaks in volume-targeted pressure support noninvasive ventilation: a bench study. *Respir Care.* (2015) 60:191–200. doi: 10.4187/respcare.03413
52. Lujan M, Pomares X. Noninvasive mechanical ventilation. Reflections on home monitoring. *Arch Bronconeumol.* (2014) 50:85–6. doi: 10.1016/j.arbr.2013.11.003
53. Teschler H, Stampa J, Ragette R, Konietzko N, Berthon-Jones M. Effect of mouth leak on effectiveness of nasal bilevel ventilatory assistance and sleep architecture. *Eur Respir J.* (1999) 14:1251–7. doi: 10.1183/09031936.99.14612519
54. Lujan M, Sogo A, Pomares X, Monso E, Sales B, Blanch L. Effect of leak and breathing pattern on the accuracy of tidal volume estimation by commercial home ventilators: a bench study. *Respir Care.* (2013) 58:770–7. doi: 10.4187/respcare.02010
55. Sogo A, Montanya J, Monso E, Blanch L, Pomares X, Lujan M. Effect of dynamic random leaks on the monitoring accuracy of home mechanical ventilators: a bench study. *BMC Pulm Med.* (2013) 13:75. doi: 10.1186/1471-2466-13-75
56. Contal O, Adler D, Borel JC, Espa F, Perrig S, Rodenstein D, et al. Impact of different backup respiratory rates on the efficacy of noninvasive positive pressure ventilation in obesity hypoventilation syndrome: a randomized trial. *Chest.* (2013) 143:37–46. doi: 10.1378/chest.11-2848
57. Fanfulla F, Taurino AE, Lupo ND, Trentin R, D'Ambrosio C, Nava S. Effect of sleep on patient/ventilator asynchrony in patients undergoing chronic non-invasive mechanical ventilation. *Respir Med.* (2007) 101:1702–7. doi: 10.1016/j.rmed.2007.02.026
58. Guo YF, Sforza E, Janssens JP. Respiratory patterns during sleep in obesity-hypoventilation patients treated with nocturnal pressure support: a preliminary report. *Chest.* (2007) 131:1090–9. doi: 10.1378/chest.06-1705
59. Ramsay M. Patient ventilator asynchrony and sleep disruption during non-invasive ventilation. *J Thorac Dis.* (2018) 10(Suppl. 1):S80–85. doi: 10.21037/jtd.2017.11.31
60. Vrijsen B, Buyse B, Belge C, Vanpee G, Van Damme P, Testelmans D. Randomized cross-over trial of ventilator modes during non-invasive ventilation titration in amyotrophic lateral sclerosis. *Respirology.* (2017) 22:1212–8. doi: 10.1111/resp.13046
61. Georges M, Adler D, Contal O, Espa F, Perrig S, Pepin JL, et al. Reliability of apnea-hypopnea index measured by a home bi-level pressure support ventilator versus a polysomnographic assessment. *Respir Care.* (2015) 60:1051–6. doi: 10.4187/respcare.03633
62. Fernandez Alvarez R, Rabec C, Rubinos Cuadrado G, Cascon Hernandez JA, Rodriguez P, Georges M, et al. Monitoring noninvasive ventilation in patients with obesity hypoventilation syndrome: comparison between ventilator built-in software and respiratory polygraphy. *Respiration.* (2017) 93:162–9. doi: 10.1159/000454954
63. Gonzalez-Bermejo J, Perrin C, Janssens JP, Pepin JL, Mroue G, Leger P, et al. Proposal for a systematic analysis of polygraphy or polysomnography for identifying and scoring abnormal events occurring during non-invasive ventilation. *Thorax.* (2012) 67:546–52. doi: 10.1136/thx.2010.142653
64. Ramsay M, Mandal S, Suh ES, Steier J, Douiri A, Murphy PB, et al. Parasternal electromyography to determine the relationship between patient-ventilator asynchrony and nocturnal gas exchange during home mechanical ventilation set-up. *Thorax.* (2015) 70:946–52. doi: 10.1136/thoraxjnl-2015-206944
65. Crescimanno G, Canino M, Marrone O. Asynchronies and sleep disruption in neuromuscular patients under home noninvasive ventilation. *Respir Med.* (2012) 106:1478–85. doi: 10.1016/j.rmed.2012.05.013
66. Berry RB, Chediak A, Brown LK, Finder J, Gozal D, Iber C, et al. Best clinical practices for the sleep center adjustment of noninvasive positive pressure ventilation (NPPV) in stable chronic alveolar hypoventilation syndromes. *J Clin Sleep Med.* (2010) 6:491–509. doi: 10.5664/jcsm.27941
67. Vrijsen B, Chatwin M, Contal O, Derom E, Janssens JP, Kampelmacher MJ, et al. Hot topics in noninvasive ventilation: report of a working group at the international symposium on sleep-disordered breathing in leuven, belgium. *Respir Care.* (2015) 60:1337–62. doi: 10.4187/respcare.03796
68. Adler D, Perrig S, Takahashi H, Espa F, Rodenstein D, Pepin JL, et al. Polysomnography in stable COPD under non-invasive ventilation to reduce patient-ventilator asynchrony and morning breathlessness. *Sleep Breath.* (2012) 16:1081–90. doi: 10.1007/s11325-011-0605-y
69. Windisch W, Freidel K, Schucher B, Baumann H, Wiebel M, Matthys H, et al. The Severe Respiratory Insufficiency (SRI) Questionnaire: a specific measure of health-related quality of life in patients receiving home mechanical ventilation. *J Clin Epidemiol.* (2003) 56:752–9. doi: 10.1016/S0895-4356(03)00088-X
70. Majorski DS, Schwarz SB, Magnet FS, Ahmad R, Mathes T, Windisch W. The Severe Respiratory Insufficiency Application (SRI App): a pilot randomised controlled trial. *Thorax.* (2021) 76:832–4. doi: 10.1136/thoraxjnl-2020-216319
71. Dupuis-Lozeron E, Gex G, Pasquina P, Bridevaux PO, Borel JC, Soccal PM, et al. Development and validation of a simple tool for the assessment of home noninvasive ventilation: the S(3)-NIV questionnaire. *Eur Respir J.* (2018) 52:1801182. doi: 10.1183/13993003.011822018
72. Zigmond AS, Snaith RP. The hospital anxiety and depression scale. *Acta Psychiatr Scand.* (1983) 67:361–70. doi: 10.1111/j.1600-0447.1983.tb09716.x
73. Georges M, Rabec C, Monin E, Aho S, Beltramo G, Janssens JP, et al. Monitoring of noninvasive ventilation: comparative analysis of different strategies. *Respir Res.* (2020) 21:324. doi: 10.1186/s12931-020-01586-8
74. Borel JC, Gonzalez-Bermejo J. Is it still relevant to consider polysomnography as essential for noninvasive ventilation titration? *Eur Respir J.* (2019) 53:1900619. doi: 10.1183/13993003.00619-2019
75. Bauman KA, Kurili A, Schmidt SL, Rodriguez GM, Chiodo AE, Sitrin RG. Home-based overnight transcutaneous capnography/pulse oximetry for diagnosing nocturnal hypoventilation associated

with neuromuscular disorders. *Arch Phys Med Rehabil.* (2013) 94:46–52. doi: 10.1016/j.apmr.2012.08.215
76. Duiverman ML, Huberts AS, van Eykern LA, Bladder G, Wijkstra PJ. Respiratory muscle activity and patient-ventilator asynchrony during different settings of noninvasive ventilation in stable hypercapnic COPD: does high inspiratory pressure lead to respiratory muscle unloading? *Int J Chron Obstruct Pulmon Dis.* (2017) 12:243–57. doi: 10.2147/COPD.S119959
77. Borel JC, Palot A, Patout M. Technological advances in home non-invasive ventilation monitoring: reliability of data and effect on patient outcomes. *Respirology.* (2019) 24:1143–51. doi: 10.1111/resp.13497
78. van den Biggelaar RJM, Hazenberg A, Cobben NAM, Gaytant MA, Vermeulen KM, Wijkstra PJ. A randomized trial of initiation of chronic noninvasive mechanical ventilation at home vs in-hospital in patients with neuromuscular disease and thoracic cage disorder: the dutch homerun trial. *Chest.* (2020) 158:2493–501. doi: 10.1016/j.chest.2020.07.007
79. Hazenberg A, Kerstjens HA, Prins SC, Vermeulen KM, Wijkstra PJ. Initiation of home mechanical ventilation at home: a randomised controlled trial of efficacy, feasibility and costs. *Respir Med.* (2014) 108:1387–95. doi: 10.1016/j.rmed.2014.07.008
80. Ando H, Ashcroft-Kelso H, Halhead R, Chakrabarti B, Young CA, Cousins R, et al. Experience of telehealth in people with motor neurone disease using noninvasive ventilation. *Disabil Rehabil Assist Technol.* (2021) 16:490–6. doi: 10.1080/17483107.2019.1659864
81. Lopes de Almeida JP, Pinto A, Pinto S, Ohana B, de Carvalho M. Economic cost of home-telemonitoring care for BiPAP-assisted ALS individuals. *Amyotroph Lateral Scler.* (2012) 13:533–7. doi: 10.3109/17482968.2012.703675
82. Pinto A, Almeida JP, Pinto S, Pereira J, Oliveira AG, de Carvalho M. Home telemonitoring of non-invasive ventilation decreases healthcare utilisation in a prospective controlled trial of patients with amyotrophic lateral sclerosis. *J Neurol Neurosurg Psychiatry.* (2010) 81:1238–42. doi: 10.1136/jnnp.2010.206680
83. Manis E, Cheng H, Shelgikar AV. Elevated residual apnea-hypopnea index on continuous positive airway pressure download after transition to full-face mask. *Ann Am Thorac Soc.* (2021) 18:524–6. doi: 10.1513/AnnalsATS.202006-725CC
84. Pepin JL, Bailly S, Tamisier R. Big data in sleep apnoea: opportunities and challenges. *Respirology.* (2020) 25:486–94. doi: 10.1111/resp.13669
85. Liu D, Armitstead J, Benjafield A, Shao S, Malhotra A, Cistulli PA, et al. Trajectories of emergent central sleep apnea during CPAP therapy. *Chest.* (2017) 152:751–60. doi: 10.1016/j.chest.2017.06.010
86. Cistulli PA, Armitstead J, Pepin JL, Woehrle H, Nunez CM, Benjafield A, et al. Short-term CPAP adherence in obstructive sleep apnea: a big data analysis using real world data. *Sleep Med.* (2019) 59:114–6. doi: 10.1016/j.sleep.2019.01.004
87. Patel SR, Bakker JP, Stitt CJ, Aloia MS, Nouraie SM. Age and sex disparities in adherence to CPAP. *Chest.* (2021) 159:382–9. doi: 10.1016/j.chest.2020.07.017
88. Cantero C, Pasquina P, Dao MD, Cedraschi C, Adler D, Plojoux J, et al. Impact of confinement in patients under long-term noninvasive ventilation during the first wave of the SARS-CoV-2 pandemic: a remarkable resilience. *Respiration.* (2021) 100:909–17. doi: 10.1159/000516327
89. Pepin JL, Daabek N, Bailly S, Tamisier R, Attias D, Pathak A. Adherence to continuous positive airway pressure hugely improved during COVID-19 lockdown in France. *Am J Respir Crit Care Med.* (2021) 204:1103–6. doi: 10.1164/rccm.202103-0803LE

18

Interaction Between CD34+ Fibrocytes and Airway Smooth Muscle Promotes IL-8 Production and Akt/PRAS40/mTOR Signaling in Asthma

Ting-Yu Lin[1,2], Po-Jui Chang[1,2], Chun-Yu Lo[1,2], Yu-Lun Lo[1,2], Chih-Teng Yu[1,2], Shu-Min Lin[1,2], Chih-His Scott Kuo[1,2] and Horng-Chyuan Lin[1,2]*

[1] Department of Thoracic Medicine, Chang Gung Memorial Hospital, Taipei, Taiwan, [2] College of Medicine, Chang Gung University, Taoyuan, Taiwan

Correspondence:
Ting-Yu Lin
yuebaoyuebao@gmail.com

Background: The circulating progenitor cells of fibroblasts (fibrocytes) have been shown to infiltrate the airway smooth muscle compartment of asthma patients; however, the pathological significance of this discovery has yet to be elucidated. This study established a co-culture model of airway smooth muscle cells (ASMCs) and fibrocytes from asthmatic or normal subjects to evaluate innate cytokine production, corticosteroid responses, and signaling in ASMCs.

Methods: CD34+ fibrocytes were purified from peripheral blood of asthmatic (Global Initiative for Asthma treatment step 4–5) and normal subjects and cultured for 5~7 days. In a transwell plate, ASMCs were co-cultured with fibrocytes at a ratio of 2:1, ASMCs were cultured alone (control condition), and fibrocytes were cultured alone for 48 h. Measurements were obtained of interleukin-8 (IL-8), IL-6, IL-17, thymic stromal lymphopoietin, and IL-33 levels in the supernatant and IL-33 levels in the cell lysate of the co-culture. Screening for intracellular signaling in the ASMCs after stimulation was performed using condition medium from the patients' co-culture (PtCM) or IL-8. mRNA and western blot analysis were used to analyze AKT/mTOR signaling in ASMCs stimulated via treatment with PtCM or IL-8.

Results: Compared with ASMCs cultured alone, IL-8 levels in the supernatant and IL-33 levels in the ASMCs lysate were significantly higher in samples co-cultured from asthmatics, but not in those co-cultured from normal subjects. Corticosteroid-induced suppression of IL-8 production was less pronounced in ASMCs co-cultured with fibrocytes from asthma patients than in ASMCs co-cultured from normal subjects. ASMCs stimulated using PtCM and IL-8 presented elevating activated AKT substrate PRAS40. Treatment with IL-8 and PtCM increased mRNA expression of mTOR and P70S6 kinases in ASMCs. Treatment with IL-8 and PtCM also significantly increased phosphorylation of AKT and mTOR subtract S6 ribosomal protein in ASMCs.

Conclusion: The interaction between ASMCs and fibrocytes from asthmatic patients was shown to increase IL-8 and IL-33 production and promote AKT/mTOR signaling in

ASMCs. IL-8 production in the co-culture from asthmatic patients was less affected by corticosteroid than was that in the co-culture from normal subjects. Our results elucidate the novel role of fibrocytes and ASMCs in the pathogenesis of asthma.

Keywords: fibrocytes, airway smooth muscle cells, interleukin-8, interleukin-33, PRAS40, mTOR, AKT, asthma

BACKGROUND

In asthma patients, immune cells have been shown to influence the contractic and proliferative functions of airway smooth muscle cells (ASMCs) (1, 2). Infiltration of the ASM layer of asthmatic patients by an elevated number of mast cells (3) has been shown to promote ASMC differentiation into its contractile phenotype (4). $CD4^+$ T cells within the ASM layer have also been shown to promote ASMC proliferation (5, 6). ASMCs are the source of inflammatory mediators perpetuating chronic inflammation (7). An increase in ASM mass is a feature of asthmatic airways and the cellular mechanism underlying ASMC proliferation, such as phosphatidylinositol 3-kinase or AKT-mammalian target of rapamycin (mTOR) (8, 9).

One study reported on the migration and infiltration of $CD34^+$ progenitor cells into the ASM compartment in asthmatic patients (10). These circulating progenitor cells, referred to as fibrocytes, co-express hematopoietic stem cell marker CD34, collagen 1, and panhematopoietic marker CD45, but do not express CD14 (11, 12). In $CD34^+$ cells from the blood of asthmatic patients, fibrocytes have been shown to produce proinflammatory and profibrotic mediators under type 2 cytokine stimulation (13). Nonetheless, few studies have addressed the pathological significance of fibrocytes infiltration in the ASM layer. Two studies demonstrated that fibrocytes promoted inflammatory cytokine production and gel contraction when co-cultured with ASMCs. However, fibrocytes did not affect the proliferation or apoptosis of ASMCs (14, 15). A number of questions still need to be addressed. For example, do the suppressive effects of corticosteroids differ between asthmatic patients and normal subjects? Do fibrocytes affect upstream proliferative signaling in ASMCs, despite previous reports that fibrocytes did not affect the proliferation of ASMCs in terms of Ki67 or cell size?

In the current study, we addressed these questions by establishing a co-culture model by which to evaluate the interactions between ASMCs and $CD34^+$ fibrocytes, respectively, from asthmatic patients and normal subjects. We analyzed the asthma-related expression of innate inflammatory cytokines and the suppressive effects of corticosteroids. Array screening of active signaling in ASMCs revealed that the AKT-mTOR pathway may be activated when co-cultured with asthmatic fibrocytes.

Abbreviations: ASMCs, Airway smooth muscle cells; IL, Interleukin; mTOR, Mammalian target of rapamycin; PtCM, Condition medium from patients' co-culture; GINA, Global Initiative for Asthma; PBMCs, Peripheral blood mononuclear cells; TSLP, Thymic stromal lymphopoietin; PS6K, P70S6 kinase; S6RP, S6 ribosomal protein; PRAS40, Proline-rich AKT substrate of 40 kDa.

MATERIALS AND METHODS

Subjects

Thirty asthma patients and ten normal subjects were recruited (**Table 1**). The asthma patients presented a consistent history including one or more of the following: (1) >12% improvement in forced expiratory volume in 1 s (FEV1) after administration of bronchodilator; (2) PC20 of methacholine test <8 mg/mL; (3) Diurnal variation of peak expiratory flow >20%. Patients in the current study were undergoing treatment in accordance with 2016 Global Initiative for Asthma (GINA) guidelines levels 4–5. Subjects were non-smokers or ex-smokers with a previous smoking history of <10 pack-years and free from respiratory or systemic infections in the previous 2 months. All subjects provided informed consent and the study protocol was approval by the Chang Gung Medical Foundation Institutional Review Board (No. 103-6844A3).

Isolation of $CD34^+$ Fibrocytes From Peripheral Blood Mononuclear Cells

Fibrocytes were separated in accordance with published methods with slight modifications (13, 16, 17). Briefly, peripheral blood mononuclear cells (PBMCs) were isolated from whole blood using Ficoll-Paque (GE Healthcare, Bio-science AB, Uppsala, Sweden) density gradient centrifugation. Mononuclear cells were harvested, washed, and resuspended in Iscove's modified Dulbecco's medium. Magnetic positive selection of CD34 was performed sequentially in accordance with manufacturer instructions (Miltenyi Biotec, Auburn, CA). Monocytes/macrophages were further depleted by negative selection of CD14. Cells isolated via immunomagnetic selection were cultured with DMEM containing 30% fibrocytes (FCS), 1% BSA, and stem cell factor (50 ng/mL). Non-adherent cells were removed within 48 h and adherent cells were cultured for an additional 5–7 days. The purity (> 90%) of fibrocytes was determined via immunofluorescence staining for CD34, CD45, and Col-I via flow cytometry (**Figure 1A**).

Culturing Airway Smooth Muscle Cells

ASMCs from normal subjects were purchased from Lonza Inc. ASMCs were maintained in DMEM with 10% FBS with 5% CO_2 at 37°C. Cells at the fourth to seventh passage were utilized in subsequent experiments. Information about the ASMCs donors were available in **Supplementary Material**.

Transwell Culturing of Airway Smooth Muscle Cells and Fibrocytes

ASMCs and FCs from patients or normal subjects were serum-starved overnight. Cells were cultured in a transwell plate (24-well culture plate; 0.4 μm pore size; Corning, Lowell, MA)

(**Figure 1B**). Co-culturing was conducted over a period of 48 h with 9.0×10^4 ASMCs in the lower well and 4.5×10^4 FCs in the upper well (i.e., cell ratio of 2:1). Note that this setup is hereafter referred to as the co-culture, which was meant to elucidate the interaction between ASMCs and FCs. We also cultured ASMCs alone in both the upper and lower wells using the same cell number ratio as a control, (hereafter referred to as ASMCs alone). We also cultured FCs alone in both the upper and lower wells using the same cell number ratio, (hereafter referred to as FCs alone). If the cultured fibrocytes were not adequate for preplanned cell numbers for co-culture, the co-culture will be processed by adjusting cell numbers with fixed ratio of lower and upper well of co-culture to 2:1. Supernatant from the cultures was assayed for interleukin-8 (IL-8), IL-6, IL-17, thymic stromal lymphopoietin (TSLP), and IL-33 using commercial ELISA kits (R&D systems and Boster Biological technology for TSLP). Cell lysate from the lower wells was also collected and assayed for IL-33 levels via ELISA. The sensitivity limit for IL-8, IL-6, IL-17, TSLP, and IL-33 was 7.5, 0.7, 15, 10, and 1.65 pg/ml, respectively. The ELISA data was presented by percentage of control. Condition medium was collected for further experiments.

Corticosteroid Suppression of Cytokine Production in Co-culture of Airway Smooth Muscle Cells and Fibrocytes

ASMCs were co-cultured with fibrocytes of asthmatic patients or normal subjects at a ratio of 2:1 in starving medium with serial doses of dexamethasone (Sigma-Aldrich; 10^{-4} to 10^{-10} M) or vehicle (DMSO) for 48 h. IL-8/IL-6 levels in the supernatant and IL-33 levels in the cell lysate from ASMCs were assessed via ELISA.

Path Scan Intracellular Signaling Array

An intracellular signaling array was used to detect the effects of IL-8 and co-culturing with fibrocytes on intracellular signaling in ASMCs. Briefly, 80% confluent ASMCs were cultured for 24 h in a 24-well plate with IL-8 (20 ng/ml) or condition medium from patient co-culture (PtCM). Cells were then harvested and lysed for 5 min with ice-cold cell lysis buffer containing a cocktail of protease inhibitors. The lysates were assayed for intracellular signaling molecules using a PathScan® Intracellular Signaling Array kit (#7323; Cell Signaling Technology). The intensity of chemiluminescent signals was quantified using a UVP biospectrum 810 imaging system (Upland, CA, United States) in accordance with the protocol outlined by the manufacturer.

Effect of Interleukin-8 and Condition Medium on AKT/Mammalian Target of Rapamycin Signaling and Cytokine Production by Airway Smooth Muscle Cells

Due to the limited number cells in the co-culture experiment, we were unable to obtain enough ASMCs for real-time reverse transcription or western blot analysis. Thus, we cultured fresh

TABLE 1 | Characteristics of recruited subjects.

	Normal subjects (*n* = 10)	Asthmatic patients (*n* = 30, GINA step 4, *n* = 23, step 5, *n* = 7)
Male, *n* (%)	4 (40.0)	20 (60.0)
Age, year	35.4 ± 4.6	58.6 ± 12.0****
Atopy, *n* (%)	2 (20.0)	16 (53.2)
Body mass index (kg/m^2)	22.2 ± 2.6	25.8 ± 4.2*
Prebronchodilator FVC, liter	3.1 ± 0.6	2.2 ± 0.7***
Prebronchodilator FVC,% of prediction	91.4 ± 3.1	74.2 ± 19.9*
Prebronchodilator FEV1, liter	2.5 ± 0.5	1.6 ± 0.5****
Prebronchodilator FEV1,% of prediction	89.4 ± 6.3	65.7 ± 21.9**
FEV1/FVC,%	80.7 ± 3.4	74.6 ± 13.8
Treatment with inhaled corticosteroid and long-acting bronchodilators, *n*	0	30 (100.0)****
Treatment with oral corticosteroid, *n*, (%)	0	3 (10.0)
Treatment with biological agent, *n*, (%)	0	2 (6.7)

*Data are expressed as means ± SEM or number of subjects with percentage (*p < 0.05, **p < 0.01, ***p < 0.001, ****p < 0.0001).*
FVC, forced vital capacity; FEV1, forced expiratory volume in 1 s.

ASMCs in the 6-well culture plate with 80% confluence to obtain cells for this experiment. PtCM was diluted with DMEM medium at a ratio of 1:3 for culturing in 6-well plate. ASMCs were then subjected to qPCR or western blot analysis after stimulation using IL-8 or PtCM.

Quantitative Real-Time Reverse Transcription

Over period of 0, 1, 2, 6, and 24 h, ASMC expression was stimulated using IL-8 (20 ng/ml) or PtCM or ASMC culture medium alone or fibrocyte culture alone for 2 h. PBS treatment as the control. Samples that underwent PBS stimulation were used as a control. Total RNA was isolated from co-cultured ASMCs using TRIzol reagent (Invitrogen, Grand Island, NY) in accordance with the manufacturer's instructions. cDNA was reverse-transcribed from isolated RNA by incubating 1 μg of DNase-treated RNA using the HiscriptIFirst Strand cDNA synthesis kit (BioNovus Life Sciences). qPCR was performed using TOOLS SuperFast SYBR Qpcr Reagent (Biotools) in a LightCycler 2.0 System (Roche Applied Science). Sequences of mTOR, P70S6 kinase (PS6K), and 18s rRNA are described in **Table 2**. Samples were denatured at 95°C for 1 min, followed by 50 cycles of annealing and extension at 95°C for 10 s, 60°C for 20 s, and 72°C for 20 s. All qPCR results were normalized to the 18s rRNA of the internal control. Data were obtained using the 2-$\Delta\Delta$Ct method using LightCycler software.

Western Blot Analysis

After treatment using IL-8 or PtCM followed by electrophoresis, proteins from ASMCs were transferred to nitrocellulose

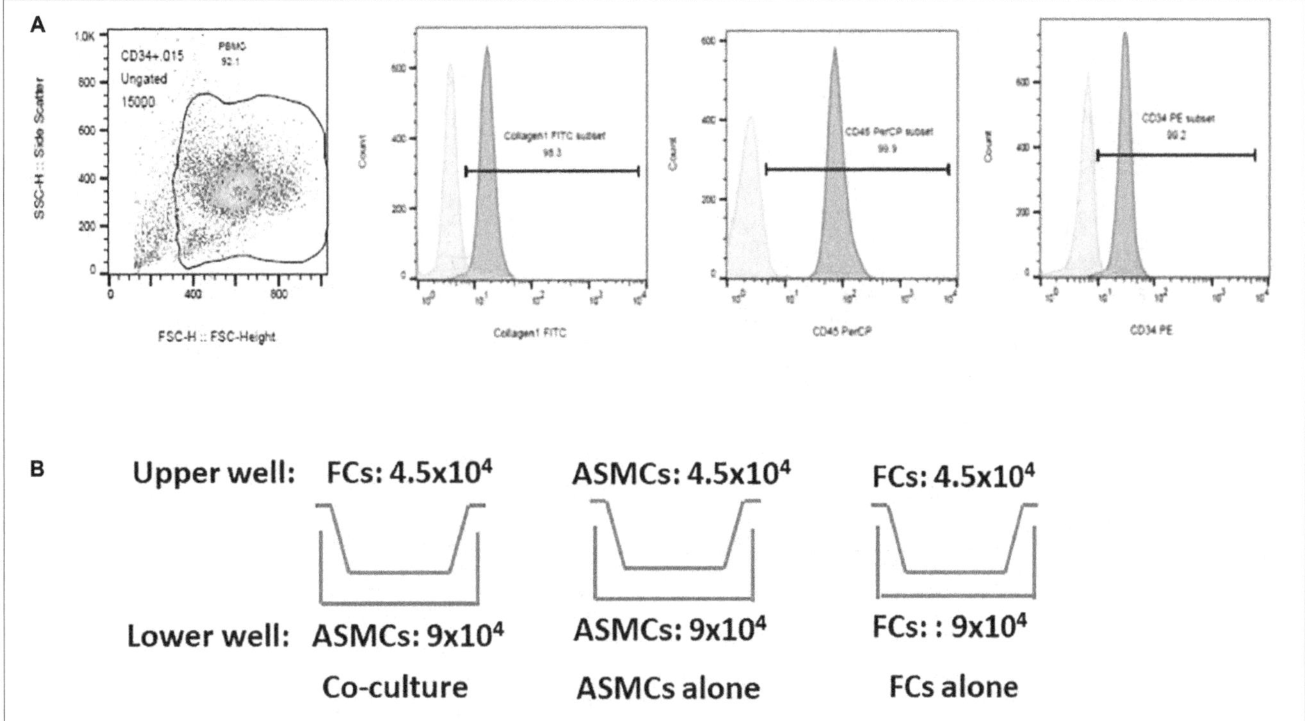

FIGURE 1 | Purification of fibrocytes (FCs) after culturing cells for 5–7 days. **(A)** Cells underwent triple positive staining (> 90% positive expression) for collagen-I, CD34 and CD45 via flow cytometry. The proportion of positive expression was defined by isotype staining. **(B)** Co-culture model of airway smooth muscle cells (ASMCs) with FCs. Co-culture: ASMCs in lower well and FCs in upper well were cultured at a cell ratio of 2:1 for 48 h. ASMCs alone were cultured in the lower and upper well at a cell ratio of 2:1 as a major control. FCs alone were cultured in the same way. Culture supernatant and cell lysates was collected from lower wells for analysis.

membranes, which were blocked with 0.1% Tween 20 in Tris-buffered saline with 5% non-fat dry milk, washed, and incubated overnight with primary antibodies. Due to the limited quantity of PtCM, we selected antibodies specific to Akt, Ser473 phospho-Akt, PARS40, Thr246 phospho-PARS40, S6 ribosomal protein and phospho-S6 ribosomal protein (Cell Signaling), and beta-actin (Millipore). Following incubation with appropriate secondary antibodies, the proteins of interest were visualized via Enhanced Chemiluminescent Assay (ECL) using horseradish peroxidase. Relevant band intensities were quantified and analyzed using a UVP ChemStudio PLUS Touch scanner (Analytik Jena AG, Jena, Germany) in conjunction with VisionWorks software (Analytik Jena AG, Jena, Germany) and Image Gauge Ver 4.0, Science Lab (FUJIFILM, Tokyo, Japan).

Statistical Analysis

Data were expressed as mean ± S.E. An unpaired two-tailed Student's *t*-test was used for single comparisons. The Chi-square test or Fisher's exact test was used to compare categorical data in cases where the sample size was small. Cytokine, mRNA, and protein levels in co-cultures were expressed in terms of fold change compared to levels in the ASMC culture alone. One way ANOVA was used with Tukey's test to compare the effect of co-culture or IL-8 stimulation with results obtained from the control group. Probability values of < 0.05 were considered significant.

TABLE 2 | Primers used for real-time RT-PCR.

Gene symbol	Sequence	Amplicon length (bp)
PS6K-Forward (F)	5′-AAgggggCTATggAAAggCAA-3′	21
PS6K-Reverse (R)	5′-AATCCACgATgAAgggATgCT-3′	21
mTOR-F	5′-gAACCTCAgggCAAgATgCT-3′	20
mTOR-R	5′-CTggTTTCCTCATTCCggCT-3′	20
18s rRNA F	5′-CTTAgAgggACAAgTggCg-3′	19
18s rRNA R	5′-AgCCTgAgCCAgTCAgTgTA-3′	20

RESULTS

Co-culturing of Airway Smooth Muscle Cells and Fibrocytes From Asthmatic Patients Increased Interleukin-8 Expression in Supernatant and Interleukin-33 Expression in Airway Smooth Muscle Cells, Compared to Culturing Airway Smooth Muscle Cells Alone

ELISA was used to analyze the supernatant from co-culturing ASMCs and fibrocytes, culturing ASMCs alone, or culturing fibrocytes alone for IL-8, IL-6, IL-17, TSLP, and IL-33 production. Culturing ASMCs with fibrocytes from asthmatic patients

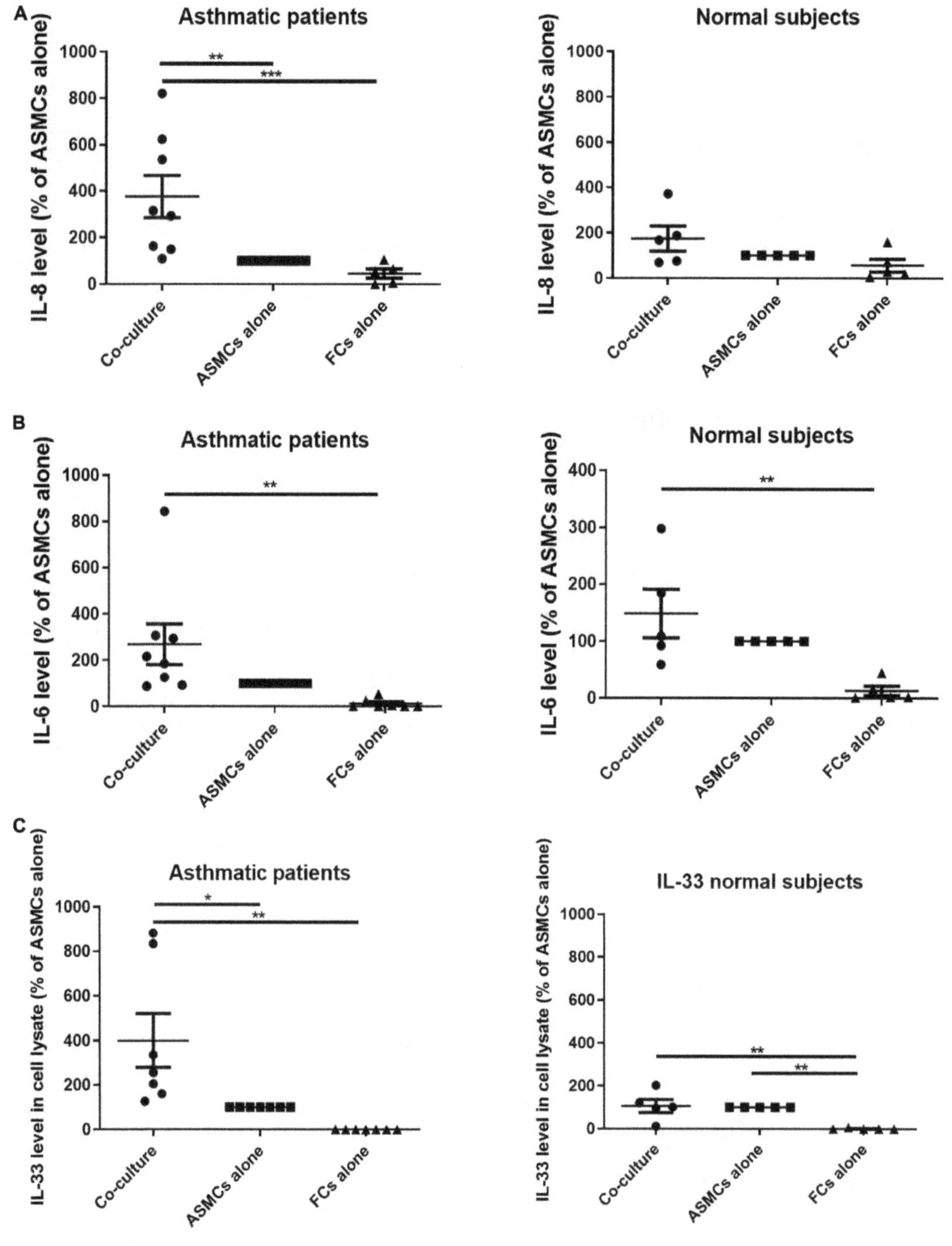

FIGURE 2 | (A) IL-8 levels and **(B)** IL-6 levels in the supernatant and **(C)** IL-33 levels in the cell lysates from the lower well in transwell experiments involving the co-culturing of ASMCs with fibrocytes, culturing ASMCs alone, and culturing fibrocytes alone. Fibrocytes were isolated from asthmatic patients or normal subjects. Cells were cultured at the same density in each well for 48 h and cytokine levels were detected using ELISA. The level of cytokines is presented as the% of ASMCs alone. $p < 0.001$, One-way ANOVA with Tukey's multiple comparison test (n = 5~8).

significantly increased IL-8 levels (**Figure 2A**), compared to culturing ASMCs alone. Note that culturing ASMCs with fibrocytes from normal subjects had no effect on IL-8 production. Co-culturing ASMCs with fibrocytes from asthmatic or normal subjects had no effect on IL-6 levels production, compared to culturing ASMCs alone (**Figure 2B**). The majority of IL-6 and IL-33 of "FC alone" were below the lowest detectable concentration. We failed to detect IL-17, TSLP, or IL-33 in the supernatant of any samples. We also checked IL-33 levels in ASMCs, due to its common accumulation in cells (18). Culturing ASMCs with fibrocytes from asthmatic patients was shown to increase the intracellular level of IL-33 in ASMCs, compared

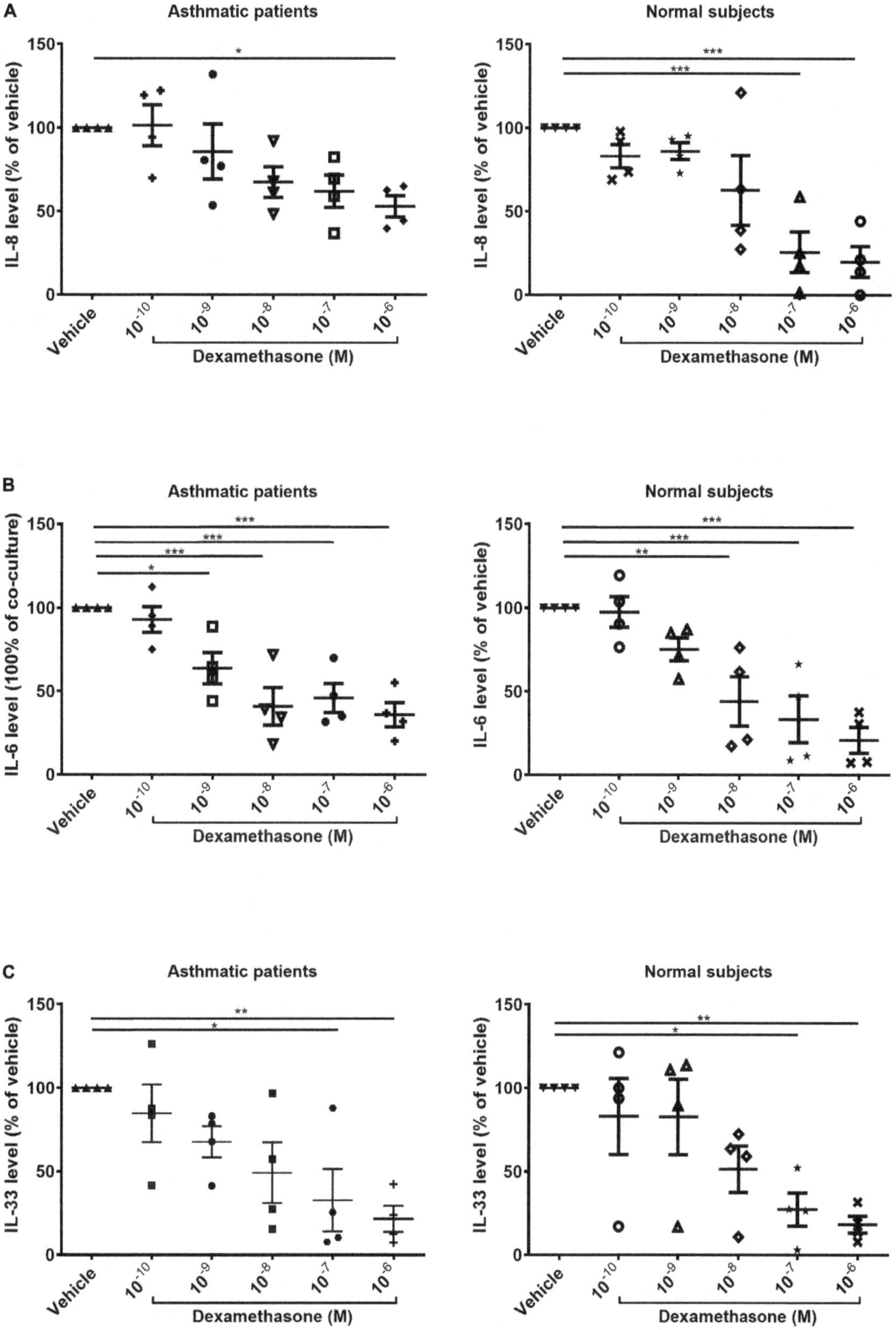

FIGURE 3 | Dexamethasone-induced suppression of **(A)** IL-8 and **(B)** IL-6 in the supernatant and **(C)** suppression of IL-33 in the cell lysates of ASMCs co-cultured with fibrocytes from asthmatic patients and normal subjects (10^{-10} to 10^{-6} mol/L, 48 h). Vehicle: DMSO of same concentration in dexamethasone solution ($n = 4$). $^*P < 0.05$; $^{**}P < 0.01$; $^{***}P < 0.001$.

to culturing ASMCs alone (**Figure 2C**). Culturing ASMCs with fibrocytes from normal subjects had no effect on IL-33 levels.

Corticosteroid-Induced Suppression of Interleukin-8 Production Was More Pronounced in Samples Co-cultured With Fibrocytes From Normal Subjects Than in Samples Co-cultured From Asthmatic Patients

We also examined the expression of IL-8 after serial dosing with dexamethasone for 48 h. In samples co-cultured with fibrocytes from normal subjects, the production of IL-8 was significantly lower when dexamethasone was administered at high concentrations (10^{-7} M and 10^{-6} M, $p < 0.001$). In samples co-cultured with fibrocytes from asthmatic patients, we observed a reduction in the production of IL-8 only when dexamethasone was administered at the highest concentration (10^{-6}M, $p < 0.05$), thereby by indicating less corticosteroid suppression on IL-8 production of co-culture from asthma patients (**Figure 3A**). Dexamethasone had a similar effect in suppressing IL-33 in ASMCs and IL-6 in the supernatant in samples co-cultured with fibrocytes from asthmatic patients as well as normal subjects (**Figures 3B,C**).

Stimulation *via* Interleukin-8 or Patients' Co-culture Increased the Phosphorylation of Proline-Rich AKT Substrate 40 kDa (PRAS40) in Airway Smooth Muscle Cells Beyond That of PBS Stimulation (Control)

Our results prompted analysis of the effects of PtCM and IL-8 on the intracellular signaling of ASMCs. We screened the phosphorylation status of signaling pathways in ASMCs after incubation with PtCM, medium of ASMCs, or FC culture alone for 24 h (**Figures 4A–C**). We observed no significantly differences between any of the samples in terms of phosphorylation; however, we observed elevate expression levels of PRAS40 in ASMCs treated with PtCM, compared to the positive control. This prompted further screening of ASMCs after stimulation by IL-8 (**Figures 4D–F**), which also exhibited high phosphorylation of PRAS40.

Note that PRAS40 is an AKT substrate known for the encoding of a key molecule connecting AKT signaling and mTOR activation (19, 20). Thus, our primary concern in subsequent experiments was the effects of IL-8 and PtCM on AKT-mTOR signaling in ASMCs.

mRNA Levels of Mammalian Target of Rapamycin and PS6K in Airway Smooth Muscle Cells Increased After Stimulation Using Patients' Co-culture or Interleukin-8

We first tested the mRNA expression of mTOR and its substrate PS6K in ASMCs. The mRNA expression of mTOR and PS6K was significantly higher in ASMCs after 2-h stimulation by IL-8 (20 ng/ml) than in PBS control samples (**Figure 5A**). We then treated ASMCs with PtCM, ASMC or fibrocyte condition medium, or PBS control for 2 h (**Figure 5B**). The mRNA expression of mTOR was significantly higher in ASMCs stimulated using PtCM than in PBS control samples. We also observed increases in PS6K expression in ASMCs following stimulation using PtCM (increasing trend; $p = 0.09$).

Condition Medium From Patient Co-cultures Promoted AKT Phosphorylation in Airway Smooth Muscle Cells and Interleukin-8 Promoted PARS40 Phosphorylation in Airway Smooth Muscle Cells

Western blot analysis was used to test the active status of AKT/mTOR signaling in ASMCs following IL-8 stimulation (for various durations) or PtCM (for 6 h) (**Figure 6A**). PtCM was shown to promote the phosphorylation of AKT in ASMCs (**Figure 6B**). IL-8 was shown to promote the phosphorylation of PRAS40 after 15-min stimulation (**Figure 6C**). We observed an increase in the phosphorylation of S6RP in ASMCs after stimulation using IL-8 or PtCM for 6 h (**Figure 6D**).

DISCUSSION

Co-culturing ASMCs with fibrocytes from asthmatic patients was shown to increase IL-8 expression in supernatant and IL-33 expression in ASMCs, compared to culturing ASMCs alone. Note that co-culturing ASMCs with fibrocytes from normal subjects had no effect. The effect of corticosteroid on IL-8 production was less pronounced in ASMCs co-cultured with fibrocytes from asthmatic patients than in ASMCs co-cultured from normal subjects. Treating ASMCs with the condition medium of co-culture from asthmatic patients or IL-8 was shown to induce the mRNA expression of mTOR and its substrate PS6K in ASMCs. Treating ASMCs with the condition medium of co-culture from asthmatic patients was shown to increase the phosphorylation of AKT and mTOR downstream signaling S6RP in ASMCs. Treating ASMCs with IL-8 alone was shown the enhance the phosphorylation of PRAS40 in ASMCs. Our work provides novel findings pertaining to the effects of corticosteroids and the proliferative signaling of AKT-PRAS40-mTOR in ASMCs co-cultured with fibrocytes from asthma patients.

IL-8 in the airways of individuals with neutrophilic asthma responds poorly to corticosteroids (21, 22). There are a limited number of treatment option specific to neutrophilic asthma, and the mechanism underlying IL-8 production in such cases is crucial to the development of new treatment regimes. Our observation of increased IL-8 expression with lower corticosteroid-induced IL-8 suppression suggests that fibrocytes have a paracrine effect on ASMCs in asthmatic patients (**Figures 2A, 3A**). Our results are comparable to those obtained in a similar previous study (14), which reported the involvement of NF-κB and ERK1/2 signaling in IL-8 production. In future

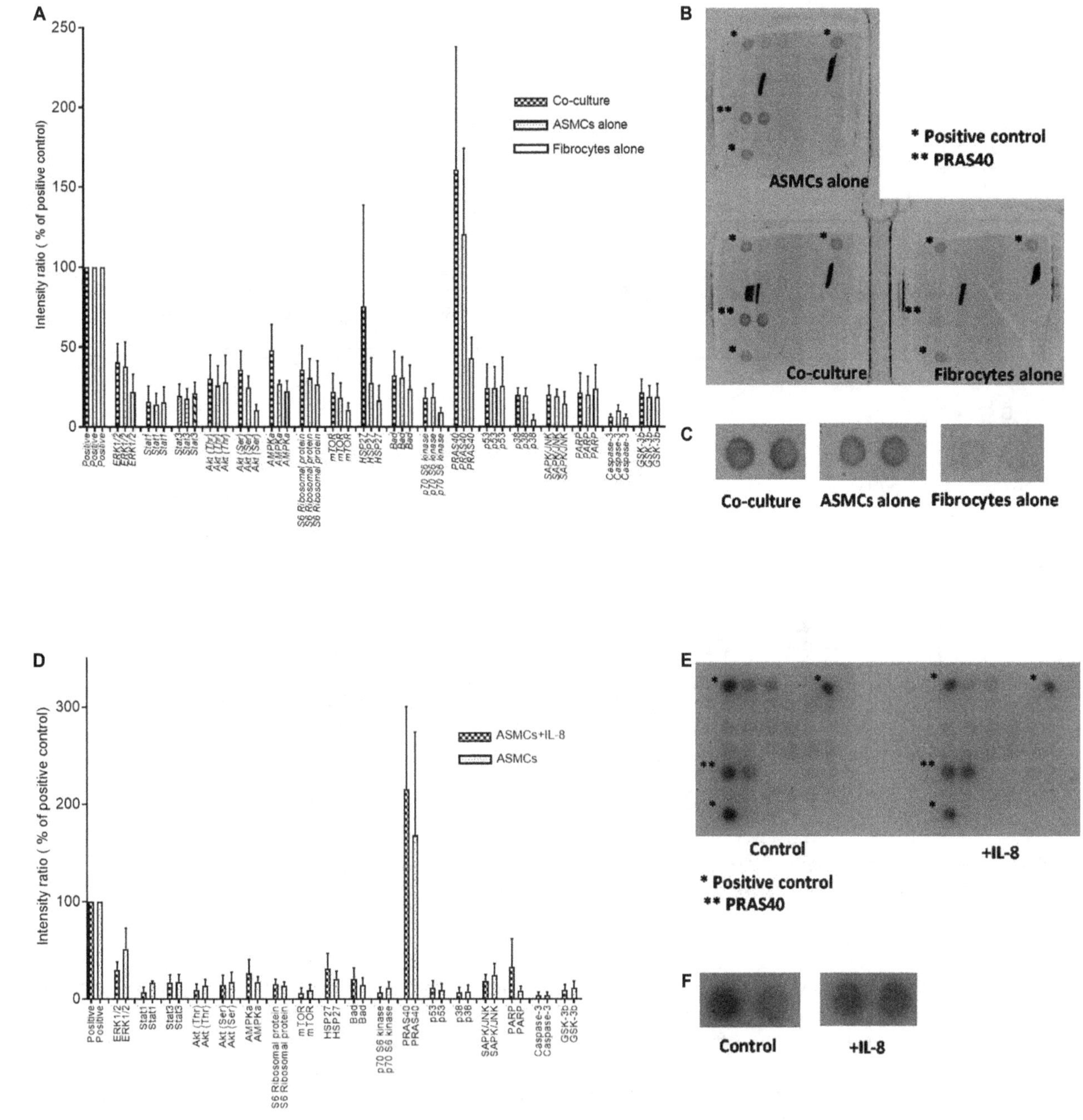

FIGURE 4 | (A) Intracellular signaling activation in ASMCs after 24-h stimulation by condition medium from co-culturing ASMCs and fibrocytes from asthmatic patients, culturing ASMCs alone, or culturing fibrocytes alone; (n = 3). **(B)** The density of all signaling in ASMCs detected by array. Each signaling was done by duplication. *: positive control. **: PRAS40. **(C)** The enlarged picture of activation of PRAS40 in ASMCs stimulated with condition medium of co-culture, culturing ASMCs alone or culturing fibrocytes alone. The expression of PRAS40 in ASMCs treated with co-cultured condition medium was higher than that of the positive control. **(D)** Intracellular signaling activation in ASMCs after stimulation by IL-8 (n = 3). **(E)** The density of all signaling in ASMCs detected by array. Each signaling was done by duplication. *: positive control. **: PRAS40. **(F)** The enlarged picture of activation of PRAS40 in ASMCs stimulated with or without IL-8. Similarly, we observed relatively high PRAS40 phosphorylation in ASMCs after IL-8 stimulation.

studies, it would be interesting to explore the cell source of IL-8 in co-culture and signaling involved in the less corticosteroid suppression on IL-8 production.

In **Figure 3A**, we showed the reduced level of IL-8 in the ASMCs co-cultured with fibrocytes from asthma after steroid treatment by comparison to the vehicle treatment. The vehicle and the steroid treatments were done in the same co-culture experiment from the same subject. The result showed the level of IL-8 of co-culture with steroid treatment was lower than co-culture without steroid treatment (their own control) with statistically significant despite higher IL-8 production in co-culture of asthma patients and lower IL-8 production in that

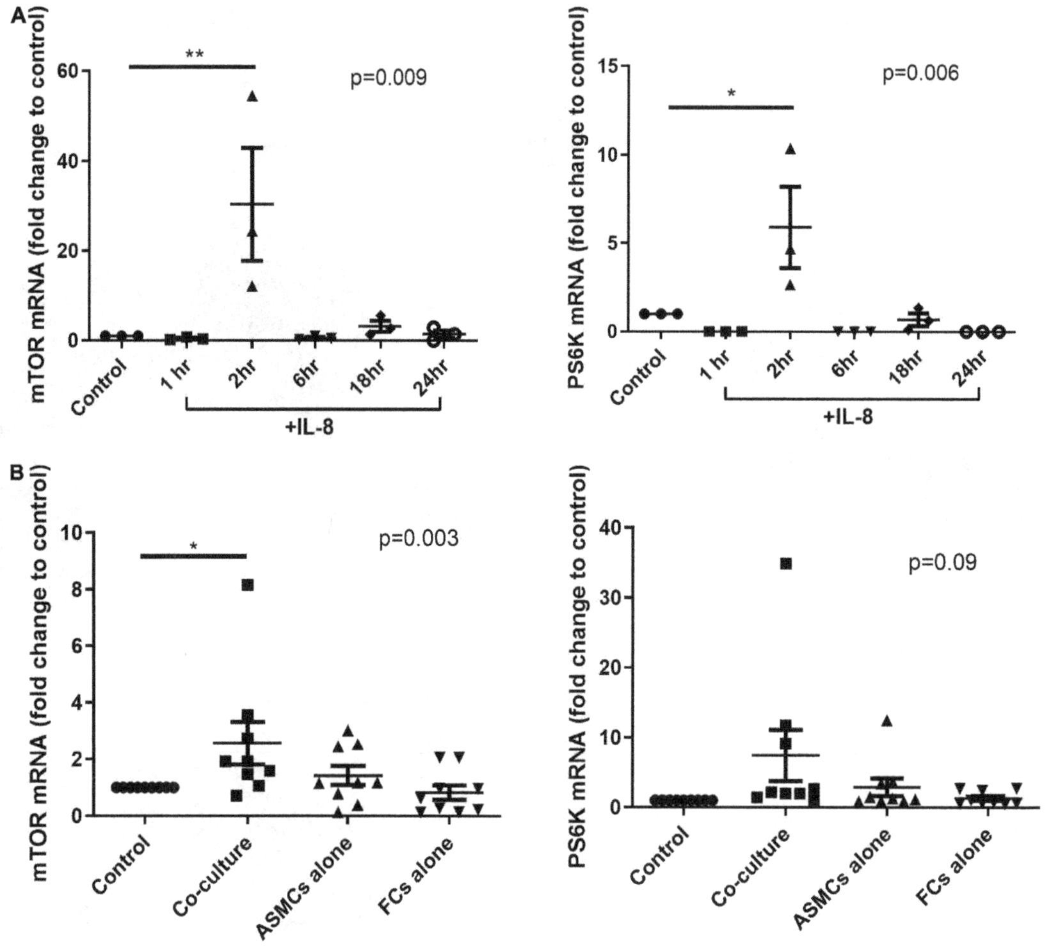

FIGURE 5 | mRNA expression of mTOR or PS6K in ASMCs after **(A)** IL-8 stimulation for 1, 2, 6, 18, and 24 h or **(B)** treatment with diluted condition medium co-cultured with fibrocytes from asthmatic patients, ASMCs cultured alone, or fibrocytes cultured alone for 2 h. PBS as the control. $^*p < 0.05$, One-way ANOVA with Tukey's multiple comparison test (n = 3~9). $^{**}P < 0.01$.

of normal subjects (Co-culture vs. ASMCs alone, **Figure 2A**). By showing the suppression effect on IL-8 occurred only at the highest concentration of steroid in co-culture of asthma patients, compared with the suppression at relative lower concentration of steroid in that of normal subjects (**Figure 3A**), and the pattern of IL-33 suppression by steroid was no different between asthma patients or normal subjects (**Figure 3C**), which was also higher IL-33 production in co-culture of asthma than that of normal subjects (Co-culture vs. ASMC alone, **Figure 2C**), we could tell the different steroid suppressive effects on IL-8 production between co-culture of asthma and normal subjects. However, the reduced effect of steroids on IL-8 secretion in ASMCs co-cultured with fibrocytes from asthmatics cannot be totally excluded the effects of increased secretion of IL-8 in co-culture of asthma. Further ELISA with actual concentration and more subject numbers are required for explore the steroid suppressive effect on high concentration IL-8 production in co-culture of asthma. However, the present study demonstrated the different pathological effects in co-culture between asthma patients and normal subjects.

Our observation of increased IL-33 in the lysate of ASMCs co-cultured with fibrocytes of asthmatic patients has not previously been reported (**Figure 2C**). Researchers have previously reported that increased IL-33 expression in ASM bundles of asthmatic airway is correlated with airway hyperresponsiveness (23, 24). In the current study, we discovered a potential source of IL-33 in asthmatic airways resulting from an interaction between ASMCs and fibrocytes. Unlike the current study, researchers previously reported that corticosteroids did not suppress IL-33 transcription in TNF-α stimulated ASMC cultures (24), due perhaps to differences in experiment design, such as the source of ASMCs and disease severity.

Signaling screen arrays revealed high PARS40 phosphorylation levels in ASMCs incubated with PtCM or IL-8 (**Figure 4**). PARS40 is a AKT substrate and key regulatory at the crossover point of AKT–mTOR transduction pathways (19). PRAS40 has been shown to inhibit the activity of the mTOR complex 1 (mTORC1) by preventing its binding to PS6K and 4E-BP1 (25). Active PS6K also phosphorylates S6RP to promote protein synthesis (26). Studies have shown that

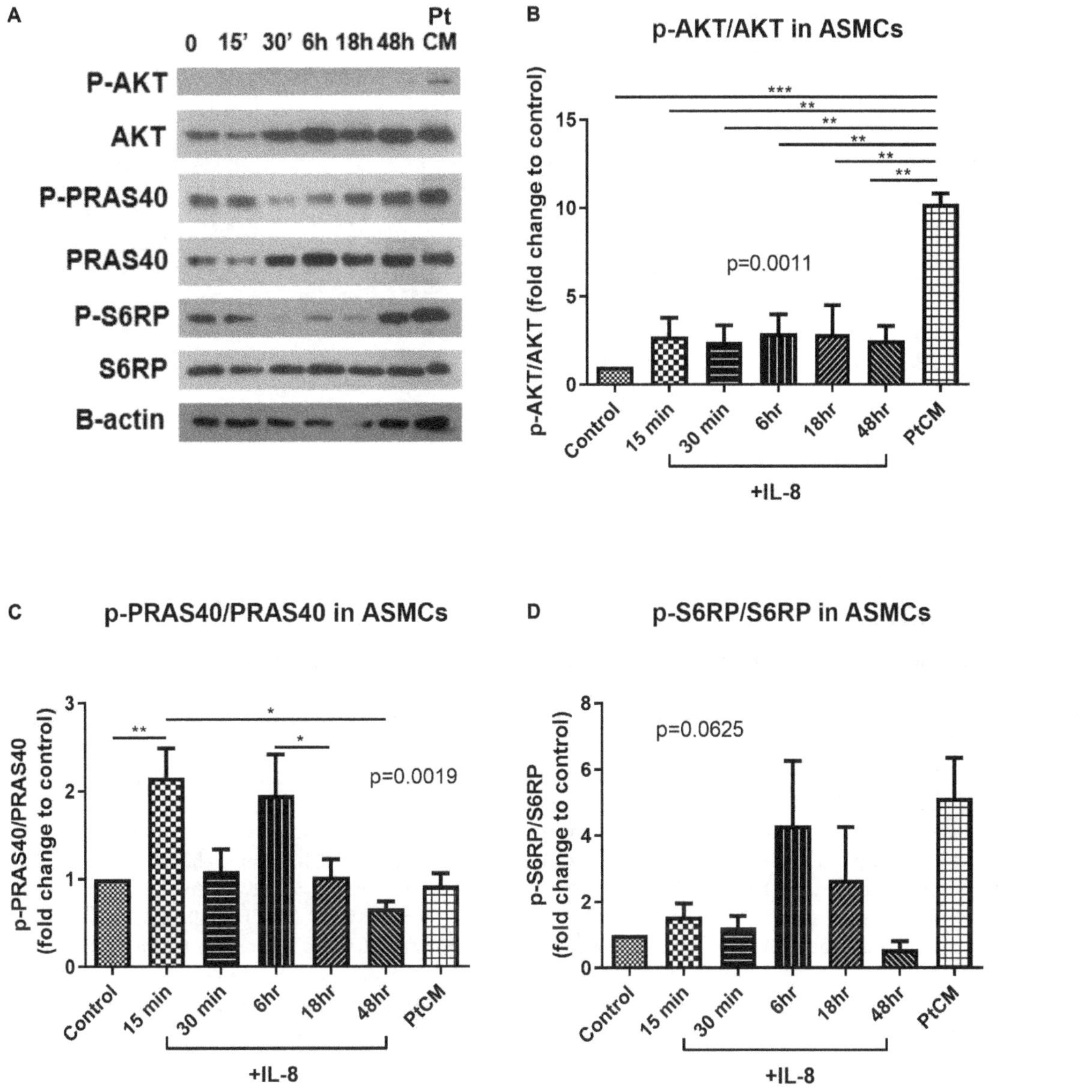

FIGURE 6 | AKT-PRAS40-mTOR in ASMCs co-cultured with IL-8 or condition medium. **(A)** ASMCs were stimulated using IL-8 (20 ng/ml) at various time points: 15′, 30′, 6, 18, and 48 h or condition medium from ASMC co-cultured with FCs from patients (Pt CM, 3:1 dilution with culture medium. 6 h treatment). **(B)** Phosphorylation status of AKT, **(C)** PRAS40 and **(D)** ribosomal protein S6 (S6RP) in ASMCs following stimulation by IL-8 or PtCM (n = 5~6). $^{*}P < 0.05$; $^{**}P < 0.01$; $^{***}P < 0.001$.

AKT is able to phosphorylate PRAS40 directly, resulting in the dissociation of PRAS40 from mTORC1 and the activation of mTOR function to promote cell growth (19, 27). It also has been shown that IL-8 can promote AKT-mTOR signaling pathways in a tissue specific manner (28). For example, IL-8 has been shown to promote the proliferation of prostate cancer through the activation of AKT-mTOR, resulting in the downstream phosphorylation of 4E-BP1 and PS6K, which could be abrogated by rapamycin (29). Similar phenomena have been observed in breast cancer cells, neutrophils, and ASMCs (9, 30–32). Based on the fact that co-culturing with fibrocytes from asthma patients significantly increased IL-8 expression levels in the supernatant, it was reasonable to explore the AKT-PRAS40-mTOR signaling. The elevated mRNA expression of mTOR and PS6K in ASMCs after stimulation with PtCM or IL-8 confirmed the reasonableness of this line of inquiry and is comparable with another study of cell line (33) (**Figure 5**).

In western blot analysis, 6-h incubation with PtCM induced strong AKT phosphorylation in ASMCs (**Figure 6B**). We observed a trend of increased downstream S6RP phosphorylation (**Figure 6D**); however, we observed no difference in the phosphorylation of PRAS40 (**Figure 6C**). The reasons for this are no doubt multifactorial. First, PtCM was the mixture of

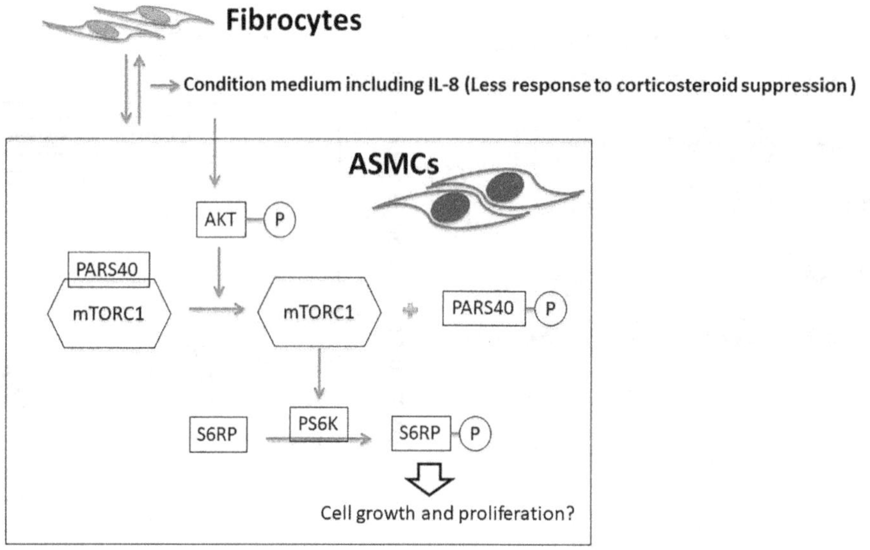

FIGURE 7 | Proposed model of ASMC remodeling by fibrocytes in asthma patients via the axis of IL-8-AKT-PARS40-mTORC1. Interaction between fibrocytes and ASMCs increases the production of IL-8 in asthmatic airways, and corticosteroid-induced suppression of IL-8 production is reduced. IL-8 stimulation activating the axis of AKT-PARS40-mTORC1 in ASMC may contribute the downstream processes involved in ASMC proliferation/growth.

IL-8, IL-6 and other factors unchecked. It is possible that unknown factors promoted effects downstream from mTOR under the complex interactions involved in this co-culture model. Therefore, the effect of IL-8 was different from that of Pt CM. Furthermore, we did not perform serial time-point experiments on PtCM stimulation as was done for IL-8 stimulation, due to the limited availability of condition medium. Specific testing for IL-8 stimulation revealed a significant increase in the phosphorylation of PRAS40 in ASMCs in as little as 15 min (**Figure 6C**), which may compensate for missing part of the PtCM stimulation experiment. Besides, the change of p-PRAS40 is different from that on S6RP. The activation of S6RP is the downstream signaling of mTOR after phosphorylated PRAS40 relieving the inhibitory constraint on mTORC1 activity. This can be one explanation for the earlier activation of PRAS40 (up to 15 min, **Figure 6B**) and the activation of S6RP occurred around 6 h or earlier time point we did not check (between 40 min and 6 h, **Figure 6D**).

Taken together, we propose remodeling the IL-8-AKT-PARS40-mTOR axis in ASMCs interacting with fibrocytes in cases of asthma (**Figure 7**). It is possible that IL-8 production via ASMC-fibrocyte interaction initiates mTOR activation, resulting in the proliferation of ASMCs. Note that no previous studies have provided evidence of proliferation or hypertrophy in ASMCs co-cultured with fibrocytes (14, 15). This could perhaps be explained by the fact that *in vitro* co-culture models interfere mTOR with downstream signaling and/or ASMC proliferation.

The study has a number of limitations. First, we obtained $CD34^{+}$ fibrocytes from patients; however, the ASMCs were purchased from a commercial supplier (i.e., they were not from the patients who provided the PBMCs). Note that simultaneous airway and blood sampling from the same subject and then growing a sufficient number of cells *in vitro* is challenging. Our use of commercial supply of cells made it possible to explore the underling molecular mechanism and consider further studies pertaining to the complex cellular interactions between FCs and ASMCs in cases of asthma. Second, we were constrained by the limited availability of FCs from patient blood, which limited the number of corresponding ASMCs for Quantitative Real-Time Reverse Transcription (rtPCR) and western blot experiments. mRNA level of some molecular markers, like IL-8, IL-6, or PRAS40 should be check in the future studies. Third, we also used PtCM to stimulate ASMCs instead of directly observing AKT-PRAS40-mTOR signaling in the ASMCs. Thus, the PtCM had to be diluted to cover the ASMC culture, which may have attenuated the effects. Nonetheless, even dilute PtCM promoted a significant increase in the expression of mTOR mRNA and p-AKT in ASMCs as well as increases in PS6K mRNA and p-S6RP expression. This suggests that PtCM has distinct biological effects on AKT-PRAS40-mTOR signaling in ASMCs.

CONCLUSION

In conclusion, the interaction between ASMCs and fibrocytes from asthmatic patients was shown to increase IL-8 and IL-33 production. Corticosteroid-induced suppression of IL-8 production was less pronounced in the co-culture from asthma patients than from normal subjects. Corticosteroid-induced suppression of IL-8 production was more pronounced in samples co-cultured with fibrocytes from normal subjects than in samples co-cultured from asthmatic patients. Furthermore, IL-8 and conditioned medium co-cultured with fibrocytes from patients promoted AKT/mTOR signaling in ASMCs. Our results elucidate the novel role of fibrocytes and ASMCs in the process of inflammation and remodeling. These results may also inspire the development of novel treatments for asthma.

AUTHOR CONTRIBUTIONS

T-YL: conceptualization, data curation, investigation, formal analysis, and writing—original draft. P-JC: data curation, resources, and formal analysis. C-YL, Y-LL, C-TY, S-ML, C-HK, and H-CL: data curation and resources. All authors contributed to the article and approved the submitted version.

REFERENCES

1. Chung KF. Airway smooth muscle cells: contributing to and regulating airway mucosal inflammation? *Eur Respir J.* (2000) 15:961–8. doi: 10.1034/j.1399-3003.2000.15e26.x
2. Hirst SJ, Walker TR, Chilvers ER. Phenotypic diversity and molecular mechanisms of airway smooth muscle proliferation in asthma. *Eur Respir J.* (2000) 16:159–77. doi: 10.1034/j.1399-3003.2000.16a28.x
3. Brightling CE, Bradding P, Symon FA, Holgate ST, Wardlaw AJ, Pavord ID. Mast-cell infiltration of airway smooth muscle in asthma. *N Engl J Med.* (2002) 346:1699–705.
4. Woodman L, Siddiqui S, Cruse G, Sutcliffe A, Saunders R, Kaur D, et al. Mast cells promote airway smooth muscle cell differentiation via autocrine up-regulation of TGF-beta 1. *J Immunol.* (2008) 181:5001–7. doi: 10.4049/jimmunol.181.7.5001
5. Ramos-Barbon D, Presley JF, Hamid QA, Fixman ED, Martin JG. Antigen-specific $CD4^+$ T cells drive airway smooth muscle remodeling in experimental asthma. *J Clin Invest.* (2005) 115:1580–9. doi: 10.1172/JCI19711
6. Ramos-Barbon D, Fraga-Iriso R, Brienza NS, Montero-Martinez C, Verea-Hernando H, Olivenstein R, et al. T cells localize with proliferating smooth muscle alpha-$actin^+$ cell compartments in asthma. *Am J Respir Crit Care Med.* (2010) 182:317–24. doi: 10.1164/rccm.200905-0745OC
7. Howarth PH, Knox AJ, Amrani Y, Tliba O, Panettieri RA Jr, Johnson M. Synthetic responses in airway smooth muscle. *J Allergy Clin Immunol.* (2004) 114:S32–50. doi: 10.1016/j.jaci.2004.04.041
8. Bara I, Ozier A, Tunon de Lara JM, Marthan R, Berger P. Pathophysiology of bronchial smooth muscle remodelling in asthma. *Eur Respir J.* (2010) 36:1174–84. doi: 10.1183/09031936.00019810
9. Zhou L, Goldsmith AM, Bentley JK, Jia Y, Rodriguez ML, Abe MK, et al. 4E-binding protein phosphorylation and eukaryotic initiation factor-4E release are required for airway smooth muscle hypertrophy. *Am J Respir Cell Mol Biol.* (2005) 33:195–202. doi: 10.1165/rcmb.2004-0411OC
10. Saunders R, Siddiqui S, Kaur D, Doe C, Sutcliffe A, Hollins F, et al. Fibrocyte localization to the airway smooth muscle is a feature of asthma. *J Allergy Clin Immunol.* (2009) 123:376–84. doi: 10.1016/j.jaci.2008.10.048
11. Pilling D, Fan T, Huang D, Kaul B, Gomer RH. Identification of markers that distinguish monocyte-derived fibrocytes from monocytes, macrophages, and fibroblasts. *PLoS One.* (2009) 4:e7475. doi: 10.1371/journal.pone.0007475
12. Schmidt M, Sun G, Stacey MA, Mori L, Mattoli S. Identification of circulating fibrocytes as precursors of bronchial myofibroblasts in asthma. *J Immunol.* (2003) 171:380–9. doi: 10.4049/jimmunol.171.1.380
13. Bellini A, Marini MA, Bianchetti L, Barczyk M, Schmidt M, Mattoli S. Interleukin (IL)-4, IL-13, and IL-17A differentially affect the profibrotic and proinflammatory functions of fibrocytes from asthmatic patients. *Mucosal Immunol.* (2012) 5:140–9. doi: 10.1038/mi.2011.60
14. Lin TY, Venkatesan N, Nishioka M, Kyoh S, Al-Alwan L, Baglole CJ, et al. Monocyte-derived fibrocytes induce an inflammatory phenotype in airway smooth muscle cells. *Clin Exp Allergy.* (2014) 44:1347–60. doi: 10.1111/cea.12421
15. Saunders R, Kaur D, Desai D, Berair R, Chachi L, Thompson RD, et al. Fibrocyte localisation to the ASM bundle in asthma: bidirectional effects on cell phenotype and behaviour. *Clin Transl Immunology.* (2020) 9:e1205. doi: 10.1002/cti2.1205
16. Bianchetti L, Marini MA, Isgro M, Bellini A, Schmidt M, Mattoli S. IL-33 promotes the migration and proliferation of circulating fibrocytes from patients with allergen-exacerbated asthma. *Biochem Biophys Res Commun.* (2012) 426:116–21. doi: 10.1016/j.bbrc.2012.08.047
17. Phillips RJ, Burdick MD, Hong K, Lutz MA, Murray LA, Xue YY, et al. Circulating fibrocytes traffic to the lungs in response to CXCL12 and mediate fibrosis. *J Clin Invest.* (2004) 114:438–46. doi: 10.1172/JCI20997
18. Carriere V, Roussel L, Ortega N, Lacorre DA, Americh L, Aguilar L, et al. IL-33, the IL-1-like cytokine ligand for ST2 receptor, is a chromatin-associated nuclear factor in vivo. *Proc Natl Acad Sci USA.* (2007) 104:282–7. doi: 10.1073/pnas.0606854104
19. Manning BD, Cantley LC. AKT/PKB signaling: navigating downstream. *Cell.* (2007) 129:1261–74. doi: 10.1016/j.cell.2007.06.009
20. Wang H, Zhang Q, Wen Q, Zheng Y, Lazarovici P, Jiang H, et al. Proline-rich Akt substrate of 40kDa (PRAS40): a novel downstream target of PI3k/Akt signaling pathway. *Cell Signal.* (2012) 24:17–24. doi: 10.1016/j.cellsig.2011.08.010
21. Gibson PG, Simpson JL, Saltos N. Heterogeneity of airway inflammation in persistent asthma : evidence of neutrophilic inflammation and increased sputum interleukin-8. *Chest.* (2001) 119:1329–36. doi: 10.1378/chest.119.5.1329
22. Wood LG, Baines KJ, Fu J, Scott HA, Gibson PG. The neutrophilic inflammatory phenotype is associated with systemic inflammation in asthma. *Chest.* (2012) 142:86–93. doi: 10.1378/chest.11-1838
23. Kaur D, Gomez E, Doe C, Berair R, Woodman L, Saunders R, et al. IL-33 drives airway hyper-responsiveness through IL-13-mediated mast cell: airway smooth muscle crosstalk. *Allergy.* (2015) 70:556–67. doi: 10.1111/all.12593
24. Prefontaine D, Lajoie-Kadoch S, Foley S, Audusseau S, Olivenstein R, Halayko AJ, et al. Increased expression of IL-33 in severe asthma: evidence of expression by airway smooth muscle cells. *J Immunol.* (2009) 183:5094–103. doi: 10.4049/jimmunol.0802387
25. Wang L, Harris TE, Roth RA, Lawrence JC Jr. PRAS40 regulates mTORC1 kinase activity by functioning as a direct inhibitor of substrate binding. *J Biol Chem.* (2007) 282:20036–44. doi: 10.1074/jbc.M702376200
26. Laplante M, Sabatini DM. mTOR signaling in growth control and disease. *Cell.* (2012) 149:274–93. doi: 10.1016/j.cell.2012.03.017
27. Volkers M, Toko H, Doroudgar S, Din S, Quijada P, Joyo AY, et al. Pathological hypertrophy amelioration by PRAS40-mediated inhibition of mTORC1. *Proc Natl Acad Sci USA.* (2013) 110:12661–6. doi: 10.1073/pnas.1301455110
28. Waugh DJ, Wilson C. The interleukin-8 pathway in cancer. *Clin Cancer Res.* (2008) 14:6735–41. doi: 10.1158/1078-0432.ccr-07-4843
29. MacManus CF, Pettigrew J, Seaton A, Wilson C, Maxwell PJ, Berlingeri S, et al. Interleukin-8 signaling promotes translational regulation of cyclin D in androgen-independent prostate cancer cells. *Mol Cancer Res.* (2007) 5:737–48. doi: 10.1158/1541-7786.MCR-07-0032
30. Abraham RT. Chemokine to the rescue: interleukin-8 mediates resistance to PI3K-pathway-targeted therapy in breast cancer. *Cancer Cell.* (2012) 22:703–5. doi: 10.1016/j.ccr.2012.11.012
31. Juvekar A, Wulf GM. Closing escape routes: inhibition of IL-8 signaling enhances the anti-tumor efficacy of PI3K inhibitors. *Breast Cancer Res.* (2013) 15:308. doi: 10.1186/bcr3400
32. Knall C, Worthen GS, Johnson GL. Interleukin 8-stimulated phosphatidylinositol-3-kinase activity regulates the migration of human neutrophils independent of extracellular signal-regulated kinase and p38 mitogen-activated protein kinases. *Proc Natl Acad Sci USA.* (1997) 94:3052–7. doi: 10.1073/pnas.94.7.3052
33. Tabatabaian F, Dougherty K, Di Fulvio M, Gomez-Cambronero J. Mammalian target of rapamycin (mTOR) and S6 kinase down-regulate phospholipase D2 basal expression and function. *J Biol Chem.* (2010) 285:18991–9001. doi: 10.1074/jbc.M110.111542

19

The Potential Roles of Exosomes in Chronic Obstructive Pulmonary Disease

Nan Wang [1†], Qin Wang [2†], Tiantian Du [3], Abakundana Nsenga Ariston Gabriel [3], Xue Wang [4], Li Sun [1], Xiaomeng Li [1], Kanghong Xu [1], Xinquan Jiang [1] and Yi Zhang [5*]*

[1] School of Public Health, Shandong First Medical University and Shandong Academy of Medical Sciences, Taian, China, [2] Department of Anesthesiology, Qilu Hospital, Shandong University, Jinan, China, [3] Department of Clinical Laboratory, Cheeloo College of Medicine, The Second Hospital, Shandong University, Jinan, China, [4] Department of Pharmacy, Binzhou Medical University Hospital, Binzhou, China, [5] Respiratory and Critical Care Medicine Department, Qilu Hospital, Shandong University, Jinan, China

***Correspondence:**
Xinquan Jiang
taianjxq@163.com
Yi Zhang
cnzhang1@126.com

† These authors have contributed equally to this work

Currently, chronic obstructive pulmonary disease (COPD) is one of the most common chronic lung diseases. Chronic obstructive pulmonary disease is characterized by progressive loss of lung function due to chronic inflammatory responses in the lungs caused by repeated exposure to harmful environmental stimuli. Chronic obstructive pulmonary disease is a persistent disease, with an estimated 384 million people worldwide living with COPD. It is listed as the third leading cause of death. Exosomes contain various components, such as lipids, microRNAs (miRNAs), long non-coding RNAs(lncRNAs), and proteins. They are essential mediators of intercellular communication and can regulate the biological properties of target cells. With the deepening of exosome research, it is found that exosomes are strictly related to the occurrence and development of COPD. Therefore, this review aims to highlight the unique role of immune-cell-derived exosomes in disease through complex interactions and their potentials as potential biomarkers new types of COPD.

Keywords: exosomes, COPD, immune cell, biomarker, treatment

INTRODUCTION

Chronic obstructive pulmonary disease (COPD) is a common chronic airway disease, characterized by irreversible, progressive airflow limitation, and repeated airway inflammation, which seriously affects the patient's breathing and interferes with the patient's life and work (1, 2). There are several viewpoints in COPD's pathogenesis, such as oxidative stress, epigenetics, cell aging, apoptosis, chronic inflammation, protease/antiprotease, and linear green body function (3). Environmental factors and genetic mutations play a role in it. Exposure to cigarette smoking(CS), whether active smoking or second-hand smoke, is the leading risk factor to get COPD (4, 5). Environmental pollution and occupational chemical exposure in some developing countries, are essential factors causing COPD (6). Exposure to indoor air pollution can affect unborn babies and is a risk factor for chronic obstructive pulmonary disease. According to the World Health Organization (WHO), COPD is the third leading cause of death globally. Statistical projections state that by 2040, the annual death toll will reach 4.4 million, and 90% of chronic obstructive pulmonary disease deaths will be more in both low-income and middle-income countries (7, 8). The airway epithelium CS events such as the first contact, long-term exposure to CS can induce epithelial cells to produce pro-inflammatory medium, senescence-associated secretory phenotype (MCP-1, IL-1, IL-6, IL-8), damage-associated molecular patterns (receptor for advanced glycation end-products, heat shock proteins, S100 proteins, high-mobility group box), the media which is released into the pulmonary and systemic circulation (9, 10), can stimulate the damage to the lung parenchyma, alveolar damage, and promote the development of COPD (11). Current treatment methods for COPD can only slow down the loss of lung function and cannot reverse the deterioration of lung structure and function. Therefore, it is essential to understand the molecular mechanism of COPD's occurrence and development and optimize the clinical treatment strategy. Various studies support the fact that exosomes containing miRNA, lncRNA, and proteins that are involved in the pathogenesis of COPD (12, 13), many exosomes, including miR-101, miR-223, miR-144, and miR-1274a act by influencing the molecular pathways associated with the pathogenesis of COPD which includes Kras, Notch, Smad, and TGF-β (14). Besides, these molecules are potential candidates for the early diagnosis and treatment of COPD. There are much-emerging shreds of evidence reporting that increased or decreased exosomes' expressions are a common feature of various lung diseases, including COPD (15). Takahashi et al. reported that changes in exosome numbers could predict a patient's physiological outcomes. For example, exosomes derived from bronchial endothelial cells were increased significantly in stable COPD (SCOPD), which were also increased in acute exacerbation COPD (AECOPD) (16).

Exosomes can maintain the stability of the intracellular environment (17). However, they can also get involved in different functions of the recipient cells (18). Direct exposure to a harmful stimulus (e.g., CS, air pollutants, and infection) may affect the nucleic acid load of lung-derived exosomes and participate in the progress of lung diseases (19). It was also found that exosomes may cause COPD pathological disturbances, that include chronic inflammation, oxidative stress, multiple organ dysfunction, epigenetic changes, cell apoptosis, aging, and diseases related to linear green body dysfunction (20, 21), and this proves that exosomes may act as a promising biomarker for the diagnosis of COPD (14). This is because, during the progression of COPD disease, COPD patients will produce a large number of exosomes, and can be isolated from sputum (22), plasma (23, 24), bronchial lavage fluid (BALF) (25), which suggests that exosomes considered as potential non-invasive diagnostic tools for COPD. This review first introduces the biological characteristics and functions of exosomes, introduces the role of exosomes in mediating intercellular communication and regulating immune cells in COPD, and finally clarifies the recent progress of exosomes in auxiliary clinical diagnosis and treatment of COPD.

MAIN COMPONENTS OF EXOSOMES

Biological Characteristics of Exosomes

Exosomes are membrane vesicles with a bilayer lipid of about 30–150 nm in diameter, produced by early and late endosomes, and eventually, form multivesicular bodies (MVB) (26). A variety of cells releases these vesicles, such as structure cells (epithelial cells, endothelial cells, and alveolar I and II, alveolar macrophages, fibroblasts), and immune cells (B and T lymphocytes, macrophages, dendritic cells) (3). CD9, CD63, CD81, and CD82 proteins from the peripheral membrane are fused during release into the extracellular space. These proteins are considered markers of exosomes (27). Besides, endosome markers also include heat shock 70 kDa protein 4 (Hsp70), MHC classes I and II, ALG-2 interacting protein X (Alix), and tumor susceptibility gene 101 (Tsg101) (28, 29).

The Genetic Material in Exosomes

The main components of exosomes are protein and lipid, genetic material including DNA, mRNA, miRNA, lncRNA, and metabolites (30, 31). Among them, miRNA is a highly studied regulatory molecule. It has found that a small non-coding RNA between 19 and 25 nucleotides in length together with silencing the 3′-untranslated region (3′UTR) of the target mRNA, negatively regulates its expression at the transcriptional and post-transcriptional levels, which in return affects various cellular functions such as proliferation, apoptosis, differentiation, and emergency resistance. The events mentioned above also affect biological processes that include autophagy, inflammatory response, cellular senescence, tissue remodeling, immune regulation, and angiogenesis (32, 33). These processes usually involve the level of multiple genes. Besides, the length of the lncRNA is over 200 nucleotides, and located in the nucleus, transcripted by RNA polymerase II, but cannot make reaction with proteins; lncRNA has been shown to participate in mRNA splicing after transcription and protein translation process, usually expresses the tissue specificity and cell specificity, and in the maintenance of steady-state (34). More information about these two types of RNA is summarized in **Table 1**.

Biological Functions of Exosomes

Exosomes can transmit information to target cells in three ways: (1) Interact with the cell surface through receptors; (2) Endocytosis; (3) The direct fusion of outer cell membrane and

---

Abbreviations: AECOPD, acute exacerbation chronic obstructive pulmonary disease; A1AT, alpha one anti-trypsin; Alix, ALG-2 interacting protein X; AM, alveolar macrophages; BALF, bronchial lavage fluid; CAMP, cyclic adenosine monophosphate; CCN1, protein cysteine-rich angiogenic protein 61; CCR10, chemokine receptor 10; COPD, chronic obstructive pulmonary disease; COX2, cyclooxygenase-2; CS, cigarette smoking; CSE, cigarette smoke extract; DC, dendritic cells; ECM, extracellular matrix; EMT, epithelial-mesenchymal transition; FAIM, Fas apoptosis inhibitory molecule Hsp70: heat shock 70 kDa protein 4; FEV1, forced expiratory volume in 1 s; FEV1/FVC, forced expiratory volume in 1 s/forced vital capacity; FFMI, fat-free body mass index; HBECs, human bronchial epithelial cells; HPMECs, human pulmonary microvascular endothelial cells; HRV, human rhinovirus; ICSs, Inhalation corticosteroids; lncRNA, long non-coding RNA; MAP3K, mitogen-activated protein kinase kinase kinase; MC, mast cells; miRNA, microRNA; MMP, matrix metalloproteinase protein; MVB, multivesicular bodies; Mϕ, macrophages; NE, neutrophilic elastase; NK:17, natural killer cells; NTHI, non-typeable Hemophilus influenza; NOR, neuron-derived orphan receptor; PASMCs, pulmonary artery smooth muscle cells; SCOPD, stable chronic obstructive pulmonary disease; SOCS, suppressor of cytokine signaling; siRNA, Small interfering RNA; STAT, signal transducer and activator of transcription; TGF-β, transforming growth factor β; TNFR2, tumor necrosis factor receptor 2; Trop, Trophoblast cells surface antigen; Tsg101, tumor susceptibility gene 101; TUG1, taurine-upregulated gene 1; UCHL1, ubiquitin C-terminal hydrolase; WHO, World Health Organization.

plasma membrane as it is shown in **Figure 1**. Briefly, exosomes' primary function is to transport essential substances and mediate communication between cells (35). This biological effect unit regulates the properties of target cells (36, 37). More evidence shows that exosomes are involved in different respiratory diseases, including COPD (38). In airway physiology, exosomes from alveolar macrophages, epithelial cells, and endothelial cells affect the disease's progress in controlling the stability of the intracellular environment and changing the function of receptor cells (39). Under normal circumstances, exosomes are highly stable in biological fluids due to the bilayer protection of lipids. High-throughput sequencing technology can detect highly sensitive and highly specific exosomes. A large amount of exosome secretion can be detected in various biological fluids, such as sputum, blood, BALF, urine, pleural effusion, ascites, synovial fluid, and breast milk (40). This makes exosomes potentially valuable for the diagnosis, prognosis, and treatment of respiratory diseases.

TABLE 1 | miRNA vs. lncRNA.

	miRNA	lncRNA
Source	Pri-miRNA	Multiple sources
Length	19–25 nt	>200 nt
Protein coding	no	no
Regulatory target	mRNA 3′UTR	Proteins, RNAs, and DNAs
Effect	Up-regulate or downregulate mRNA	Up-regulate or downregulate target
Mechanisms	Inhibits gene expression at the transcriptional and post-transcriptional levels	Maintain the dynamic balance of cells and tissues and regulate inflammation

miRNA, microRNA; lncRNA, long non-coding RNAs.

THE CLINICALLY RELEVANT ROLES OF EXOSOMES IN COPD

Chronic obstructive pulmonary disease is a chronic inflammatory respiratory disease characterized by irreversible airflow limitations caused by prolonged exposure to cigarette smoke or harmful irritants. Multiple studies have demonstrated that exosomes play an essential role in the occurrence and progression of COPD, including inflammation of the lung parenchyma and surrounding small airways (chronic bronchitis), degeneration of lung tissue (emphysema), and remodeling of small airways, leading to decreased lung function (41). The related exosomes miRNAs and lncRNAs involved in COPD's development and progression are summarized in **Figure 2**.

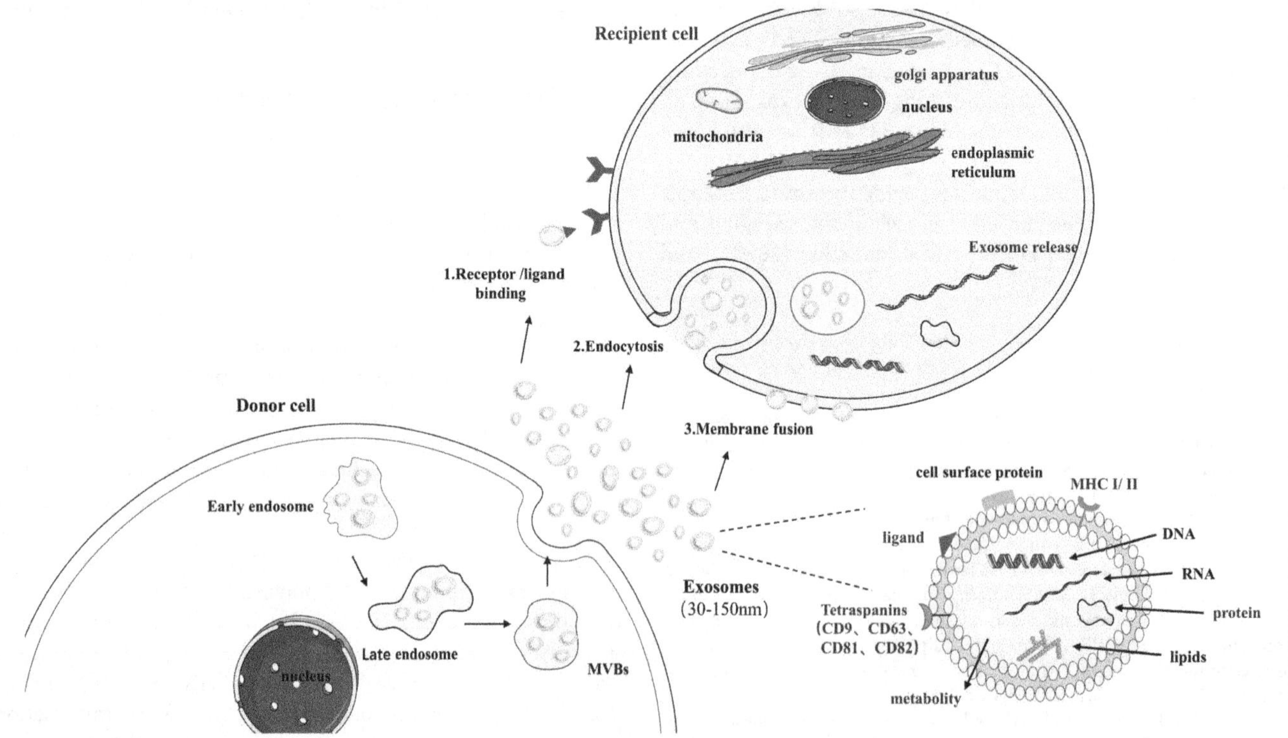

FIGURE 1 | Exosome in cell communication. Exosomes are nanovesicles (30–150 nm) that originate formed by early endosomes, late endosomes, and ultimately multivesicular bodies (MVB). Exosomes contain a variety of proteins, lipids, DNA, RNA, and metabolites. The cell body's surface includes major histocompatibility complex (MHC I/II), Tetraspanins (CD9, CD63, CD81, CD82), cell surface proteins ligand. This confers them with functional features. Exosomes can transmit information to target cells by: (1) binding to the cell surface by ligand, (2) endocytosis, (3) direct fusion of extracellular with plasma membranes.

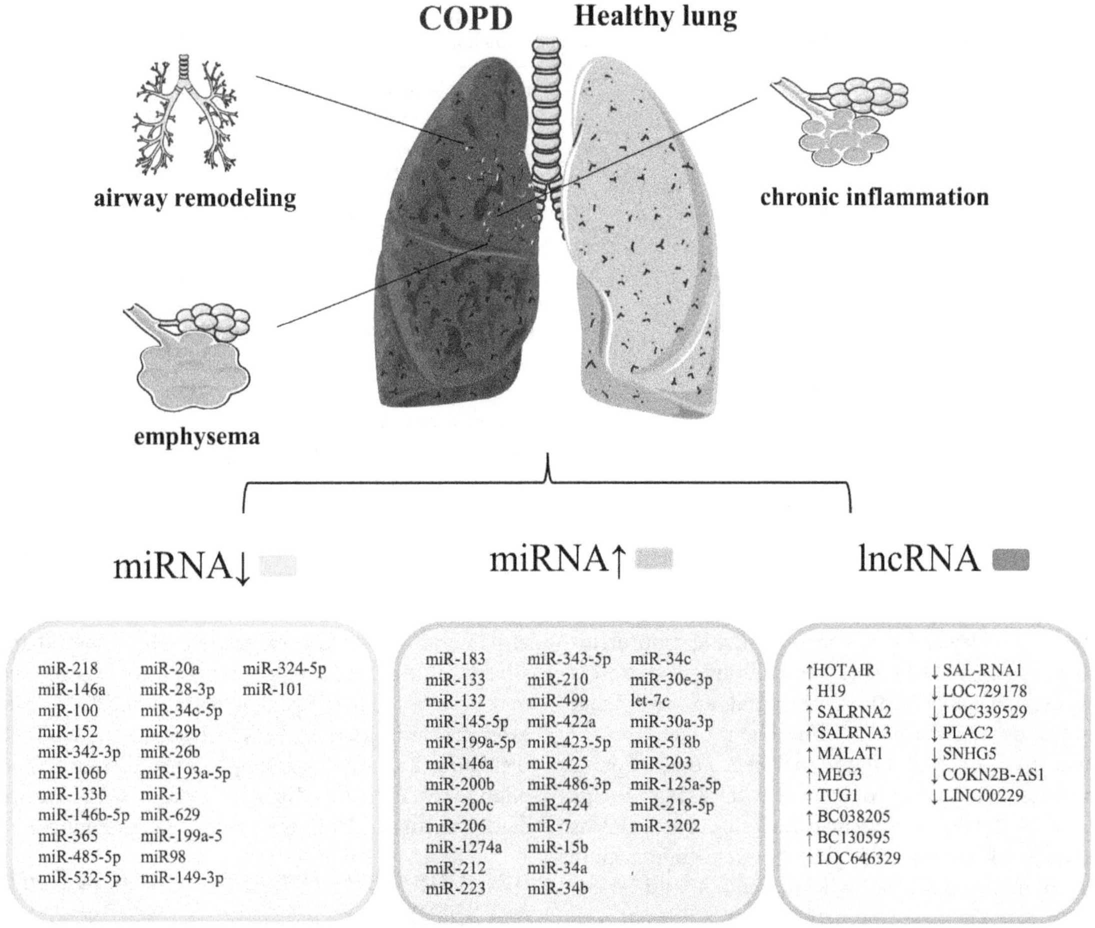

FIGURE 2 | COPD's pathological features are chronic inflammation of the lung parenchyma and surrounding airways, emphysema, and narrowing. Remodeling of the small airways, and exosomes are closely related to the course of this cases. List of previously reported miRNA associated with COPD. COPD, chronic obstructive pulmonary disease. Summary data are based on the following references (4, 14, 15, 42–52) for miRNAs and (53–56) for lncRNAs.

The Role of Exosomes in the Pathogenesis of COPD

Exosomes and Chronic Airway Inflammation

Cordazzo et al. reported that cigarette smoke extract (CSE) could induce exosomes to be released from mononuclear cells, induce bronchial epithelial cells to produce IL8, monocyte chemoattractant protein-1, and up-regulate CD542, thereby promoting inflammation (57). Also, Tan et al. believe that inflammation and exosomes increase in patients with COPD Relevant, they used Exo ELISA kits to compare the levels of $CD9^+$ exosomes in COPD patients and healthy controls, and found that the levels of COPD patients were significantly higher (58). Moon et al. believe that exosomes rich in COPD-related protein cysteine-rich angiogenic protein 61 (CCN1) can be cleaved after CS exposure. CCN1 allows inflammatory signaling to the far end of the lung. Interaction with integrin 7 in pulmonary epithelial cells activates the secretion of matrix metalloproteinase protein (MMP-1) in pulmonary epithelial cells, thereby promoting the release of vascular endothelial growth factor and IL-8.Il-8 promotes neutrophil infiltration into the lung parenchyma and causes inflammation (59). Besides, after CSE treatment, MEG3 up-regulated in 16HBE cells of COPD patients can release the expressions of inflammatory factors IL1, IL6, and TNF by regulating HSA-Mir-218, thus inducing inflammation and cell apoptosis.

Exosomes and Emphysema

Emphysema is characterized by decreased airway elasticity, hyperinflation, and swelling of the terminal bronchioles (60). Ezzie et al. believe that transforming growth factor β (TGF-β) suggested changes in miRNA expression, such as miR-223 and miR-15b. After knocking out the transforming growth factor TGF R-II in mouse lung epithelial cells, they showed emphysema signs (14). Van Pottelberge et al. analyzed miRNA expression in sputum samples from 32 subjects using qPCR. The results showed that the expression of miR-125b and let-7C in PATIENTS with COPD was lower than that in healthy non-smokers. Low let-7C expression was negatively correlated with the concentration of tumor necrosis factor receptor 2(TNFR2) (42).

TABLE 2 | List of miRNAs potentially associated with COPD pathogenesis.

miRNA	Expression	Target	Function/pathogenesis	References
miR-210	↑	ATG7	Promoted myofibroblast differentiation in primary lung fibroblasts control autophagy	(63)
miR-144	↑	CFTR, IRF7	Regulate inflammatory and antiviral responses in COPD	(43)
miR-101	↑	CFTR, MKP1		
miR-223	↑	TGF-β	TGF-β signal activation is associated with emphysema	(14)
miR-15b	↑	SMAD7	TGF-β inhibitory primary intracellular signal smad2/3/4	(14)
miR-218	↓	NF-κB	Up-regulates the expression of several pro-inflammatory cytokines by AEC, including IL-6 and CXCL8.	(65)
miR-128-5p	↓	apoptotic processes	Participate in the epithelial damage and remodeling in COPD	(44)
miR-181d	↑	and growth factor pathways		(43)
miR-1274a	↑	FOXO4	Probably related to oxidative stress or cellular aging in COPD	(14)
miR-1	↓	AKT	COPD-associated skeletal muscle dysfunction	(66)
miR-542-5p	↑	–		(45)
miR-542-3p				

↑Upregulation; ↓downregulation.

Furthermore, Stockley and Turne reported that glycoproteins alpha one anti-trypsin (A1AT) works by inhibiting the process of preventing excessive inflammation neutrophils and eosinophil enzymes work, and A1AT deficiency will lead to the development of emphysema (61). It was also found that in the evaluation of miRNA expression in lung tissue of patients with COPD patients with mild and moderate emphysema, moderate five miRNAs in lung samples of emphysema patients were significantly down-regulated, namely miR-34c, miR34b, miR-149, miR-133a, and miR-133b. Among them, the expression of miR-34c was significantly down-regulated (62).

Exosomes and Airway Remodeling

Long-term harmful stimuli lead to damage to airway epithelial cells, promote phenotypic changes of epithelial cells, and lead to fibrosis and airway remodeling. Fujita's research showed that CS-induced down-regulation of miR-210 could drive the differentiation of myofibroblasts in airway remodeling and inhibit the expression of ATG7 in LFS to control the autophagy process directly (63). This indicates that exosomes may contribute to the tracking of COPD differentiated fibers. miR-15b may be involved in airway remodeling by mediating TGF- related signaling pathways (15). Besides, it has also revealed that different microRNAs such as miR-224, miR-339-5p, and miR-382 are involved in COPD's pathogenesis (64), and particular pieces of information are presented in **Table 2**.

Gu's research shows that taurine-upregulated gene 1 (TUG1) expression is enhanced in COPD patients, and TUG1 inhibits the expression of miR-145-5pp/DUSP6 axis to promote airway remodelings such as TGF-β1, mucus hypersecretion, collagen 1 and α-SMA and inflammation such as increased IL-6 and pulmonary neutrophil infiltration (67). TUG1, combined with CDKN2B-AS1, can be used to predict acute exacerbation in COPD patients (68). It was found that the expressions of SAL-RNA2 and SAL-RNA3 (senescence-related genes) were significantly increased in COPD lung tissues, and the expressions of p53 and P21 were up-regulated. This shows that lncRNA in airway epithelial cells II type error control in the process of aging may be involved in the pathogenesis of COPD (53). In summary, exosomes influence COPD's occurrence and development by regulating inflammatory, emphysema, airway remodeling, and pulmonary fibrosis. MiRNAs and lncRNAs involved in the development of COPD are summarized in **Figure 2**.

Immune Cell-Derived Exosome Participate in COPD

Exosomes are recognized as tools for mediating intercellular communication and signal transduction and signaling to immune cells to regulate function. Various studies highlighted that exosomes are secreted by some types of cells, including immune cells, such as B lymphocytes (69), T lymphocytes (70), macrophages (Mϕ) (71), mast cells (MC) (30), dendritic cells (DC) (72), and 17 natural killer cells (NK) (73). Immune-cell-derived exosomes perform numerous physiological and pathological functions, including antigen presentation, immunosuppression, T-cell polarization toward Treg cells, and anti-inflammatory effects, to enhance or suppress immune activity (74). Infiltration of various immune cells, such as neutrophils and macrophages, into small airways, is a common phenomenon in COPD (75). For these reasons, in-depth research is needed to explore the role of immune-cell-derived exosomes in COPD.

Role of Macrophages and Exosomes in COPD

Alveolar macrophages (AM) form the first host defense line against infection/inhalation of harmful substances. They are one of the primary cells in the lung that produce exosomes (76). AM promotes inflammation of COPD. First, macrophage-derived exosomes induce differentiation of immature monocytes into macrophages by mediating miR-223 (77). Exosomes miR-17 and miR-221 then promote macrophage migration by mediating integrin β under sterility stimulation (78). Finally,

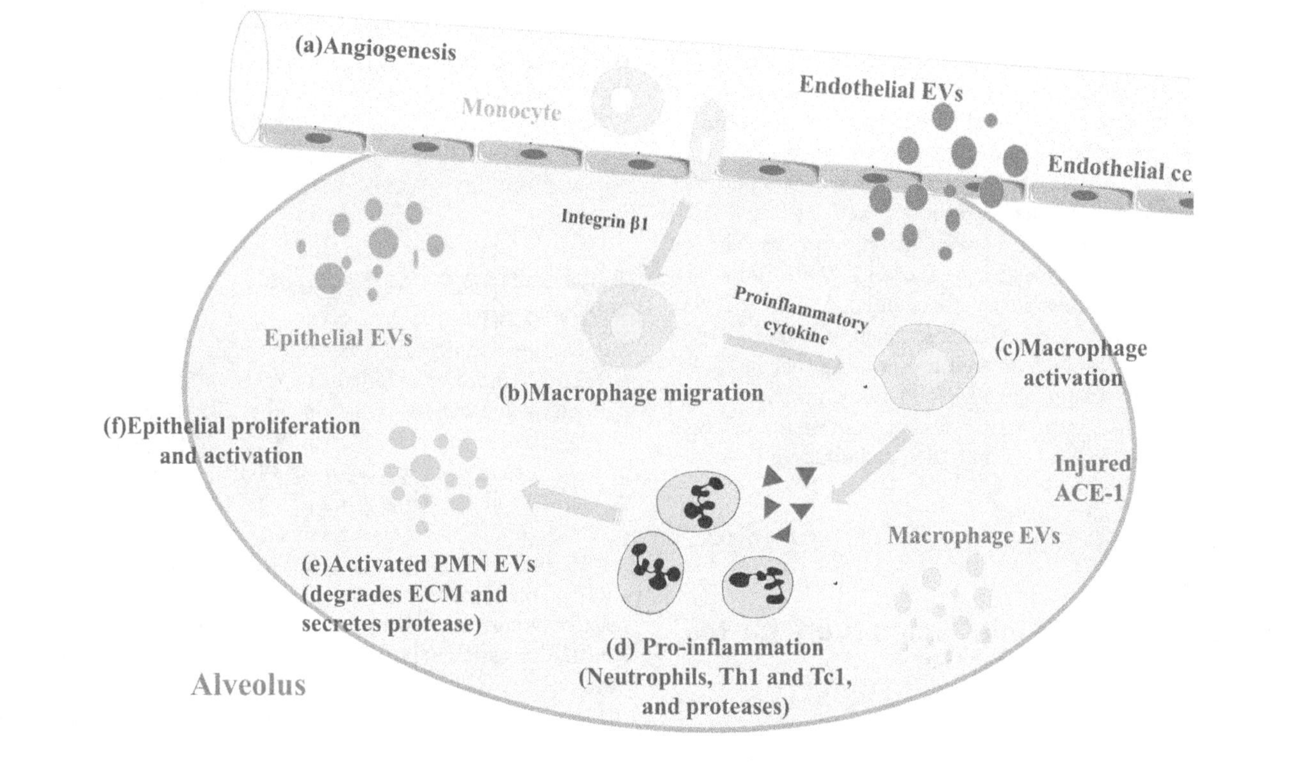

FIGURE 3 | Exosomes and macrophages promote alveolar inflammation in COPD.

exosomes miR-221 and miR-320 stimulate the secretion of pro-inflammatory cytokines, thereby activating AM (79). After a series of differentiation, migration, and activation, AM recruits neutrophils, Th1, and Tc1, to promote inflammation (32). The specific process is shown in **Figure 3**.

After CS stimulation, miRNA mediated by endothelial cells, such as miR-125a, miR-126, miR-191, were transferred to macrophages to promote apoptotic cell clearance (80). A study reported that macrophages release outside secretes body with antigen-presenting ability lower associated macrophage transfer specific immune (81). Kulshreshtha et al. found that epithelial-derived exosomes extracted from BALF of mice with COPD induced undifferentiated macrophages and proliferative effects (82). During the pathogenesis of COPD, alveolar macrophages combine with suppressor of cytokine signaling (SOCS) protein, which is taken up by alveolar epithelial cells and inhibits IFN γ-induced signal transducer and activator of transcription (STAT) (58). Also, M1 macrophages (pro-inflammatory) are the predominant cells in the peripheral blood of COPD patients, leading to pro-inflammatory factors (IL-1β, IL-12, TNF-α) and lncRNA miR-155HG are up-regulated (83). As mentioned above, the studies show that the increase of exosomes in the regulation of lung inflammation by macrophages in the lung has practical significance.

Role of Neutrophils and Exosomes in COPD

Neutrophils are a crucial component of innate immune responses in COPD, and Kristopher described a new pathogen, activated PMN (neutrophil) source of NE-rich exosomes (84). These exosomes bind and degrade the extracellular matrix (ECM) involved in COPD's pathogenesis. Mac-1 and neutrophilic elastase (NE) play essential roles in this process. NE is the surface binding protease obtained by $CD63^+/CD66b^+$ nanovesicles during PMN degranulation, and NE is resistant to A1AT. It is because of the resistance of the A1AT. The ECM targeting, the outer body of the outer body, which is more potent than the free NE biology (85), and an imbalance of the proteinase-antiprotease system are typical in COPD (86). In this system, PMN-derived NE and lung suppressor A1AT are most prominent (87). Experiments have shown that injecting enough NE into an animal's airways can cause emphysema (88). These findings show that novel exosomes derived from neutrophils participate in disease progression by breaking ECM dynamic balance through NE activity in COPD.

Role of Other Cells and Exosomes in COPD

Among mast cells, the exosomes of human mast cell line-1 overlapped with the proteins of the exosomes inhaled by the patient, suggesting that mast cells also contribute to the lung exosome pool (89). It is worth noting that exosomes from NK cells can react against NK cells and increase the cytotoxic activity and NK cells' targeting (90). Besides, exosomes released by macrophages, NK cells, and dendritic cells through a paracrine act as pro-inflammatory mediators of the innate immune system (81). Exosomes secreted by DC are associated with amplification of the immune response, and DC-based exosomes induce specific humoral responses and activation of $CD4^+T$ cells and $CD8^+T$ cells (91). As mentioned above, immune cell-derived exosomes are involved in the development and progression of COPD. Exosomes derived from circulating immune cells have immunomodulatory effects. Therefore, it has been reported that immune-cell-derived exosomes can be delivered to target cells by small molecule drugs or specific molecules to stimulate the immune system in patients to recognize and destroy lesions (90). Also, exosomes derived from circulating immune cells can serve as specific biomarkers for the severity of inflammation, which has been demonstrated in liver inflammation (92, 93). The application of exosomes derived from immune cells in immunotherapy is now considered a promising tool in COPD treatment. In conclusion, there are still many questions to be answered about the relationship between immune cells and exosomes involved in lung inflammation and injury in COPD.

CLINICAL APPLICATION OF EXOSOMES IN COPD

Exosomes as Potential Biomarkers for the Clinical Diagnosis of COPD

The study results compared healthy exosomes and exosomes released by bronchial epithelial cells in COPD patients, especially in the AECOPD, and the study reported that exosomes from AECOPD were significantly increased. Moreover, they found that by detecting exosomes' content, pulmonary endothelial cell apoptosis can be analyzed. The degree of activation and the dysfunction of endothelial cells is directly related to the severity of COPD. It is usually evaluated by forced expiratory volume in 1 s (FEV1) to track the disease's advancement (16). Lacedonia and his research team reported that the number of exosomes in sputum is negatively correlated with FEV1, similar to changes in exosome levels related to inflammation. It shows that senescent cells accumulated with age in COPD may affect the release and competition of circulating exosomes (94). Moreover, Shi et al. reported that miR-203 might be a new biomarker for COPD diagnosis; it is just because miR-203 targets P13KCA to inhibit nuclear factors light chain enhancers, which activate B cell signaling pathways significantly involved in COPD (95). Another critical study showed that evidence suggests that miR-21 has potential value in the diagnosis and treatment of COPD. The level of miR-21 in the serum of smokers and patients with COPD is significantly increased. The increased level of miR-21 is associated with the percentage of forced expiratory volume in 1 s/forced vital capacity (FEV1/FVC) (18).

Besides, comparing miR-4455 and miR-4785 in smokers and non-smokers in COPD patients, there was a significant expression difference (96). This made the two exosomal microRNAs to be considered as a potential biomarker for early diagnosis of COPD. Chronic obstructive pulmonary disease, early diagnosis, and patient monitoring are other essential factors. Based on that, researchers conducted a study. They found that miR-218-5p is another essential miRNA that plays an essential role in COPD pathogenesis and promises to be a successful candidate for diagnosing and controlling COPD patients (65). Moreover, other essential study findings showed that miR-29c and miR-126 were up-regulated in Stage III COPD patients relative to stable controls. Such results indicate that all these miRNAs may be used as screening biomarkers for COPD patients (97). As mentioned above from different studies, the findings show that exosomal miRNAs can be used as potential biomarkers for the diagnosis of COPD.

Application of Exosomes in COPD Prognosis

Studies have shown that exosomes with CD144, CD31, and CD62E are more abundant in patients with AECOPD than in patients with SCOPD, suggesting that COPD patients tend to deteriorate can be used as an indicator of prognosis (16). Ge et al. detected the expression of ANRIL in SCOPD patients, AECOPD, and the whole group. They found that the expression of ANRIL in AECOPD patients was the lowest. The expression of ANRIL in SCOPD patients was not related to the GOLD stage. In contrast, the expression of ANRIL in patients with AECOPD was negatively correlated with the GOLD stage. Most importantly, ANRIL expression in patients with AECOPD and stable COPD is negatively correlated with inflammatory cytokines such as IL1B, IL17A, TNF, and LTB4 (98). They finally concluded that lncRNA ANRIL (antisense non-coding RNA at INK4 locus) is associated with chronic diseases' occurrence and prognosis.

It is well-known that skeletal muscle weakness is a severe systemic complication of COPD, which seriously affects patients' quality of life and mobility. Lewis et al. showed that exosome miR-1 plays a crucial role in skeletal muscle dysfunction in patients with COPD, associated with smoking history, function, defatted body mass index, 6-min walking distance, and percentage of quadriceps type I muscle fibers (66). Besides, compared with healthy COPD patients with fat-free body mass index (FFMI), H19 is expressed by demethylation isolation of has-miR-519a after up-regulation increases patients' susceptibility with COPD to low FFMI (99). So far, researchers have used exosomes as a potential non-invasive biomarker for COPD that has never stopped. In short, these studies are mainly used to identify the role of exosomes in the diagnosis of COPD, providing a new basis for the early clinical diagnosis of some exosomes in COPD. Through continuous efforts, new diagnostic tools and more complete treatment methods may appear.

Exosomes Are Essential in the Treatment of COPD

COPD Treatment Using Exosomal miRNA

At present, the drugs used to treat COPD are mainly bronchodilators, which are borrowed from medications used to treat asthma. Inhalation corticosteroids (ICSs) are added to LAMA/LABA combination therapy (triple therapy), and the risk of exacerbation and death in COPD patients. However, most patients are not sensitive to steroids, and the use of large doses increases the risk of pneumonia (100). Therefore, COPD patients urgently need critical target treatment. There is also a great need for drugs to prevent the aggravation of the disease and pulmonary hypertension, plus many other COPD complications.

Sun's study reported that miR-206 expression in human pulmonary microvascular endothelial cells (HPMECs) exposed to CS was up-regulated. They also noted that both Caspase3 and HPMEC apoptosis activities were increased. There was a negative correlation between the expression levels of miR-206 and Notch3 and VEGFA mRNA levels. During their study, they concluded that miR-206 could directly target Notch3 and VEGF-A to regulate the process of COPD vascular remodeling (101). It was reported that anti-miR-27-3p could effectively reverse the inflammatory process and reduce the infiltration of neutrophils and macrophages in the lungs and the level of inflammatory cytokines in BALF. Another study aimed to determine miRNA-3202 in COPD noted that the overexpression of miR-3202 could significantly inhibit the increase of T lymphocyte IFN-γ and TNF-α levels induced by CSE while increasing the expression of Fas and FasL. The study also revealed that the high levels of miR-3202 pass target gene Fas apoptosis inhibitory molecule (FAIM) 2 to inhibit T cell apoptosis and protect human bronchial epithelial cells (HBECs). FAIM2 plays a central role in COPD's pathogenesis, inhibits T cell death, and participates in CS-induced cell apoptosis and cell wall destruction (64). Besides, it has also been found that the high levels of miR-145-5p alleviate CS-induced apoptosis and the production of pro-inflammatory cytokines by inhibiting the lytic expression of p53 and caspase339. Besides, some miR-145-5p and KLF5 inhibits CSE-induced NF-κB signal activation, thereby reducing participation in the pathogenesis of COPD (102).

Du et al. tested the expression rates of miR-181c in 34 COPD (smoking cases) patients relative to safety controls, and findings showed that miR-181c might be slightly less controlled in COPD patients than healthy control patients had never smoked. They also demonstrated that the upregulation of miR-181c might be correlated with several consequences, such as inflammatory response reduction, neutrophil invasion, reactive oxygen species formation, and inflammatory cytokine development. MiR-181c downregulation may be correlated with different consequences. They also found that miR-181c exerts its impact by attacking CCN1. The downregulation of the miR-181c could contribute to the increase in CCN1 expression in the pulmonary tissues of patients with COPD relative to stable controls. The results mentioned above show that miR-181c might be used as a therapeutic target to treat COPD patients (103). Another study also reported that the deregulation of miR-126 is correlated with ATM kinase activation, and they have also demonstrated that miR-126 levels have been decreased in the smoker and COPD endothelial blood cells relative to non-smoker subjects. These findings indicated that the reduction of miR-126 through ATM targeting might facilitate tissue aging and dysfunction in smokers and COPD subjects. This miRNA may also be seen as a new therapeutic target for treating COPD patients (104). Taken together, it is clear that exosomes play an essential role in the treatment of COPD patients.

The Treatment of COPD by Synthetic siRNA

Synthetic siRNAs' potential to treat COPD by transcriptionally down-regulating target genes' expression has been successfully

TABLE 3 | Principle, advantages and disadvantages of common exosome isolation methods.

Methods	Theory	Advantages	Disadvantages	References
Ultracentrifugation techniques (UC)	The required components are obtained according to the size and density differences of each component in the sample.	There is no need to mark the outer cut body to avoid cross contamination	High cost, Time consuming, structural failure, aggregation and lipoprotein separation are not conducive to downstream analysis	(46)
Density gradient centrifugation	Usually used in combination with the overspeed centrifuge method	Improve the purity of exosomes	The high viscosity of sucrose solution will reduce the settling velocity of exosomes and lead to long time consuming	(47)
Polymer Precipitatio	Using the method of virus extraction, exosomes is obtained by reducing the solubility of exosomes, usually using polyethylene glycol (PEG) as medium	Simple operation, short analysis time, suitable for large—dose sample treatment	Due to its low purity and recovery rate, the resulting polymer is difficult to remove and may produce false positive	(48)
Size-based isolation techniques	Based on the size differences between exosomes and other components of a biological sample	Fast, simple, low-cost and separated exosomes have complete structure and uniform size, and their biological characteristics will not be significantly affected.	Other particles of similar size are difficult to separate, resulting in reduced purity	(46)
Ultrafiltration	Ultrafiltration membranes with different molecular weight cutoffs (MWCO) were used to selectively separate the samples	The sample cost is low, the concentration efficiency is high, and the activity of the exosomes is not affected	Low purity and poor binding of the exosomes to the ultrafiltration membrane resulted in low recovery rate.	(49)
Immunoaffinity chromatography (IAC)	The specificity of antibodies and ligand is combined to separate the required exosomes from heterogeneous mixtures	The sample size required is small.It can be used for the qualitative and quantitative detection of exosomes.This method has strong specificity, high sensitivity, high purity and high yield	The preservation condition of the exosomes obtained by this method is harsh, and it is not suitable for large scale separation of the exosomes. The non-specific interference adsorption of matrix produces interfering proteins, which limits the wide application of this method.	(50)

validated in multiple animal models (105). For example, mitogen-activated protein kinase kinase kinase (MAP3K) 19 phosphorylates the nucleus of Smad2/3 Translocation and activation of NF-κB reduces lung neutrophil infiltration and BALF levels of KC (a mouse homolog of human IL-8) (106). A recent study has shown that it is caused by infection of the upper respiratory tract. Among the causes of worsening COPD, human rhinovirus (HRV) and non-typeable Hemophilus influenza (NTHI) is the most common. The combined HRV/NTHI response increased IL-17C production, and IL-17C-specific siRNA could block IL-17C and CXCL1 and neutrophil migration induced by HRV/NTHI (107). Trophoblast cells' surface antigen (Trop) 2 expressed on the basal lung compartment's multipotent progenitor cells in preventing COPD airway remodeling Surface antigen. Its specific siRNA reverses cell movement and migration of basal cell hyperplasia. Epithelial-mesenchymal transition (EMT) (108), COPD combined pulmonary hypertension is a common complication of patients, which is closely related to the high expression of the neuron-derived orphan receptor (NOR)1.NOR1 plays a role in regulating inflammation and vascular remodeling. Its specific siRNA inhibits hypoxia-induced cyclin D1 level, cell proliferation, and DNA synthesis in primary human pulmonary artery smooth muscle cells (PASMCs) (109) SI00A4, a secretory member of S100 calcium-binding protein, is highly expressed in COPD patients and mouse models and is involved in the proliferation, migration, and EMT of smooth muscle cells. HIF-1α or HIF-2α siRNA can inhibit the high expression of S100A4 (110). Based on the above facts, exosomes play a crucial role in the treatment of COPD. However, COPD is a disease caused by a variety of factors.

FUTURE DIRECTION AND THE LIMITATION

The study of exosomes vs. COPD is an emerging and rapidly evolving field where we can use exosomes to develop therapeutic tools to prevent and stop lung injury caused by COPD. However, there are still many problems to be solved, such as the lack of uniformity and standardization of exosome detection, isolation, and purification technologies. The advantages and disadvantages of exosome isolation methods are shown in **Table 3**. Secondly, the mechanism of exosome uptake by recipient cells is not fully understood. Also, collecting tissue samples from the lungs is more complicated. More in-depth studies are needed to fully understand the pathogenesis of exosomes in COPD and fully reveal the role of miRNA and lncRNA in the disease.

CONCLUSION

Chronic obstructive pulmonary disease is a heterogeneous disorder marked by airway inflammation, lung tissue damage, and airflow restriction consistent with airway remodeling. Exacerbations are a significant cause of disease development, morbidity, and death, and novel therapies and medications for COPD remain particularly crucial due to a lack of effective drugs. Exosomes are incredibly durable and practical packages of cellular material. They can transfer their bioactive loads to receiver cells across the body, influencing physiological and pathological conditions. Exosomes have considerable clinical value due to their capacity to be controlled and optimized to guide treatment. Although this review tried to highlight the latest evidence of exosomes from various cell sources as biomarkers and their potential for application in COPD treatment, in-depth researches are needed to be used in daily early diagnosis and treatment of COPD.

AUTHOR CONTRIBUTIONS

NW and QW designed and drafted the manuscript. TD, AG, XW, LS, XL, and KX discussed and revised the manuscript. All authors read and approved the final manuscript.

REFERENCES

1. Putcha N, Puhan MA, Hansel NN, Drummond MB, Boyd CM. Impact of co-morbidities on self-rated health in self-reported COPD: an analysis of NHANES 2001-2008. *COPD.* (2013) 10:324–32. doi: 10.3109/15412555.2012.744963
2. Chen Y, Wang H, Luo G, Dai X. SIRT4 inhibits cigarette smoke extracts-induced mononuclear cell adhesion to human pulmonary microvascular endothelial cells *via* regulating NF-κB activity. *Toxicol Lett.* (2014) 226:320–7. doi: 10.1016/j.toxlet.2014.02.022
3. Sundar IK, Li D, Rahman I. Small RNA-sequence analysis of plasma-derived extracellular vesicle miRNAs in smokers and patients with chronic obstructive pulmonary disease as circulating biomarkers. *J Extracell Vesicles.* (2019) 8:1684816. doi: 10.1080/20013078.2019.1684816
4. Salimian J, Mirzaei H, Moridikia A, Harchegani AB, Sahebkar A, Salehi H. Chronic obstructive pulmonary disease: microRNAs and exosomes as new diagnostic and therapeutic biomarkers. *J Res Med Sci.* (2018) 23:27. doi: 10.4103/jrms.JRMS_1054_17
5. Chen Y, Luo H, Kang N, Guan C, Long Y, Cao J, et al. Beraprost sodium attenuates cigarette smoke extract-induced apoptosis in vascular endothelial cells. *Mol Biol Rep.* (2012) 39:10447–57. doi: 10.1007/s11033-012-1924-1
6. GBD 2015 Chronic Respiratory Disease Collaborators. Global, regional, and national deaths, prevalence, disability-adjusted life years, and years lived with disability for chronic obstructive pulmonary disease and asthma, 1990-2015: a systematic analysis for the Global Burden of Disease Study 2015. *Lancet Respir Med.* (2017) 5:691–706. doi: 10.1016/S2213-2600(17)30293-X
7. GBD 2017 Causes of Death Collaborators. Global, regional, and national age-sex-specific mortality for 282 causes of death in 195 countries and territories, 1980-2017: a systematic analysis for the Global Burden of Disease Study 2017. *Lancet.* (2018) 392:1736–88. doi: 10.1016/S0140-6736(18)32203-7
8. Rabe KF, Watz H. Chronic obstructive pulmonary disease. *Lancet.* (2017) 389:1931–40. doi: 10.1016/S0140-6736(17)31222-9
9. Pouwels SD, Heijink IH, ten Hacken NH, Vandenabeele P, Krysko DV, Nawijn MC, et al. DAMPs activating innate and adaptive immune responses in COPD. *Mucosal Immunol.* (2014) 7:215–26. doi: 10.1038/mi.2013.77
10. Kumar M, Seeger W, Voswinckel R. Senescence-associated secretory phenotype and its possible role in chronic obstructive pulmonary disease. *Am J Respir Cell Mol Biol.* (2014) 51:323–33. doi: 10.1165/rcmb.2013-0382PS
11. Yao H, Rahman I. Current concepts on oxidative/carbonyl stress, inflammation and epigenetics in pathogenesis of chronic obstructive pulmonary disease. *Toxicol Appl Pharmacol.* (2011) 254:72–85. doi: 10.1016/j.taap.2009.10.022
12. Gomez-Cabrero D, Menche J, Vargas C, Cano I, Maier D, Barabási AL, et al. From comorbidities of chronic obstructive pulmonary disease to identification of shared molecular mechanisms by data integration. *BMC Bioinformatics.* (2016) 17(Suppl. 15):441. doi: 10.1186/s12859-016-1291-3

13. Hobbs BD, Hersh CP. Integrative genomics of chronic obstructive pulmonary disease. *Biochem Biophys Res Commun.* (2014) 452:276–86. doi: 10.1016/j.bbrc.2014.07.086
14. Ezzie ME, Crawford M, Cho JH, Orellana R, Zhang S, Gelinas R, et al. Gene expression networks in COPD: microRNA and mRNA regulation. *Thorax.* (2012) 67:122–31. doi: 10.1136/thoraxjnl-2011-200089
15. Osei ET, Florez-Sampedro L, Timens W, Postma DS, Heijink IH, Brandsma CA. Unravelling the complexity of COPD by microRNAs: it's a small world after all. *Eur Respir J.* (2015) 46:807–18. doi: 10.1183/13993003.02139-2014
16. Takahashi T, Kobayashi S, Fujino N, Suzuki T, Ota C, He M, et al. Increased circulating endothelial microparticles in COPD patients: a potential biomarker for COPD exacerbation susceptibility. *Thorax.* (2012) 67:1067–74. doi: 10.1136/thoraxjnl-2011-201395
17. Njock MS, Cheng HS, Dang LT, Nazari-Jahantigh M, Lau AC, Boudreau E, et al. Endothelial cells suppress monocyte activation through secretion of extracellular vesicles containing antiinflammatory microRNAs. *Blood.* (2015) 125:3202–12. doi: 10.1182/blood-2014-11-611046
18. Xu H, Ling M, Xue J, Dai X, Sun Q, Chen C, et al. Exosomal microRNA-21 derived from bronchial epithelial cells is involved in aberrant epithelium-fibroblast cross-talk in COPD induced by cigarette smoking. *Theranostics.* (2018) 8:5419–33. doi: 10.7150/thno.27876
19. Maes T, Cobos FA, Schleich F, Sorbello V, Henket M, De Preter K, et al. Asthma inflammatory phenotypes show differential microRNA expression in sputum. *J Allergy Clin Immunol.* (2016) 137:1433–46. doi: 10.1016/j.jaci.2016.02.018
20. Lerner CA, Sundar IK, Rahman I. Mitochondrial redox system, dynamics, and dysfunction in lung inflammaging and COPD. *Int J Biochem Cell Biol.* (2016) 81:294–306. doi: 10.1016/j.biocel.2016.07.026
21. Sundar IK, Yao H, Rahman I. Oxidative stress and chromatin remodeling in chronic obstructive pulmonary disease and smoking-related diseases. *Antioxid Redox Signal.* (2013) 18:1956–71. doi: 10.1089/ars.2012.4863
22. Porro C, Lepore S, Trotta T, Castellani S, Ratclif L, Battaglino A, et al. Isolation and characterization of microparticles in sputum from cystic fibrosis patients. *Respir Res.* (2010) 11:94. doi: 10.1186/1465-9921-11-94
23. Caby MP, Lankar D, Vincendeau-Scherrer C, Raposo G, Bonnerot C. Exosomal-like vesicles are present in human blood plasma. *Int Immunol.* (2005) 17:879–87. doi: 10.1093/intimm/dxh267
24. Ohtani N, Hara E. Roles and mechanisms of cellular senescence in regulation of tissue homeostasis. *Cancer Sci.* (2013) 104:525–30. doi: 10.1111/cas.12118
25. Admyre C, Grunewald J, Thyberg J, Gripenbäck S, Tornling G, Eklund A, et al. Exosomes with major histocompatibility complex class II and co-stimulatory molecules are present in human BAL fluid. *Eur Respir J.* (2003) 22:578–83. doi: 10.1183/09031936.03.00041703
26. van Niel G, D'Angelo G, Raposo G. Shedding light on the cell biology of extracellular vesicles. *Nat Rev Mol Cell Biol.* (2018) 19:213–28. doi: 10.1038/nrm.2017.125
27. Cocucci E, Meldolesi J. Ectosomes and exosomes: shedding the confusion between extracellular vesicles. *Trends Cell Biol.* (2015) 25:364–72. doi: 10.1016/j.tcb.2015.01.004
28. Escola JM, Kleijmeer MJ, Stoorvogel W, Griffith JM, Yoshie O, Geuze HJ. Selective enrichment of tetraspan proteins on the internal vesicles of multivesicular endosomes and on exosomes secreted by human B-lymphocytes. *J Biol Chem.* (1998) 273:20121–7. doi: 10.1074/jbc.273.32.20121
29. Yoshioka Y, Konishi Y, Kosaka N, Katsuda T, Kato T, Ochiya T. Comparative marker analysis of extracellular vesicles in different human cancer types. *J Extracell Vesicles.* (2013) 18:2. doi: 10.3402/jev.v2i0.20424
30. Keerthikumar S, Chisanga D, Ariyaratne D, Al Saffar H, Anand S, Zhao K, et al. ExoCarta: a web-based compendium of exosomal cargo. *J Mol Biol.* (2016) 428:688–92. doi: 10.1016/j.jmb.2015.09.019
31. Pathan M, Fonseka P, Chitti SV, Kang T, Sanwlani R, Van Deun J, et al. Vesiclepedia 2019: a compendium of RNA, proteins, lipids and metabolites in extracellular vesicles. *Nucleic Acids Res.* (2019) 47:D516–9. doi: 10.1093/nar/gky1029
32. Hough KP, Chanda D, Duncan SR, Thannickal VJ, Deshane JS. Exosomes in immunoregulation of chronic lung diseases. *Allergy.* (2017) 72:534–44. doi: 10.1111/all.13086
33. Nana-Sinkam SP, Acunzo M, Croce CM, Wang K. Extracellular vesicle biology in the pathogenesis of lung disease. *Am J Respir Crit Care Med.* (2017) 196:1510–8. doi: 10.1164/rccm.201612-2457PP
34. De Smet EG, Mestdagh P, Vandesompele J, Brusselle GG, Bracke KR. Non-coding RNAs in the pathogenesis of COPD. *Thorax.* (2015) 70:782–91. doi: 10.1136/thoraxjnl-2014-206560
35. Raposo G, Stoorvogel W. Extracellular vesicles: exosomes, microvesicles, and friends. *J Cell Biol.* (2013) 200:373–83. doi: 10.1083/jcb.201211138
36. Mathieu M, Martin-Jaular L, Lavieu G, Théry C. Specificities of secretion and uptake of exosomes and other extracellular vesicles for cell-to-cell communication. *Nat Cell Biol.* (2019) 21:9–17. doi: 10.1038/s41556-018-0250-9
37. Kalluri R, LeBleu VS. The biology, function, and biomedical applications of exosomes. *Science.* (2020) 367:eaau6977. doi: 10.1126/science.aau6977
38. Kubo H. Extracellular vesicles in lung disease. *Chest.* (2018) 153:210–6. doi: 10.1016/j.chest.2017.06.026
39. Fujita Y, Kosaka N, Araya J, Kuwano K, Ochiya T. Extracellular vesicles in lung microenvironment and pathogenesis. *Trends Mol Med.* (2015) 21:533–42. doi: 10.1016/j.molmed.2015.07.004
40. Simpson RJ, Jensen SS, Lim JW. Proteomic profiling of exosomes: current perspectives. *Proteomics.* (2008) 8:4083–99. doi: 10.1002/pmic.200800109
41. Wahlund CJE, Eklund A, Grunewald J, Gabrielsson S. Pulmonary extracellular vesicles as mediators of local and systemic inflammation. *Front Cell Dev Biol.* (2017) 5:39. doi: 10.3389/fcell.2017.00039
42. Van Pottelberge GR, Mestdagh P, Bracke KR, Thas O, van Durme YM, Joos GF, et al. MicroRNA expression in induced sputum of smokers and patients with chronic obstructive pulmonary disease. *Am J Respir Crit Care Med.* (2011) 183:898–906. doi: 10.1164/rccm.201002-0304OC
43. Molina-Pinelo S, Pastor MD, Suarez R, Romero-Romero B, González De la Peña M, Salinas A, et al. MicroRNA clusters: dysregulation in lung adenocarcinoma and COPD. *Eur Respir J.* (2014) 43:1740–9. doi: 10.1183/09031936.00091513
44. Cao Z, Zhang N, Lou T, Jin Y, Wu Y, Ye Z, et al. MicroRNA-183 down-regulates the expression of BKCaβ1 protein that is related to the severity of chronic obstructive pulmonary disease. *Hippokratia.* (2014) 18:328–32.
45. Donaldson A, Natanek SA, Lewis A, Man WD, Hopkinson NS, Polkey MI, et al. Increased skeletal muscle-specific microRNA in the blood of patients with COPD. *Thorax.* (2013) 68:1140–9. doi: 10.1136/thoraxjnl-2012-203129
46. Savarimuthu Francis SM, Davidson MR, Tan ME, Wright CM, Clarke BE, Duhig EE, et al. MicroRNA-34c is associated with emphysema severity and modulates SERPINE1 expression. *BMC Genomics.* (2014) 15:88. doi: 10.1186/1471-2164-15-88
47. Gelb AF, Hogg JC, Müller NL, Schein MJ, Kuei J, Tashkin DP, et al. Contribution of emphysema and small airways in COPD. Chest. 1996;109(2):353-9. doi: 10.1378/chest.109.2.353
48. Grimson A, Farh KK, Johnston WK, Garrett-Engele P, Lim LP, Bartel DP. MicroRNA targeting specificity in mammals: determinants beyond seed pairing. *Mol Cell.* (2007) 27:91–105. doi: 10.1016/j.molcel.2007.06.017
49. Halappanavar S, Nikota J, Wu D, Williams A, Yauk CL, Stampfli M. IL-1 receptor regulates microRNA-135b expression in a negative feedback mechanism during cigarette smoke-induced inflammation. *J Immunol.* (2013) 190:3679–86. doi: 10.4049/jimmunol.1202456
50. Mizuno S, Bogaard HJ, Gomez-Arroyo J, Alhussaini A, Kraskauskas D, Cool CD, et al. MicroRNA-199a-5p is associated with hypoxia-inducible factor-1α expression in lungs from patients with COPD. *Chest.* (2012) 142:663–72. doi: 10.1378/chest.11-2746
51. Schembri F, Sridhar S, Perdomo C, Gustafson AM, Zhang X, Ergun A, et al. MicroRNAs as modulators of smoking-induced gene expression changes in human airway epithelium. *Proc Natl Acad Sci USA.* (2009) 106:2319–24. doi: 10.1073/pnas.0806383106
52. Xie L, Wu M, Lin H, Liu C, Yang H, Zhan J, et al. An increased ratio of serum miR-21 to miR-181a levels is associated with the early pathogenic process of chronic obstructive pulmonary disease in asymptomatic heavy smokers. *Mol Biosyst.* (2014) 10:1072–81. doi: 10.1039/C3MB70564A
53. Gu C, Li Y, Liu J, Ying X, Liu Y, Yan J, et al. LncRNA-mediated SIRT1/FoxO3a and SIRT1/p53 signaling pathways regulate type II alveolar epithelial cell senescence in patients with chronic obstructive pulmonary disease. *Mol Med Rep.* (2017) 15:3129–34. doi: 10.3892/mmr.2017.6367
54. Tang W, Shen Z, Guo J, Sun S. Screening of long non-coding RNA and TUG1 inhibits proliferation with TGF-β induction in patients with COPD. *Int J Chron Obstruct Pulmon Dis.* (2016) 11:2951–64. doi: 10.2147/COPD.S109570

55. Bi H, Zhou J, Wu D, Gao W, Li L, Yu L, et al. Microarray analysis of long non-coding RNAs in COPD lung tissue. *Inflamm Res.* (2015) 64:119–26. doi: 10.1007/s00011-014-0790-9
56. Poulet C, Njock MS, Moermans C, Louis E, Louis R, Malaise M, et al. Exosomal long non-coding RNAs in lung diseases. *Int J Mol Sci.* (2020) 21:3580 doi: 10.3390/ijms21103580
57. Cordazzo C, Petrini S, Neri T, Lombardi S, Carmazzi Y, Pedrinelli R, et al. Rapid shedding of proinflammatory microparticles by human mononuclear cells exposed to cigarette smoke is dependent on Ca2+ mobilization. *Inflamm Res.* (2014) 63:539–47. doi: 10.1007/s00011-014-0723-7
58. Tan DBA, Armitage J, Teo TH, Ong NE, Shin H, Moodley YP. Elevated levels of circulating exosome in COPD patients are associated with systemic inflammation. *Respir Med.* (2017) 132:261–4. doi: 10.1016/j.rmed.2017.04.014
59. Moon HG, Kim SH, Gao J, Quan T, Qin Z, Osorio JC, et al. CCN1 secretion and cleavage regulate the lung epithelial cell functions after cigarette smoke. *Am J Physiol Lung Cell Mol Physiol.* (2014) 307:L326–37. doi: 10.1152/ajplung.00102.2014
60. Kanazawa H, Yoshikawa J. Elevated oxidative stress and reciprocal reduction of vascular endothelial growth factor levels with severity of COPD. *Chest.* (2005) 128:3191–7. doi: 10.1378/chest.128.5.3191
61. Stockley RA, Turner AM. α-1-Antitrypsin deficiency: clinical variability, assessment, and treatment. *Trends Mol Med.* (2014) 20:105–15. doi: 10.1016/j.molmed.2013.11.006
62. Disayabutr S, Kim EK, Cha SI, Green G, Naikawadi RP, Jones KD, et al. miR-34 miRNAs regulate cellular senescence in type II alveolar epithelial cells of patients with idiopathic pulmonary fibrosis. *PLoS ONE.* (2016) 11:e0158367. doi: 10.1371/journal.pone.0158367
63. Fujita Y, Araya J, Ito S, Kobayashi K, Kosaka N, Yoshioka Y, et al. Suppression of autophagy by extracellular vesicles promotes myofibroblast differentiation in COPD pathogenesis. *J Extracell Vesicles.* (2015) 4:28388. doi: 10.3402/jev.v4.28388
64. Shen W, Liu J, Fan M, Wang S, Zhang Y, Wen L, et al. MiR-3202 protects smokers from chronic obstructive pulmonary disease through inhibiting FAIM2: an *in vivo* and *in vitro* study. *Exp Cell Res.* (2018) 362:370–7. doi: 10.1016/j.yexcr.2017.11.038
65. Conickx G, Mestdagh P, Avila Cobos F, Verhamme FM, Maes T, Vanaudenaerde BM, et al. MicroRNA profiling reveals a role for microRNA-218-5p in the pathogenesis of chronic obstructive pulmonary disease. *Am J Respir Crit Care Med.* (2017) 195:43–56. doi: 10.1164/rccm.201506-1182OC
66. Lewis A, Riddoch-Contreras J, Natanek SA, Donaldson A, Man WD, Moxham J, et al. Downregulation of the serum response factor/miR-1 axis in the quadriceps of patients with COPD. *Thorax.* (2012) 67:26–34. doi: 10.1136/thoraxjnl-2011-200309
67. Gu W, Yuan Y, Wang L, Yang H, Li S, Tang Z, et al. Long non-coding RNA TUG1 promotes airway remodelling by suppressing the miR-145-5p/DUSP6 axis in cigarette smoke-induced COPD. *J Cell Mol Med.* (2019) 23:7200–9. doi: 10.1111/jcmm.14389
68. Ge J, Geng S, Jiang H. Long noncoding RNAs antisense noncoding RNA in the INK4 locus (ANRIL) correlates with lower acute exacerbation risk, decreased inflammatory cytokines, and mild GOLD stage in patients with chronic obstructive pulmonary disease. *J Clin Lab Anal.* (2019) 33:e22678. doi: 10.1002/jcla.22678
69. Buschow SI, van Balkom BW, Aalberts M, Heck AJ, Wauben M, Stoorvogel W. MHC class II-associated proteins in B-cell exosomes and potential functional implications for exosome biogenesis. *Immunol Cell Biol.* (2010) 88:851–6. doi: 10.1038/icb.2010.64
70. Barnes PJ. Immunology of asthma and chronic obstructive pulmonary disease. *Nat Rev Immunol.* (2008) 8:183–92. doi: 10.1038/nri2254
71. Mittelbrunn M, Sánchez-Madrid F. Intercellular communication: diverse structures for exchange of genetic information. *Nat Rev Mol Cell Biol.* (2012) 13:328–35. doi: 10.1038/nrm3335
72. Sobo-Vujanovic A, Munich S, Vujanovic NL. Dendritic-cell exosomes cross-present Toll-like receptor-ligands and activate bystander dendritic cells. *Cell Immunol.* (2014) 289:119–27. doi: 10.1016/j.cellimm.2014.03.016
73. Lunding L, Wegmann M. NK cells in asthma exacerbation. *Oncotarget.* (2015) 6:19932–3. doi: 10.18632/oncotarget.4841
74. Zhang B, Yin Y, Lai RC, Lim SK. Immunotherapeutic potential of extracellular vesicles. *Front Immunol.* (2014) 5:518. doi: 10.3389/fimmu.2014.00518
75. Wang Y, Xu J, Meng Y, Adcock IM, Yao X. Role of inflammatory cells in airway remodeling in COPD. *Int J Chron Obstruct Pulmon Dis.* (2018) 13:3341–8. doi: 10.2147/COPD.S176122
76. Lefkowitz DL, Lefkowitz SS. Macrophage-neutrophil interaction: a paradigm for chronic inflammation revisited. *Immunol Cell Biol.* (2001) 79:502–6. doi: 10.1046/j.1440-1711.2001.01020.x
77. Ismail N, Wang Y, Dakhlallah D, Moldovan L, Agarwal K, Batte K, et al. Macrophage microvesicles induce macrophage differentiation and miR-223 transfer. *Blood.* (2013) 121:984–95. doi: 10.1182/blood-2011-08-374793
78. Lee H, Zhang D, Wu J, Otterbein LE, Jin Y. Lung epithelial cell-derived microvesicles regulate macrophage migration *via* microRNA-17/221-induced integrin β(1) recycling. *J Immunol.* (2017) 199:1453–64. doi: 10.4049/jimmunol.1700165
79. Lee H, Zhang D, Zhu Z, Dela Cruz CS, Jin Y. Epithelial cell-derived microvesicles activate macrophages and promote inflammation via microvesicle-containing microRNAs. *Sci Rep.* (2016) 6:35250. doi: 10.1038/srep35250
80. Serban KA, Rezania S, Petrusca DN, Poirier C, Cao D, Justice MJ, et al. Structural and functional characterization of endothelial microparticles released by cigarette smoke. *Sci Rep.* (2016) 6:31596. doi: 10.1038/srep31596
81. Yáñez-Mó M, Siljander PR, Andreu Z, Zavec AB, Borràs FE, Buzas EI, et al. Biological properties of extracellular vesicles and their physiological functions. *J Extracell Vesicles.* (2015) 4:27066. doi: 10.3402/jev.v4.27066
82. Kulshreshtha A, Ahmad T, Agrawal A, Ghosh B. Proinflammatory role of epithelial cell-derived exosomes in allergic airway inflammation. *J Allergy Clin Immunol.* (2013) 131:1194–203, 203.e1–14. doi: 10.1016/j.jaci.2012.12.1565
83. Li N, Liu Y, Cai J. LncRNA MIR155HG regulates M1/M2 macrophage polarization in chronic obstructive pulmonary disease. *Biomed Pharmacother.* (2019) 117:109015. doi: 10.1016/j.biopha.2019.109015
84. Van Eeden SF, Hogg JC. Immune-modulation in chronic obstructive pulmonary disease: current concepts and future strategies. *Respiration.* (2020) 99:550–65. doi: 10.1159/000502261
85. Genschmer KR, Russell DW, Lal C, Szul T, Bratcher PE, Noerager BD, et al. Activated PMN exosomes: pathogenic entities causing matrix destruction and disease in the lung. *Cell.* (2019) 176:113–26.e15. doi: 10.1016/j.cell.2018.12.002
86. Laurell CB, Eriksson S. The electrophoretic α1-globulin pattern of serum in α1-antitrypsin deficiency. 1963. *COPD.* (2013) 10(Suppl. 1):3–8. doi: 10.3109/15412555.2013.771956
87. Sng JJ, Prazakova S, Thomas PS, Herbert C. MMP-8, MMP-9 and neutrophil elastase in peripheral blood and exhaled breath condensate in COPD. *COPD.* (2017) 14:238–44. doi: 10.1080/15412555.2016.1249790
88. Senior RM, Tegner H, Kuhn C, Ohlsson K, Starcher BC, Pierce JA. The induction of pulmonary emphysema with human leukocyte elastase. *Am Rev Respir Dis.* (1977) 116:469–75. doi: 10.1164/arrd.1977.116.3.469
89. Veerappan A, Thompson M, Savage AR, Silverman ML, Chan WS, Sung B, et al. Mast cells and exosomes in hyperoxia-induced neonatal lung disease. *Am J Physiol Lung Cell Mol Physiol.* (2016) 310:L1218–32. doi: 10.1152/ajplung.00299.2015
90. Wen C, Seeger RC, Fabbri M, Wang L, Wayne AS, Jong AY. Biological roles and potential applications of immune cell-derived extracellular vesicles. *J Extracell Vesicles.* (2017) 6:1400370. doi: 10.1080/20013078.2017.1400370
91. Qazi KR, Gehrmann U, Domange Jordö E, Karlsson MC, Gabrielsson S. Antigen-loaded exosomes alone induce Th1-type memory through a B-cell-dependent mechanism. *Blood.* (2009) 113:2673–83. doi: 10.1182/blood-2008-04-153536
92. Julich H, Willms A, Lukacs-Kornek V, Kornek M. Extracellular vesicle profiling and their use as potential disease specific biomarker. *Front Immunol.* (2014) 5:413. doi: 10.3389/fimmu.2014.00413
93. Kornek M, Lynch M, Mehta SH, Lai M, Exley M, Afdhal NH, et al. Circulating microparticles as disease-specific biomarkers of severity of inflammation in patients with hepatitis C or nonalcoholic steatohepatitis. *Gastroenterology.* (2012) 143:448–58. doi: 10.1053/j.gastro.2012.04.031

94. Lacedonia D, Carpagnano GE, Trotta T, Palladino GP, Panaro MA, Zoppo LD, et al. Microparticles in sputum of COPD patients: a potential biomarker of the disease? *Int J Chron Obstruct Pulmon Dis.* (2016) 11:527–33. doi: 10.2147/COPD.S99547
95. Shi L, Xin Q, Chai R, Liu L, Ma Z. Ectopic expressed miR-203 contributes to chronic obstructive pulmonary disease *via* targeting TAK1 and PIK3CA. *Int J Clin Exp Pathol.* (2015) 8:10662–70.
96. Wang R, Li M, Zhou S, Zeng D, Xu X, Xu R, et al. Effect of a single nucleotide polymorphism in miR-146a on COX-2 protein expression and lung function in smokers with chronic obstructive pulmonary disease. *Int J Chron Obstruct Pulmon Dis.* (2015) 10:463–73. doi: 10.2147/COPD.S74345
97. Kara M, Kirkil G, Kalemci S. Differential expression of microRNAs in chronic obstructive pulmonary disease. *Adv Clin Exp Med.* (2016) 25:21–6. doi: 10.17219/acem/28343
98. Devadoss D, Long C, Langley RJ, Manevski M, Nair M, Campos MA, et al. Long noncoding transcriptome in chronic obstructive pulmonary disease. *Am J Respir Cell Mol Biol.* (2019) 61:678–88. doi: 10.1165/rcmb.2019-0184TR
99. Lewis A, Lee JY, Donaldson AV, Natanek SA, Vaidyanathan S, Man WD, et al. Increased expression of H19/miR-675 is associated with a low fat-free mass index in patients with COPD. *J Cachexia Sarcopenia Muscle.* (2016) 7:330–44. doi: 10.1002/jcsm.12078
100. Mei D, Tan WSD, Tay Y, Mukhopadhyay A, Wong WSF. Therapeutic RNA strategies for chronic obstructive pulmonary disease. *Trends Pharmacol Sci.* (2020) 41:475–86. doi: 10.1016/j.tips.2020.04.007
101. Sun Y, An N, Li J, Xia J, Tian Y, Zhao P, et al. miRNA-206 regulates human pulmonary microvascular endothelial cell apoptosis via targeting in chronic obstructive pulmonary disease. *J Cell Biochem.* (2019) 120:6223–36. doi: 10.1002/jcb.27910
102. Sørheim IC, Johannessen A, Gulsvik A, Bakke PS, Silverman EK, DeMeo DL. Gender differences in COPD: are women more susceptible to smoking effects than men? *Thorax.* (2010) 65:480–5. doi: 10.1136/thx.2009.122002
103. Du Y, Ding Y, Chen X, Mei Z, Ding H, Wu Y, et al. MicroRNA-181c inhibits cigarette smoke-induced chronic obstructive pulmonary disease by regulating CCN1 expression. *Respir Res.* (2017) 18:155. doi: 10.1186/s12931-017-0639-1
104. Paschalaki KE, Zampetaki A, Baker JR, Birrell MA, Starke RD, Belvisi MG, et al. Downregulation of microRNA-126 augments DNA damage response in cigarette smokers and patients with chronic obstructive pulmonary disease. *Am J Respir Crit Care Med.* (2018) 197:665–8. doi: 10.1164/rccm.201706-1304LE
105. Dua K, Wadhwa R, Singhvi G, Rapalli V, Shukla SD, Shastri MD, et al. The potential of siRNA based drug delivery in respiratory disorders: recent advances and progress. *Drug Dev Res.* (2019) 80:714–30. doi: 10.1002/ddr.21571
106. Boehme SA, Franz-Bacon K, Ludka J, DiTirro DN, Ly TW, Bacon KB. MAP3K19 is overexpressed in COPD and is a central mediator of cigarette smoke-induced pulmonary inflammation and lower airway destruction. *PLoS ONE.* (2016) 11:e0167169. doi: 10.1371/journal.pone.0167169
107. Jamieson KC, Traves SL, Kooi C, Wiehler S, Dumonceaux CJ, Maciejewski BA, et al. Rhinovirus and bacteria synergistically induce IL-17C release from human airway epithelial cells to promote neutrophil recruitment. *J Immunol.* (2019) 202:160–70. doi: 10.4049/jimmunol.1800547
108. Liu Q, Li H, Wang Q, Zhang Y, Wang W, Dou S, et al. Increased expression of TROP2 in airway basal cells potentially contributes to airway remodeling in chronic obstructive pulmonary disease. *Respir Res.* (2016) 17:159. doi: 10.1186/s12931-016-0463-z
109. Wang CG, Li C, Lei W, Jiang JH, Huang JA, Zeng DX. The association of neuron-derived orphan receptor 1 with pulmonary vascular remodeling in COPD patients. *Int J Chron Obstruct Pulmon Dis.* (2018) 13:1177–86. doi: 10.2147/COPD.S151820
110. Reimann S, Fink L, Wilhelm J, Hoffmann J, Bednorz M, Seimetz M, et al. Increased S100A4 expression in the vasculature of human COPD lungs and murine model of smoke-induced emphysema. *Respir Res.* (2015) 16:127. doi: 10.1186/s12931-015-0284-5

20

Characteristics and Prognostic Factors of Pulmonary Fibrosis After COVID-19 Pneumonia

Elisabetta Cocconcelli[1†], *Nicol Bernardinello*[1†], *Chiara Giraudo*[2], *Gioele Castelli*[1], *Adelaide Giorgino*[2], *Davide Leoni*[3], *Simone Petrarulo*[1], *Anna Ferrari*[3], *Marina Saetta*[1], *Annamaria Cattelan*[3], *Paolo Spagnolo*[1] and *Elisabetta Balestro*[1*]

[1] Respiratory Disease Unit, Department of Cardiac, Thoracic, Vascular Sciences and Public Health, University of Padova and Padova City Hospital, Padova, Italy, [2] Department of Medicine, Institute of Radiology, University of Padova and Padova City Hospital, Padova, Italy, [3] Division of Infectious and Tropical Diseases, University of Padova and Padova City Hospital, Padova, Italy

***Correspondence:**
Elisabetta Balestro
elisabetta.balestro@aopd.veneto.it

†These authors share first authorship

Background: Few is known about the long-term pulmonary sequelae after COVID-19 infection. Hence, the aim of this study is to characterize patients with persisting pulmonary sequelae at follow-up after hospitalization. We also aimed to explore clinical and radiological predictors of pulmonary fibrosis following COVID-19.

Methods: Two hundred and 20 consecutive patients were evaluated at 3–6 months after discharge with high-resolution computed tomography (HRCT) and categorized as recovered (REC) or not recovered (NOT-REC). Both HRCTs at hospitalization ($HRCT_0$), when available, and $HRCT_1$ during follow-up were analyzed semiquantitatively as follows: ground-glass opacities (alveolar score, AS), consolidations (CONS), and reticulations (interstitial score, IS).

Results: A total of 175/220 (80%) patients showed disease resolution at their initial radiological evaluation following discharge. NOT-REC patients (45/220; 20%) were mostly older men [66 (35–85) years vs. 56 (19–87); $p = 0.03$] with a longer in-hospital stay [16 (0–75) vs. 8 (1–52) days; $p < 0.0001$], and lower P/F at admission [233 (40–424) vs. 318 (33–543); $p = 0.04$]. Moreover, NOT-REC patients presented, at hospital admission, higher ALV [14 (0.0–62.0) vs. 4.4 (0.0–44.0); $p = 0.0005$], CONS [1.9 (0.0–26.0) vs. 0.4 (0.0–18.0); $p = 0.0064$], and IS [11.5 (0.0– 29.0) vs. 0.0 (0.0–22.0); $p < 0.0001$] compared to REC patients. On multivariate analysis, the presence of CONS and IS at $HRCT_0$ was independent predictors of radiological sequelae at follow-up [OR 14.87 (95% CI: 1.25–175.8; $p = 0.03$) and 28.9 (95% CI: 2.17–386.6; $p = 0.01$, respectively)].

Conclusions: In our population, only twenty percent of patients showed persistent lung abnormalities at 6 months after hospitalization for COVID-19 pneumonia. These patients are predominantly older men with longer hospital stay. The presence of reticulations and consolidation on HRCT at hospital admission predicts the persistence of radiological abnormalities during follow-up.

Keywords: SARS-CoV-2, coronavirus disease 2019, pulmonary fibrosis, high-resolution computed tomography, pulmonary sequelae

BACKGROUND

Coronavirus disease 2019 (COVID-19), which is caused by the severe acute respiratory syndrome coronavirus 2 (SARS-CoV-2), has infected more than 130 million people worldwide. COVID-19 leads to respiratory manifestations that can range from mild flu-like symptoms such as fever, cough, and fatigue to severe respiratory failure requiring intensive care (1, 2).

Data from previous pandemics caused by coronaviruses suggested that there may be pulmonary sequelae in one-third of patients at 12 weeks after discharge (3, 4).

Some recent studies tried to characterize radiological sequelae after COVID-19 pneumonia (5, 6). This condition, which is referred to as "post-COVID syndrome," still lacks a universally agreed definition (7). On May 2020, a document of the British Thoracic Society (BTS) proposed an algorithm on post-discharge management of patients with COVID-19 and distinguished two groups of interest: patients with severe pneumonia and patients with mild-to-moderate pneumonia (8). Following up on this document, George and colleagues suggested a structured respiratory follow-up for patients with clinico-radiological confirmation of COVID-19 pneumonia (9). Importantly, they proposed patients with severe pneumonia undergo a full clinical assessment at 12 weeks with a chest X-ray whereas patients with persisting radiological abnormalities should undergo a high-resolution computed tomography (HRCT) scan. In this regard, the role of chest X-ray and HRCT in disease management both during hospitalization and follow-up is well established (10, 11). Han and coauthors recently reported that fibrotic-like changes on CT performed at 6 months during follow-up persist in approximately one-third of patients with COVID-19 (12), but the data on long-term pulmonary sequelae in this patient population remain scarce. The aim of this study is to characterize, among patients hospitalized for COVID-19 pneumonia, those presenting persisting pulmonary sequelae during follow-up, and to define which clinical and radiological features are predictive of persistent radiological abnormalities.

MATERIALS AND METHODS

Study Population and Study Design

We prospectively collected patients evaluated at the post-COVID clinic of the University Hospital of Padova between June and December 2020. The patients evaluated at the post-COVID clinic were initially admitted to the Division of Infectious and Tropical Diseases of the University Hospital of Padova between February and September 2020 for SARS-CoV-2 infection confirmed by the real-time polymerase chain reaction (RT-PCR) at nasopharyngeal swab.

Among all patients evaluated, we specifically followed up every 3 months those presenting a COVID-19-related severe disease according to the WHO criteria ($n = 220$) (13). Demographics and clinical data at hospital admission [symptoms, gas exchange values (paO_2/FiO_2)] and during hospitalization [days of hospital stay, maximal FiO_2 (FiO_2 max) needed, level of care, treatment] were collected. Comorbidities were categorized as cardiovascular diseases (CVDs), respiratory diseases, metabolic diseases (including diabetes mellitus, obesity, and dyslipidemia), autoimmune diseases, and oncologic diseases (including lung, prostate, pancreatic, breast, and colon cancer). Based on patient's clinical conditions during hospitalization, we distinguished those requiring a low- (LIMC) and high-intensity medical care (HIMC), as previously described (14).

Radiological Evaluation

At follow-up, HRCT was available for the entire study population ($HRCT_1$) whereas at hospital admission, it was available in only a subgroup of patients ($HRCT_0$) ($n = 79$, 36%). The HRCTs were performed by a 64 slice Siemens Somatom Sensation (Siemens Healthcare, Erlangen, Germany) applying a slice thickness $\leq$0.5 mm.

According to the presence or absence of radiological abnormalities on $HCRT_1$, the study population was categorized as recovered patients (REC, $n = 175$) or not recovered patients (NOT-REC, $n = 45$).

Two expert thoracic radiologists (CG and AG), who were blinded to clinical data and timing of HRCTs, scored the images independently using a composite semiquantitative scale. This represented a modification of the previously reported scoring systems standardized by our group (13). Specifically, ground-glass opacities (GGO) (alveolar score, AS), consolidations (CONS), and reticulations (interstitial score, IS) were analyzed. For each lung lobe, the two radiologists assessed the extent of AS, CONS, and IS using a scale from 0 to 100 and estimated extent to the nearest 2%. The result was expressed as the mean value of the five lobes in AS, CONS, and IS. The level of interobserver agreement was obtained for each patient as a mean of 5 lobes and for each radiological abnormality (AS, CONS, and IS) and expressed as Cohen's k value. Disagreement between radiologists was resolved by consensus.

Statistical Analysis

Categorical variables were described as absolute (n) and relative values (%), whereas continuous variables were described as median and range. To compare demographic and clinical data between REC and NOT-REC patients, chi-square test and Fisher's exact test ($n < 5$) for categorical variables and Mann–Whitney U tests for continuous variables were used, as appropriate.

To compare radiological scores at $HRCT_1$ in NOT-REC patients, Mann–Whitney U test for continuous variables was used, whereas Wilcoxon signed-rank test was used to compare radiological scores between $HRCT_0$ and $HRCT_1$. A univariate logistic regression analysis, followed by a regression model adjusted for gender, pack-years, paO_2/FiO_2 at admission, degree of medical care (high or low), and FiO_2 max, was performed to detect the predictive factors of radiologic sequelae (NOT-REC)

Abbreviations: IPF, idiopathic pulmonary fibrosis; FVC, forced vital capacity; HRCT, high-resolution computed tomography; REC, recovered; NOT-REC, not recovered; AS, alveolar score; CONS, consolidations; IS, interstitial score; COVID-19, Coronavirus disease 2019; SARS-CoV-2, severe acute respiratory syndrome coronavirus 2; RT-PCR, real- time polymerase chain reaction; LIMC, low-intensity medical care; HIMC, high-intensity medical care; BMI, body mass index; CVDs, cardiovascular diseases; TLC, total lung capacity; DLCO, diffusing capacity of the lung for carbon monoxide.

TABLE 1 | Baseline demographics and clinical features of the overall population evaluated at post-COVID clinic, and of the two subgroups categorized according to the presence of radiological recovery during the follow-up period.

	Overall population (n = 220)	REC (n = 175; 80%)	NOT−REC (n = 45; 20%)	*P* value
Male—*n (%)*	115 (52)	86 (49)	29 (64)	0.06
Age at admission—*years*	59 (19–87)	56 (19–87)	66 (35–85)	<0.0001
Smoking history—*pack-years*	0 (0–67)	0 (0–67)	0 (0–60)	0.07
Current—*n (%)*	15 (7)	10 (6)	5 (11)	0.20
Former—*n (%)*	70 (32)	54 (31)	16 (36)	0.54
Nonsmokers—*n (%)*	135 (61)	111 (63)	24 (53)	0.21
BMI—(kg/m^2)	26 (18–39)	27 (18–39)	26 (21–35)	0.35
Cardiovascular diseases—*n* (%)	98 (45)	72 (41)	26 (58)	0.04
Respiratory diseases—*n* (%)	39 (18)	30 (17)	9 (20)	0.65
Autoimmune diseases—*n* (%)	36 (16)	25 (14)	11 (24)	0.10
Metabolic diseases—*n* (%)	102 (4)	78 (45)	24 (53)	0.29
Oncologic diseases—*n* (%)	25 (11)	17 (8)	8 (18)	0.12
PaO_2 / FiO_2 at admission	314 (33–543)	318 (33–543)	233 (40–424)	0.04
FiO_2max during hospitalization—%	28 (21–100)	27 (21–100)	45 (21–100)	<0.0001
Hospitalization—days	9 (0–75)	8 (1–52)	16 (0–75)	<0.0001
Low degree of care—*n* (%)	163 (74)	138 (79)	25 (56)	0.002
High degree of care—*n* (%)	57 (26)	37 (21)	20 (44)	

Values are expressed as numbers and (%) or median and range, as appropriate. To compare demographics between recovery (REC) and not recovery (NOT-REC), chi-square test and Fisher's t-test (n < 5) for categorical variables and Mann–Whitney t-test for continuous variables were used.

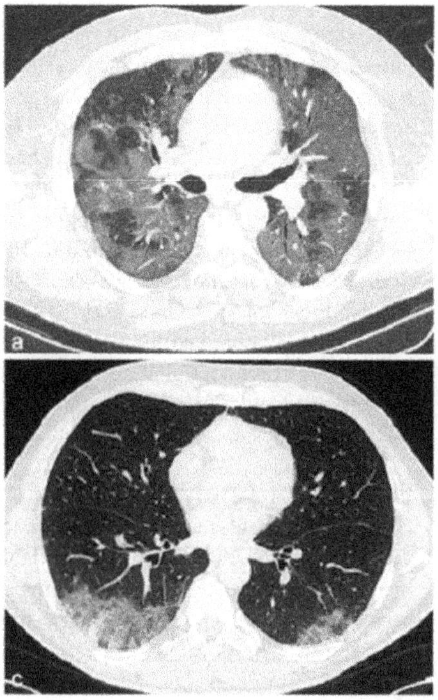

FIGURE 1 | Chest CT features of two patients with COVID-19 pneumonia at different time points: hospitalization and 6 months after discharge. Chest CT images of a 58-year-old male patient with COVID-19, not recovery patient **(a,b)**. The first CT performed at admission shows bilateral areas of ground-glass opacities in a peripheral distribution **(a)**, and after 6 months from discharge, CT shows persistent of interlobular septal thickening with peripheral distribution **(b)**. Chest CT images of a 51-year-old male patient with COVID-19, recovery patient **(c,d)**. The first CT shows, at admission, a small consolidation at the right lower lobe accompanied by ground-glass opacities in both lower lobes **(c)**, and after 6 months from discharge, no residual abnormalities were observed **(d)**.

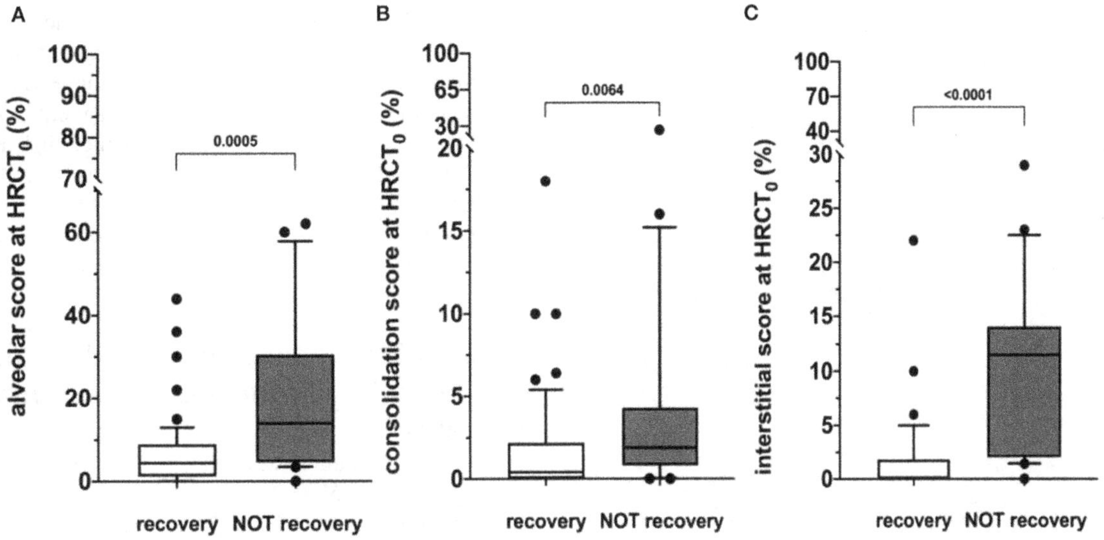

FIGURE 2 | HRCT scores during hospitalization (HRCT0) of the two subgroups categorized according to the presence of radiological recovery [recovery (REC) or NOT-recovery (NOT-REC)] at follow-up period. Horizontal bars represent median values; bottom and top of each box plot 25th and 75th; brackets show 10th and 90th percentiles; and circles represent outliers. White boxes indicate values for recovery group and gray boxes not recovery group. **(A)** ALV [14.0 (0.0–62.0) vs. 4.4 (0.0–44.0); $p = 0.0005$]; **(B)** CONS [1.9 (0.0–26.0 vs. 0.4 (0.0–18.0); $p = 0.0064$]; **(C)** INT [11.5 (0.0–29.0) vs. 0.0 (0.0–22.0); $p < 0.0001$].

TABLE 2 | HRCT scores during hospitalization (HRCT$_0$) of the overall population evaluated at post-COVID clinic and of the two subgroups categorized according to the presence of radiological recovery during the follow-up period.

	Overall population ($n = 220$)	REC ($n = 175$; 80%)	NOT−REC ($n = 45$; 20%)	*p*-value
Alveolar score−%	5.0 (0.0–62)	4.4 (0.0–44.0)	14.0 (0.0–62.0)	0.0005
Consolidations−%	0.8 (0.0–26.0)	0.4 (0.0–18.0)	1.9 (0.0–26.0)	0.006
Interstitial score−%	0.8 (0.0–29.0)	0.0 (0.0–22.0)	11.5 (0.0–29.0)	<0.0001

Values are expressed as median and range, as appropriate. To compare HRCT scores at hospitalization (HRCT$_0$) between recovery (REC) and not recovery (NOT-REC), Mann–Whitney t-test for continuous variables was used.

at follow-up. All data were analyzed using SPSS Software version 25.0 (US: IBM Corp., New York, NY, USA). p-Values < 0.05 were considered statistically significant. The graphs were obtained using the statistical package GraphPad Prism 7.0 (GraphPad Software, Inc., La Jolla, CA, USA).

Ethics Statement

The study protocol complies with the ethical guidelines of the 1975 Declaration of Helsinki, and in agreement with national regulation on observational studies, it was notified and approved by the local ethics committee (number: 46430/03.08.2020) and the need for patient's informed consent was waived.

RESULTS

Clinical Evaluation at Hospital Admission and During Hospitalization

Two hundred and 20 patients with COVID-19 pneumonia evaluated at the post-COVID clinic were included in the study (**Table 1**). A total of 115 patients (52%) were men, with a median age of 59 years (range 19–84) and body mass index (BMI) 26 (18–39). The most prevalent comorbidities were CVDs ($n = 98$, 45%), followed by the chronic respiratory diseases (18%). Based on the presence of radiological sequelae on HRCT performed at follow-up (HRCT$_1$), 175 (80%) patients were categorized as REC and 45 (20%) as NOT-REC (**Figure 1**). Baseline demographic and clinical data of REC and NOT-REC patients are summarized in **Table 1**.

No differences in sex, smoking history, or BMI were observed between the two groups, with a prevalence of men in NOT-REC compared to REC (64 vs. 49%, respectively). NOT-REC patients were significantly older compared to REC [66 (35–85) vs. 56 (19–87) years; $p < 0.0001$]. CVDs were significantly more frequent in NOT-REC compared to REC [26 (58%) vs. 72 (41%); $p = 0.04$] whereas autoimmune, metabolic, and oncologic diseases did not differ between the two groups. Symptoms before hospital admission were also similar, except for a higher proportion of patients presenting with dyspnea in NOT-REC compared to REC group [33 (73%) vs. 64 (37%); $p < 0.0001$] (**Supplementary Table 1**).

At hospital admission, NOT-REC had a worse gas exchange with a lower PiO_2/FiO_2 ratio than REC [233 (40–424) vs. 318 (33543); $p = 0.04$]. In addition, compared to REC, during hospitalization, NOT-REC required more frequently

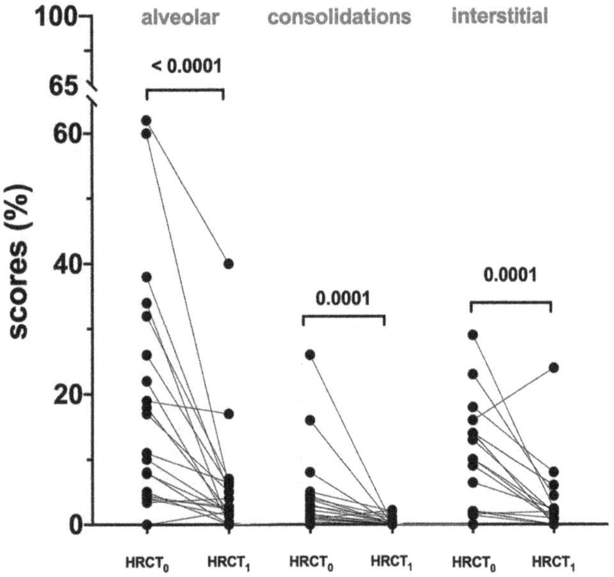

FIGURE 3 | HRCT scores of the not recovery population (NOT-REC) from HRCT0 to HRCT1: ALV. [from 14 (0.0–62.0) to 2.6 (0.0–40.0); $p < 0.0001$], CONS [from 1.9 (0.0–26.0) to 0.0 (0.0–2.2); $p = 0.0001$] and INT [1.5 (0.0–29.0) to 1.4 (0.0–24.0)].

high-intensity medical care (HIMC) (20, 44 vs. 37, 21%; $p = 0.002$), higher FiO_2 max [45 (21–100) vs. 27 (21–100); $p < 0.0001$], and longer in-hospital stay [16 (0–75) vs. 8 (1–52) days; $p < 0.0001$].

The majority of patients were admitted during the first SARS-CoV-2 wave when no standardized protocols existed for treatment of hospitalized patients. NOT-REC patients were more frequently treated with hydroxychloroquine ($n = 37$, 82 vs. 111, 63%; $p = 0.01$), antibiotics other than ceftriaxone and azithromycin ($n = 25$, 56 vs. 44, 25%; $p < 0.0001$), remdesevir ($n = 7$, 16 vs. 10, 6%, $p = 0.02$), tocilizumab ($n = 8$, 18 vs. 12, 7%; $p = 0.02$), and steroids ($n = 27$, 60 vs. 74, 42%; $p = 0.03$) compared to REC. Conversely, the two groups did not differ with regard to the use of ceftriaxone, azithromycin, lopinovir/ritonavir, and hyperimmune plasma (**Supplementary Table 2**). At discharge, a similar proportion of patients in both groups were prescribed steroids.

Clinical, Functional, and Radiologic Evaluation at Follow-Up

Patients were evaluated at post-COVID clinic at regular 3-month intervals after discharge. At first evaluation, NOT-REC patients presented more frequently a modified Medical Research Council (mMRC) scores of 1 and 2 compared to REC [15 (33%) vs. 22 (13%), $p = 0.0009$ and 7 (16%) vs. 3 (2%), $p < 0.0001$, respectively]. In the overall population, pulmonary function tests (PFTs) revealed a median forced vital capacity (FVC) of 3.40 liters (L) (range 1.40–7.96), 96%pred. and a median total lung capacity (TLC) of 5.36 L (3.63–8.09), 89% pred. within the normal range. Likewise, NOT-REC patients showed preserved lung volumes within normal range (**Supplementary Table 3**). A number of 32 patients out of 220 (14.5%) had an abnormal diffusing capacity of the lung for carbon monoxide (DLco) at the 6-month follow-up, which occurred in those with persistent interstitial lung abnormalities (NOT-REC patients). At follow-up CT ($HRCT_1$), NOT-REC patients presented higher ALV [2.8 (0.0–40.0)] compared to CONS [0.0 (0.0–2.0); $p < 0.0001$] and IS [0.6 (0.0–24.0); $p < 0.0001$] (**Supplementary Figure 1**). Overall, the interobserver agreement between the two radiologists with regard to change in AS, CONS, and IS was good (Cohen's kappa = 0.79 for AS, k = 0.88 for CONS, and k = 0.81 for IS).

Longitudinal Evaluation of Radiologic Manifestation: From Hospitalization to Follow-Up

At hospital admission, HRCT ($HRCT_0$) was available for 79/220 (36%) patients. ALV [5.0 (0.0–62.0)] was significantly more prevalent compared to CONS [0.8 (0.0–26.0); $p < 0.0001$] and IS [0.8 (0.0–29.0); $p < 0.0001$]. When this patient subgroup was stratified in NOT-REC and REC, NOT-REC patients ($n = 20$) had at hospital admission higher ALV [14.0 (0.0–62.0) vs. 4.4 (0.0–44.0); $p = 0.0005$] (**Figure 2A**), CONS [1.9 (0.0–26.0 vs. 0.4 (0.0–18.0); $p = 0.0064$] (**Figure 2B**), and IS [11.5 (0.0–29.0) vs. 0.0 (0.0–22.0); $p < 0.0001$] (**Figure 2C**) compared to REC patients ($n = 59$) (**Table 2**). Finally, when comparing $HRCT_0$ with $HRCT_1$, we observed that in NOT-REC patients, ALV [from 14 (0.0–62.0) to 2.6 (0.0–40.0); $p < 0.0001$], CONS [from 1.9 (0.0–26.0) to 0.0 (0.0–2.2); $p = 0.0001$], and IS [1.5 (0.0–29.0) to 1.4 (0.0–24.0)] decreased significantly (**Figure 3**).

Prognostic Factors for Radiological Sequelae at Follow-Up

Univariate analysis showed that older age, a prolonged in-hospital stay, a lower $PiO2/FiO_2$ at hospital admission, cardiovascular comorbidities, a higher degree of medical care, a higher FiO_2 max, and higher ALV, CONS, and INT scores at $HRCT_0$, not use of hydroxychloroquine, antibiotics other than azithromycin and ceftriaxone, tocilizumab, remdesevir, and systemic steroids are associated with persistent radiological abnormalities at follow-up. Multivariate analysis revealed that CONS [OR: 20.6 (95%CI: 1. −301.2); $p = 0.02$] and IS score [23.0 (1.4–377.2); $p = 0.02$] are independent predictors of radiological sequelae at follow-up (**Table 3**).

Finally, on multivariate analysis adjusted for gender, pack-years, PiO_2/FiO_2 ratio at admission, degree of care (high or low), and FiO_2 max, both CONS and IS at $HRCT_0$ are independent predictors of radiological sequelae at follow-up with an OR of 14.87 (95% CI: 1.25–175.8; $p = 0.03$) and 28.9 (95% CI: 2.17–386.6; $p = 0.01$), respectively (**Table 4**).

DISCUSSION

In our study, we demonstrated that only a significant minority of patients hospitalized for COVID-19 pneumonia has persistent radiological abnormalities at follow-up. Patients who did not recover are mainly elder men, with a more severe gas exchange

TABLE 3 | Predictive factors of radiological sequelae at follow-up in patients hospitalized for SARS-COV-2-related pneumonia.

	Univariate analysis		Multivariate analysis	
	OR (95% IC)	***p***	**OR (95% IC)**	***p***
Sex				
Female	Ref.	-	-	-
Male	1.87 (0.95–3.69)	0.07	-	-
Age—years				
<59	Ref.	-	Ref.	-
≥59	2.99 (1.47–6.08)	0.002	0.81 (0.10–6.39)	0.84
BMI—(kg/m^2)				
<26	Ref.	-	-	-
≥26	0.80 (0.41–1.58)	0.52	-	-
Smoking history–*pack–years*				
=0	Ref.	-	-	-
>0	1.56 (0.79–3.10)	0.19	-	-
Hospitalization—*days*				
<9	Ref.	-	Ref.	-
≥9	4.77 (2.15–10.5)	<0.0001	12.77 (0.65–248.8)	0.09
PiO_2/FiO_2 at admission				
<314	Ref.	-	Ref.	-
≥314	0.33 (0.13–0.80)	0.01	1.24 (0.13–11.46)	0.84
CVD				
No	Ref.	-	Ref.	-
Yes	1.95 (1.00–3.80)	0.04	1.40 (0.15–12.48)	0.76
Respiratory diseases				
No	Ref.	-	-	-
Yes	1.20 (0.52–2.77)	0.65	-	-
Autoimmune diseases				
No	Ref.	-	-	-
Yes	1.94 (0.87–4.32)	0.11	-	-
Metabolic diseases				
No	Ref.	-	-	-
Yes	1.42 (0.73–2.74)	0.29	-	-
Oncologic diseases				
No	Ref.	-	-	-
Yes	2.01 (0.80–5.01)	0.13	-	-
Degree of care				
Low	Ref.	-	Ref.	-
High	2.98 (1.49–5.95)	0.002	1.35 (0.13–13.12)	0.79
FiO_2 max—%				
<28	Ref.	-	Ref.	-
≥28	3.25 (1.54–6.80)	0.002	1.01 (0.07–16.2)	0.99
Alveolar score HRCT0—%				
<7	Ref.	-	Ref.	-
≥7	4.0 (1.33–11.98)	0.01	0.74 (0.09–5.99)	0.78
Consolidations HRCT0—%				
<0.8	Ref.	-	Ref.	-
≥0.8	6.29 (1.66–23.87)	0.007	20.6 (1.40–301.2)	0.02
Interstitial score HRCT0—%				
<1.4	Ref.	-	Ref.	-
≥1.4	41.2 (5.1–331.8)	<0.0001	23.0 (1.40–377.2)	0.02
Hidroxicloroquina				
Yes	Ref 2.66 (1.17–6.07)	0.02	Ref 1.26 (0.18–8.82)	0.80
No				
Azithromycin				
Yes	Ref.	-	-	-
No	0.76 (0.39–1.47)	0.41	-	-
Ceftriaxone				
Yes	Ref.	-	-	-
No	1.74 (0.89–3.40)	0.10	-	-
Other antibiotics				
Yes	Ref.	-	Ref.	-
No	3.72 (1.88–7.34)	<0.0001	4.87 (0.52–45.7)	0.16
Lopinovir/Ritonavir				
Yes	Ref.	-	-	-
No	1.49 (0.75–2.94)	0.24	-	-
Remdesevir				
Yes	Ref.	-	Ref.	-
No	3.03 (1.08–8.49)	0.03	12.5 (0.41–3.85)	0.14
Glutathione				
Yes	Ref.	-	-	-
No	0.22 (0.09–1.75)	0.15	-	-
Tocilizumab				
Yes	Ref.	-	Ref. 0.6 (0.03–11.1)	-
No	2.93 (1.12–7.69)	0.02		0.73
Plasma				
Yes	Ref.	-	-	-
No	1.49 (0.37–5.86)	0.56	-	-
Steroids during hospitalization				
Yes	Ref.	-	Ref. 1.04 (0.09	-
No	2.04 (1.05–3.99)	0.03	– 11.6)	0.97

Values are expressed as OR (95%CI). Logistic regression analysis was used to determine the relationship of clinical data with radiological sequelae at follow-up.

impairment at hospital admission and a more severe clinical course during hospitalization. Interestingly, the presence of reticulation and consolidation at admission was predictive of persistent interstitial changes at follow-up.

To date, few studies have reported on the follow-up of patients hospitalized for COVID-19 pneumonia (5, 6). Different approaches based on disease severity have been proposed with the aim to standardize patients' follow-up. Specifically, the British Thoracic Society guidelines for management of post-COVID-19 syndrome distinguished patients with severe pneumonia requiring intensive care from patients with mild-to-moderate

TABLE 4 | Multivariate analysis for factors independently associated with radiological sequelae at follow-up in patients hospitalized for SARS-COV-2-related pneumonia.

	Multivariate analysis*	
	OR (95% IC)	***p***
Alveolar score HRCT0—%		
<7	Ref. 1.80 (0.39-–8.20)	-
≥7		−0.44
Consolidations HRCT0—%		
<0.8	Ref. 14.87 (1.25-–175.8)	-
≥0.8		−0.03
Interstitial score HRCT0—%		
<1.4	Ref. 28.9 (2.17-–386.6)	-
≥1.4		**-0.01**

*Values are expressed as OR (95%CI). Univariate and multivariate-adjusted odds ratio for radiological NOT recovery according to radiological patterns during hospitalization ($HRCT_0$). *Adjusted for gender, pack-years, PiO_2/FiO_2 ratio at admission, degree of care (high or low), FiO_2 max.*

pneumonia treated in a medical ward or at home (4). However, it is becoming increasingly clear that radiological changes following COVID-19 pneumonia do not resolve completely in a large minority of patients (5, 15). Some studies have started to use CT to assess the presence of long-term lung abnormalities. A recent work from the Chongqing University Three Gorges Hospital evaluated 41 patients and showed that in most patients, the chest CT lesions were no longer present at 7 months after discharge, whereas older patients with severe comorbidities were more prone to develop fibrosis. (16). From the Wuhan cohort, Han and colleagues investigated 114 patients with severe pneumonia according to the WHO criteria (12) and observed fibrotic changes in one-third of them at the 6-month follow-up. Of note, on multivariate analysis, they found that a higher baseline/initial CT lung involvement score (>18 in a score of 25) was independently associated with fibrotic-like changes in the lung (12). Huang and colleagues conducted a cohort study that included 353 patients who were enrolled between January and May 2020 who underwent HRCT at follow-up after discharge. They found that more than 50% of the patients had residual lung abnormalities. Moreover, they found that disease severity in the acute phase was independently associated with the percentage change of CT score in a multivariable analysis (17).

In our hospital, the first patients with COVID-19 pneumonia were admitted in February 2020 and were evaluated in the post-COVID clinic in June 2020. We enrolled prospectively patients diagnosed with COVID-19 pneumonia according to the WHO criteria. Two hundred and 20 patients were evaluated at 3 months after discharge and every 3 months thereafter, according to the current guidelines (8). We found that as many as 20% of our entire patient population had radiological pulmonary sequelae at follow-up. This percentage is lower than that observed in previous studies (12, 17), but our patients' population has been followed up for a longer period of time, thus allowing non-fibrotic pulmonary abnormalities to clear. Patients who did not recover (NOT-REC) were older, mostly men and with worse disease impairment both at admission and during hospitalization compared to patients without radiological sequelae at follow-up. Specifically, NOT-REC patients had a lower PiO_2/FiO_2 ratio at admission and a more severe clinical course. Moreover, NOT-REC patients who required higher maximal FiO_2 during hospital stay were more often treated in a high-intensive care setting and required a longer in-hospital stay, consistent with the findings from the Wuhan cohort (17). Furthermore, we have shown that, in NOT-REC patients, the HRCT performed at hospital admission is more likely to display ground-glass opacities, consolidations, and reticulation. These data suggest that the risk of pulmonary sequelae may be related to the severity of the acute illness and to the intensity of care needed. This is in line with the hypothesis that a cytokine storm might contribute to the pathogenesis of COVID-19 whereas its severity is associated with poor outcomes (18). However, mechanical ventilation and ventilator-induced lung injury, and high-flow oxygen therapy might also have contributed to the development of fibrotic-like changes (19, 20).

The primary aim of our study was to identify predictors of radiological sequelae following COVID-19 pneumonia. Whereas on univariate analysis age, prolonged in-hospital stay, lower $PiO2/FiO_2$ at hospital admission, cardiovascular comorbidities, higher intensity of medical care, and higher FiO_2 max, not using hydroxychloroquine, antibiotics other than azithromycin and ceftriaxone, tocilizumab, remdesevir, or systemic steroids were significantly associated with the presence of interstitial changes during follow-up, we found that higher CONS [OR: 20.6 (95%CI: 1.4–301.2); $p = 0.02$] and IS [23.0 (1.4–377.2); $p = 0.02$] at hospitalization were the only variables independently associated with the persistence of fibrotic changes at follow-up in multivariate analysis. In particular, this latter observation is consistent with that of Han and colleagues who found that a more extensive baseline or initial CT lung involvement was independently associated with permanent fibrotic-like changes in the lung (12). Additionally, the higher amount of consolidation and reticulation at admission remained significantly associated with persistent radiological abnormalities when adjusted for gender, pack-years of smoking, and PiO_2/FiO_2 ratio. However, it remains uncertain whether the fibrotic-like changes we observed represent irreversible pulmonary fibrosis, and further monitoring is warranted to answer this question.

The findings of our study should be interpreted in light of some limitations. First, this is a single-center study; however, it is among the first to analyze HRCT changes over time in a large population of patients hospitalized for COVID-19 pneumonia. In addition, we included a large proportion of patients with severe COVID-19, who are at higher risk of developing persistent lung disease. Second, the CT scan at hospital admission was available for only a subset of patients; however, the aim of our study was to characterize the radiological changes occurring over time as previously done in idiopathic pulmonary fibrosis (21) and to identify predictors of persistent radiological abnormalities.

In conclusion, in our study, about 20% of patients with COVID-19 pneumonia had radiological sequelae at follow-up. Patients who did not fully recover showed a more severe impairment at hospital admission and during hospitalization. Moreover, the presence of reticulation and consolidation on the initial chest CT is predictive of persistent radiological interstitial changes at follow-up.

AUTHOR CONTRIBUTIONS

EB, EC, and PS contributed in conceptualization, writing, reviewing and editing, and supervision. EB and EC performed writing original draft—preparation, visualization, and investigation. EC, NB, CG, GC, and AG provided resources and conducted investigation. SP, GC, DL, and AF performed data curation. EB, PS, AC, and MS contributed in resources, visualization, and supervision. All authors have written, read, and approved the final version of the manuscript.

ACKNOWLEDGMENTS

The authors thank Dr. Sara Lococo (Department of Cardiac, Thoracic, Vascular Sciences, and Public Health, University of Padova and Padova City Hospital, Padova, Italy) for data collection.

REFERENCES

1. Ranard BL, Megjhani M, Terilli K, Doyle K, Claassen J, Pinsky MR, et al. Identification of endotypes of hospitalized COVID-19 patients. *Front Med.* (2021) 8:770343. doi: 10.3389/fmed.2021.770343
2. Baratella E, Bussani R, Zanconati F, Marrocchio C, Fabiola G, Braga L, et al. Radiological-pathological signatures of patients with COVID-19-related pneumomediastinum: is there a role for the Sonic hedgehog and Wnt5a pathways? *ERJ Open Res.* (2021) 7:00346-2021. doi: 10.1183/23120541.00346-2021
3. Antonio GE, Wong KT, Hui DS, Wu A, Lee N, Yuen EH, et al. Thin-section CT in patients with severe acute respiratory syndrome following hospital discharge: preliminary experience. *Radiology.* (2003) 228:810–5. doi: 10.1148/radiol.2283030726
4. Das KM, Lee EY, Singh R, Enani MA, Al Dossari K, Van Gorkom K, et al. Follow-up chest radiographic findings in patients with MERS-CoV after recovery. *Indian J Radiol Imaging.* 27:342–9. doi: 10.4103/ijri.IJRI_469_16
5. Baratella E, Ruaro B, Marrocchio C, Starvaggi N, Salton F, Giudici F, et al. Interstitial lung disease at high resolution CT after SARS-CoV-2-related acute respiratory distress syndrome according to pulmonary segmental anatomy. *J Clin Med.* (2021) 10:3985. doi: 10.3390/jcm10173985
6. Korkmaz I, Keleş F. COVID-19-Related lung involvement at different time intervals: evaluation of computed tomography images with semiquantitative scoring system and COVID-19 reporting and data system scoring. *Cureus.* (2021) 13:e18554. doi: 10.7759/cureus.18554
7. Greenhalgh T, Knight M, A'Court C, Buxton M, Husain L. Management of post-acute covid-19 in primary care. *BMJ.* (2020) 370:m3026. doi: 10.1136/bmj.m3026
8. British Thoracic Society. *Guidance on Respiratory Follow Up of Patients with a Clinico-Radiological Diagnosis of COVID-19 Pneumonia.* Available online at: https://britthoracic.org.uk/about-us/covid-19-information-forthe-respiratory-community/. (accessed: May 7, 2021).
9. George PM, Barratt SL, Condliffe R, Desai SR, Devaraj A, Forrest I, et al. Respiratory follow-up of patients with COVID-19 pneumonia. *Thorax.* (2020) 75:1009–16. doi: 10.1136/thoraxjnl-2020-215314
10. Fichera G, Stramare R, De Conti G, Motta R, Giraudo C. It's not over until it's over: the chameleonic behavior of COVID-19 over a six-day period. *Radiol Med.* (2020) 125:514–6. doi: 10.1007/s11547-020-01203-0
11. Kwee TC, Kwee RM. Chest CT in COVID-19: what the radiologist needs to know. *Radiographics.* (2020) 40:1848–65. doi: 10.1148/rg.2020200159
12. Han X, Fan Y, Alwalid O, Li N, Jia X, Yuan M, et al. Six-month follow-up Chest CT Findings after severe COVID-19 pneumonia. *Radiology.* (2021) 299:E177–86. doi: 10.1148/radiol.2021203153
13. WHO. *Clinical Management of Severe Acute Respiratory Infection When Novel Coronavirus (nCoV) Infection is Suspected: Interim Guidance.* (2020). Available online at: https://www.who.int/docs/default-source/coronaviruse/clinical-management-of-novel-cov.pdf (accessec March 13, 2020).
14. Cocconcelli E, Biondini D, Giraudo C, Lococo S, Bernardinello N, Fichera G, et al. Clinical features and chest imaging as predictors of intensity of care in patients with COVID-19. *J Clin Med.* (2020) 9:2990. doi: 10.3390/jcm9092990
15. Spagnolo P, Balestro E, Aliberti S, Cocconcelli E, Biondini D, Casa GD, et al. Pulmonary fibrosis secondary to COVID-19: a call to arms? *Lancet Respir Med.* (2020) 8:750–752. doi: 10.1016/S2213-2600(20)30222-8
16. Liu M, Lv F, Huang Y, Xiao K. Follow-up study of the chest CT characteristics of Covid-19 survivors seven months after recovery. *Front Med (Lausanne).* (2021) 8:636298. doi: 10.3389/fmed.2021.636298
17. Huang C, Huang L, Wang Y, Li X, Ren L, Gu X, et al. 6-month consequences of COVID-19 in patients discharged from hospital: a cohort study. *Lancet.* (2021) 397:220–32. doi: 10.1016/S0140-6736(20)32656-8
18. Fajgenbaum DC, June CH. Cytokine Storm. *N Engl J Med.* (2020) 383:2255–73. doi: 10.1056/NEJMra2026131
19. Beitler JR, Malhotra A, Thompson BT. Ventilator-induced Lung Injury. *Clin Chest Med.* (2016) 37:633–46. doi: 10.1016/j.ccm.2016.07.004
20. Bates JH, Smith BJ, Allen GB. Computational models of ventilator induced lung injury and surfactant dysfunction. *Drug Discov Today Dis Models.* (2015) 15:17–22. doi: 10.1016/j.ddmod.2014.02.005
21. Balestro E, Cocconcelli E, Giraudo C, Polverosi R, Biondini D, Lacedonia D, et al. High-resolution CT change over time in patients with idiopathic pulmonary fibrosis on antifibrotic treatment. *J Clin Med.* (2019) 8:1469. doi: 10.3390/jcm8091469

21

Transcriptome Analysis of Peripheral Blood Mononuclear Cells in Pulmonary Sarcoidosis

Keiichiro Yoshioka [1†], Hironori Sato [2,3†], Takeshi Kawasaki [1], Daisuke Ishii [1], Takuro Imamoto [1], Mitsuhiro Abe [1], Yoshinori Hasegawa [2], Osamu Ohara [2], Koichiro Tatsumi [1] and Takuji Suzuki [1]*

[1] Department of Respirology, Graduate School of Medicine, Chiba University, Chiba, Japan, [2] Department of Applied Genomics, Kazusa DNA Research Institute, Chiba, Japan, [3] Department of Pediatrics, Graduate School of Medicine, Chiba University, Chiba, Japan

***Correspondence:**
Takeshi Kawasaki
kawatake@chiba-u.jp

† These authors have contributed equally to this work and share first authorship

Background: Sarcoidosis is a granulomatous systemic disease of unknown etiology. Mononuclear cells such as macrophages or lymphocytes in lung tissue and hilar or mediastinal lymph nodes have been recognized to play an essential role in granuloma formation in pulmonary sarcoidosis. Peripheral blood mononuclear cells (PBMCs) consist of several immunocompetent cells and have been shown to play a mechanistic role in the pathogenesis of sarcoidosis. However, the genetic modifications that occur in bulk PBMCs of sarcoidosis remain to be elucidated.

Purpose: This study aimed to explore the pathobiological markers of sarcoidosis in PBMCs by comparing the transcriptional signature of PBMCs from patients with pulmonary sarcoidosis with those of healthy controls by RNA sequencing.

Methods: PBMC samples were collected from subjects with pulmonary sarcoidosis with no steroid/immunosuppressant drugs ($n = 8$) and healthy controls ($n = 11$) from August 2020 to April 2021, and RNA sequencing was performed with the PBMC samples.

Results: Principal component analysis using RNA sequencing datasets comparing pulmonary sarcoidosis with healthy controls revealed that the two groups appeared to be differentiated, in which 270 differentially expressed genes were found in PBMCs between sarcoidosis and healthy controls. Enrichment analysis for gene ontology suggested that some biological processes related to the pathobiology of sarcoidosis, such as cellular response to interleukin (IL)-1 and IFN-γ, regulation of IL-6 production, IL-8 secretion, regulation of mononuclear cell migration, and response to lipopolysaccharide, were involved. Enrichment analysis of the KEGG pathway indicated the involvement of tumor necrosis factor (TNF), toll-like receptor signaling, IL-17 signaling pathways, phagosomes, and ribosomes. Most of the genes involved in TNF and IL-17 signaling pathways and phagosomes were upregulated, while most of the ribosome-related genes were downregulated.

Conclusion: The present study demonstrated that bulk gene expression patterns in PBMCs were different between patients with pulmonary sarcoidosis and healthy controls. The changes in the gene expression pattern of PBMCs could reflect the existence of sarcoidosis lesions and influence granuloma formation in sarcoidosis. These new findings are important to strengthen our understanding of the etiology and pathobiology of sarcoidosis and indicate a potential therapeutic target for sarcoidosis.

Keywords: RNA sequencing, transcriptome analysis, pulmonary sarcoidosis, peripheral blood mononuclear cell, granuloma formation

INTRODUCTION

Sarcoidosis is a systemic granulomatous disease of unknown etiology that can cause dysfunction in various organs. The development of sarcoidosis can be influenced by genetic factors, environmental stimulation, and foreign or self-antigens (1). Granuloma formation is initiated by the accumulation of antigen-presenting cells, such as activated monocytes/macrophages and $CD4^+$ Th cells. Granulomas consist of monocyte-derived epithelioid and giant cells encircled by various immune-competent cells such as CD4 + helper T (Th) cells, CD8 T cells, fibroblasts, regulatory T cells, and B lymphocytes (2). A variety of agents can be phagocytosed by antigen-presenting cells of monocytes/macrophages, leading to the activation of immune cells including T cells. Activated $CD4^+$ Th cells then differentiate into Th1 cells, secreting primarily interleukin (IL)-2 and IFN-γ (3). Th1 cells have been shown to play a key role in granuloma formation in sarcoidosis. Recently, IFN-γ-derived Th17.1 cells have also been suggested to be involved in sarcoidosis (4). In any case, mononuclear cells such as monocytes/macrophages or lymphocytes have been recognized to play a central mechanistic role in granuloma formation in sarcoidosis. However, the mechanisms and general epidemiology of sarcoidosis remain unclear.

Peripheral blood mononuclear cells (PBMCs) comprise immunocompetent cells, which are mainly classified into two cell types: monocytes and lymphocytes. Monocytes are defined as $CD14^+$ cells in PBMCs (5), which can be further categorized into three populations with different functions by the combination of CD14 expression level and CD16 expression: $CD14^{++}CD16^-$ classical, $CD14^{++}CD16^+$intermediate, and $CD14^+CD16^+$non-classical monocytes. Lymphocytes can be mainly categorized into three groups: T, B, and natural killer cells, and each population is known to comprise cells with wide variation in functional roles (6, 7). As such, PBMCs, consisting of various cell types, are considered to play important roles in immune-related diseases, including sarcoidosis.

Omics is a recently developed analysis method that encompasses genomics, epigenomics, transcriptomics, proteomics, and metabolomics, and has already been widely used to understand polygenic and phenotypically diverse diseases. In particular, transcriptomics has also been applied to understand the pathogenesis of sarcoidosis at the levels of PBMCs, monocytes, regulatory T cells, and single cells of PBMCs, to explore specific genetic expressions of mRNAs or microRNAs that might explain disease progression and distinguish it from other diseases (8, 9).

A previous study showed that gene expression in PBMCs was different between sarcoidosis patients and healthy controls (10); however, some data included in the analysis were from sarcoidosis patients who received steroids and/or immunosuppressant drugs. Therefore, the transcriptome status may be largely affected by drugs that mask some notable differences between sarcoidosis patients and healthy controls. Taking this into consideration, it would be worth performing transcriptome analysis comparing healthy controls with sarcoidosis patients who do not take steroids or immunosuppressant drugs.

Therefore, this study aimed to explore the pathobiological significance of PBMCs in sarcoidosis by comparing the transcriptional signature of PBMCs from healthy controls with that from pulmonary sarcoidosis subjects not receiving steroids and/or immunosuppressant drugs.

MATERIALS AND METHODS

Subjects

This study was approved by the Human Ethics Committee of Chiba University (protocol number 2083). PBMCs were collected from patients diagnosed with pulmonary sarcoidosis and from healthy controls between August 2020 and April 2021 at Chiba University Hospital. Patients with pulmonary sarcoidosis were diagnosed according to the recommendations of the ATS/ERS/WASOG statement (11), and all patients who had no histopathological confirmation of granulomas were excluded from the present study.

Isolation of PBMC

Peripheral blood was collected using a BD Vacutainer CPT Cell Preparation Tube with sodium citrate according to the manufacturer's protocol (#362760) (Becton, Dickinson and Company, NJ, USA). Briefly, the tubes containing blood were centrifuged at 1,500 rpm at room temperature for 20 min. After centrifugation, the plasma was removed from the uppermost layer. The PBMC layer was transferred to 15 ml conical tubes, washed with PBS twice, followed by the addition of Isogen (Nippongene, Tokyo, Japan), and then stored at −80°C.

Total RNA Extraction, mRNA Library Preparation, and 3'RNA-Seq

Total RNA was extracted from 1.0 to 2.0×10^6 PBMCs, and each sample was transferred to 1.0 ml isogen reagent (Life Technologies, Carlsbad, CA, USA). The solution was vigorously vortexed and incubated at room temperature for 5 min. The solution was then centrifuged after adding chloroform, and the aqueous phase was carefully transferred to a new tube, following which 10 mg glycogen (Life Technologies) was added as a co-precipitant. RNA was precipitated by adding 600 μL

TABLE 1 | Characteristics of samples.

Pulmonary sarcoidosis

Samples	Male/female	Age	Stage	Organ involvements	Smoking history
No.1	Female	76	3	Eye, heart	None
No.2	Male	56	1	Heart	None
No.3	Male	47	3	None	None
No.4	Female	68	3	Heart, liver, kidney	Yes
No.5	Female	59	2	None	Yes
No.6	Female	43	1	None	None
No.7	Male	62	1	None	Yes
No.8	Female	49	2	None	Yes

Healthy controls

Samples	Male/female	Age	Smoking history
No.1	Male	42	None
No.2	Male	31	None
No.3	Female	34	None
No.4	Female	58	None
No.5	Female	45	None
No.6	Female	46	None
No.7	Female	48	None
No.8	Female	43	None
No.9	Male	66	None
No.10	Female	37	None
No.11	Female	40	None

Pulmonary sarcoidosis vs. healthy controls

	Pulmonary sarcoidosis	Healthy controls	*P*-value
Age	58.1 ± 11.5	44.5 ± 10.2	0.01*
Gender (male/female)	3/5	3/8	1.0#

**Student's t-test.*
#Fisher's exact test.

of isopropyl alcohol. The RNA pellet was washed once with 75% ethanol and then dissolved in 10 μL RNase-free water. The concentration and quality of the RNA were verified using a Qubit fluorometer (Life Technologies) and an Agilent 2100 bioanalyzer, respectively. Purified total RNA (200 ng) was used for RNA library preparation, according to the instructions of the Quant Seq 3' mRNA-seq library preparation kit FWD for Illumina (Lexogen, Vienna, Austria). The RNA libraries were sequenced on an Illumina NextSeq 500 system with 75-nt-long reads.

3' RNA-Seq Data Analysis

RNA-seq count data were analyzed using the iDEP.92 (integrated differential expression and pathway analysis online tools: the details of analysis are described in the following website (http://bioinformatics.sdstate.edu/idep92/) and published paper (12). Briefly, expression matrix was pre-processed by filtering more than 0.5 counts per million per sample (pseudo count 4) and converted to Ensemble gene IDs, which are used internally to identify genes. These data were used for principal component analysis (PCA) and hierarchical clustering. RNA-seq count data after the filtration were normalized using EdgeR, an R/Bioconductor package connected to iDEP.92. In addition, DEGs from two group comparisons were obtained using the DESeq2 package with a threshold of false discovery rate (FDR) < 0.05, and fold-change > 2 or < 0.5. For enrichment analysis of the DEGs, gene set enrichment analysis (GSEA) was used to perform Gene Ontology (GO) analysis and Kyoto Encyclopedia of Genes and Genomes (KEGG) pathway analysis.

Statistical Analysis

The age characteristics of the samples are expressed as means ± standard deviations. Student's *t*-test was used for age comparisons. We compared the samples for gender characteristics using Fisher's exact test. Statistical significance was set at $P < 0.05$.

RESULTS

Differential Gene Expression and Pathway Analysis in PBMC

The present study included two groups: subjects comprising 8 patients with pulmonary sarcoidosis and 11 healthy controls. The subjects' demographics are shown in **Table 1**. Four patients with pulmonary sarcoidosis had a smoking history, and none were on immunosuppressive medication. All pulmonary sarcoidosis patients had lung involvement with chest radiograph stages 1, 2, or 3. There was a significant difference in age between patients with pulmonary sarcoidosis and healthy controls ($p < 0.05$).

We prepared RNA-seq libraries from mRNA isolated from the PBMCs of subjects with pulmonary sarcoidosis and healthy controls. The RNA integrity number values of all samples were >8, and 26,472 genes from mRNA were obtained. After additional quality control methods, 18,139 genes were retained as DEGs for further analyses. Next, the count data obtained by RNA-seq were processed and analyzed using iDEP.92.

PCA enables us to project samples into two-dimensional space (12). We performed PCA by comparing gene expression levels using count data between patients with pulmonary sarcoidosis and healthy controls. The results showed that the two groups appeared to be divided, as shown in **Figure 1**. Next, we compared the DEGs in PBMCs between patients with pulmonary sarcoidosis and healthy controls using DEseq2. **Figure 2** shows the distribution of log_2-fold change and FDR expression levels for the 18,139 genes expressed in these samples by volcano plotting with 270 DEGs (FDR < 0.05 and fold-change > 2 or < 0.5) highlighted in color. **Figure 3** shows the heat map of the 270 DEGs, with 156 genes downregulated, and 114 genes upregulated in PBMCs of pulmonary sarcoidosis patients compared to healthy controls; the blue bar indicates genes that are upregulated in

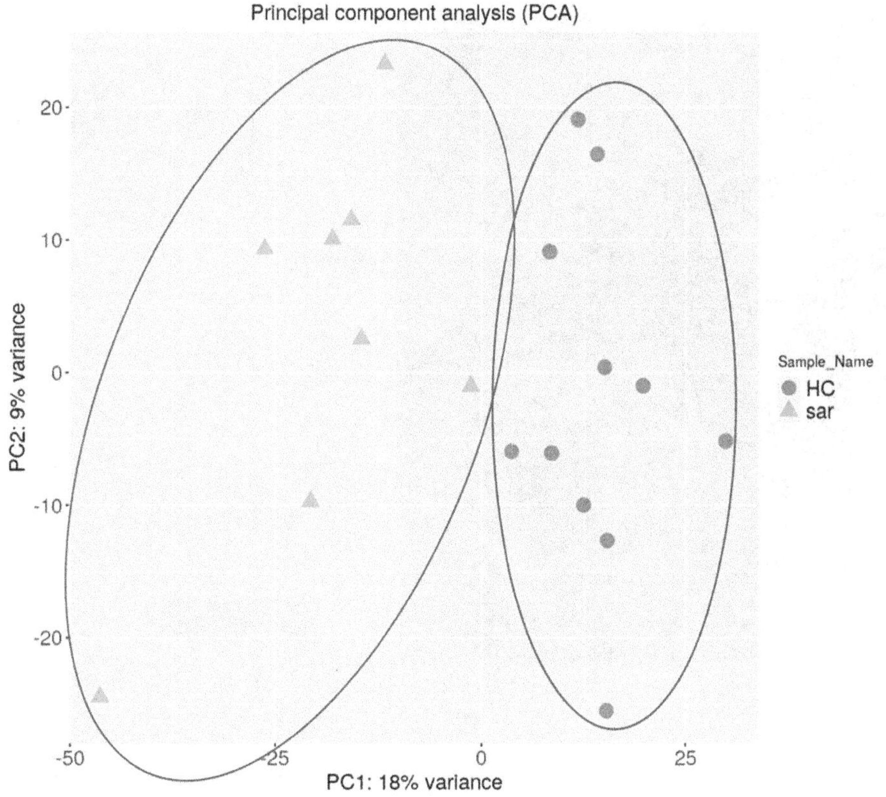

FIGURE 1 | Principal component analysis (PCA). Principal component analysis (PCA) shows that two groups of pulmonary sarcoidosis and healthy controls are well-differentiated.

healthy controls, while the yellow bar indicates genes that are upregulated in patients with pulmonary sarcoidosis.

To explore the pathways that are modulated in PBMCs of pulmonary sarcoidosis compared to that of healthy controls, we performed enrichment analysis (GO analysis and KEGG pathway analysis) using GSEA (FDR < 0.05, and fold-change > 2 or < 0.5). As shown in **Table 2A**, GO analysis revealed that various biological processes were enriched, such as "Cellular response to interleukin-1 (IL-1)" "Cellular response to IFN-γ," "Positive regulation of interleukin-6 (IL-6) production," "interleukin-8 (IL-8) secretion," "Mononuclear cell migration," "Regulation of mononuclear cell migration" and "response to lipopolysaccharide." As shown in **Table 2B**, KEGG pathway analysis revealed that multiple pathways that include "TNF signaling pathways," "IL-17 signaling pathways," and "Toll-like receptor signaling pathways," "Phagosome" and "Ribosome" were enriched; the majority of the genes involved in TNF, IL-17, and Toll-like receptor signaling pathways, and phagosome were upregulated (**Figures 4–7**), while most genes involved in ribosome pathway were downregulated (**Figure 8**).

Significant difference in mean age between sarcoidosis and healthy controls was detected (**Table 1**). Age is a very important factor that could influence the transcriptional signatures, therefore, additional transcriptome analysis was performed focusing on age by comparing the data of younger age ($n =$ 4) with those of older age ($n = 4$) (mean age: 49 ± 4.6 vs. 67 ± 6.5, $p < 0.05$) to see if the findings described above become biologically irrelevant. PCA was performed by comparing gene expression patterns between older and younger patients with

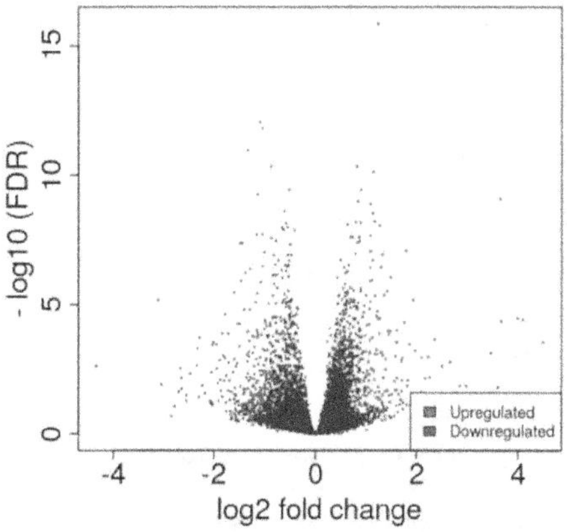

FIGURE 2 | Volcano plotting of differentially expressed genes (DEGs). The distribution of log_2-fold change and FDR expression level for the 18,139 genes are shown in volcano plotting. Dots highlighted in color are 270 DEGs between pulmonary sarcoidosis and healthy controls.

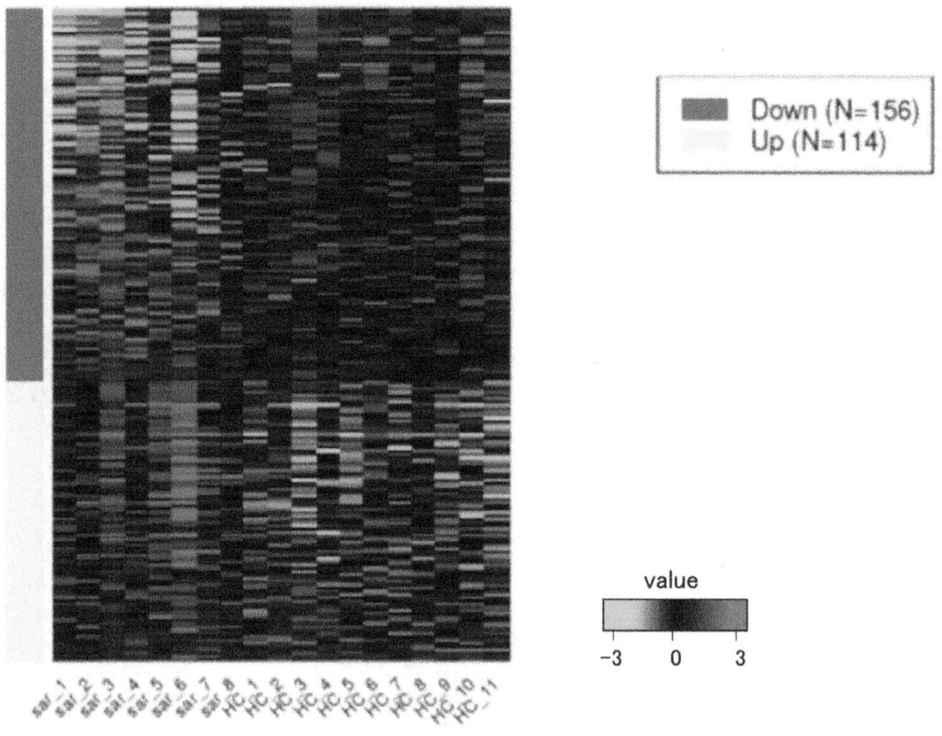

FIGURE 3 | Heatmap of DEGs. The heatmap shows the DEGs between pulmonary sarcoidosis vs. healthy controls. Red bars represent high expression and green bars represent low expression.

TABLE 2 | Enrichment analysis of transcriptomic data (pulmonary sarcoidosis vs. healthy controls).

A. Gene ontology (biological process): relevant terms were excerpted	
Term (gene ontology: biological process) with upregulated genes	***P*-value**
Cellular response to interleukin-1	1e-03
Response to lipopolysaccharide	1e-03
Cellular response to interferon-gamma	1e-03
Regulation of interleukin-1 beta production	1e-03
Positive regulation of interleukin-6 production	1e-03
Interleukin-8 secretion	1e-03
Mononuclear cell migration	1e-03
Regulation of mononuclear cell migration	1e-03
B. KEGG pathway: relevant terms were excerpted	
Term (KEGG pathway) with upregulated genes	***P*-value**
TNF signaling pathway	5.6e-04
IL-17 signaling pathway	5.6e-04
Toll-like receptor signaling pathway	5.6e-04
Phagosome	5.6e-04
Term (KEGG pathway) with downregulated genes	***P*-value**
Ribosome	1.2e-03

pulmonary sarcoidosis. The results showed that the two groups appeared to be undifferentiated, as shown in **Figure S1**. Of the 18,139 genes expressed in these samples, only two DEGs was detected (FDR < 0.05 and fold-change > 2 or < 0.5) and no term was detected by enrichment analysis (GO analysis and KEGG pathway analysis).

Sex difference is also a very important factor that could influence the transcriptional signatures. Therefore, additional transcriptome analysis was performed focusing on gender by comparing the data of females ($n = 5$) with those of males ($n = 3$) to see if the findings described above become biologically irrelevant. PCA was performed by comparing gene expression patterns between the male and female patients with pulmonary sarcoidosis. The results showed that the two groups appeared to be divided, as shown in **Figure S2**. Of the 18,139 genes expressed in these samples, only 14 DEGs were detected (FDR < 0.05 and fold-change > 2 or < 0.5) and terms of "Protein demethylation" and "Oxygen transport" was enriched by GO analysis.

Multiorgan involvements were observed in 3 out of 8 pulmonary sarcoidosis patients (**Table 1**), therefore, additional transcriptome analysis was performed by comparing data of patients with multiorgan involvements ($n = 3$) with those having only pulmonary lesion ($n = 5$) to clarify if differences in transcriptome of PBMCs exist between them. The results of PCA showed that the two groups appeared to be undifferentiated, as shown in **Figure S3**. Next, we compared the DEGs in PBMCs between the two groups. Of the 18,139 genes expressed in these samples, only five DEGs was detected as downregulated (FDR < 0.05 and fold-change > 2 or < 0.5) and terms of "Antibiotic catabolic process" and "Oxygen transport" were enriched by GO analysis.

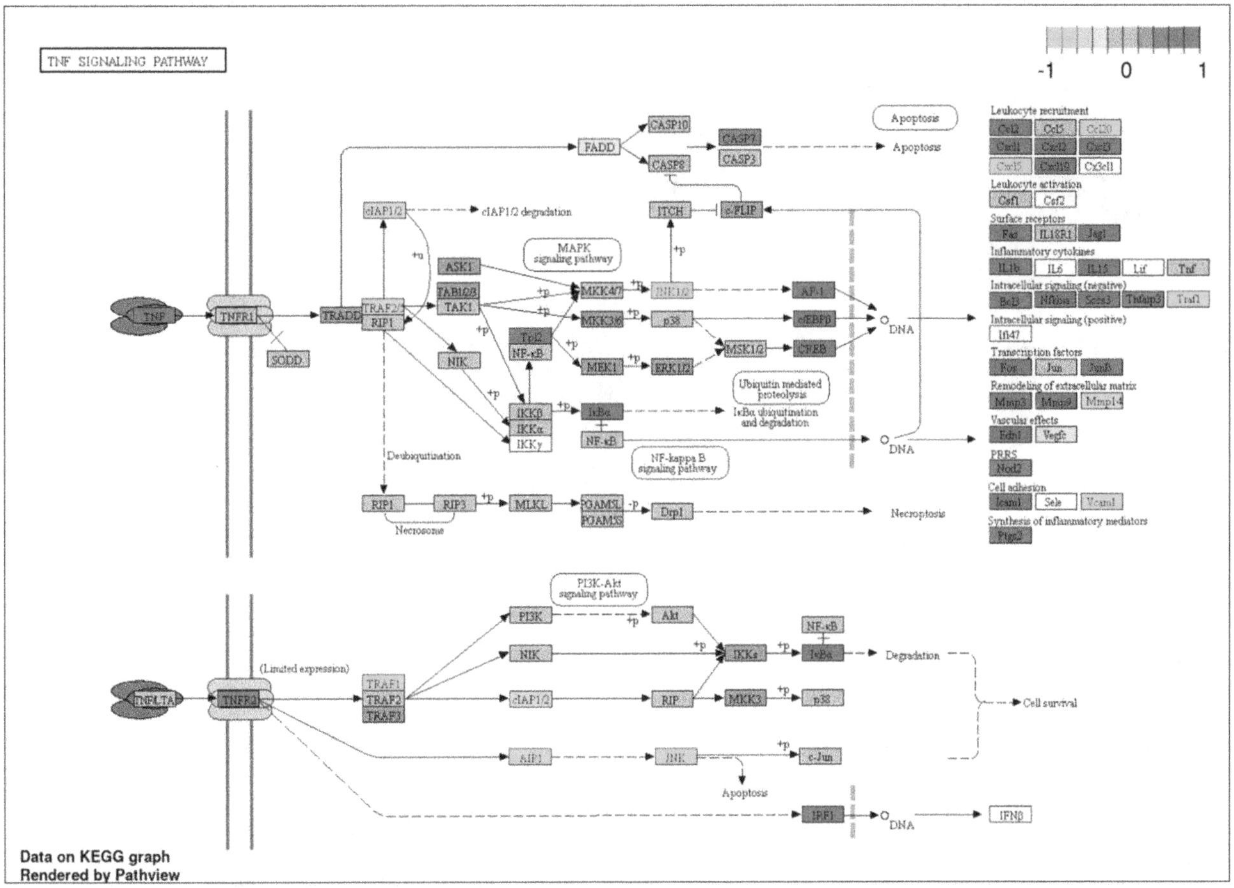

FIGURE 4 | Genes involved in tumor necrosis factor (TNF) signaling pathway in pulmonary sarcoidosis peripheral blood mononuclear cells (PBMCs) by Kyoto Encyclopedia of Genes and Genomes (KEGG). A graphical illustration of KEGG pathway analysis of DEGs (log_2-fold change with FDR < 0.05) related to TNF signaling pathway in pulmonary sarcoidosis PBMCs. The color intensity corresponds to the levels of upregulation (red) or downregulation (green) of the DEGs in pulmonary sarcoidosis PBMCs.

DISCUSSION

In the present study, transcriptome analysis indicated that gene expression profiles differ in PBMC level between pulmonary sarcoidosis and healthy controls, probably reflecting the pathobiological state with granuloma formation. To our knowledge, the present study revealed, for the first time, the potential difference in gene expression profiles of PBMCs between healthy controls and pulmonary sarcoidosis without the influence of any immunomodulatory drugs such as steroids and/or immunosuppressant drugs. The present gene expression study using heterogeneous cell mixtures lacks insight into cell type-specific immune dysregulation. However, bulk RNA evaluation at the PBMC level could reflect some aspects of the clinical phenotype as a final product of cell-cell interactions among blood immune cells. Of note, changes in transcriptome of lots of mediators and pathways that were reported to be related to sarcoidosis, were detected in PBMC levels.

The present study revealed that 270 genes were differentially expressed in PBMCs between subjects with pulmonary sarcoidosis and healthy controls. Enrichment analysis with GO analysis revealed that various biological pathways were enriched such as "Cellular response to IL-1," "Cellular response to IFN-γ," "Positive regulation of IL-6," "IL-8 secretion," "Mononuclear cell migration," "Regulation of mononuclear cell migration," and "Response to lipopolysaccharide (LPS)," all of which are reported to be in relation to granuloma formation in sarcoidosis lesion (**Table 2A**). In addition, enrichment analysis with KEGG pathway analysis showed that genes involved in TNF, IL-17 and toll-like receptor signaling, and phagosomes were mostly upregulated, while ribosome-related genes were mostly downregulated (**Table 2B**). The terms that were led by enrichment analysis in the present study were not described in a previous study that performed transcriptome analysis with PBMC to compare healthy controls with pulmonary sarcoidosis patients (10). One of the reasons could be that some transcriptome data of sarcoidosis patients were from those who received steroids and/or immunosuppressant drugs (10). Therefore, the results of the present study could provide notable new insights into the sarcoidosis research field as

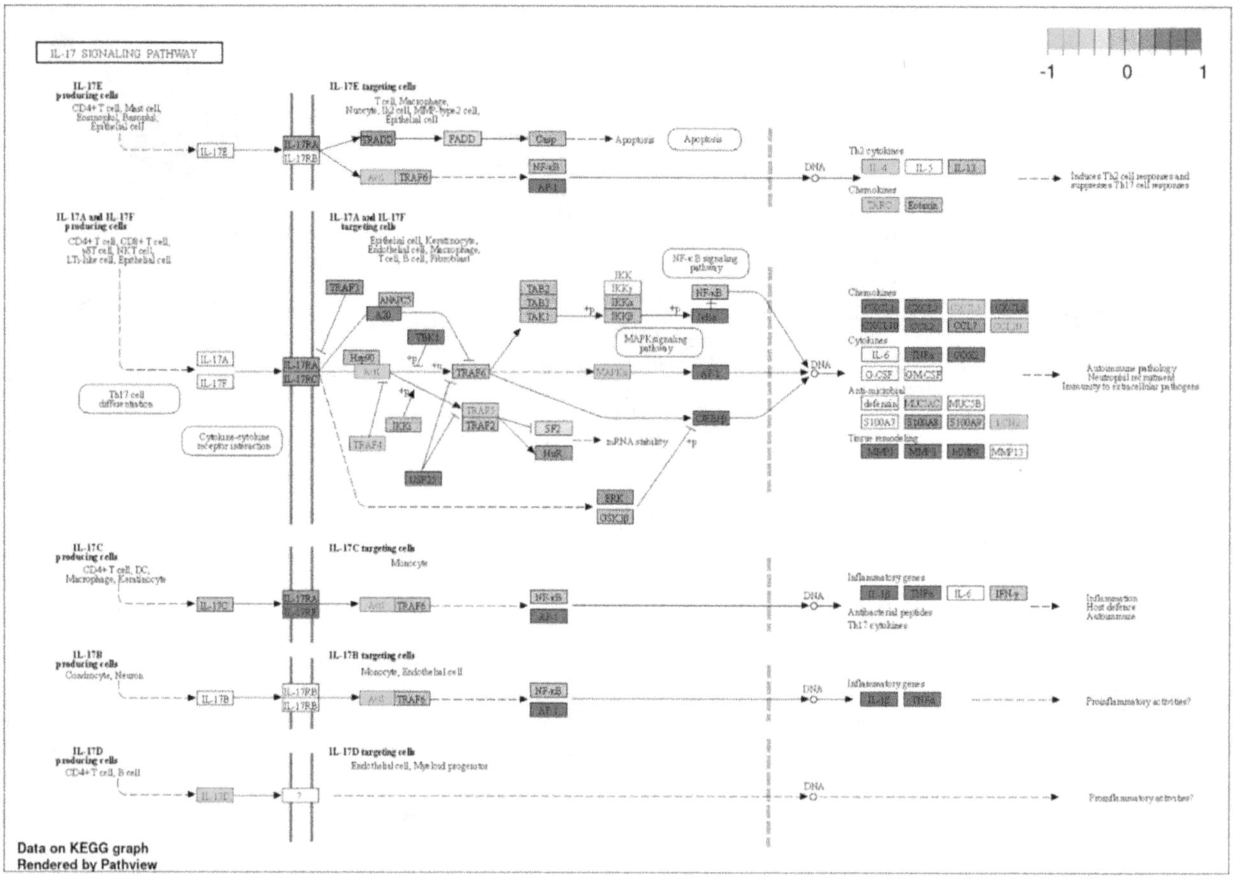

FIGURE 5 | Genes involved in interleukin (IL)-17 signaling pathway in pulmonary sarcoidosis PBMCs by KEGG. A graphical illustration of KEGG pathway analysis of DEGs (log_2-fold change with FDR < 0.05) related to the IL-17 signaling pathway in pulmonary sarcoidosis PBMCs.

transcriptome analysis was performed with DEGs in sarcoidosis patients who did not receive anti-inflammatory drugs such as steroids and/or immunosuppressant drugs. Our results also suggest that steroids or immunosuppressant drugs may certainly suppress the pro-inflammatory signals at PBMC level in pulmonary sarcoidosis.

First, the terms "Cellular response to IL-1," and "TNF signaling pathway" were listed in this study (**Table 2**; **Figure 4**). In sarcoidosis, unstimulated sarcoid-derived alveolar macrophages have been shown to intrinsically produce increased amounts of IL-1 and TNF-α (13, 14). IL-1 is a cytokine with potent pro-inflammatory properties implicated in the pathogenesis of sarcoidosis (15). TNF has also been shown to play a pivotal role in orchestrating innate inflammatory responses, leading to granuloma formation (16). Together, the results of the present study support those of previous studies that indicate a central role of IL-1 and TNF signaling in sarcoidosis.

Next, "IL-17 signaling pathway" was listed in this study (**Table 2B**; **Figure 5**). IL-17 has been designated as IL-17A, a founding member of the IL-17 cytokine family, which are produced by human Th17 cells. IL-17 induces the mobilization, recruitment, and activation of neutrophils and triggers the production of proinflammatory cytokines and chemokines by a broad range of cellular targets, including epithelial cells, endothelial cells, and macrophages (17–19). Regarding IL-17 in sarcoidosis, it was reported that the primary Th17-cytokine, IL-17A, is an important mediator of granuloma formation and maturation (20). In addition, it was also reported that IL-17A could potentiate IFN-γ-induced giant cell formation (21), and can stimulate TNF-α production by macrophages (22). The results of the current study support previous reports that suggest a central role for IL-17 signaling in sarcoidosis.

The terms "Response to lipopolysaccharide" and "Toll-like signaling pathway" were listed in this study (**Tables 2A,B**; **Figure 6**). LPS is the major outer surface membrane component present in almost all gram-negative bacteria and acts as an extremely strong stimulator of innate or natural immunity in diverse eukaryotic species ranging from insects to humans. Sarcoidosis is generally thought to occur when genetically susceptible individuals are exposed to disease-related antigens, triggering a Th1-dominant immune response that eventually leads to the formation of granulomas. LPS has been identified in the lungs of sarcoidosis patients, and PBMCs of sarcoidosis patients show hypersensitivity reactions when stimulated with

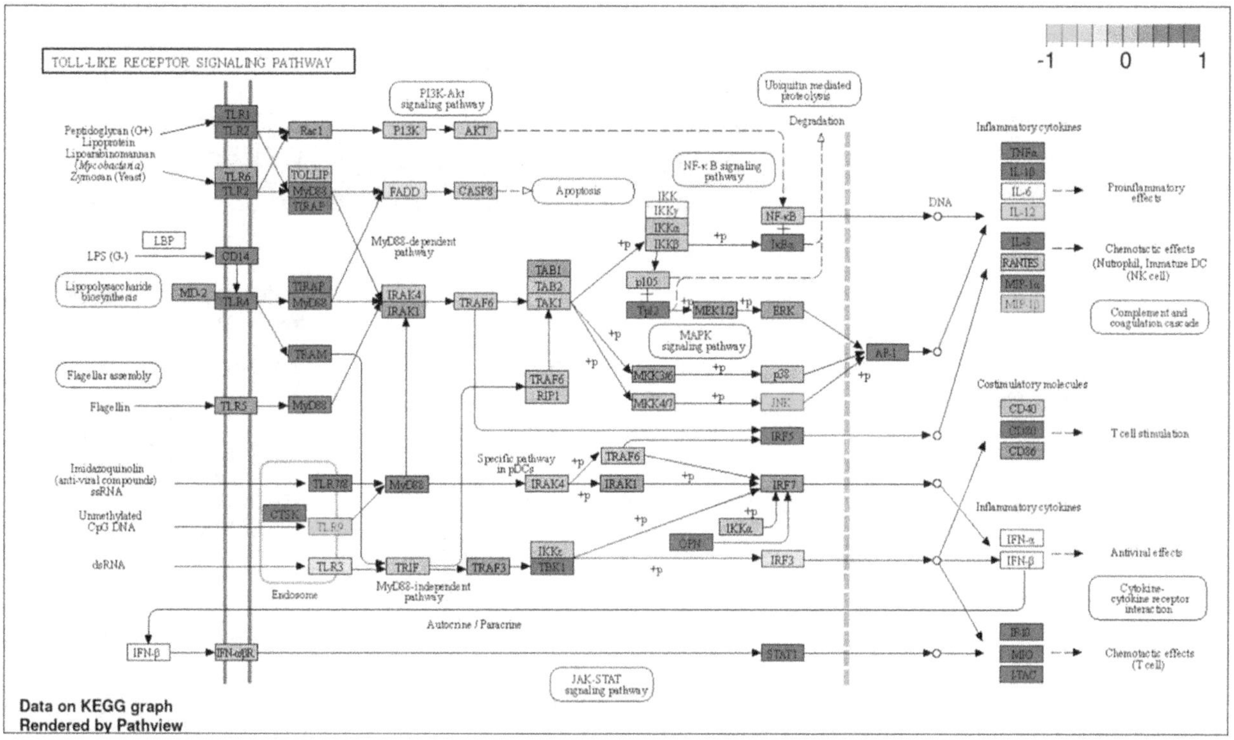

FIGURE 6 | Genes involved in Toll-like receptor signaling pathway in pulmonary sarcoidosis PBMCs by KEGG. A graphical illustration of KEGG pathway analysis of DEGs (log_2-fold change with FDR < 0.05) related to the Toll-like receptor signaling pathway in pulmonary sarcoidosis PBMCs.

LPS (23). Furthermore, LPS is known to induce a Th1-based immune response that promotes IFN-γ, a key cytokine involved in granuloma formation in sarcoidosis (24, 25). The present study showed upregulation of many genes related to the "Toll-like receptor signaling pathway," indicating that altered gene expression is important in the activation of pattern recognition receptors and signaling molecules (**Figure 6**). Granulomatous inflammation is thought to be a dysregulated antigenic response to unknown environmental exposure in genetically susceptible individuals (26). Together, the present study supports previous reports that suggest possible major mechanistic roles for the innate immune signaling pathway in granuloma formation.

Next, the terms "Cellular response to IFN-γ," "Cellular response to IL-6," and "IL-8 secretion" were listed in the GO analysis (**Table 2A**). IFN-γ was originally identified as a "macrophage-activating factor," and macrophages are a major physiological target for IFN-γ action (27). The activation of macrophages in sarcoid lesions is thought to be driven by Th1 cell immune responses and mediated by several cytokines, including IFN-γ. IFN-γ is a cytokine that is primarily produced by cells of the immune system, including innate-like lymphocyte populations, such as natural killer (NK) cells and innate lymphoid cells (ILCs), and adaptive immune cells, such as Th1 cells and $CD8^+$ cytotoxic T cells (28). IFN-γ is also derived from Th17.1 cells, which may have an important role in sarcoidosis (4). IL-6 induces the development of Th17 cells from naïve T cells together with transforming growth factor β (TGF-β) and inhibits anti-inflammatory regulatory T cells (29). IL-8 is a potent chemokine for neutrophils and is also chemotactic for T cells (30), and previous report suggests that this chemokine might be involved in delayed hypersensitivity reactions (31). Together, the results of the present study support previous studies that suggest possible central roles for IFN-γ, IL-6, and IL-8 in sarcoidosis.

The terms "mononuclear cell migration" and "regulation of mononuclear cell migration" were listed in the GO analysis (**Table 2A**). "Mononuclear cell migration" or "regulation of mononuclear cell migration" refers to the action of mononuclear cells moving to the tissues and organs that require functions of the immune system. In sarcoidosis, Garman et al. reported altered expression of genes important for activation (pattern recognition receptors and signaling molecules) and migration (adhesion molecules and chemokine receptors) in monocytes isolated from sarcoidosis patients compared to those from controls (32). Cells in the peripheral blood are thought to be directly involved in the formation of granulomas in the lungs. Monocytes in the blood, along with antigen-presenting cells present in tissues such as dendritic cells and alveolar macrophages, act as sentinels to detect potential threats to the host, leaving the vascular space and patrolling in the interstitial spaces of the lung (33). The results of the present study support previous reports that indicate the importance of PBMC migration for granuloma formation in pulmonary sarcoidosis.

Next, the term "Phagosome" was listed in the KEGG pathway analysis (**Table 2B**; **Figure 7**). Phagocytosis is a cellular process

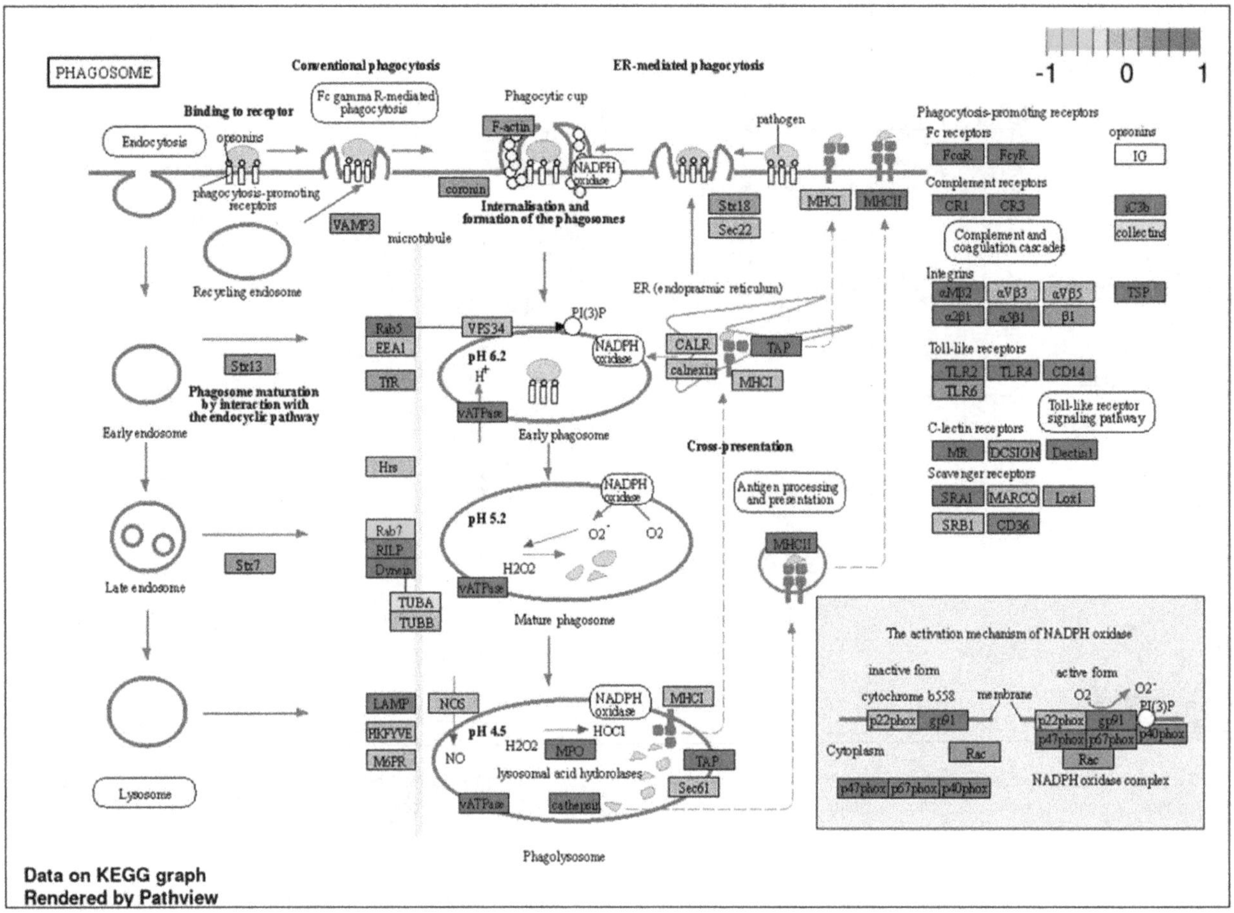

FIGURE 7 | Genes involved in phagosome signaling pathway in pulmonary sarcoidosis PBMCs by KEGG. A graphical illustration of KEGG pathway analysis of DEGs ($\log_2$-fold change with FDR < 0.05) related to phagosome signaling pathway in pulmonary sarcoidosis PBMCs.

that ingests and eliminates particles, including microorganisms, foreign substances, and apoptotic cells. It is an essential process in tissue homeostasis, and macrophages and monocytes are the dedicated cells for this process. The suggested upregulation in phagocytosis supports the notion that the development of lung sarcoidosis may be associated with the response to an unknown external exposure requiring antigen processing and presentation. Taken together, it would be reasonable to see that the phagosome-related genes were mostly upregulated at PBMC levels.

Finally, the term "Ribosome" was listed in the KEGG pathway analysis (**Table 2B**; **Figure 8**). Ribosome biogenesis is an extremely energetically expensive cellular process that has long been linked to human health and disease. Taljera et al. recently reported that RNA-seq analysis of monocytes from sarcoidosis patients showed that pathways associated with ribosomes were downregulated, similar to the results of the present study (34). Together, downregulation of ribosomal constituent proteins in PBMCs, including monocyte levels, could be related to the pathobiological state of sarcoidosis. However, it remains unclear how ribosomes are involved in the pathogenesis of sarcoidosis; therefore, further studies are needed to clarify the role of ribosomes in the etiology of pulmonary sarcoidosis.

The current study indicates functional roles of PBMCs, including monocytes, the so-called circulating precursors of macrophages, in the etiology and pathobiology of pulmonary sarcoidosis. However, this study had several limitations. First, this study was conducted in a single center in Japan, and the sample size was small, which potentially limited the generalizability of findings in the current study. Attention should also be paid to the fact that sarcoidosis group is very heterogeneous in terms of different stages at chest radiograph findings. The subjects' nationality would affect the genetic risk of developing sarcoidosis. Our previous study on assessing the incidence of concurrent sarcoid-like granuloma in patients with malignancy indicated that Japanese subjects were less likely to have stage 2, 3, and 4 sarcoidosis than Americans (OR 0.31, 95% CI 0.13–0.72, p = 0.007) and were less likely to develop sarcoid-like granulomas within 5 years of cancer diagnosis (OR 0.31, 95% CI 0.13–0.72, p = 0.006) (35). The ethnicity of Japanese patients, which may make it difficult for sarcoidosis granulomas to form, might influence the results of this study. It is well known that sarcoidosis

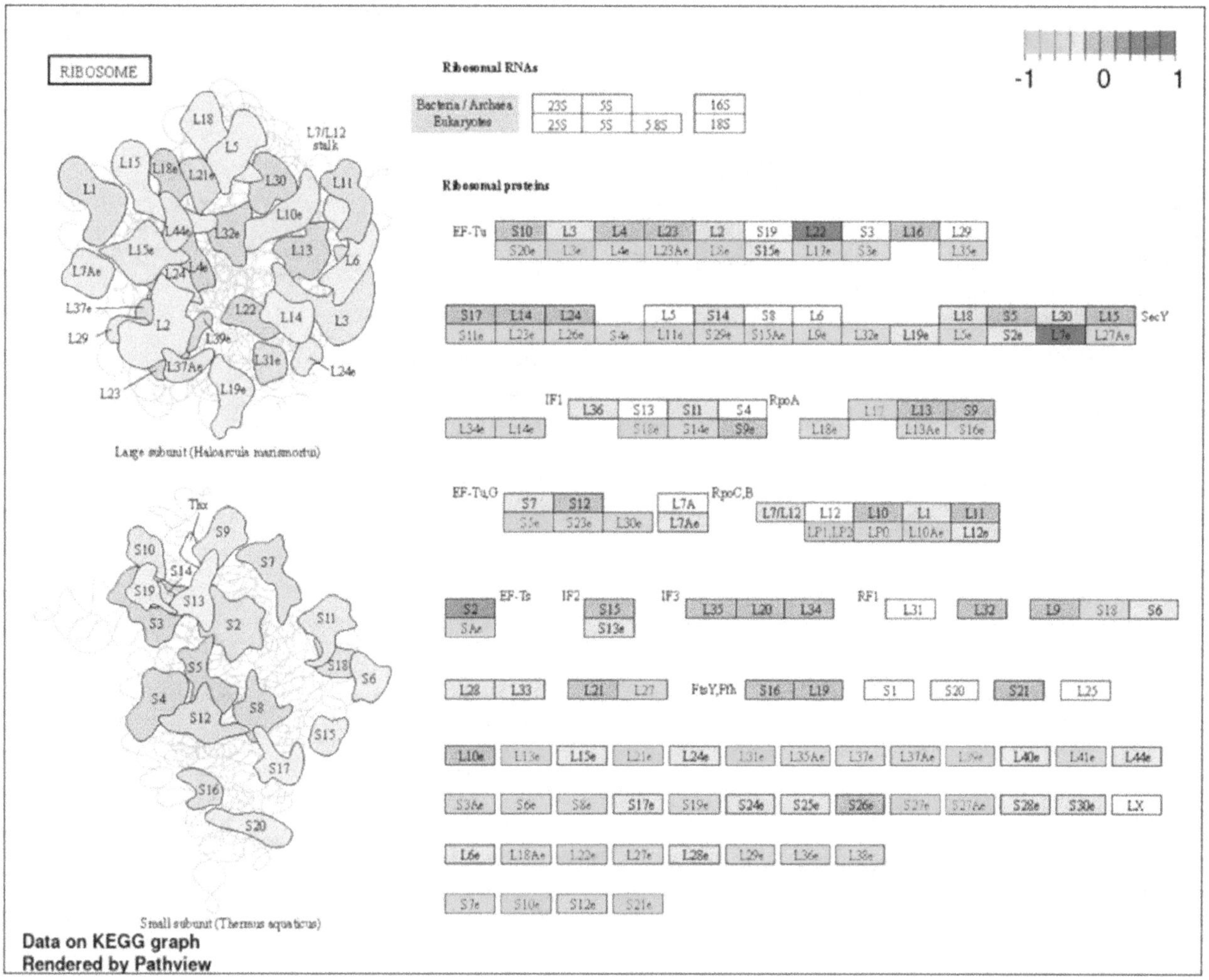

FIGURE 8 | Genes involved in ribosomal pathway in pulmonary sarcoidosis PBMCs by KEGG. A graphical illustration of KEGG pathway analysis of DEGs (log_2-fold change with FDR < 0.05) related to ribosomal signaling pathway in pulmonary sarcoidosis PBMCs.

is a polygenic, multifactorial disease (36). Many association studies have attempted to identify genetic susceptibility in sarcoidosis, and various genes have been found to increase the risk of developing sarcoidosis, including chemokine receptors, tumor necrosis factor (TNF)-α, and several HLA loci and MHC class II antigens (37). Therefore, careful interpretation of the transcriptional signature, as well as genetic linkage analysis, is required considering ethnicity. Second, this study shows the characteristics of PBMC gene expression at the time of diagnosis in patients with pulmonary sarcoidosis and was not intended to explore the relationship between transcriptome expression and prognosis of sarcoidosis. Third, we showed that gene expression of cytokines such as TNF and IL-17 was upregulated in patients with pulmonary sarcoidosis, but we did not confirm that by measuring interleukin levels in PBMCs or lung tissue. Therefore, further studies are needed to validate the mechanistic roles of PBMCs in sarcoidosis.

In the present study, additional transcriptome sub-analyses were performed to see apparent influence of differences in age, sex, and the lesions, although the sample number in each group was small (**Figures S1–S3**). The results showed that no same term as that shown in **Tables 2A,B** was detected in the three types of comparison by enrichment analysis (GO and KEGG pathway analysis), potentially implying that age and sex have no apparent influence on developing pulmonary sarcoidosis, and other than transcriptome signature in PBMCs may be more relevant to multiorgan involvement. However, it needs to be further evaluated with more samples to form a firm conclusion.

In conclusion, the current study suggests that bulk gene expression patterns in PBMCs are different between healthy controls and patients with pulmonary sarcoidosis. Most of the terms from enrichment analysis in the present study were different from those in a previous study that performed transcriptome analysis of PBMC comparing healthy controls with pulmonary sarcoidosis patients, more than half of whom received anti-inflammatory drugs. The changes in gene expression patterns of PBMCs could reflect the existence of sarcoidosis lesions and have an influence on granuloma formation in sarcoidosis. These new findings are important to strengthen our understanding of the etiology and pathobiology of sarcoidosis and indicate a potential therapeutic target for sarcoidosis.

AUTHOR CONTRIBUTIONS

TK and KT: conceptualization. KY, TK, DI, TI, and MA: data curation. KY, HS, TK, YH, and OO: formal analysis and methodology. KT: funding acquisition. KY, HS, TK, and KT: investigation. TK, KT, and TS: project administration. OO, KT, and TS: supervision. KY and HS: visualization. KY and TK: writing - original draft. TK, OO, KT, and TS: writing - review and editing. All authors contributed to the article and approved the submitted version.

ACKNOWLEDGMENTS

We are grateful to Sumina Atarashi, Tomoko Misawa, and Akiko Moriya for technical advice or assistance, and to Chieko Handa, Tamie Hirano, and Mika Sakurai for administrative support. We would like to thank Editage (www.editage.com) for English language editing.

SUPPLEMENTARY MATERIAL

Figure S1 | Principal component analysis (PCA). Principal component analysis (PCA) shows that two groups in pulmonary sarcoidosis are undifferentiated between older patients and younger patients.

Figure S2 | Principal component analysis (PCA). Principal component analysis (PCA) shows that two groups in pulmonary sarcoidosis appeared to be differentiated between female and male.

Figure S3 | Principal component analysis (PCA). Principal component analysis (PCA) shows that two groups in pulmonary sarcoidosis are undifferentiated between patients with multiorgan involvement and those with only pulmonary lesions.

REFERENCES

1. Moller DR, Rybicki BA, Hamzeh NY, Montgomery CG, Chen ES, Drake W, et al. Genetic, immunologic, and environmental basis of sarcoidosis. *Ann Am Thoracic Soc.* (2017) 14 (Suppl. 6):S429–36. doi: 10.1513/AnnalsATS.201707-565OT
2. Baughman RP, Culver DA, Judson MA. A concise review of pulmonary sarcoidosis. *Am J Respir Crit Care Med.* (2011) 183:573–81. doi: 10.1164/rccm.201006-0865CI
3. Iannuzzi MC, Rybicki BA, Teirstein AS. Medical progress. *Sarcoidosis N Eng J Med.* (2007) 357:2153–65. doi: 10.1056/NEJMra071714
4. Ramstein J, Broos CE, Simpson LJ, Ansel KM, Sun SA, Ho ME, et al. IFN-γ-producing T-helper 17.1 cells are increased in sarcoidosis and are more prevalent than T-helper type 1 cells. *Am J Respir Crit Care Med.* (2016) 193:1281–91. doi: 10.1164/rccm.201507-1499OC
5. Wong KL, Yeap WH, Tai JJY, Ong SM, Dang TM, Wong SC. The three human monocyte subsets: implications for health and disease. *Immunol Res.* (2012) 53:41–57. doi: 10.1007/s12026-012-8297-3
6. Milioglou I, Kalaitzidou I, Ladomenou F. Interpretation of lymphocyte subset counts by the general pediatrician. *Pediatr Int.* (2019) 61:16–22. doi: 10.1111/ped.13701
7. Wang F, Nie J, Wang H, Zhao Q, Xiong Y, Deng L, et al. Characteristics of peripheral lymphocyte subset alteration in COVID-19 pneumonia. *J Infect Dis.* (2020) 221:1762–9. doi: 10.1093/infdis/jiaa150
8. Jazwa A, Kasper L, Bak M, Sobczak M, Szade K, Jozkowicz A, et al. Differential inflammatory microRNA and cytokine expression in pulmonary sarcoidosis. *Archivum immunologiae et therapiae experimentalis.* (2015) 63:139–46. doi: 10.1007/s00005-014-0315-9
9. Crouser ED, Julian MW, Crawford M, Shao G, Yu L, Planck SR, et al. Differential expression of microRNA and predicted targets in pulmonary sarcoidosis. *Biochem Biophys Res Commun.* (2012) 417:886–91. doi: 10.1016/j.bbrc.2011.12.068
10. Zhou T, Zhang W, Sweiss NJ, Chen ES, Moller DR, Knox KS, et al. Peripheral blood gene expression as a novel genomic biomarker in complicated sarcoidosis. *PLoS ONE.* (2012) 7:e44818. doi: 10.1371/journal.pone.0044818
11. Costabel U, Hunninghake G. ATS/ERS/WASOG statement on sarcoidosis. Sarcoidosis statement committee. American thoracic society. European respiratory society. World association for sarcoidosis and other granulomatous disorders. *Eur Respir J.* (1999) 14:735–7. doi: 10.1034/j.1399-3003.1999.14d02.x
12. Ge SX, Son EW, Yao R. iDEP: an integrated web application for differential expression and pathway analysis of RNA-Seq data. *BMC bioinformatics.* (2018) 19:1–24. doi: 10.1186/s12859-018-2486-6
13. Hunninghake GW. Release of interleukin-1 by alveolar macrophages of patients with active pulmonary sarcoidosis. *Am Rev Respir Dis.* (1984) 129:569–72.
14. Bachwich PR, Lynch JP, 3rd, Larrick J, Spengler M, Kunkel SL. Tumor necrosis factor production by human sarcoid alveolar macrophages. *Am J Pathol.* (1986) 125:421–5.
15. Rolfe MW, Standiford TJ, Kunkel SL, Burdick MD, Gilbert AR, Moore S, et al. Interleukin-1 receptor antagonist expression in sarcoidosis. *Am Rev Respir Dis.* (1993) 148:1378. doi: 10.1164/ajrccm/148.5.1378
16. Sasaki M, Namioka Y, Ito T, Izumiyama N, Fukui S, Watanabe A, et al. Role of ICAM-1 in the aggregation and adhesion of human alveolar macrophages in response to TNF-alpha and INF-gamma. *Mediat Inflam.* (2001) 10:309–13. doi: 10.1080/09629350120102325
17. Moseley T, Haudenschild DR, Rose L, Reddi AH. Interleukin-17 family and IL-17 receptors. *Cytokine Growth Factor Rev.* (2003) 14:155–74. doi: 10.1016/S1359-6101(03)00002-9
18. Kolls JK, Lindén A. Interleukin-17 family members and inflammation. *Immunity.* (2004) 21:467–76. doi: 10.1016/j.immuni.2004.08.018
19. Weaver CT, Hatton RD, Mangan PR, Harrington LE. IL-17 family cytokines and the expanding diversity of effector T cell lineages. *Annu Rev Immunol.* (2007) 25:821–52. doi: 10.1146/annurev.immunol.25.022106.141557
20. Yoshida YO, Umemura M, Yahagi A, O'Brien RL, Ikuta K, Kishihara K, et al. Essential role of IL-17A in the formation of a mycobacterial infection-induced granuloma in the lung. *J Immunol.* (2010) 184:4414–22. doi: 10.4049/jimmunol.0903332
21. Coury F, Annels N, Rivollier A, Olsson S, Santoro A, Speziani C, et al. Langerhans cell histiocytosis reveals a new IL-17A–dependent pathway of dendritic cell fusion. *Nat Med.* (2008) 14:81–7. doi: 10.1038/nm1694
22. Jovanovic DV, Di Battista JA, Martel-Pelletier J, Jolicoeur FC, He Y, Zhang M, et al. IL-17 stimulates the production and expression of proinflammatory cytokines, IL-β and TNF-α, by human macrophages. *J Immunol.* (1998) 160:3513–21.
23. Kelly DM, Greene CM, Meachery G, O'Mahony M, Gallagher PM, Taggart CC, et al. Endotoxin up-regulates interleukin-18: potential role for gram-negative colonization in sarcoidosis. *Am J Respir Crit Care Med.* (2005) 172:1299–307. doi: 10.1164/rccm.200411-1594OC
24. Le J, Lin JX, Henriksen-DeStefano D, Vilcek J. Bacterial lipopolysaccharide-induced interferon-gamma production: roles of interleukin 1 and interleukin 2. *J Immunol.* (1986) 136:4525–30.
25. Ringkowski S, Thomas PS, Herbert C. Interleukin-12 family cytokines and sarcoidosis. *Front Pharmacol.* (2014) 5:233. doi: 10.3389/fphar.2014.00233
26. Drent M, Crouser ED, Grunewald J. Challenges of sarcoidosis and its management. *New Engl J Med.* (2021) 385:1018–32. doi: 10.1056/NEJMra2101555

27. Hu X, Ivashkiv LB. Cross-regulation of signaling pathways by interferon-γ: implications for immune responses and autoimmune diseases. *Immunity.* (2009) 31:539–50. doi: 10.1016/j.immuni.2009.09.002
28. Ivashkiv LB. IFNγ: signalling, epigenetics and roles in immunity, metabolism, disease and cancer immunotherapy. *Nat Rev Immunol.* (2018) 18:545–58. doi: 10.1038/s41577-018-0029-z
29. Kimura A, Kishimoto T. IL-6: regulator of Treg/Th17 balance. *Eur J Immunol.* (2010) 40:1830–5. doi: 10.1002/eji.201040391
30. Pease JE, Sabroe I. The role of interleukin-8 and its receptors in inflammatory lung disease: implications for therapy. *Am J Respir Med Drugs Devices Other Interv.* (2002) 1:19–25. doi: 10.1007/BF03257159
31. Larsen CG, Thomsen MK, Gesser B, Thomsen PD, Deleuran BW, Nowak J, et al. The delayed-type hypersensitivity reaction is dependent on IL-8. Inhibition of a tuberculin skin reaction by an anti-IL-8 monoclonal antibody. *J Immunol.* (1995) 155:2151–7.
32. Garman L, Pelikan RC, Rasmussen A, Lareau CA, Savoy KA, Deshmukh US, et al. Single cell transcriptomics implicate novel monocyte and T cell immune dysregulation in sarcoidosis. *Front Immunol.* (2020) 11:567342. doi: 10.3389/fimmu.2020.567342
33. Jakubzick C, Gautier EL, Gibbings SL, Sojka DK, Schlitzer A, Johnson TE, et al. Minimal differentiation of classical monocytes as they survey steady-state tissues and transport antigen to lymph nodes. *Immunity.* (2013) 39:599–610. doi: 10.1016/j.immuni.2013.08.007
34. Talreja J, Farshi P, Alazizi A, Luca F, Pique-Regi R, Samavati L. RNA-sequencing identifies novel pathways in sarcoidosis monocytes. *Sci Rep.* (2017) 7:1–10. doi: 10.1038/s41598-017-02941-4
35. Brito-Zeron P, Kostov B, Superville D, Baughman RP, Ramos-Casals M. Geoepidemiological big data approach to sarcoidosis: geographical and ethnic determinants. *Clin Exp Rheumatol.* (2019) 37:1052–64.
36. Calender A, Weichhart T, Valeyre D, Pacheco Y. Current insights in genetics of sarcoidosis: functional and clinical impacts. *J Clin Med.* (2020) 9:2633. doi: 10.3390/jcm9082633
37. Iannuzzi MC, Rybicki BA. Genetics of sarcoidosis: candidate genes and genome scans. *Proc Am Thoracic Soc.* (2007) 4:108–16. doi: 10.1513/pats.200607-141JG

22

A Novel Normalized Cross-Correlation Speckle-Tracking Ultrasound Algorithm for the Evaluation of Diaphragm Deformation

Xiong Ye [1,2], *Zhi Liu* [3], *Ying Ma* [4], *Ye Song* [4], *Lihua Hu* [4], *Jianwen Luo* [3] *and Hui Xiao* [5*]

[1] *School of Clinical Medicine, Shanghai University of Medicine & Health Sciences, Shanghai, China,* [2] *National Medical Products Administration (NMPA) Key Laboratory for Respiratory and Anaesthetic Equipment, Shanghai, China,* [3] *Department of Biomedical Engineering, School of Medicine, Tsinghua University, Beijing, China,* [4] *Department of Ultrasound, Shanghai University of Medicine and Health Sciences Affiliated Zhoupu Hospital, Shanghai, China,* [5] *Department of Respiratory and Critical Care Medicine, Shanghai General Hospital, Shanghai Jiaotong University, Shanghai, China*

***Correspondence:**
Hui Xiao
xiaohui771210@163.com

Objectives: To develop a two-dimensional normalized cross-correlation (NCC)-based ultrasonic speckle-tracking algorithm for right diaphragm deformation analysis.

Methods: Six healthy and eight mechanical ventilation patients were enrolled in this study. Images were acquired by a portable ultrasound system in three sections. DICOM data were processed with NCC to obtain the interframe/cumulative vertical and horizontal displacements, as well as the global strain of the right diaphragm, with continuous tracking and drift correction.

Results: The NCC algorithm can track the contraction and relaxation of the right diaphragm by following the respiratory movement continuously. For all three sections, the interframe and accumulated horizontal displacements were both significantly larger than the corresponding vertical displacements (interframe p values: 0.031, 0.004, and 0.000; cumulative p values: 0.039, 0.001, and <0.0001). For the global strain of the right diaphragm, there was no significant difference between each pair of sections (all $p > 0.05$), regardless of whether the horizontal interval of the initial diaphragm point was 1, 3, 5, or 10 times in the sampling interval.

Conclusions: This study developed a novel diaphragm deformation ultrasound imaging method. This method can be used to estimate the diaphragm interframe/accumulated displacement in the horizontal and vertical directions and the global strain on three different imaging planes, and it was found that the strain was not sensitive to the imaging plane.

Keywords: diaphragm, deformation, ultrasound, speckle tracking, strain

KEYPOINTS

- We developed a two-dimensional normalized cross-correlation-based ultrasound speckle-tracking algorithm as a novel method for diaphragm deformation analysis.
- The interpolation of both the radiofrequency signals and cross-correlation function algorithm can be used to track the contraction and relaxation of the right diaphragm with respiratory movement continuously in the horizontal and vertical directions.

INTRODUCTION

The diaphragm is a thin (2–4 mm), movable, dome-shaped, muscular-fibrous structure with a central tendon that separates the thorax from the abdomen and maintains the pressure gradient between those two cavities (1). It is also a vital organ that plays a major role in maintaining ventilation for mammals, as it provides ~80% of the volume capacity for respiration (2). Diaphragm contractility and relaxation occur throughout an individual's life span without resting, not even during sleep; its importance is almost equal to that of the heart, if without normal movement of the diaphragm, life as it is currently known would not be possible (2). The phrenic nerve (PhN), which emerges mainly from the fourth cervical nerve root and partly from the third and fifth nerve roots, maintains the function of the human diaphragm (3). Unilateral PhN injury in most young people without lung pathology is well-tolerated, but in patients with chronic obstructive pulmonary disease, emphysema, or other lung disease may produce symptoms even with mild exertion. Bilateral diaphragmatic paralysis is usually always symptomatic, and the patient may be symptomatic even at rest (4), due to accessory muscles for respiration can compensate only in the short term (5, 6). Protecting the PhN is important because ipsilateral PhN damage significantly reduces the expiratory lung volume, gas exchange, and exercise capacity (7–9). There are various causes of PhN injury, such as cardiac or neck surgery, trauma, pneumonectomy, lung tumors, lung or liver transplantation, metabolic disorders, chronic lung diseases, as well as many systemic diseases, such as multiple sclerosis, that can lead to diaphragm paralysis and ultimately respiratory failure. The use of ice slush is an independent risk factor for PhN dysfunction in patients undergoing cardiac surgery with hypothermic cardiopulmonary bypass (10). Among intensive care unit (ICU) patients, 70% of those with sepsis and multiple organ failure will develop diaphragm dysfunction, which can lead to difficulty in weaning from mechanical ventilation and a prolonged ICU stay (11, 12). Although there are many clinical situations in which the diaphragm can be damaged, the assessment of diaphragm function is often fairly under-recognized (13, 14). The main reason is that there has never been a convenient and accurate method to evaluate the deformation and elastic characteristics of the diaphragm, and there is still a lack of real-time and non-invasive tools for monitoring diaphragm activity at the bedside (15), although such monitoring is sometimes necessary. Currently, Twitch transdiaphragm pressure following magnetic stimulation of the PhN is the gold standard for the non-volitional assessment of diaphragm function (16). Other methods to assess diaphragm function often have little diagnostic value, such as chest X-rays (17), or involve radiation exposure and are difficult to perform at the bedside, as is the case for computed tomography (CT) and magnetic resonance imaging (MRI). Ultrasound is the only non-invasive, radiation-free, portable, and safe diagnostic method with which to directly assess diaphragm motor function in various clinical departments (18–20). Accordingly, many related studies have been published in recent years based on M- and B-mode ultrasound, but the results of each study are quite different. Moreover, M-mode ultrasound provides a one-dimensional measurement of moving tissue along the ultrasound propagation beam. When tissue concurrently moves laterally, this vector cannot be captured (21); consequently, M-mode cannot reflect the true motion of locomotive organs. B-mode ultrasound can only reflect structural information and cannot provide details regarding the elastic characteristics of tissues. Furthermore, both B- and M-mode ultrasound depends on the angle of incidence of the ultrasound beam and requires the operator to have experience.

The ultrasound speckle-tracking imaging technique can provide tissue deformation and more dimensional motion information, such as radial, longitudinal, and circular vectors, which has been successfully used to assess myocardial strain. In 2013, we proposed the concept of diaphragm deformation analysis and used commercial myocardial speckle-tracking software to evaluate diaphragm strain in healthy volunteers (22). Hatam et al. (23) and Orde et al. (24) also used myocardial strain analysis software to evaluate diaphragm strain. All of the above studies were performed using the algorithm designed specifically for myocardium. Currently, in commercial myocardial strain analysis software, analysis of the region of interest is triggered by the R wave of the electrocardiogram, and the analytical process lasts until aortic valve closure. The entire duration of myocardial strain analysis is ~0.02 s, which is much shorter than the duration of inspiration in one respiratory cycle. It is obvious that for the direct analysis of diaphragm deformation using myocardial strain software, the mode of triggering and the duration of the analysis are not consistent with the physiological characteristics of respiration. One potential solution for this limitation is to develop a new specialized algorithm that makes the analytical process cover the entire breathing process or the inspiration phase to fully evaluate the dynamics of the diaphragm (22).

In this study, according to respiratory physiology, we developed a novel speckle-tracking algorithm [i.e., normalized cross-correlation (NCC) algorithm (25)] to evaluate the kinetic characteristics (i.e., displacement and strain) of the right diaphragm first and then carried out a preliminary clinical study in 14 volunteers.

Abbreviations: BMI, Body mass index; C T, Computed tomography; DICOM, Digital imaging and communications in medicine; GS, Global strain; MRI, Magnetic resonance imaging; MV, Mechanical ventilation; NCC, Normalized cross-correlation; PhN, Phrenic nerve; ICU, Intensive care unit; Interp_Both, Interpolation of both the radiofrequency signals and cross-correlation function; ROI, Region of interest; SIMV, Synchronized intermittent mandatory ventilation.

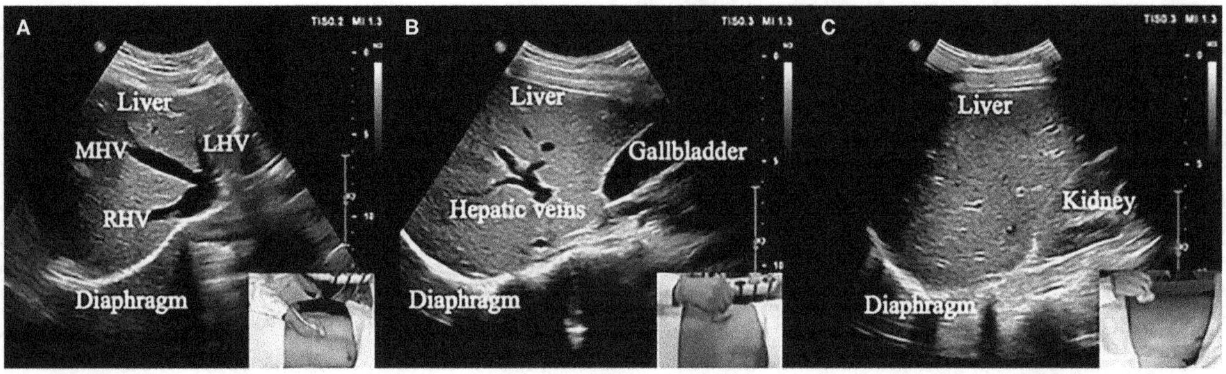

FIGURE 1 | (A) Section I: Oblique section of the lower right costal arch through the second hepatic portal with the left hepatic vein (LHV), middle hepatic vein (MHV), and right hepatic vein (RHV) as anatomical markers. **(B)** Section II: Oblique section of the right intercostal passage through the first hepatic portal with the inferior vena cava, hepatic vein, and gallbladder as anatomical markers. **(C)** Section III: Sagittal section of the liver and right kidney with the right kidney and hepatorenal space as anatomical markers.

METHODS

Participants

Six healthy subjects and eight mechanical ventilation patients (a total of 14 participants) were prospectively enrolled in this study. The healthy subjects were examined in the supine position during normal quiet breathing, and the invasive mechanical ventilation patients were lying in bed at a 35-degree angle. The tidal volume of mechanical ventilation was measured with a spirometer for healthy subjects and was obtained from machine settings for mechanical ventilation patients. All of our mechanical ventilation patients were kept in an intubated state using a synchronized intermittent mandatory ventilation model. The ethics committee of the Shanghai University of Medicine & Health Sciences approved this study, and written consent was obtained from all participants.

Design of Diaphragm Ultrasound Scanning Sections

Movement of the diaphragm in three sections (**Figure 1**) was assessed by ultrasound using a 3–5-MHz convex-array probe and a LOGIQ V2 ultrasound machine (General Electric Healthcare, Horton, Norway). Twenty-second dynamic digital imaging and communications in medicine (DICOM) images were saved for subsequent ultrasound speckle-tracking imaging analysis. To achieve the desired high-quality boundary of the right diaphragm (26), the dynamic range (e.g., 45–65 dB) was selected based on the clinical application and the patient's condition.

1) Section I: Oblique section of the right costal arch through the second hepatic portal (**Figure 1A**).
2) Section II: Oblique section of the right intercostal passage through the first hepatic portal (**Figure 1B**).
3) Section III: Sagittal section of the liver and right kidney (**Figure 1C**).

Basic Process of Tracking Diaphragm Deformation

The specific process of diaphragm deformation can be found in **Figure 2A**. For the normalized cross-correlation-based speckle-tracking method (i.e., lateral interpolation of both the radiofrequency signals and cross-correlation function (Interp_Both), please kindly refer to the study by Liu Z and his colleagues (27).

Establishment of the Region of Interest (ROI) on Diaphragm Ultrasound

The ROI was set up with four initial points on the diaphragm with 1-, 3-, 5-, and 10-fold (a, b, c, and d) horizontal sampling spacing, as shown in **Figure 2B**.

Definition of Diaphragm Displacement and Strain

Diaphragm Displacement

The peak-to-peak value of the overall interframe/cumulative vertical and horizontal displacement was extracted as the displacement of the right diaphragm in one breathing cycle by taking the mean and median displacement of all points in the diaphragm ROI (**Figure 3A**).

Global Diaphragm Strain

The Euclidean distance between each two adjacent points in the ROI was calculated, which can be considered to be approximately equal to the initial length of the diaphragm (i.e., the length of the green segment shown in **Figure 3**), and it is marked as L0. Continuous tracking of these initial points and calculation of the sum of their distances can yield the length of the diaphragm at a certain time, which is recorded as Lt (**Figure 3B**). The global strain (GS) of the diaphragm can then be calculated by the following formula (1).

$$GS = \frac{Lt - L0}{L0} * 100\% \qquad (1)$$

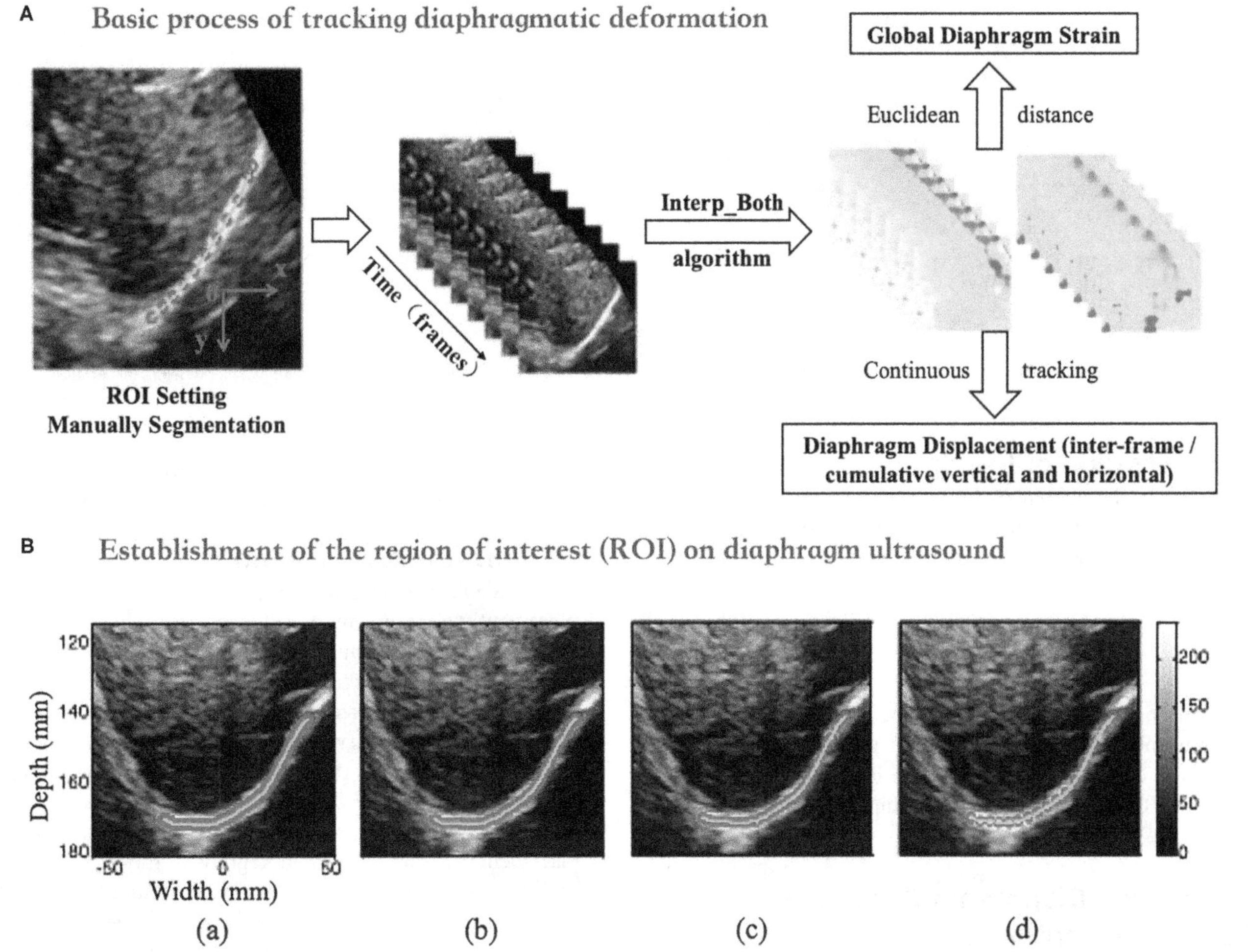

FIGURE 2 | (A) Flow chart of diaphragm speckle tracking. **(B)** ROI (initial point) of the diaphragm based on 1- (a), 3- (b), 5- (c), and 10-fold (d) horizontal sampling spacing.

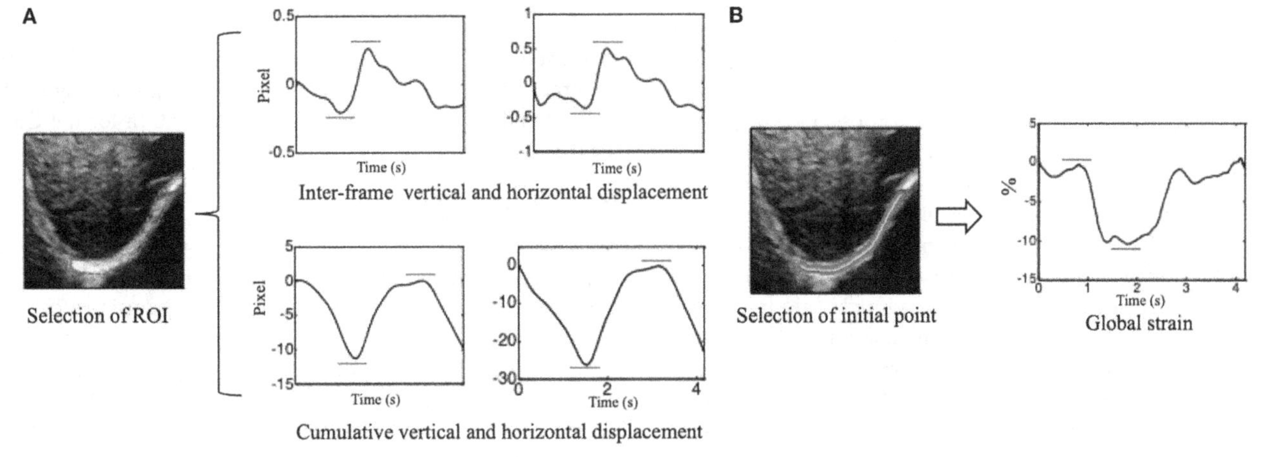

FIGURE 3 | (A) Vertical (left side) and horizontal (right side) of inter-frame and cumulative displacement of the right diaphragm in one breathing cycle and schematics of peak-to-peak value extraction. **(B)** Time-dependent global strain curves of the right diaphragm and schematic of peak-to-peak value extraction.

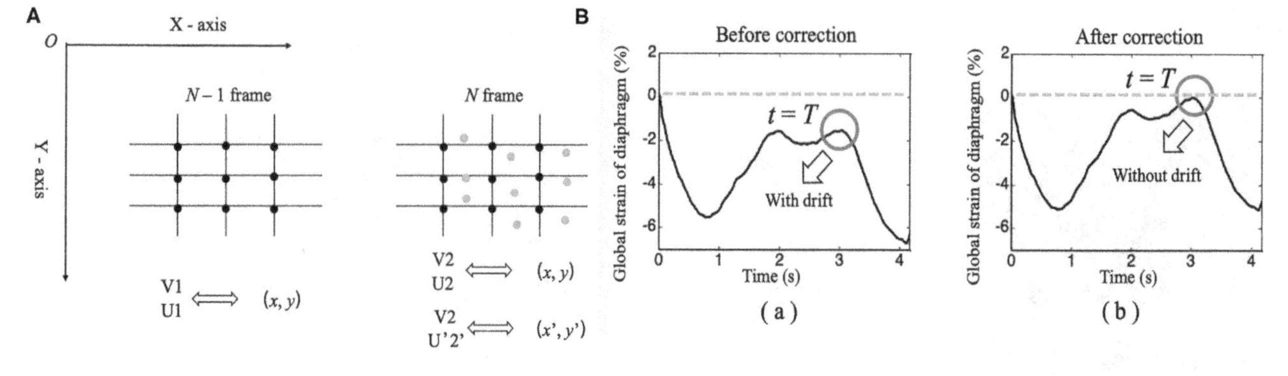

FIGURE 4 | (A) Diagram of the continuous tracking algorithm. **(B)** Changes in the global strain curves of the diaphragm correction with time before (a) and after (b).

Normalization of Interframe Displacement

To eliminate the influence of the frame rate on the estimation of the interframe displacement, the interframe displacement was normalized with the following formula (2).

$$D\_norm = \frac{FR}{FR\ max} * D \quad (2)$$

D_norm and D denote the interframe displacement after and before normalization, respectively. FR is the acquisition frame rate of the data used to calculate the interframe displacement D, while FRmax refers to the maximum of all data acquisition frame rates.

Continuous Diaphragm Deformation Tracking Algorithm (Figure 4A)

1) When calculating the interframe displacement, the selected grid points are represented by black dots. The coordinates of the black dots are assumed to be (x, y), while the vertical and horizontal displacements are represented by V1 (U1) and V2 (U2), respectively, which are obtained from the N-1 and N frames and the N and N+1 frames, respectively.
2) Because the diaphragm is moving at all times during breathing, the selected grid point (i.e., black dot) in frame N-1 has moved to a new position (i.e., green dot) in frame N when calculating the displacement, and its coordinates are assumed to be (x', y'); here, x'= x + U1 and y'= y + V1.
3) We can interpolate linearly the vertical and horizontal displacements of the green dots based on the displacements of the black dots in frame N and express them as V2' and U2'.
4) Finally, when frame N-1 changes to frame N, the interframe vertical displacement of the diaphragm changes from V1 to V2' (instead of V2), the interframe horizontal displacement of the diaphragm changes from U1 to U2' (instead of U2), the cumulative vertical displacement of the diaphragm changes from V1 to V1 + V2', and the cumulative horizontal displacement of the diaphragm changes from U1 to U1 + U2'. Similarly, the GS of the diaphragm can be obtained by applying the above process to continuously track the position of the initial points of the diaphragm, followed by calculating the Euclidean distances between the adjacent points, summing the distances, and applying formula (1).

Drift Correction Algorithm

An unavoidable problem in continuous tracking is that the displacement or strain curve will drift with the increase in frame number (time), which occurs due to estimation error accumulation in the tracking process (28). Therefore, a drift correction algorithm is used to compensate for the drift in the displacement or strain curve. The process of drift correction is described as follows. First, the movement cycle of the diaphragm with respiration was determined by M-mode ultrasonography, which was assumed to be T. Then, the distribution of the displacement or strain of the diaphragm with time was assumed to be S (t). Displacement or strain begins to accumulate at $t = 0$, and S (T) should return to the original position when $t = T$ [i.e., S (T) = 0]. However, due to error accumulation, S (T) is usually not zero. Therefore, to correct the drift of displacement or strain, we adopted formula (3), as follows.

$$S\_corr\ (t) = \begin{cases} S\ (t) - \frac{S(T)}{T} * t,\ 0 \leq t \leq T \\ S\ (t) - S\ (T),\ t \geq T \end{cases} \quad (3)$$

In formula (3), S_corr(t), and S(t) represent the displacement or strain after and before correction, respectively. **Figure 4B** shows the drift correction effect of this algorithm for the GS of the diaphragm.

Data Analysis

After correcting the drift, the peak-to-peak values of displacement and strain were extracted to evaluate diaphragm function, and statistical analyses were performed using SPSS 19.0 software (SPSS, Inc., Chicago, IL, USA). All values are shown as the mean ± standard deviation. Descriptive analyses were performed for all investigated variables, and the D'Agostino-Pearson test was used to test for normality. The unpaired t-test and non-parametric tests were used to analyze the results of differences in the displacement or strain of the right diaphragm between the two groups, and one-way ANOVA was used for comparing three groups according to data characteristics.

Bartlett's test was used to analyze statistical significance, which was defined as $P < 0.05$.

RESULTS

Baseline Characteristics of the Subjects

Diaphragm ultrasound images were acquired from six healthy subjects during quiet spontaneous breathing and eight ICU patients under mechanical ventilation, all of whom were males. The baseline characteristics of all subjects are described in **Table 1**.

Continual Tracking of Diaphragm Movement

Figure 5 shows the results of continuous tracking of the diaphragm ROI during one breathing cycle based on lateral interpolation of both the radiofrequency signals and the cross-correlation function (Interp_Both) algorithm. The ROI of the diaphragm was obtained by manual segmentation at $t = 0$ s. In addition, the ROI of the diaphragm at $t = 1.31$ s was significantly shorter than that at $t = 0$ s, which indicates that the diaphragm was contracting during the inspiratory phase. Then, the diaphragm ROI began to stretch slowly from $t = 1.31$ s to $t = 2.60$ s, which indicated passive relaxation of the diaphragm during the expiratory phase. Most importantly, at the end of the expiratory phase ($t = 3.03$ s), the ROI of the diaphragm essentially returned to the initial position and shape ($t = 0$ s).

TABLE 1 | Baseline characteristics of 14 subjects (mean ± SD).

Variable	Healthy subjects (*N* = 6)	MV patents (*N* = 8)	*P*
Age (years)	56 ± 8.2	51 ± 3.6	0.061
BMI (kg/m^2)	21 ± 5.3	23 ± 2.8	0.084
Tidal volume (ml)	520 ± 17.3	450 ± 38.2	0.102
Ventilation mode	-	SIMV	-

BMI, body mass index; MV, mechanical ventilation; SIMV, synchronized intermittent mandatory ventilation.

Displacement of the Diaphragm

On ultrasound imaging of the three different sections, there were no significant differences in the peak-to-peak values of the vertical or horizontal displacement and strain of the diaphragm based on the median and mean in the same section, and the *P* values were all >0.05. Therefore, the following results of this study were compared according to the median values.

Figure 6 depicts the horizontal and vertical interframe (**Figure 6A**) and cumulative (**Figure 6B**) displacements of the right diaphragm for the same sections. The red and blue boxes represent the horizontal and vertical displacements of sections I, II, and III, respectively. The interframe and cumulative horizontal displacements of sections I, II, and III were significantly greater than the vertical displacements. In terms of significant differences, the *P* values for the differences between the interframe horizontal and vertical displacements of sections I, II, and III were 0.031, 0.004, and 0.000, respectively, while those for the cumulative horizontal and vertical displacements of sections I, II, and III were 0.039, 0.001, and <0.0001, respectively.

GS of the Diaphragm

Table 2 is based on the differential distribution of the GS of the right diaphragm for the three imaging sections estimated by selecting the initial point of the diaphragm at different sampling intervals. **Table 2** shows that when different horizontal intervals were selected to estimate the GS of the diaphragm, the

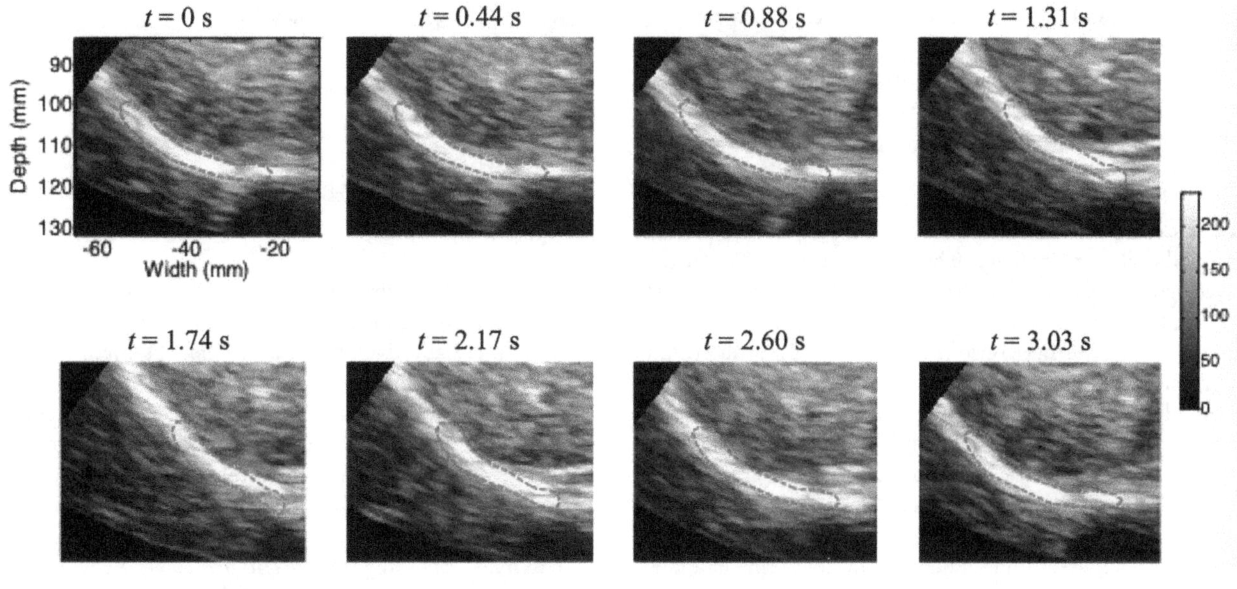

FIGURE 5 | Movement of the diaphragm tracked during one breathing cycle based on the Interp_Both algorithm (red circle, ROI).

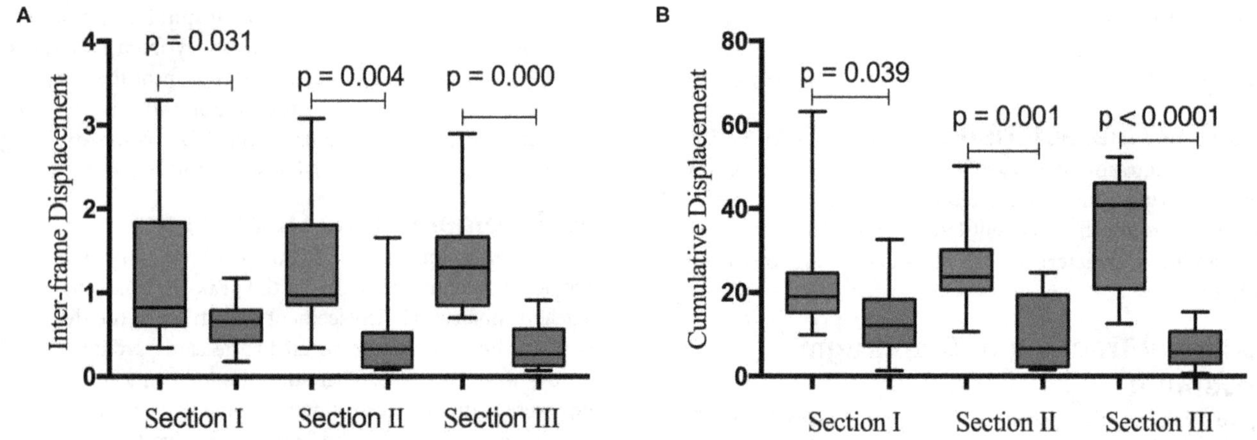

FIGURE 6 | Difference between inter-frame horizontal (red bar) and vertical (blue bar) displacement **(A)** and cumulative horizontal (red bar) and vertical (blue bar) displacement **(B)** of the right diaphragm for the same ultrasound imaging sections.

strain values were slightly different. However, after testing the difference in the strain between each pair of sections by one-way ANOVA, it was found that the GS of the diaphragm did not differ significantly by section ($P > 0.05$), regardless of whether the horizontal sampling interval of the initial diaphragm point was 1, 3, 5, or 10 (**Table 3**).

TABLE 2 | GS of the right diaphragm determined by selecting the initial point of the ROI based on the horizontal sampling spacing of 1, 3, 5, and 10 for three sections ($N = 14$).

Horizontal sampling spacing	ANOVA summary		Bartlett's test	
	F (dfn, dfd)	P	Bartlett's statistic	P
1	0.309 (2, 32)	0.737	10.54	0.005
3	0.793 (2, 32)	0.641	10.81	0.005
5	1.664 (2, 32)	0.205	23.7	<0.0001
10	1.441 (2, 32)	0.252	16.24	0.000

TABLE 3 | GS of the right diaphragm determined by selecting the initial point of the ROI based on the horizontal sampling spacing of 5 for the three sections ($N = 14$).

Section	GS (%) (Mean ± SD)	95% CI	*F* (dfn, dfd)	*P*
I	7.89 ± 2.46	6.40 - 9.38		0.218
II	12.9 ± 10.94	5.95 – 19.85	1.602 (2, 31)	
III	10.07 ± 4.00	7.00 – 13.14		

DISCUSSION

The diaphragm is widely distributed between the thoracic and abdominal regions as the main respiratory muscle pump, including the crural, dorsocostal, midcostal, and ventrocostal regions and the zone of apposition (29). The diaphragm has important physiological functions; thus, evaluating and monitoring changes in its function in the clinic is necessary (30, 31). In ultrasound strain imaging, the displacement and deformation of tissue are estimated using pre- and post-compression imaging data (32). The mechanics of the interaction between the diaphragm and the load are well-understood, but the force-length properties of the diaphragm are non-linear, and algebraic analysis of the interaction is ineffective (33). Ultrasound speckle is granular and textured in appearance due to the backscattered echoes of either randomly or coherently distributed scatterers in tissue. The statistical properties of the received echo speckle signals have been shown to depend on the density and spatial distribution of scatters.

In this study, we developed a new Interp_Both algorithm for ultrasound speckle-tracking imaging of the right diaphragm, and the deformation characteristics of the diaphragm were analyzed successfully by this method. Our previous research showed that Interp_Both with a small interpolation factor (e.g., 3–5) yields the best tradeoff between the estimation accuracy and the time required for computation, thus suggesting such a factor for lateral motion estimation in the case of a low line density (i.e., <2.8 lines/mm) (27). All of the ultrasound data of the right diaphragm that we collected had a low line density. The entire process of active contraction in the inspiratory phase and passive relaxation in the expiratory phase of the right diaphragm could be observed, as shown in **Figure 5**. The vertical and horizontal movements of the right diaphragm during one respiratory cycle could successfully be tracked continuously. The drift phenomenon could be completely removed from the corrected strain curve by applying the drift correction algorithm. To our knowledge, this is the first study in which a newly designed Interp_Both algorithm based on diaphragm anatomy and respiratory physiology was used to analyze diaphragm deformation. Referencing the standard sections used in liver ultrasonography, we defined three sections of the right diaphragm, which were marked by the three hepatic veins (section I), the inferior vena cava and gallbladder (section II), and the right kidney (section III). According to our newly developed algorithm, the deformation information of these three diaphragm sections was analyzed in 6 normal persons and 8 patients under mechanical ventilation. We used the peak-to-peak values of the instantaneous and cumulative horizontal and vertical displacements and the GS of the right diaphragm as indexes of diaphragm kinetics. The dynamic index of strain reflects the internal characteristics and provides insight into the elastic properties of tissues in either active or passive contraction processes.

This work yielded several interesting findings. First, the instantaneous horizontal displacement was larger than the vertical displacement at both the interframe and cumulative level for the same section, as shown in **Figure 6**, which indicates that the diaphragm moves horizontally more than vertically in the inspiratory period. Understanding regional diaphragm mechanics and kinematics is very important; however, no studies have shown how the diaphragm moves in different directions during the breathing cycle. Brooke Greybeck and his team studied four dogs and showed that the volume displacement of the diaphragm was heterogeneous and dependent on regional muscle shortening, posture and level of muscle activation (34). Another finding was that the GS of the diaphragm obtained for the three sections did not differ significantly ($P > 0.05$), regardless of whether the horizontal sampling interval of the initial diaphragm point was 1, 3, 5, or 10. This shows that for the diaphragm strain, the section selected has little effect. Furthermore, the initial points of the diaphragm ROI determined with different sampling spacings at different levels have little influence on the final results, which indicates that the selection of imaging sections may not be so strict when calculating the GS of the diaphragm. Although the concept of diaphragm strain in this study is consistent with previous studies (22–24), the results are not comparable due to the completely different algorithm used.

There are some limitations to this study. First, although we have established a new method for diaphragm deformation analysis, the number of samples used for verification was small. Second, the good contrast of the right diaphragm ultrasound images makes it possible to set the ROI, but ultrasound images are probably the most difficult medical images to use for segmentation during image recognition and tracking. Before the ROI set up, we manually segmented the diaphragm images according to the dynamic B- and M-mode ultrasound images, which led to a reduction in the tracking quality. In further research on diaphragm deformation, sensors could be added to display the respiratory waveform on the ultrasound equipment and allow automatic segmentation of the image with the starting point of the inspiratory phase curve as the trigger point for analysis. Because the left diaphragm does not have as nice an acoustic window as the right diaphragm (due to the liver), it is difficult to obtain an ideal image of the left diaphragm. We have not yet attempted to conduct a deformation tracking analysis on the left diaphragm but will in future studies.

CONCLUSIONS

In summary, a novel ultrasound algorithm for deformation (displacement and strain) imaging of the diaphragm based on cross-correlation was developed in our study, and the peak-to-peak values of instantaneous and cumulative displacement and GS were proposed as kinetic indexes of diaphragm function. Differences in the interframe and cumulative vertical and horizontal displacements of the right diaphragm and the GS among three different sections were analyzed. The results show greater horizontal than vertical movement of the diaphragm in each section, and the GS of the diaphragm was not sensitive to the imaging section, which will help reduce the difficulty of choosing the section when performing strain imaging of the diaphragm in the future. In subsequent studies, more clinical data need to be collected to further explore the value and significance of this new technology.

AUTHOR CONTRIBUTIONS

XY, HX, ZL, and JL contributed to the design of the study, analysis of the data, and drafting of the manuscript. XY, YM, YS, and LH contributed to obtaining the ultrasound images. All authors critically revised the paper and agreed to be accountable for all aspects of the work.

ACKNOWLEDGMENTS

The authors would like to thank our patients, who willingly gave their time to participate in this research.

REFERENCES

1. Downey R. Anatomy of the normal diaphragm. *Thorac Surg Clin.* (2011) 21:273–9. doi: 10.1016/j.thorsurg.2011.01.001
2. Maish MS. The diaphragm. *Surg Clin North Am.* (2010) 90:955–68. doi: 10.1016/j.suc.2010.07.005
3. Fell SC. Surgical anatomy of the diaphragm and the phrenic nerve. *Chest Surg Clin N Am.* (1998) 8:281–94.
4. Shahid Z, Burns B. *Anatomy, Abdomen and Pelvis, Diaphragm.* Treasure Island, FL: StatPearls (2020).
5. Kokatnur L, Rudrappa M. Diaphragmatic Palsy. *Diseases.* (2018) 6:E16. doi: 10.3390/diseases6010016
6. Mandoorah S, Mead T. Phrenic nerve injury. Treasure Island, FL: StatPearls (2019).
7. Burns J, Dunning J. Is the preservation of the phrenic nerve important after pneumonectomy? *Interact Cardiovasc Thorac Surg.* (2011) 12:47–50. doi: 10.1510/icvts.2010.248583
8. Kocher GJ, Mauss K, Carboni GL, Hoksch B, Kuster R, Ott SR, et al. Effect of phrenic nerve palsy on early postoperative lung function after pneumonectomy: a prospective study. *Ann Thorac Surg.* (2013) 96:2015–20. doi: 10.1016/j.athoracsur.2013.07.006
9. Ugalde P, Miro S, Provencher S, Quevillon M, Chau L, Deslauriers DR, et al. Ipsilateral diaphragmatic motion and lung function in long-term pneumonectomy patients. *Ann Thorac Surg.* (2008) 86:1745–51. discussion 1751–42. doi: 10.1016/j.athoracsur.2008.05.081
10. Dimopoulou I, Daganou M, Dafni U, Karakatsani A, Khoury M, Geroulanos S, et al. Phrenic nerve dysfunction after cardiac operations: electrophysiologic evaluation of risk factors. *Chest.* (1998) 113:8–14. doi: 10.1378/chest.113.1.8

11. Watson AC, Hughes PD, Louise Harris M, Hart N, Ware RJ, Wendon J, et al. Measurement of twitch transdiaphragmatic, esophageal, and endotracheal tube pressure with bilateral anterolateral magnetic phrenic nerve stimulation in patients in the intensive care unit. *Crit Care Med.* (2001) 29:1325–31. doi: 10.1097/00003246-200107000-00005
12. Doorduin J, van Hees HW, van der Hoeven JG, Heunks LM. Monitoring of the respiratory muscles in the critically ill. *Am J Respir Crit Care Med.* (2013) 187:20–7. doi: 10.1164/rccm.201206-1117CP
13. McCool FD, Tzelepis GE. Dysfunction of the diaphragm. *N Engl J Med.* (2012) 366:932–42. doi: 10.1056/NEJMra1007236
14. Nason LK, Walker CM, McNeeley MF, Burivong W, Fligner CL, Godwin JD. Imaging of the diaphragm: anatomy and function. *Radiographics.* (2012) 32:E51–70. doi: 10.1148/rg.322115127
15. Zambon M, Greco M, Bocchino S, Cabrini L, Beccaria PF, Zangrillo A. Assessment of diaphragmatic dysfunction in the critically ill patient with ultrasound: a systematic review. *Intensive Care Med.* (2017) 43:29–38. doi: 10.1007/s00134-016-4524-z
16. Spiesshoefer J, Henke C, Herkenrath SD, Randerath W, Brix T, Görlich D, et al. Noninvasive prediction of twitch transdiaphragmatic pressure: insights from spirometry, diaphragm ultrasound, and phrenic nerve stimulation studies. *Respiration.* (2019) 98:301–11. doi: 10.1159/000501171
17. Chetta A, Rehman AK, Moxham J, Carr DH, Polkey MI. Chest radiography cannot predict diaphragm function. *Respir Med.* (2005) 99:39–44. doi: 10.1016/j.rmed.2004.04.016
18. Nekludova GV, Avdeev SN. Possibilities of ultrasound research of the diaphragm. *Ter Arkh.* (2019) 91:86–92. doi: 10.26442/00403660.2019.03.000129
19. Sferrazza Papa GF, Pellegrino GM, Di Marco F, Imeri G, Brochard L, Goligher E, et al. A review of the ultrasound assessment of diaphragmatic function in clinical practice. *Respiration.* (2016) 91:403–11. doi: 10.1159/000446518
20. Vetrugno L, Guadagnin GM, Barbariol F, Langiano N, Zangrillo A, Bove T. Ultrasound imaging for diaphragm dysfunction: a narrative literature review. *J Cardiothorac Vasc Anesth.* (2019) 33:2525–36. doi: 10.1053/j.jvca.2019.01.003
21. Goutman SA, Hamilton JD, Swihart B, Foerster B, Feldman EL, Rubin JM. Speckle tracking as a method to measure hemidiaphragm excursion. *Muscle Nerve.* (2017) 55:125–7. doi: 10.1002/mus.25380
22. Ye X, Xiao H, Bai W, Liang Y, Chen M, Zhang S. Two-dimensional strain ultrasound speckle tracking as a novel approach for the evaluation of right hemidiaphragmatic longitudinal deformation. *Exp Ther Med.* (2013) 6:368–72. doi: 10.3892/etm.2013.1133
23. Hatam N, Goetzenich A, Rossaint R, et al. A novel application for assessing diaphragmatic function by ultrasonic deformation analysis in noninvasively ventilated healthy young adults. *Ultraschall Med.* (2014) 35:540–6. doi: 10.1055/s-0034-1366090
24. Orde SR, Boon AJ, Firth DG, Villarraga HR, Sekiguchi H. Diaphragm assessment by two dimensional speckle tracking imaging in normal subjects. *BMC Anesthesiol.* (2016) 16:43. doi: 10.1186/s12871-016-0201-6
25. Luo J, Konofagou E. A fast normalized cross-correlation calculation method for motion estimation. *IEEE Trans Ultrason Ferroelectr Freq Control.* (2010) 57:1347–57. doi: 10.1109/TUFFC.2010.1554
26. Lee Y, Kang J, Yoo Y. Automatic dynamic range adjustment for ultrasound B-mode imaging. *Ultrasonics.* (2015) 56:435–43. doi: 10.1016/j.ultras.2014.09.012
27. Liu Z, Huang C, Luo J. A systematic investigation of lateral estimation using various interpolation approaches in conventional ultrasound imaging. *IEEE Trans Ultrason Ferroelectr Freq Control.* (2017) 64:1149–60. doi: 10.1109/TUFFC.2017.2705186
28. Rivaz H, Boctor EM, Choti MA, Hager GD. Ultrasound elastography using multiple images. *Med Image Anal.* (2014) 18:314–29. doi: 10.1016/j.media.2013.11.002
29. De Troyer A, Boriek AM. Mechanics of the respiratory muscles. *Compr Physiol.* (2011) 1:1273–300. doi: 10.1002/cphy.c100009
30. Bertoni M, Spadaro S, Goligher EC. Monitoring patient respiratory effort during mechanical ventilation: lung and diaphragm-protective ventilation. *Crit Care.* (2020) 24:106. doi: 10.1186/s13054-020-2777-y
31. Schepens T, Fard S, Goligher EC. Assessing diaphragmatic function. *Respir Care.* (2020) 65:807–19. doi: 10.4187/respcare.07410
32. Lopata RG, Nillesen MM, Hansen HH, Gerrits IH, Thijssen JM, de Korte CL. Performance evaluation of methods for two-dimensional displacement and strain estimation using ultrasound radio frequency data. *Ultrasound Med Biol.* (2009) 35:796–812. doi: 10.1016/j.ultrasmedbio.2008.11.002
33. Wilson TA, De Troyer A. Diagrammatic analysis of the respiratory action of the diaphragm. *J Appl Physiol.* (2010) 108:251–5. doi: 10.1152/japplphysiol.00960.2009
34. Greybeck B, Lu R, Ramanujam A, Adeyeye M, Wettergreen M, Wynd S, et al. Regional diaphragm volume displacement is heterogeneous in dogs. *Am J Physiol Regul Integr Comp Physiol.* (2017) 312:R443–50. doi: 10.1152/ajpregu.00270.2016

Permissions

All chapters in this book were first published by Frontiers; hereby published with permission under the Creative Commons Attribution License or equivalent. Every chapter published in this book has been scrutinized by our experts. Their significance has been extensively debated. The topics covered herein carry significant findings which will fuel the growth of the discipline. They may even be implemented as practical applications or may be referred to as a beginning point for another development.

The contributors of this book come from diverse backgrounds, making this book a truly international effort. This book will bring forth new frontiers with its revolutionizing research information and detailed analysis of the nascent developments around the world.

We would like to thank all the contributing authors for lending their expertise to make the book truly unique. They have played a crucial role in the development of this book. Without their invaluable contributions this book wouldn't have been possible. They have made vital efforts to compile up to date information on the varied aspects of this subject to make this book a valuable addition to the collection of many professionals and students.

This book was conceptualized with the vision of imparting up-to-date information and advanced data in this field. To ensure the same, a matchless editorial board was set up. Every individual on the board went through rigorous rounds of assessment to prove their worth. After which they invested a large part of their time researching and compiling the most relevant data for our readers.

The editorial board has been involved in producing this book since its inception. They have spent rigorous hours researching and exploring the diverse topics which have resulted in the successful publishing of this book. They have passed on their knowledge of decades through this book. To expedite this challenging task, the publisher supported the team at every step. A small team of assistant editors was also appointed to further simplify the editing procedure and attain best results for the readers.

Apart from the editorial board, the designing team has also invested a significant amount of their time in understanding the subject and creating the most relevant covers. They scrutinized every image to scout for the most suitable representation of the subject and create an appropriate cover for the book.

The publishing team has been an ardent support to the editorial, designing and production team. Their endless efforts to recruit the best for this project, has resulted in the accomplishment of this book. They are a veteran in the field of academics and their pool of knowledge is as vast as their experience in printing. Their expertise and guidance has proved useful at every step. Their uncompromising quality standards have made this book an exceptional effort. Their encouragement from time to time has been an inspiration for everyone.

The publisher and the editorial board hope that this book will prove to be a valuable piece of knowledge for researchers, students, practitioners and scholars across the globe.

List of Contributors

Beatrice Aramini, Valentina Masciale, Daniel Bianchi, Beatrice Manfredini and Uliano Morandi
Division of Thoracic Surgery, Department of Medical and Surgical Sciences, University of Modena and Reggio Emilia, Modena, Italy

Federico Banchelli and Roberto D'Amico
Department of Medical and Surgical Sciences, Center of Statistic, University of Modena and Reggio Emilia, Modena, Italy

Federica Bertolini and Massimo Dominici
Division of Oncology, Department of Medical and Surgical Sciences, University of Modena and Reggio Emilia, Modena, Italy

Antonino Maiorana
Department of Medical and Surgical Sciences, Institute of Pathology, University of Modena and Reggio Emilia, Modena, Italy

Wei-Chih Liao, Chih-Yen Tu and Wu-Huei Hsu
Division of Pulmonary and Critical Care Medicine, Department of Internal Medicine, China Medical University Hospital, Taichung, Taiwan
School of Medicine, China Medical University, Taichung, Taiwan

Cheng-Li Lin
Management Office for Health Data, China Medical University Hospital, Taichung, Taiwan

Te-Chun Shen
Division of Pulmonary and Critical Care Medicine, Department of Internal Medicine, China Medical University Hospital, Taichung, Taiwan
School of Medicine, China Medical University, Taichung, Taiwan
Intensive Care Unit, Chu Shang Show Chwan Hospital, Nantou, Taiwan

Te-Chun Hsia
Division of Pulmonary and Critical Care Medicine, Department of Internal Medicine, China Medical University Hospital, Taichung, Taiwan

Pere Trias-Sabrià, Maria Molina-Molina, Jordi Dorca, Salud Santos and Guillermo Suárez-Cuartin
Respiratory Department, Hospital Universitari de Bellvitge, Institut d'Investigació Biomèdica de Bellvitge (IDIBELL), L'Hospitalet de Llobregat, Spain
Universitat de Barcelona-Campus Bellvitge, L'Hospitalet de Llobregat, Spain

Eduard Dorca Duch
Pathology Department, Hospital Universitari de Bellvitge, Institut d'Investigació Biomèdica de Bellvitge (IDIBELL), L'Hospitalet de Llobregat, Spain

Samantha Aso, Marta Díez-Ferrer, Alfredo Marín Muñiz and Jaume Bordas-Martínez
Respiratory Department, Hospital Universitari de Bellvitge, Institut d'Investigació Biomèdica de Bellvitge (IDIBELL), L'Hospitalet de Llobregat, Spain

Joan Sabater
Universitat de Barcelona-Campus Bellvitge, L'Hospitalet de Llobregat, Spain
Critical Care Department, Hospital Universitari de Bellvitge, Institut d'Investigació Biomèdica de Bellvitge (IDIBELL), L'Hospitalet de Llobregat, Spain

Patricio Luburich, Belén del Rio and Xavier Solanich
Radiology Department, Hospital Universitari de Bellvitge, Institut d'Investigació Biomèdica de Bellvitge (IDIBELL), L'Hospitalet de Llobregat, Spain

Yong Liu, Jian Liu and Liang Huang
Department of Emergency, The First Affiliated Hospital of Nanchang University, Nanchang, China

Hanying Liu, Shenghua Sun and Chun Liu
Department of Respiratory Diseases, The 3rd Xiangya Hospital, Central South University, Changsha, China

Ying Zhang
Transplantation Center, The 3rd Xiangya Hospital, Central South University, Changsha, China

Guiyang Chen
Department of Cardiology, Hunan Aerospace Hospital, Changsha, China

Jiangang Wang
Department of Health Management, The 3rd Xiangya Hospital, Central South University, Changsha, China

Fengyi Chen
Vision Medicals Co. Ltd, Guangzhou, China

Quan Zhuang
Transplantation Center, The 3rd Xiangya Hospital, Central South University, Changsha, China
Research Center of National Health Ministry on Transplantation Medicine, Changsha, China

Yu-Che Lee
Department of Medicine, University at Buffalo-Catholic Health System, Buffalo, NY, United States

Ko-Yun Chang
Division of Chest Medicine, Taichung Veterans General Hospital, Taichung, Taiwan

Mehdi Mirsaeidi
Division of Pulmonary and Critical Care and Sleep Medicine, University of Florida College of Medicine, Jacksonville, FL, United States

Yadan Wang
Ruibiao (Wuhan) Biotechnology Co. Ltd., Wuhan

Weijie Li and Guizuo Wang
Department of Respiratory and Critical Care Medicine, Shaanxi Provincial People's Hospital, Xi'an, China

Taehee Kim and Hayoung Choi
Division of Pulmonary, Allergy, and Critical Care Medicine, Department of Internal Medicine, Hallym University Kangnam Sacred Heart Hospital, Hallym University College of Medicine, Seoul, South Korea

Jai Hoon Yoon
Department of Gastroenterology, Hanyang University Hospital, Seoul, South Korea

Bumhee Yang
Division of Pulmonary and Critical Care Medicine, Department of Internal Medicine, Chungbuk National University Hospital, Chungbuk National University College of Medicine, Cheongju, South Korea

Jiin Ryu
Biostatistical Consulting and Research Lab, Medical Research Collaborating Center, Hanyang University, Seoul, South Korea

Chang Ki Yoon
Department of Ophthalmology, Seoul National University Hospital, Seoul, South Korea

Youlim Kim
Division of Pulmonary and Allergy, Department of Internal Medicine, Konkuk University Hospital, School of Medicine, Konkuk University, Seoul, South Korea

Jang Won Sohn and Hyun Lee
Division of Pulmonary Medicine and Allergy, Department of Internal Medicine, Hanyang University College of Medicine, Seoul, South Korea

Yu-Chih Wu and Feng-Ming Yang
School of Respiratory Therapy, College of Medicine, Taipei Medical University, Taipei, Taiwan

Sung-Po Hsu
Department of Physiology, School of Medicine, College of Medicine, Taipei Medical University, Taipei, Taiwan
Graduate Institute of Medical Sciences, College of Medicine, Taipei Medical University, Taipei, Taiwan

Meng-Chun Hu and Yu-Ting Lan
Graduate Institute of Physiology, National Taiwan University College of Medicine, Taipei, Taiwan

Edward T. H. Yeh
Department of Internal Medicine, University of Arkansas for Medical Sciences, Little Rock, AK, United States
Winthrop P. Rockefeller Cancer Institute, University of Arkansas for Medical Sciences, Little Rock, AK, United States

Sandra Elena-Pérez and David Hansoe Heredero-Jung
Department of Clinical Biochemistry, University Hospital of Salamanca, Salamanca, Spain

Asunción García-Sánchez and Miguel Estravís
Allergic Disease Research Group IIMD-01, Institute for Biomedical Research of Salamanca, Salamanca, Spain
Department of Biomedical Sciences and Diagnostics, University of Salamanca, Salamanca, Spain
Network for Cooperative Research in Health - RETICS ARADyAL, Carlos III Health Institute, Madrid, Spain

Maria J. Martin
Allergic Disease Research Group IIMD-01, Institute for Biomedical Research of Salamanca, Salamanca, Spain
Network for Cooperative Research in Health - RETICS ARADyAL, Carlos III Health Institute, Madrid, Spain

Jacinto Ramos-González
Department of Pneumology, University Hospital of Salamanca, Salamanca, Spain

Juan Carlos Triviño
Sistemas Genómicos, Paterna, Spain

María Isidoro-García
Department of Clinical Biochemistry, University Hospital of Salamanca, Salamanca, Spain
Allergic Disease Research Group IIMD-01, Institute for Biomedical Research of Salamanca, Salamanca, Spain
Network for Cooperative Research in Health - RETICS ARADyAL, Carlos III Health Institute, Madrid, Spain
Department of Medicine, University of Salamanca, Salamanca, Spain

Catalina Sanz
Allergic Disease Research Group IIMD-01, Institute for Biomedical Research of Salamanca, Salamanca, Spain
Network for Cooperative Research in Health - RETICS ARADyAL, Carlos III Health Institute, Madrid, Spain
Department of Microbiology and Genetics, University of Salamanca, Salamanca, Spain

Ignacio Dávila
Allergic Disease Research Group IIMD-01, Institute for Biomedical Research of Salamanca, Salamanca, Spain
Department of Biomedical Sciences and Diagnostics, University of Salamanca, Salamanca, Spain
Network for Cooperative Research in Health - RETICS ARADyAL, Carlos III Health Institute, Madrid, Spain
Department of Allergy, University Hospital of Salamanca, Salamanca, Spain

Hyun Lee
Division of Pulmonary Medicine and Allergy, Department of Internal Medicine, Hanyang University College of Medicine, Seoul, South Korea

Hayoung Choi
Division of Pulmonary, Allergy, and Critical Care Medicine, Department of Internal Medicine, Hallym University Kangnam Sacred Heart Hospital, Hallym University College of Medicine, Seoul, South Korea

Yong Suk Jo
Division of Pulmonary and Critical Care Medicine, Department of Internal Medicine, Seoul St. Mary's Hospital, College of Medicine, The Catholic University of Korea, Seoul, South Korea

Qianqian Chen, Hui Kong, Xu Qi, Wenqiu Ding, Ningfei Ji, Chaojie Wu, Mao Huang and Weiping Xie
Department of Respiratory and Critical Care Medicine, The First Affiliated Hospital of Nanjing Medical University, Nanjing, China

Chaolin Huang and Wenjuan Wu
Division of Intensive Care Unit, Wuhan Jin Yin-tan Hospital, Wuhan, China

Yun Liu
Department of Medical Informatics, School of Biomedical Engineering and Informatics, Nanjing Medical University, Nanjing, China

Jinhai Tang
Department of General Surgery, The First Affiliated Hospital of Nanjing Medical University, Nanjing, China

Xiaoxue Liu, Sumaira Mubarik, Fang Wang, Yafeng Wang, Fang Shi and Haoyu Wen
Department of Epidemiology and Biostatistics, School of Public Health, Wuhan University, Wuhan, China

Yong Yu
School of Public Health and Management, University of Medicine, Shiyan, China

Chuanhua Yu
Department of Epidemiology and Biostatistics, School of Public Health, Wuhan University, Wuhan, China
Global Health Institute, Wuhan University, Wuhan, China

Jing Li, Xiaoying Wei, Daxiong Zeng and Junhong Jiang
Department of Medicine, Respiratory, Emergency and Intensive Care Medicine, The Affiliated Dushu Lake Hospital of Soochow University, Suzhou, China

Shanle Yan
Department of Rheumatology and Immunology, The Affiliated Dushu Lake Hospital of Soochow University, Suzhou, China,

Xiaohui Zhang, Chuanyun You, Shenhua Chen and Ling Gu
Department of Medicine, Respiratory, Emergency and Intensive Care Medicine, The First Affiliated Hospital of Soochow University, Suzhou, China

Mengqi Xiang
Department of Medical Oncology, Sichuan Cancer Hospital, Medical School, University of Electronic Science and Technology of China, Chengdu, China

Chuanhua Zhang
Department of Thoracic Surgery, Sichuan Cancer Hospital, Medical School, University of Electronic Science and Technology of China, Chengdu, China

Mahmood Yaseen Hachim
College of Medicine, Mohammed Bin Rashid University of Medicine and Health Sciences, Dubai, United Arab Emirates
Sharjah Institute for Medical Research, College of Medicine, University of Sharjah, Sharjah, United Arab Emirates

Noha Mousaad Elemam, Rakhee K. Ramakrishnan and Thenmozhi Venkatachalam
Sharjah Institute for Medical Research, College of Medicine, University of Sharjah, Sharjah, United Arab Emirates

Laila Salameh
Rashid Hospital, Dubai Health Authority, Dubai, United Arab Emirates

Ronald Olivenstein
Meakins-Christie Laboratories, McGill University, Montreal, QC, Canada

Ibrahim Yaseen Hachim and Rabih Halwani
Sharjah Institute for Medical Research, College of Medicine, University of Sharjah, Sharjah, United Arab Emirates
Department of Clinical Sciences, College of Medicine, University of Sharjah, Sharjah, United Arab Emirates

Bassam Mahboub
Rashid Hospital, Dubai Health Authority, Dubai, United Arab Emirates
Department of Clinical Sciences, College of Medicine, University of Sharjah, Sharjah, United Arab Emirates

Saba Al Heialy
College of Medicine, Mohammed Bin Rashid University of Medicine and Health Sciences, Dubai, United Arab Emirates
Meakins-Christie Laboratories, McGill University, Montreal, QC, Canada

Qutayba Hamid
Sharjah Institute for Medical Research, College of Medicine, University of Sharjah, Sharjah, United Arab Emirates
Meakins-Christie Laboratories, McGill University, Montreal, QC, Canada
Department of Clinical Sciences, College of Medicine, University of Sharjah, Sharjah, United Arab Emirates

Rifat Hamoudi
Sharjah Institute for Medical Research, College of Medicine, University of Sharjah, Sharjah, United Arab Emirates
Department of Clinical Sciences, College of Medicine, University of Sharjah, Sharjah, United Arab Emirates
Division of Surgery and Interventional Science, UCL, London, United Kingdom

Jean-Paul Janssens
Division of Pulmonary Diseases, Department of Medicine, Geneva University Hospitals, Geneva, Switzerland
Hôpital de La Tour, Centre Cardio-Respiratoire, Geneva, Switzerland
Faculty of Medicine, University of Geneva, Geneva, Switzerland

Chloé Cantero
Service de Pneumologie, Hôpital Pitié-Salpêtrière AP-HP - Sorbonne Université, Paris, France

Patrick Pasquina
Division of Pulmonary Diseases, Department of Medicine, Geneva University Hospitals, Geneva, Switzerland

Marjolaine Georges and Claudio Rabec
Pulmonary Department and Respiratory Critical Care Unit, University Hospital Dijon, Dijon, France

Ting-Yu Lin, Po-Jui Chang, Chun-Yu Lo, Yu-Lun Lo, Chih-Teng Yu, Shu-Min Lin, Chih-His Scott Kuo and Horng-Chyuan Lin
Department of Thoracic Medicine, Chang Gung Memorial Hospital, Taipei, Taiwan
College of Medicine, Chang Gung University, Taoyuan, Taiwan

Nan Wang, Li Sun, Xiaomeng Li, Kanghong Xu and Xinquan Jiang
School of Public Health, Shandong First Medical University and Shandong Academy of Medical Sciences, Taian, China

Qin Wang
Department of Anesthesiology, Qilu Hospital, Shandong University, Jinan, China

Tiantian Du and Abakundana Nsenga Ariston Gabriel
Department of Clinical Laboratory, Cheeloo College of Medicine, The Second Hospital, Shandong University, Jinan, China

Xue Wang
Department of Pharmacy, Binzhou Medical University Hospital, Binzhou, China

Yi Zhang
Respiratory and Critical Care Medicine Department, Qilu Hospital, Shandong University, Jinan, China

Elisabetta Cocconcelli, Nicol Bernardinello, Gioele Castelli, Simone Petrarulo, Marina Saetta, Paolo Spagnolo and Elisabetta Balestro
Respiratory Disease Unit, Department of Cardiac, Thoracic, Vascular Sciences and Public Health, University of Padova and Padova City Hospital, Padova, Italy

Chiara Giraudo and Adelaide Giorgino
Department of Medicine, Institute of Radiology, University of Padova and Padova City Hospital, Padova, Italy

Davide Leoni, Anna Ferrari and Annamaria Cattelan
Division of Infectious and Tropical Diseases, University of Padova and Padova City Hospital, Padova, Italy

Keiichiro Yoshioka, Takeshi Kawasaki, Daisuke Ishii, Takuro Imamoto, Mitsuhiro Abe, Koichiro Tatsumi and Takuji Suzuki
Department of Respirology, Graduate School of Medicine, Chiba University, Chiba, Japan

Hironori Sato
Department of Applied Genomics, Kazusa DNA Research Institute, Chiba, Japan
Department of Pediatrics, Graduate School of Medicine, Chiba University, Chiba, Japan

Yoshinori Hasegawa and Osamu Ohara
Department of Applied Genomics, Kazusa DNA Research Institute, Chiba, Japan

Xiong Ye
School of Clinical Medicine, Shanghai University of Medicine & Health Sciences, Shanghai, China
National Medical Products Administration (NMPA) Key Laboratory for Respiratory and Anaesthetic Equipment, Shanghai, China

Zhi Liu and Jianwen Luo
Department of Biomedical Engineering, School of Medicine, Tsinghua University, Beijing, China

Ying Ma, Ye Song and Lihua Hu
Department of Ultrasound, Shanghai University of Medicine and Health Sciences Affiliated Zhoupu Hospital, Shanghai, China

Hui Xiao
Department of Respiratory and Critical Care Medicine, Shanghai General Hospital, Shanghai Jiaotong University, Shanghai, China

Index

Printed in the USA
CPSIA information can be obtained
at www.ICGtesting.com
JSHW061324061223
53387JS00005B/32

9 798887 405865